T0073794

THE NETTER COLLECTION

OF MEDICAL ILLUSTRATIONS

Cardiovascular System

3rd Edition

VOLUME 8

A compilation of paintings prepared by **FRANK H. NETTER, MD**

Authored by

Jamie B. Conti, MD, FACC
Professor and Chair of Medicine
American Heart Association Eminent Scholar
University of Florida College of Medicine
Gainesville, Florida

C. Richard Conti, MD, MACC, FESC, FAHA
Emeritus Professor of Medicine
University of Florida College of Medicine
Gainesville, Florida

Additional Illustrations by

Carlos A.G. Machado, MD

CONTRIBUTING ILLUSTRATORS
John A. Craig, MD
Tiffany S. DaVanzo, MA, CMI
DragonFly Media
Anita Impagliazzo, MA, CMI
Kristen W. Marzejon, CMI
James A. Perkins, MS, MFA

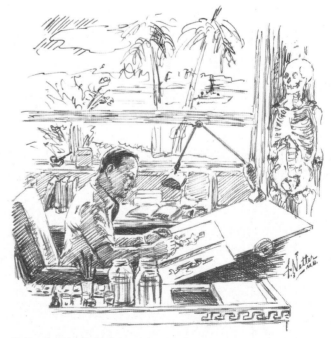

Self portrait by Dr. Netter

ELSEVIER

ELSEVIER
1600 John F. Kennedy Blvd.
Suite 1600
Philadelphia, Pennsylvania

THE NETTER COLLECTION OF MEDICAL ILLUSTRATIONS:
CARDIOVASCULAR SYSTEM, VOLUME 8, THIRD EDITION   ISBN: 978-0-323-88129-6

Copyright © 2025 by Elsevier, Inc. All rights reserved, including those for text and data mining, AI training, and similar technologies.

No part of this publication may be reproduced or transmitted in any form or by any means, electronic or mechanical, including photocopying, recording, or any information storage and retrieval system, without permission in writing from the publisher. Details on how to seek permission, further information about the Publisher's permissions policies and our arrangements with organizations such as the Copyright Clearance Center and the Copyright Licensing Agency, can be found at our website: http://elsevier.com/permissions.

Permission to use Netter Art figures may be sought through the website http://NetterImages.com or by emailing Elsevier's Licensing Department at H.Licensing@elsevier.com.

This book and the individual contributions contained in it are protected under copyright by the Publisher (other than as may be noted herein).

Notices

Knowledge and best practice in this field are constantly changing. As new research and experience broaden our understanding, changes in research methods, professional practices, or medical treatment may become necessary.

Practitioners and researchers must always rely on their own experience and knowledge in evaluating and using any information, methods, compounds, or experiments described herein. In using such information or methods they should be mindful of their own safety and the safety of others, including parties for whom they have a professional responsibility.

With respect to any drug or pharmaceutical products identified, readers are advised to check the most current information provided (i) on procedures featured or (ii) by the manufacturer of each product to be administered, to verify the recommended dose or formula, the method and duration of administration, and contraindications. It is the responsibility of practitioners, relying on their own experience and knowledge of their patients, to make diagnoses, to determine dosages and the best treatment for each individual patient, and to take all appropriate safety precautions.

To the fullest extent of the law, neither the Publisher nor the authors, contributors, or editors, assume any liability for any injury and/or damage to persons or property as a matter of products liability, negligence or otherwise, or from any use or operation of any methods, products, instructions, or ideas contained in the material herein.

Publisher: Elyse O'Grady
Senior Content Strategist: Marybeth Thiel
Publishing Services Manager: Catherine Jackson
Senior Project Manager/Specialist: Carrie Stetz
Book Design: Patrick Ferguson

Printed in India

Last digit is the print number: 9 8 7 6 5 4 3 2 1

Working together
to grow libraries in
developing countries

www.elsevier.com • www.bookaid.org

"Clarification is the goal. No matter how beautifully it is painted, a medical illustration has little value if it does not make clear a medical point."

Frank H. Netter, MD

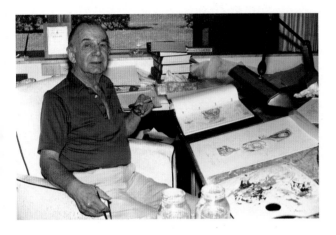

Dr. Frank Netter at work.

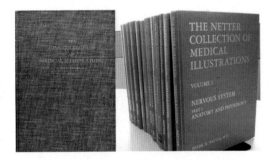

The single-volume "Blue Book" that preceded the multivolume Netter Collection of Medical Illustrations series, affectionately known as the "Green Books."

The Netter Collection
OF MEDICAL ILLUSTRATIONS
3rd Edition

Dr. Frank Netter created an illustrated legacy unifying his perspectives as physician, artist, and teacher. Both his greatest challenge and greatest success was charting a middle course between artistic clarity and instructional complexity. That success is captured in *The Netter Collection,* beginning in 1948 when the first comprehensive book of Netter's work was published by CIBA Pharmaceuticals. It met with such success that over the following 40 years the collection was expanded into an 8-volume series—with each title devoted to a single body system. Between 2011 and 2016, these books were updated and rereleased. Now, after another decade of innovation in medical imaging, renewed focus on patient-centered care, conscious efforts to improve inequities in healthcare and medical education, and a growing understanding of many clinical conditions, including multisystem effects of COVID-19, we are happy to make available a third edition of Netter's timeless work enhanced and informed by modern medical knowledge and context.

Inside the classic green covers, students and practitioners will find hundreds of original works of art. This is a collection of the human body in pictures—Dr. Netter called them *pictures,* never paintings. The latest expert medical knowledge is anchored by the sublime style of Frank Netter that has guided physicians' hands and nurtured their imaginations for more than half a century.

Noted artist-physician Carlos Machado, MD, the primary successor responsible for continuing the Netter tradition, has particular appreciation for the Green Book series. "*The Reproductive System* is of special significance for those who, like me, deeply admire Dr. Netter's work. In this volume, he masters the representation of textures of different surfaces, which I like to call 'the rhythm of the brush,' since it is the dimension, the direction of the strokes, and the interval separating them that create the illusion of given textures: organs have their external surfaces, the surfaces of their cavities, and texture of their parenchymas realistically represented. It set the style for the subsequent volumes of *The Netter Collection*—each an amazing combination of painting masterpieces and precise scientific information."

This third edition could not exist without the dedication of all those who edited, authored, or in other ways contributed to the second edition or the original books, nor, of course, without the excellence of Dr. Netter. For this third edition, we also owe our gratitude to the authors, editors, and artists whose relentless efforts were instrumental in adapting these classic works into reliable references for today's clinicians in training and in practice. From all of us with the Netter Publishing Team at Elsevier, thank you.

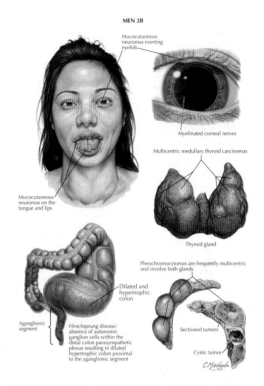

An illustrated plate painted by Carlos Machado, MD.

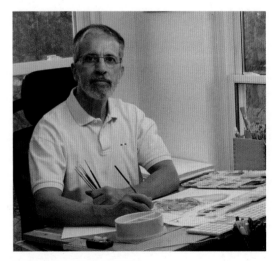

Dr. Carlos Machado at work.

DEDICATION

This edition is dedicated to my father, who taught me and many generations of cardiologists the love of learning, the love of all things cardiovascular, and to always ask why. He was an extraordinary teacher, writer, and father. This work is his final contribution to cardiovascular literature and to the cardiovascular community as a whole. He worked on this volume until the day of his death. I hope you will treasure it as I do.

Jamie B. Conti, MD, FACC

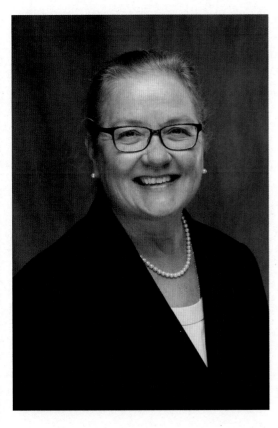

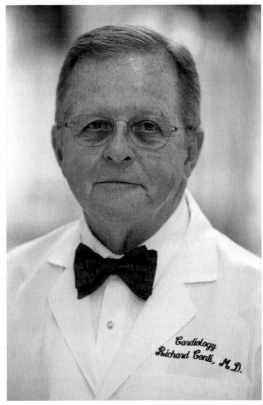

Jamie B. Conti, MD, FACC, holds the Palm Beach Heart Association Eminent Scholar Endowed Chair and is Professor of Medicine, Chair of the Department of Medicine at the University of Florida College of Medicine. She graduated from Buchholz High School in Gainesville, Florida, cum laude from Harvard University, and from the University of Florida College of Medicine in 1987. She did her internship in internal medicine at Georgetown University, followed by a residency at Emory University. She pursued a cardiology and clinical cardiac electrophysiology fellowship at the University of Florida and subsequently joined the cardiology faculty. In 2008 she became the chief of the Division of Cardiovascular Diseases and then chair of Internal Medicine in 2019.

Her honors and awards include the American College of Cardiology (ACC) Proctor Harvey Teaching Award in 1998; election to the American Clinical and Climatologic Association in 2006; election to the Association of University Cardiologists in 2006; and election to the Alpha Omega Alpha Society in 2010. She was also the recipient of the 2002 Distinguished Service Award, ACC, Florida Chapter; the 2007 Chapter Recognition Award, ACC; the 2008 Distinguished Service Award, ACC Florida Chapter; and the 2011 Founders Award, ACC, Florida Chapter. She was elected governor of the ACC from 2005 to 2008.

C. Richard Conti, MD, MACC, FESC, FAHA, previously held the Palm Beach Heart Association Eminent Scholar Endowed Chair (Clinical Cardiology) and was Professor of Medicine and Adjunct Professor of Physiology at the University of Florida College of Medicine. He was a distinguished 1952 graduate of Central Catholic High School in Allentown, Pennsylvania, a 1956 Phi Beta Kappa graduate of Lehigh University, and a 1960 Alpha Omega Alpha graduate of Johns Hopkins University School of Medicine. He received his medical training on the Osler Medical Service of the Johns Hopkins Hospital and his cardiology training at Johns Hopkins Hospital. He then served on the cardiology faculty at that institution from 1968 through 1974 when, at the age of 39 years, he became Professor of Medicine and Director of the Cardiovascular Division at the University of Florida.

Dr. Conti was president of the ACC; received an honorary fellowship from the College of Medicine of South Africa; was elected to the Johns Hopkins University Society of Scholars; and received a Docteur Honoris Causa from the University of Marseilles. Dr. Conti was selected for the Gifted Teacher Award by the ACC and received the Italian Society of Cardiology Distinguished Mentor and Scientist Award. He served for 24 years as Editor in Chief of the international journal *Clinical Cardiology* and served 10 years as Editor in Chief of the ACC audio journal *ACCEL* from 1999 to 2010. In addition, he was founding Editor in Chief for the international journal *Cardiovascular Innovations and Applications.*

He died on February 21, 2022, leaving a hole in the hearts of his family and the entire cardiovascular community.

PREFACE FROM THE SECOND EDITION

Unfortunately, I did not have the good fortune to know Dr. Netter personally, but as I read the introduction written years ago by his wife, Vera Netter, I got the distinct impression that, as she put it, "He was genius at what he did."

When I first received my copy of *The Heart*, by Frank Netter, in the 1960s (first printing, 1969) I was greatly impressed by the quality of the illustrations and the accompanying text. From the outset it was apparent that this was not a textbook of cardiovascular medicine and surgery. If one needed to know the details to perform a procedure or an operation, books that are dedicated to those subjects must be consulted. This book is an effective companion to textbooks of cardiovascular medicine and surgery or electronic resources specific to cardiovascular subjects. I find the illustrations particularly useful as teaching aids when trying to get across to medical students and young physicians the principles of cardiovascular disease.

In 2012 I accepted the challenge and undertook the task to update the book at the request of the publisher, Elsevier.

I very quickly came to realize that I was not quite as smart as I thought I was about cardiovascular matters. So, on many occasions, I informally consulted with many friends about several old and new topics contained in the original version of *The Heart*. Because the text accompanying the illustrations was written in the 1960s, an update was needed because of the many changes in cardiovascular disease diagnosis and therapy. Despite this requirement, the original artwork is spectacular and remains so. Several medical artists working with Dr. Netter also contributed illustrations that I have included in this new edition.

Several important new diagnostic and therapeutic concepts have evolved since the initial 1969 publication. For example, cardiac ultrasound is not mentioned in the early edition, nor are four major imaging methods now used: computed tomographic imaging, magnetic resonance imaging, nuclear imaging, and angiography. Thus a new section has been added on imaging because imaging plays a major role in modern diagnosis and therapy of cardiac disease. Several new therapeutic areas have been added, including the medical therapy of acute myocardial infarction, heart failure, arrhythmias, pacing strategies including biventricular pacing, and cardiac resynchronization therapy in patients with heart failure.

Although coronary artery surgery was mentioned in the first edition, coronary artery bypass graft surgery with saphenous vein grafts or with internal thoracic artery bypass of stenotic epicardial lesions, as we know it now, is new. Valve surgery also has changed. Although the initial illustrations of early valve surgery using the Starr Edwards ball-valve prosthesis, Beall valve, and Hufnagel valve were important in the evolution of valve replacement, these procedures are no longer performed. Thus I have added illustrations of currently used valve prostheses for aortic valve disease, mitral valve, and tricuspid valve problems. In addition, interventional procedures that affect valve function are introduced, such as transcutaneous aortic valve replacement (TAVR).

C. Richard Conti, MD, MACC, FESC, FAHA
November 2013

The 2013 edition of Netter's *The Heart*, now titled *Cardiovascular System*, was composed of six sections, including anatomy, physiology and pathophysiology, cardiac imaging, cardiac embryology, congenital heart disease, and acquired heart disease (Section 6). Section 6 is a large section that includes subsections on acute coronary syndromes, new information on treatment of cardiopulmonary arrest, syncope, sudden cardiac death in young athletes, HIV/AIDS and the heart, sleep apnea, endocrine disorders and the heart, and collagen vascular diseases and the heart.

In 2022, my father and I embarked on updating the 2012 edition. We added newer techniques of imaging, current therapeutic options, and identified knowledge gaps. My father was editing this edition actively until the day he died. Cardiology was his passion, and this volume is his last contribution to the world of cardiovascular medicine.

I am deeply grateful to Carrie Stetz, Marybeth Thiel, and Elyse O'Grady at Elsevier for their oversight, help, and direction of this work. Their gracious guidance made our edits more meaningful and the task of updating this volume a pleasure. My father and I hope you enjoy the new edition.

Jamie B. Conti, MD, FACC
July 2022

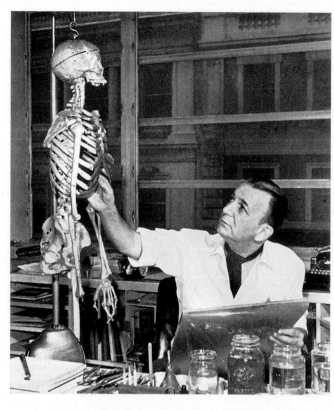

What's it like to be married to a genius? I can tell you—it's wonderful! My genius doesn't act the way people think a genius is supposed to act. He is a very simple, warm personality who enjoys the ordinary everyday things of life. Indeed, he is so taken up with these matters—with me, with the children, his friends, the stock market, his golf—that I often wonder how he manages to create all the pictures he does. On occasion, when he has completed a large series of pictures, I have asked him, "Frank, how did you manage to do all these?" He has answered me, "You know, darling, the difficult thing about making medical pictures is not the painting at all but rather the study, the thinking, the planning, the creation of a picture so that it says something. Once I have the picture in my mind it is easy to put it on paper." I know that he is thinking about his pictures in the middle of the night when he tosses about restlessly in bed, in the midst of a conversation when he becomes a little detached, or on the golf course when occasionally he makes a poor shot. I know also when he is troubled by a particularly difficult problem; then he sits very quietly and withdrawn, curling a forelock of his hair. But, once the problem is solved, he becomes his usual outgoing, friendly self again.

We travel considerably in quest of the knowledge that my husband pictorializes, and it is always amazing to me, after having been told of the very great scientist we are to meet, to find the scientist is more impressed in having the opportunity of meeting him. It is this humility and unconsciousness of his own great gift that endears him to so many. At these meetings it is also very interesting to note the great scientist's surprise to find that this artist can converse with him on his own plane regardless of whether the subject is neurophysiology, thoracic surgery, anatomy, biochemistry, orthopedics, or any other phase of medical science. They are always amazed to see how quickly he grasps the essence of the subject and organization his presentation. The immediate relaxation and response is electric. Most fascinating to me, however, is to see the glow of satisfaction which invariably suffuses the face of the consultant when he sees his lifework graphically depicted and clarified by the pencil and brush of my husband's. In most instances these associations have led to long, sincere friendships.

Frank also loves languages—and they come to him very naturally—but time will never permit him to really study seriously. Once, when we were in Switzerland, he was somewhat troubled because he learned that the two doctors he had wished to consult that morning at the university spoke no English. That evening I went a little early to meet him at the hospital, expecting to have my ear filled with his frustration at communicating, when, through the door, I was dumbfounded to hear a most familiar voice speaking Italian as though he had never been out of Italy. He says that if he drinks Chianti he can talk Italian, if he drinks champagne he can talk French, if he eats knockwurst he can talk German. (They must have served Chianti!)

In English, Frank is very articulate. He is often asked to speak at various medical assemblies because people seem to want to know about his unusual career. Unfortunately, he cannot accept most of these invitations because of time limitations. When he does agree to speak, I become nervous as the day of the address approaches and I see him making no preparation. Just before the meeting he will sit down for 15 minutes and plan what he will say! He believes that too much preparation makes a speech stilted and dull. Then he gets up on the rostrum and delights his audience with philosophy, narrative, and humor as he speaks extemporaneously.

We live in Manhattan in an apartment overlooking the East River. In the spring I decorate the terrace with colorful plants, but the pride of the terrace is the tomatoes that my husband cultivates and nurtures all spring and summer and then serves with his barbecued steaks. Frank is an early riser but cannot begin the day before the newspaper is delivered so he can see how "Dick Tracy" and his other cartoon friends have fared. His studio is on the lower floor of our duplex, and his usual day there beings at 8 in the morning and lasts to 4 in the afternoon, but when he is under pressure he may keep going till 6 or later. In his early days he would often work until 3 or 4 in the morning and sometimes right through the night, but now he abhors such hours and refuses to work at night regardless of the pressure. His work attire surprises even me sometimes. It consists of a pair of paint-stained slacks and bright plaid shirt and, to my horror, he often neglects to change when he has an outside appointment and ventures forth in this attire with simply the addition of a jacket, even though his closets are full of clothes. On one occasion, when one of the many aspiring students who come to ask his counsel appeared at the house, Frank opened the door in his customary work attire and the young man looked at him and said, "I have an appointment with your father, Dr. Netter." When Frank told him that he was Dr. Netter, his mouth fell open and he said, "But with all those drawings and books I though you would be an old man." Frank got a real chuckle out of that.

The letters received from all parts of the world in all languages, even from behind the "Iron Curtain," attest to the great utility of these books and give Frank the strength and desire to go on to the next one, vowing to make each better than the last to the end that those who use them may have the final word in pictorial medicine as it has been given to him.

Vera Netter

With each volume that I have undertaken in *The CIBA Collection of Medical Illustrations*, I have vowed at the outset to execute it with great expedition and simplicity. But in every case the task has proved to be much more complex and difficult than I had anticipated. As I became involved and absorbed in the subject matter, many facets of the various topics came to light that demanded pictorialization. Just as when a skin diver plunges beneath the surface of a calm sea, he does not realize what a myriad of hidden phenomena are to come into his view, so have I repeatedly discovered new and marvelous worlds beneath the superficial concepts. But, in the case of this volume on the heart, these factors have been even more pronounced. They were amplified by the fact that the sea of knowledge in which I was swimming kept continuously rising and expanding. New facts were being discovered, new concepts evolved, new methods and techniques developed. I had difficulty in keeping abreast of them with my studies as well as with my pencil and brush. But the exploration was always stimulating and inspiring—so much so that I might have gone on indefinitely expanding, revising, and adding, with the result that the book might never have appeared. I therefore had to call a halt, although I am aware that, even as this book goes to press, the pace of progress is accelerating.

The rate of this acceleration becomes evident in the light of a multitude of accomplishments. Somewhat less than 350 years ago, William Harvey established the concept of the circulation of the blood, and, since that epochal event, more has been learned about the circulatory system than in the 350,000 years preceding it. In 1902 William Einthoven devised the string galvanometer, and shortly thereafter it was applied, by Sir James Mackenzie and by Sir Thomas Lewis, to the study of the heartbeat, based on the fundamental studies of the cardiac conduction system of Gaskell. Thus modern cardiology was born some 65 years ago. But it continued to grow and mature, nurtured by many, many men and women who are too numerous to mention here. Finally came the advent of cardiac surgery, given tremendous impetus, within the past two decades, by the practical application of extracorporeal circulation. And, just before this book went to press, the first cardiac transplants were performed and we were able to include something about them herein. Thus although our knowledge of heart function and heart disease may seem slow in the perspective of a man's lifetime, it has been extremely rapid and, indeed, geometrically accelerating in the light of human history. It is significant also that as each new step forward was made, it necessitated going back and restudying fundamentals. The advent of cardiac surgery necessitated a restudy of heart anatomy; the correction of cardiac anomalies called for a reappraisal of embryology; the discovery of new drugs impelled a deeper analysis of cardiac physiology.

But progress has not ceased. On the contrary, it moves constantly onward at an ever-increasing pace. In the preparation of this volume it has been a great pleasure as well as a great intellectual stimulation to have collaborated with so many men who are catalyzing this progress. And so I herewith express my appreciation to these, my collaborators. Without them, this book would, of course, have been impossible; with them, it was a joy and a great adventure. To have met them, to have come to know them, to have worked with them was a memorable experience. I thank them all for the time they gave me, for the knowledge they imparted to me, for the material with which they supplied me, and, above all, for the friendship which they extended to me.

One collaborator in particular, however, I must single out, namely, Dr. L.H.S. Van Mierop, who has become simply "Bob" to me. Here is a man, warm and friendly by nature, forthright and simple in demeanor, yet imbued with an insatiable quest for truth and the comprehension of fundamentals. And his great talents have enabled him to follow this latter bent, so that he is at once clinician, anatomist, embryologist, investigator, student, and teacher. Because of his contributions, I believe that the sections on embryology and congenital heart disease are both original and classic.

I wish to thank also Dr. Fredrick F. Yonkman, the Editor, for the care and devotion which he gave to this work. Dr. Yonkman, Mr. A.W. Custer, and other executives of the CIBA Pharmaceutical Company have encouraged and helped me in every way possible. But the concept, and indeed the origination of this series of volumes, must be credited to the foresight and vision of Mr. Paul W. Roder of the CIBA company.

Frank H. Netter, MD

CONTRIBUTORS

AUTHORS

Jamie B. Conti, MD, FACC
Professor and Chair of Medicine
American Heart Association Eminent Scholar
University of Florida College of Medicine
Gainesville, Florida

C. Richard Conti, MD, MACC, FESC, FAHA
Emeritus Professor of Medicine
University of Florida College of Medicine
Gainesville, Florida

CONTRIBUTORS

R. David Anderson, MD, MS, FACC, FSCAI
Professor of Medicine
Director of Interventional Cardiology
Program Director, Interventional Cardiology
    Fellowship
University of Florida
Gainesville, Florida
PLATE 3.11

Juan M. Aranda Jr, MD, FACC, FHFSA
Professor and Chief, Division of Cardiovascular
    Medicine
Vice Chair of Clinical Affairs, Department of
    Medicine
American Heart Association Suncoast Endowed
    Chair
University of Florida
Gainesville, Florida
PLATES 6.133–6.134, 6.142–6.144

Michael R. Massoomi, MD
Assistant Professor of Medicine
University of Florida
Gainesville, Florida
PLATES 3.16, 6.40, 6.47

William M. Miles, MD, FACC, FHRS
Professor of Medicine
Silverstein Chair for Cardiovascular Education
University of Florida
Gainesville, Florida
IMAGING FOR PLATE 3.15

Juan R. Vilaro, MD, FACC
Associate Professor of Medicine
Division of Cardiology
Heart Transplant Medical Director
Advanced Heart Failure and Transplant Cardiology
    Fellowship Director
University of Florida
Gainesville, Florida
PLATES 6.133–6.134, 6.142–6.144

CONTENTS

ANATOMY

Plate 1.1   Cardiovascular System: VOLUME 8

LUNGS IN SITU: ANTERIOR VIEW

Thyroid gland
Trachea and inferior thyroid veins
Omohyoid, sternothyroid, and sternohyoid muscles
Common carotid artery
Manubrium of sternum
Internal jugular vein
Sternocleidomastoid muscle
Phrenic nerve
External jugular vein
Anterior scalene muscle
Costal part of parietal pleura (cut away)
Thoracic duct
Clavicle
Brachial plexus
Pectoralis major muscle
Subclavian artery and vein
Pectoralis minor muscle
Internal thoracic artery and vein
Intercostal muscles
Axillary artery and vein
Cardiac notch of left lung
Superior lobe
Middle lobe
Inferior lobe of right lung
Superior lobe
Inferior lobe of left lung
Oblique fissure
Costo-mediastinal space
Horizontal fissure of right lung
Costodia-phragmatic recess
Oblique fissure
Diaphragmatic part of parietal pleura
Musculophrenic artery
Diaphragm
Lingula of superior lobe of left lung
7th costal cartilage
Internal thoracic artery
Xiphoid process
Mediastinal part of parietal pleura
Pleural reflections
Fibrous pericardium

THORAX

Before describing the anatomy of the heart, it is helpful to review other anatomic features of the thoracic cavity and organs.

The thorax proper constitutes the upper part of the body or trunk, with a shape between a barrel and a truncated cone that is functionally favorable. Although the intrathoracic pressure is often subatmospheric, the chest wall is still able to retain its integrity by means of rather thin, lightweight skeletal elements. The thoracic cavity occupies only the upper part of the thoracic cage. The abdominal (peritoneal) cavity reaches upward as high as the lower tip of the *sternum,* affording protection to large, easily injured abdominal organs such as the liver, spleen, stomach, and kidneys.

The thoracic and abdominal cavities are separated by the dome-shaped *diaphragm,* a sheet of tissue consisting of a peripheral muscular part and a central tendinous part that closes the thoracic cavity interiorly. Superiorly, the narrow upper thoracic aperture—bounded by the upper part of the sternum, the short stout first ribs, and the body of the first thoracic vertebra (T1)—gives access to the root of the neck and is not closed by a specific structure. The thorax is bounded posteriorly by the bodies of the 12 thoracic vertebrae and the posterior portions of the ribs; anteriorly by the sternum, *costal cartilages,* and anterior portions of the ribs; and laterally by the remaining parts of the ribs. The spaces between successive ribs are bridged by the *intercostal muscles.*

The sternum (breastbone) lies anterior in the midline and superficially. The *clavicles* and the first seven pairs of ribs articulate with it. The sternum consists of three parts: the bony *manubrium* and corpus sterni and the small, cartilaginous *xiphoid process.* The clavicles articulate with the manubrium on its upper border, and the notch between these joints is the interclavicular (or suprasternal) notch. Just below the sternoclavicular joints, the cartilages of the first ribs are attached to the sternum. No joint spaces are present here. The manubrium and the body of the sternum are united by fibrocartilage. The junction between the manubrium and the body of the sternum usually forms a prominent ridge, accentuated by the two parts of the sternum forming a slight angle with each other known as the *sternal angle of Louis.* This is an important landmark because the cartilages of the second ribs articulate with the sternum at this point. The third, smallest part of the sternum is the xiphoid cartilage, a thin, spoon-shaped process attached to the lower end of the sternal body.

Most of the bony thorax is formed by the ribs, usually 12 on each side of the trunk. The ribs consist of a series of thin, curved, rather elastic bones that articulate posteriorly with the thoracic vertebrae and terminate anteriorly in the costal cartilages. The first seven pairs of ribs attach to the sternum by means of their cartilages, whereas the eighth, ninth, and tenth pairs articulate with each other and do not reach the sternum. The eleventh and twelfth pairs are small and poorly developed, ending in free cartilaginous tips. The ribs are thickest posteriorly; they flatten out and widen as they curve forward. Along the inferior and inner surface of the posterior part of each rib, a groove—the sulcus costae—affords protection to the intercostal vessels and nerve.

The first two and last two ribs differ somewhat from the previous description. The *first rib* (see Plate 1.2) is very short and relatively heavier than the other ribs. On the superior surface of the first rib, two grooves are divided by a tubercle—the tuberculum scaleni—that forms the point of insertion of the anterior scalene muscle. The groove in front of the muscle is occupied by the *subclavian vein,* whereas the *subclavian artery* follows the groove behind the tubercle. The second rib is longer than the first and resembles the other ribs except the small eleventh and twelfth ribs.

The spaces between successive ribs are occupied by *intercostal muscles* (Plate 1.1). Each external

Plate 1.2   Anatomy

THORAX (Continued)

intercostal muscle arises from the lower border of the rib above, runs obliquely downward and medially, and inserts into the upper border of the rib below. Each internal intercostal muscle arises from the lower border of the rib above and runs downward and outward to insert on the upper border of the rib below. Between these two muscle layers lie the intercostal vessels, whereas the intercostal nerves lie between the internal and the innermost intercostal muscles.

Many muscles of the upper extremities originate from the chest wall, including the *pectoralis major* (see Plate 1.1) and pectoralis minor muscles and the serratus anterior muscle, which originate from the anterior and lateral portions of the chest wall.

Several neck muscles originate from the upper rim of the thoracic cage. The *sternohyoid* and *sternothyroid* (see Plate 1.1) are thin, strap-like muscles that arise from the superior border and posterior surface of the sternum and insert into the hyoid bone and the thyroid cartilage, respectively. The *sternocleidomastoid muscle* (SCM) arises (see Plate 1.1) as a stout sternal head from the upper border of the sternum, adjacent to the sternoclavicular joint, and as a second clavicular head from the medial third of the clavicle. The interval between the two heads is usually visible as a slight depression, behind which the apex of the lung rises from the thorax into the root of the neck. Above this interval the two heads of the SCM unite to form a single muscular belly that passes obliquely upward, backward, and laterally to insert into the lateral surface of the mastoid process and occipital bone.

Superficial to the SCM, the *external jugular vein* passes perpendicularly downward from its origin at the lower border of the parotid gland, crosses the SCM, and penetrates the deep fascia of the neck to empty into the *subclavian vein*.

Of the deeper neck muscles, the three scalene muscles originate from the transverse processes of the cervical vertebrae. The *anterior scalene muscle* inserts into the scalene tubercle of the first rib; the medial scalene muscle also attaches to the upper surface of the first rib but more posteriorly. The *posterior scalene muscle* inserts on the second rib. The components of the cervical nerve plexus emerge from the groove between the anterior and middle scalene muscles. The anterior scalene muscle is crossed laterally and anteriorly by the *phrenic nerve*, which originates from the cervical plexus and runs downward and behind the subclavian vein to enter the thoracic cavity. The groove between the anterior and middle scalene muscles widens inferiorly to form a triangular opening through which emerge the components of the *brachial plexus* and the *subclavian artery*. After ascending from the thoracic cavity, the subclavian artery crosses the upper surface of the first rib, lying in the groove posterior to

the scalene muscle, and enters the axilla. The subclavian vein runs parallel to the subclavian artery but in front of the anterior scalene muscle.

Deep in the lower portion of the neck under the SCM, a narrow space is bordered anteriorly by the *omohyoid* and strap muscles, posteriorly by the anterior scalene muscle and prevertebral fascia, and medially by the pharynx, esophagus, trachea, and thyroid gland (see Plate 1.1). In this space, the common carotid artery, internal jugular vein, and vagus nerve are enclosed in a

common connective tissue sheath; the jugular vein runs most superficially and the vagus nerve lies beneath, between the common carotid artery and internal jugular veins. On the left side, the *thoracic duct* (see Plate 1.1) crosses over the subclavian artery and runs anteriorly to empty into the proximal subclavian vein.

Blood for the chest wall is supplied by the intercostal arteries and the *internal thoracic* (internal mammary) *arteries*. After originating from the *aorta*, the posterior intercostal arteries cross the vertebral bodies and enter

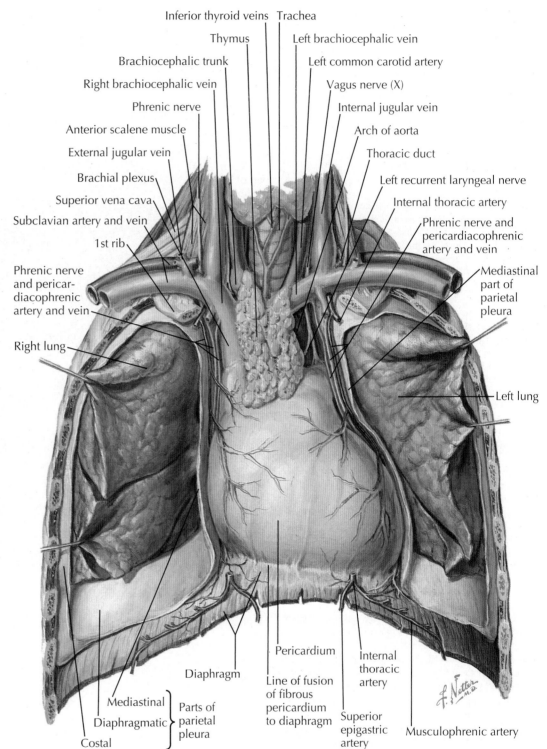

HEART IN SITU

Inferior thyroid veins — Trachea
Thymus — Left brachiocephalic vein
Brachiocephalic trunk — Left common carotid artery
Right brachiocephalic vein — Vagus nerve (X)
Phrenic nerve — Internal jugular vein
Anterior scalene muscle — Arch of aorta
External jugular vein — Thoracic duct
Brachial plexus — Left recurrent laryngeal nerve
Superior vena cava — Internal thoracic artery
Subclavian artery and vein — Phrenic nerve and pericardiacophrenic artery and vein
1st rib — Mediastinal part of parietal pleura
Phrenic nerve and pericardiacophrenic artery and vein —
Right lung — Left lung
Pericardium — Internal thoracic artery
Diaphragm — Line of fusion of fibrous pericardium to diaphragm
Mediastinal — Parts of parietal pleura
Diaphragmatic —
Costal — Superior epigastric artery — Musculophrenic artery

Plate 1.3

Cardiovascular System: VOLUME 8

MEDIASTINUM: CROSS SECTION

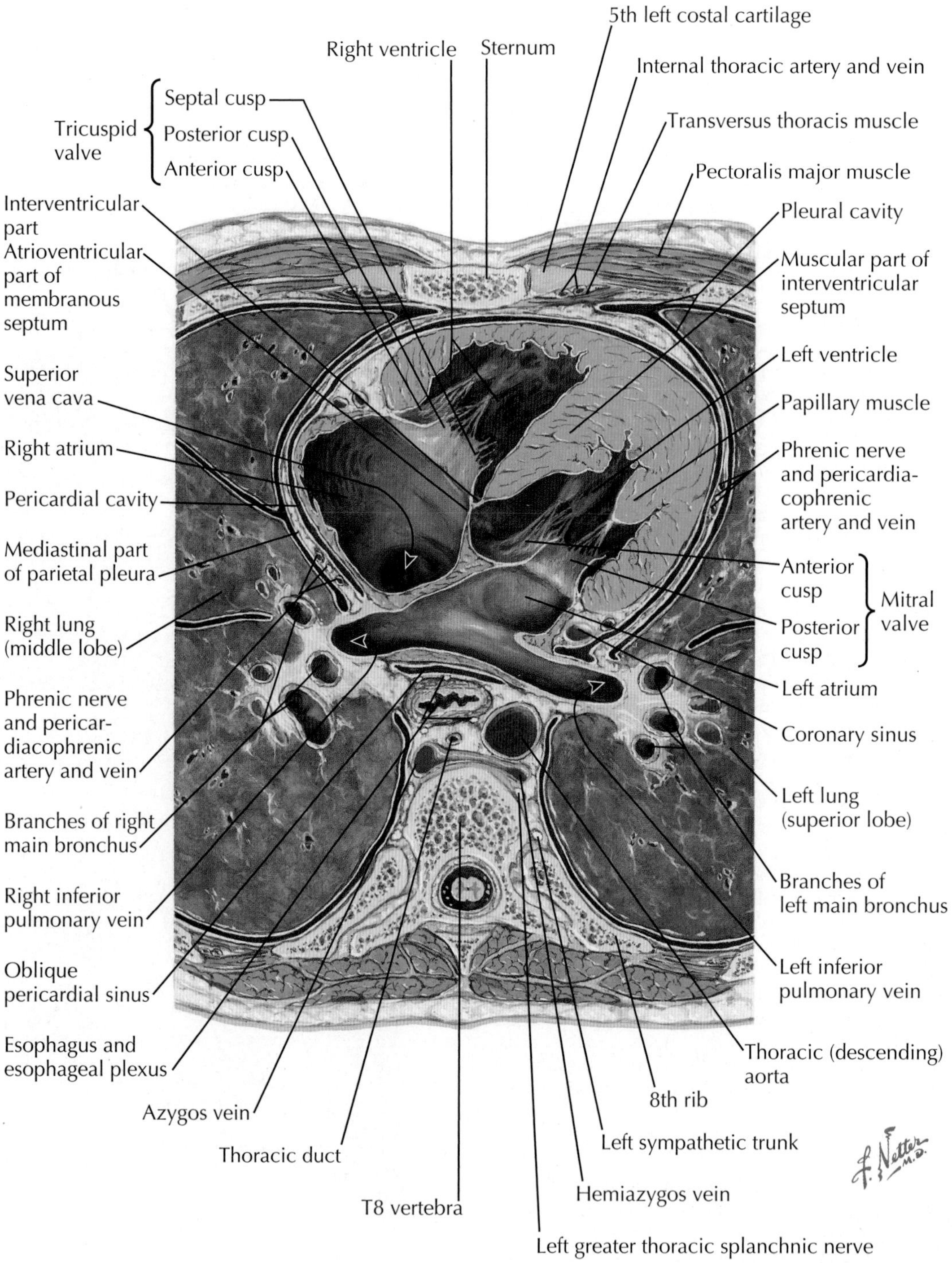

Labels (clockwise):
5th left costal cartilage
Right ventricle
Sternum
Internal thoracic artery and vein
Transversus thoracis muscle
Tricuspid valve — Septal cusp, Posterior cusp, Anterior cusp
Pectoralis major muscle
Interventricular part
Atrioventricular part of membranous septum
Pleural cavity
Muscular part of interventricular septum
Superior vena cava
Left ventricle
Papillary muscle
Right atrium
Pericardial cavity
Phrenic nerve and pericardiacophrenic artery and vein
Mediastinal part of parietal pleura
Mitral valve — Anterior cusp, Posterior cusp
Right lung (middle lobe)
Left atrium
Phrenic nerve and pericardiacophrenic artery and vein
Coronary sinus
Branches of right main bronchus
Left lung (superior lobe)
Right inferior pulmonary vein
Branches of left main bronchus
Oblique pericardial sinus
Left inferior pulmonary vein
Esophagus and esophageal plexus
Thoracic (descending) aorta
Azygos vein
8th rib
Thoracic duct
Left sympathetic trunk
T8 vertebra
Hemiazygos vein
Left greater thoracic splanchnic nerve

f. Netter

THORAX (Continued)

their corresponding intercostal spaces, passing along the inferior border of the ribs between the internal and external intercostal muscles. The vessels are well protected posteriorly by the subcostal groove. The internal thoracic arteries originate from the inferior surface of the subclavian arteries and run downward, lateral to, and (for a short distance) with the *phrenic nerve*, reaching the posterior surface of the anterior chest wall. The arteries continue their downward course for approximately 0.25 inches laterally to the edges of the sternum, dividing just above the diaphragm into their two terminal branches: the *musculophrenic* and *superior epigastric arteries*. Along their course the internal thoracic arteries give rise to branches to the *thymus*, mediastinum, and *pericardium* posteriorly; to the perforating branches to the skin and subcutaneous tissues anteriorly; and finally to the lateral branches that pass along the rib cartilages and anastomose with the posterior intercostal arteries.

The veins of the thoracic wall correspond in their course with the arteries. The 10 lower intercostal veins on the right enter the *azygos vein*, and the upper two intercostal veins enter either the azygos or the *brachiocephalic* (innominate) vein. The lower intercostal veins on the left side enter the *hemiazygos* or *accessory hemiazygos vein*. The three left superior intercostal veins enter the left brachiocephalic vein by a common stem, the left superior intercostal vein.

The chest wall receives its nerve supply from the intercostal nerves, which accompany the intercostal vessels.

Most of the thoracic cavity is occupied by the two *lungs*, each of which is enclosed by its *pleura*. Each pleura forms a closed sac invaginated by the lung so that part of it covers (and is adherent to) the inner surface of the chest wall, the diaphragm, and the mediastinum, known as the *costal*, the *diaphragmatic*, and the *mediastinal* pleura, respectively, and collectively as the parietal pleura (see Plate 1.2). That part of the mediastinal pleura that covers the pericardium is called the *pericardial pleura*; the remainder (visceral pleura) covers the lung. The virtual space between the visceral and parietal pleurae contains a tiny amount of clear fluid. The *pleural reflections* (see Plate 1.1), between the costal and diaphragmatic portions of the parietal pleura, lie lower than the corresponding lower edge of the lung. The resulting space normally is not completely filled by the lung, even on deep inspiration, and is called the *recessus costodiaphragmaticus*.

The *right lung* consists of three lobes—the superior, middle, and inferior lobes—and is somewhat larger than the *left lung*, which has two—the superior and inferior lobes (see Plate 1.1). The smaller size of the left lung results from the eccentric position of the heart, which encroaches on the *left pleural cavity*. The two pleural cavities almost meet behind the upper *sternum*,

but the left costomediastinal reflection deviates laterally below the fourth rib cartilage, exposing a small triangular portion of the pericardium that is not covered by pleura. At the same level, the anteroinferior portion of the left superior lobe recedes even more, leaving a portion of the pericardial pleura that is not covered by lung tissue.

The central space between the two pleural cavities is the mediastinum. The mediastinum is divided arbitrarily into superior, anterior, middle, and posterior mediastina. The shallow anterior mediastinum contains a portion of

the *left internal thoracic vessels* and the vestigial *transverse thoracic muscle*. The superior mediastinum contains the thymus (see Plate 1.2), which largely disappears by about age 12 years, leaving a small pad of fat and areolar tissue, and the brachiocephalic veins, which join each other on the right to form the *superior vena cava* (see Plate 1.5). Posterior to the brachiocephalic veins, the phrenic and vagus nerves descend from the neck. The *phrenic nerves*, accompanied by the *pericardiacophrenic vessels*, run laterally, anterior to the lung roots and along the pericardium, until they reach the diaphragm.

Plate 1.4

Anatomy

PERICARDIAL SAC

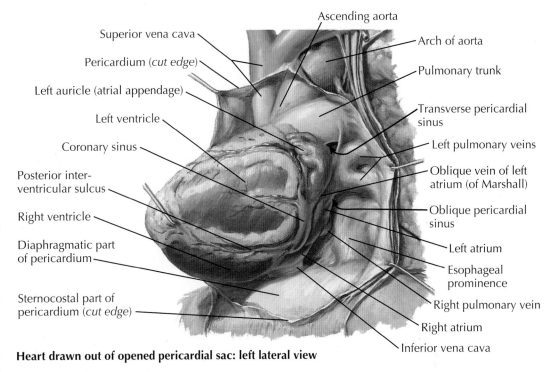

Heart drawn out of opened pericardial sac: left lateral view

THORAX (Continued)

The *aortic arch* ascends from the heart into the superior mediastinum, almost reaches the upper border of the manubrium sterni, courses obliquely backward and to the left over the left main *bronchus,* and continues as the *descending aorta* downward, anteriorly, and slightly to the left of the vertebral column. Originating from the convexity of the arch, from the proximal to the distal position, are the brachiocephalic, left common carotid, and subclavian arteries.

The *right vagus nerve* (see Plate 1.5) passes between the subclavian artery and vein and gives off the right recurrent nerve, which loops around the subclavian artery to ascend along the trachea. The *left vagus nerve* runs between the subclavian vein and the aortic arch, giving rise to the *left recurrent nerve* (see Plate 1.5), which similarly loops around the arch to ascend along the trachea.

The trachea descends from the neck behind the aortic arch and bifurcates into right and left main bronchi at the level of the sternal angle. Behind the trachea runs the normally collapsed *esophagus* (Plate 1.4), joined by the vagus nerves just beyond the branching of the recurrent nerves from the vagi. Behind the esophagus, between the azygos vein and the descending aorta, the *thoracic duct* (see Plate 1.2) ascends, coursing behind the aortic arch to enter the neck, where it empties into the left subclavian vein.

Against the necks of the ribs, the *sympathetic trunks* descend from the neck, first giving off the *greater thoracic splanchnic nerve* (major splanchnic nerve; see Plate 1.3) at about the level of the sixth rib and then the *minor* or *lesser* and *lowest thoracic splanchnic nerves.*

The posterior mediastinum is a shallow space containing the lower portions of the esophagus, vagus nerves, descending aorta, azygos and hemiazygos veins, thoracic duct, and sympathetic nerve chains. The remaining and largest part of the mediastinum, the middle mediastinum, contains the *pericardium,* heart, lung roots, and *phrenic nerves.*

The *pericardial cavity* is the third serous cavity contained in the chest, with the two pleural cavities. The pericardial cavity is conical in shape, with the base of the cone lying posteriorly to the right and the apex anteriorly to the left. It completely invests the heart and the proximal portions of the great vessels. As with the pleura, a visceral portion of the pericardium is distinguished overlying the heart and proximal great vessels, usually called the *epicardium,* as is a parietal portion. The inferior part of the parietal pericardium is densely adherent to the middle tendinous part of the diaphragm. Most of the lateral and anterior portions are contiguous but not normally adherent to the pleura. A small triangular part of the anterior portion of the parietal pericardium lies directly behind the

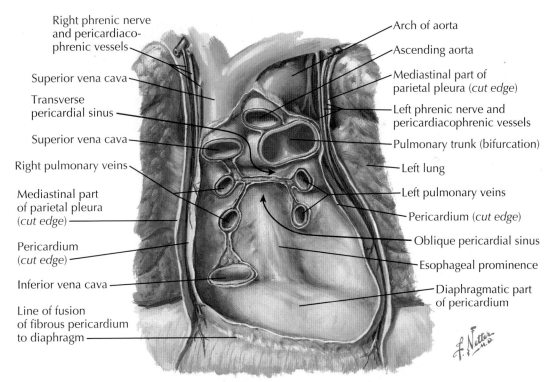

Pericardial sac with heart removed: anterior view

sternum, separated only by areolar and fatty tissue (endothoracic fascia) and the transverse thoracic muscle.

The great vessels enter and leave the pericardial cavity at its base. A curved, transversely running passageway between the arterial and venous poles of the heart is called the *transverse pericardial sinus.* Posteriorly, a blind recess of the pericardial cavity is bordered by the pericardial reflection between the pulmonary veins and

inferior vena cava, called the *oblique pericardial sinus.* Small recesses exist between the *superior* and *inferior pulmonary veins* on each side and behind the *fold of the left vena cava* (ligament of Marshall), a small crease of pericardium running from the left aspect of the pulmonary trunk to the left atrium, between the neck of the left auricle and the left pulmonary veins. The left vena cava fold contains the vestigial remains of the left common cardinal vein.

Plate 1.5

Cardiovascular System: VOLUME 8

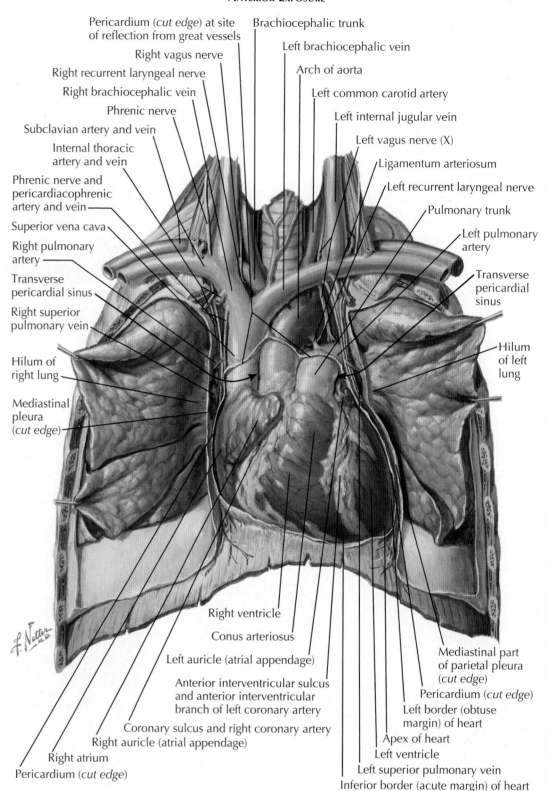

ANTERIOR EXPOSURE

Pericardium (*cut edge*) at site of reflection from great vessels
Brachiocephalic trunk
Right vagus nerve
Left brachiocephalic vein
Right recurrent laryngeal nerve
Arch of aorta
Right brachiocephalic vein
Left common carotid artery
Phrenic nerve
Left internal jugular vein
Subclavian artery and vein
Left vagus nerve (X)
Internal thoracic artery and vein
Ligamentum arteriosum
Phrenic nerve and pericardiacophrenic artery and vein
Left recurrent laryngeal nerve
Superior vena cava
Pulmonary trunk
Right pulmonary artery
Left pulmonary artery
Transverse pericardial sinus
Transverse pericardial sinus
Right superior pulmonary vein
Hilum of left lung
Hilum of right lung
Mediastinal pleura (*cut edge*)
Right ventricle
Conus arteriosus
Mediastinal part of parietal pleura (*cut edge*)
Left auricle (atrial appendage)
Pericardium (*cut edge*)
Anterior interventricular sulcus and anterior interventricular branch of left coronary artery
Left border (obtuse margin) of heart
Coronary sulcus and right coronary artery
Apex of heart
Right auricle (atrial appendage)
Left ventricle
Right atrium
Left superior pulmonary vein
Pericardium (*cut edge*)
Inferior border (acute margin) of heart

EXPOSURE OF THE HEART

STERNOCOSTAL ASPECT

Within the *pericardium* lies the heart, a hollow, muscular, four-chambered organ suspended at its base by the great vessels. In situ the heart occupies an asymmetric position, with its *apex* pointing anteriorly, inferiorly, and about 60 degrees toward the left. Its four chambers are arranged in two functionally similar pairs, separated from each other by the cardiac *septum* (Plate 1.5). Each pair consists of a thin-walled atrium and a thicker-walled ventricle.

The anatomic nomenclature of the heart removes it from the body and places it on its apex; thus the cardiac septum is in a sagittal plane. This practice has led to misconceptions and difficulties in orientation among cardiologists and surgeons. On a chest radiograph, for example, the left cardiac border is formed by the left ventricle, but the right border is formed by the right atrium, not the right ventricle, which lies anterior. The major and important part of the left atrium lies directly posterior and in the midline in front of the spine and esophagus, allowing the *pulmonary veins* to be as short as possible.

On removing the anterior chest wall and opening the pericardium, most of the presenting part of the heart is formed by the right ventricle, with its exposed surface triangular in shape. The right atrium lies to the right of the right ventricle.

The term "auricle" is often improperly used instead of atrium. The true auricle is then regrettably called "auricular appendage" instead of *atrial appendage*, which is morphologically correct. The term "auricular fibrillation" is clinically incorrect and should be *atrial fibrillation*.

The right atrium and right ventricle are separated by the *right atrioventricular* (coronary) *sulcus*, through

which runs the right coronary artery, embedded in a variable amount of fat. To the left of the right ventricle, a small segment of the left ventricle is visible, separated from it by the *anterior interventricular sulcus* (groove). The *anterior interventricular* (descending) *branch* of the *left coronary artery* (Plate 1.5) lies in this groove, again embedded in fat.

Superiorly, the *pulmonary trunk* is seen originating from the right ventricle and leaving the pericardium

just before it bifurcates into its two main branches: the *right and left pulmonary arteries*. To the right of the pulmonary trunk lies the intrapericardial portion of the ascending *aorta*, the base of which is largely covered by the *right auricle* (right atrial appendage). The base of the aorta, including the first part of the right coronary artery, is surrounded by lobules of fatty tissue called *Rindfleisch folds*, the largest and uppermost of which is rather constant.

Plate 1.6   Anatomy

BASE AND DIAPHRAGMATIC SURFACES

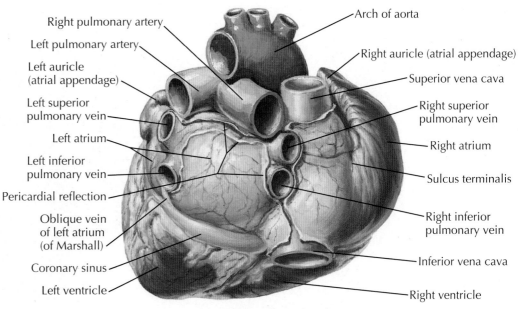

Right pulmonary artery — Arch of aorta
Left pulmonary artery — Right auricle (atrial appendage)
Left auricle (atrial appendage) — Superior vena cava
Left superior pulmonary vein — Right superior pulmonary vein
Left atrium — Right atrium
Left inferior pulmonary vein — Sulcus terminalis
Pericardial reflection — Right inferior pulmonary vein
Oblique vein of left atrium (of Marshall) — Inferior vena cava
Coronary sinus — Right ventricle
Left ventricle

Base of heart: posterior view

EXPOSURE OF THE HEART (Continued)

POSTERIOR AND DIAPHRAGMATIC ASPECTS

After removal of the heart from the pericardium, its *posterior* (basilar) and *diaphragmatic* aspects can be inspected. The *superior vena cava* (SVC) and *inferior vena cava* (IVC) enter the *right atrium,* with the long axis of both cavae inclined slightly forward and the IVC in a more medial position. A pronounced groove, the *sulcus terminalis,* separates the right aspect of the SVC from the base of the *right auricle.* As this groove descends along the posterior aspect of the right atrium, it becomes less distinct.

The *right pulmonary veins* (usually two but occasionally three) arise from the right lung and cross the right atrium posteriorly to enter the right side of the *left atrium.* The two *left pulmonary veins* enter the left side of the left atrium, sometimes by a large common stem. The posterior wall of the left atrium forms the anterior wall of the *oblique pericardial sinus.* Normally, the left atrium is not in contact with the diaphragm.

The bifurcation of the pulmonary trunk lies on the roof of the left atrium. The *left pulmonary artery* courses immediately toward the left lung, and the *right pulmonary artery* runs behind the proximal SVC and above the right pulmonary veins to the right lung.

The *aortic arch* crosses the pulmonary artery bifurcation after giving off its three main branches: the *brachiocephalic* (innominate), *left common carotid,* and *left subclavian arteries.* Variations in this pattern occur and usually are not significant.

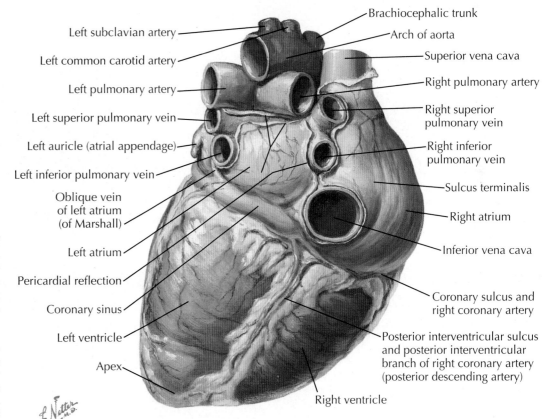

Left subclavian artery — Brachiocephalic trunk
Left common carotid artery — Arch of aorta
— Superior vena cava
Left pulmonary artery — Right pulmonary artery
Left superior pulmonary vein — Right superior pulmonary vein
Left auricle (atrial appendage) — Right inferior pulmonary vein
Left inferior pulmonary vein — Sulcus terminalis
Oblique vein of left atrium (of Marshall) — Right atrium
Left atrium — Inferior vena cava
Pericardial reflection —
Coronary sinus — Coronary sulcus and right coronary artery
Left ventricle — Posterior interventricular sulcus and posterior interventricular branch of right coronary artery (posterior descending artery)
Apex — Right ventricle

Base and diaphragmatic surface: posteroinferior view

The *coronary sinus* lies between the left atrium and the *left ventricle* in the posterior (diaphragmatic) portion of the *left atrioventricular groove* (coronary sulcus). The cardiac veins enter the coronary sinus, which has the appearance of a short, wide vein. However, its wall consists of cardiac muscle, and because of its embryonic origin, the coronary sinus should be considered a true cardiac structure. Its right extremity turns forward and upward to enter the right atrium.

The diaphragmatic surfaces of the *right ventricle* and the *left ventricle* are separated by the *posterior interventricular sulcus* (groove). This sulcus is continuous with the anterior interventricular groove just to the right of the cardiac *apex,* which in a normal heart is formed by the left ventricle. The posterior interventricular (descending) artery and middle cardiac vein lie in the posterior interventricular sulcus, embedded in fat.

Plate 1.7

Cardiovascular System: VOLUME 8

RIGHT ATRIUM AND RIGHT VENTRICLE

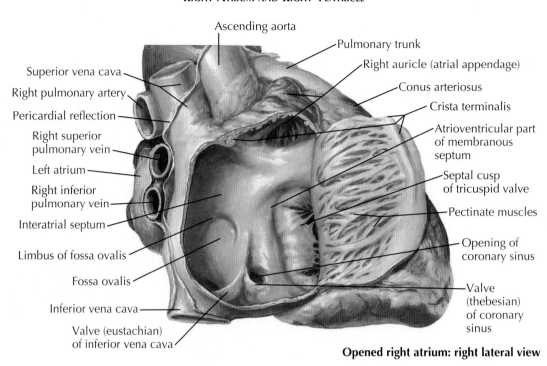

Ascending aorta
Pulmonary trunk
Superior vena cava
Right auricle (atrial appendage)
Right pulmonary artery
Conus arteriosus
Pericardial reflection
Crista terminalis
Right superior pulmonary vein
Atrioventricular part of membranous septum
Left atrium
Septal cusp of tricuspid valve
Right inferior pulmonary vein
Pectinate muscles
Interatrial septum
Opening of coronary sinus
Limbus of fossa ovalis
Fossa ovalis
Valve (thebesian) of coronary sinus
Inferior vena cava
Valve (eustachian) of inferior vena cava

Opened right atrium: right lateral view

Pericardial reflection
Pulmonary trunk
Aorta
Transverse pericardial sinus
Transverse pericardial sinus
Anterior semilunar cusp
Right semilunar cusp — Pulmonary valve
Superior vena cava
Left semilunar cusp
Right auricle (atrial appendage)
Conus arteriosus
Right atrium
Supraventricular crest
Membranous part of interventricular septum
Septal papillary muscle
Anterior cusp
Interventricular septum (muscular part)
Tricuspid valve — Septal cusp
Posterior cusp
Septomarginal trabecula (moderator band)
Chordae tendineae
Posterior papillary muscle
Anterior papillary muscle
Trabeculae carneae

Opened right ventricle: anterior view

ATRIA AND VENTRICLES

RIGHT ATRIUM

The right atrium consists of two parts: (1) a posterior smooth-walled part derived from the embryonic sinus venosus, into which enter the superior and inferior venae cavae, and (2) a thin-walled trabeculated part that constitutes the original embryonic right atrium. The two parts of the atrium are separated by a ridge of muscle. This ridge, the *crista terminalis* (Plate 1.7), is most prominent superiorly, next to the SVC orifice, and then fades out to the right of the IVC ostium. Its position corresponds to that of the *sulcus terminalis* externally (see Plate 1.6). Often described as a remnant of the embryonic right venous valve, the crista terminalis actually lies just to the right of the valve.

From the lateral aspect of the crista terminalis, a large number of *pectinate muscles* run laterally and generally parallel to each other along the free wall of the atrium. The atrial wall is paper thin and translucent between the pectinate muscles. The triangular-shaped superior portion of the right atrium—the *right auricle*—is also filled with pectinate muscles. One pectinate muscle originating from the crista terminalis is usually larger than the others and is called the *taenia sagittalis*.

The right auricle usually is not well demarcated externally from the rest of the atrium. The right auricle is a convenient, ready-made point of entry for the cardiac surgeon and is used extensively.

The anterior border of the IVC ostium is guarded by a fold of tissue, the *inferior vena cava (eustachian) valve*, which varies greatly in size and may even be absent. When large, the IVC valve is usually perforated by numerous openings, forming a delicate lace-like structure known as the *network of Chiari*. The coronary sinus enters the right atrium just anterior to the medial extremity of the IVC valve. The eustachian valve's *orifice* may also be guarded by a valve-like fold, the *coronary sinus* (thebesian) *valve*. Both IVC valves and coronary sinus valves are derived from the large, embryonic right venous valve.

The posteromedial wall of the right atrium is formed by the *interatrial septum,* which has a thin, fibrous,

central ovoid portion. The interatrial septum forms a shallow depression in the septum called the *fossa ovalis*. The remainder of the septum is muscular and usually forms a ridge around the fossa ovalis, the *limbus fossae ovalis*. A probe can be passed under the anterosuperior part of the limbus into the left atrium in some cases, and the foramen (fossa) ovalis is then "probe patent." Anteromedially, the tricuspid valve gives access to the right ventricle.

RIGHT VENTRICLE

The *right ventricular cavity* (Plate 1.7) can be divided arbitrarily into a posteroinferior inflow portion, containing the *tricuspid valve,* and an anterosuperior outflow portion, from which the *pulmonary trunk* originates. These two parts are separated by prominent muscular bands, including the *parietal band,* the *supraventricular crest* (crista supraventricularis), the *septal band,* and the *moderator band.* These bands form a

Plate 1.8

Anatomy

LEFT ATRIUM AND LEFT VENTRICLE

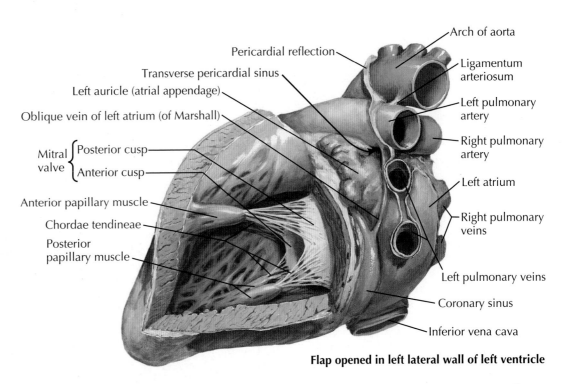

Arch of aorta
Pericardial reflection
Transverse pericardial sinus
Left auricle (atrial appendage)
Oblique vein of left atrium (of Marshall)
Ligamentum arteriosum
Left pulmonary artery
Right pulmonary artery
Left atrium
Mitral valve { Posterior cusp / Anterior cusp }
Right pulmonary veins
Anterior papillary muscle
Chordae tendineae
Posterior papillary muscle
Left pulmonary veins
Coronary sinus
Inferior vena cava

Flap opened in left lateral wall of left ventricle

Left auricle (atrial appendage)
Conus arteriosus
Arch of aorta
Aortic valve { Left semilunar cusp / Right semilunar cusp / Posterior semilunar cusp }
Left pulmonary artery
Right pulmonary artery
Mem-branous septum { Interventricular part / Atrioventricular part }
Left superior pulmonary vein
Right pulmonary veins
Muscular part of interventricular septum
Valve of foramen ovale
Left atrium
Mitral valve (cut away)
Inferior vena cava
Coronary sinus

Section through left atrium and ventricle with mitral valve cut away

ATRIA AND VENTRICLES
(Continued)

wide, almost circular orifice with no impediment to flow in the normal heart.

The wall of the inflow portion is heavily trabeculated, particularly in its most apical portion. These *trabeculae carneae* enclose a more or less elongated, ovoid opening. The outflow portion of the right ventricle, often called the infundibulum, contains only a few trabeculae. The subpulmonic area is smooth walled.

A number of *papillary muscles* anchor the *tricuspid valve cusps* to the right ventricular wall through many slender, fibrous strands called the *chordae tendineae*. Two papillary muscles, the medial and anterior, are reasonably constant in position but vary in size and shape. The other papillary muscles are extremely variable in all respects. Approximately where the crista supraventricularis joins the septal band, the small *medial papillary muscle* receives chordae tendineae from the anterior and septal cusps of the tricuspid valve. Often well developed in infants, the medial papillary muscle is almost absent in adults or is reduced to a tendinous patch. An important surgical landmark, the medial papillary muscle is also of diagnostic value to the cardiac pathologist with its interesting embryonic origin. The *anterior papillary muscle* originates from the moderator band and receives chordae from the anterior and posterior cusps of the tricuspid valve. In variable numbers, the usually small *posterior papillary muscle* and septal papillary muscle receive chordae from the posterior and medial (septal) cusps. The muscles originating from the posteroinferior border of the septal band are important in the analysis of some congenital cardiac anomalies.

The *pulmonary trunk* arises superiorly from the right ventricle and passes backward and slightly upward. It bifurcates into right and left *pulmonary arteries* (see Plate 1.7) just after leaving the pericardial cavity. A short ligament—the *ligamentum arteriosum* (Plate 1.8)—connects the upper aspect of the bifurcation to the inferior surface of the *aortic arch* (arch of

aorta; see Plate 1.6). It is a remnant of the fetal ductus arteriosus (duct of Botallo).

LEFT ATRIUM

The left atrium consists mainly of a smooth-walled sac with the transverse axis longer than the vertical and sagittal axes. On the right, two or occasionally three *pulmonary veins* enter the left atrium; on the left there

are also two (sometimes one) pulmonary veins. The wall of the left atrium is distinctly thicker than that of the right atrium. The septal surface is usually fairly smooth, with only an irregular area indicating the position of the fetal *valve of the foramen ovale*. A narrow slit may allow a probe to be passed from the right atrium to the left atrium.

The *left auricle* is a continuation of the left upper anterior part of the left atrium. The auricle's variable

Plate 1.9

Cardiovascular System: VOLUME 8

ATRIA, VENTRICLES, AND INTERVENTRICULAR SEPTUM

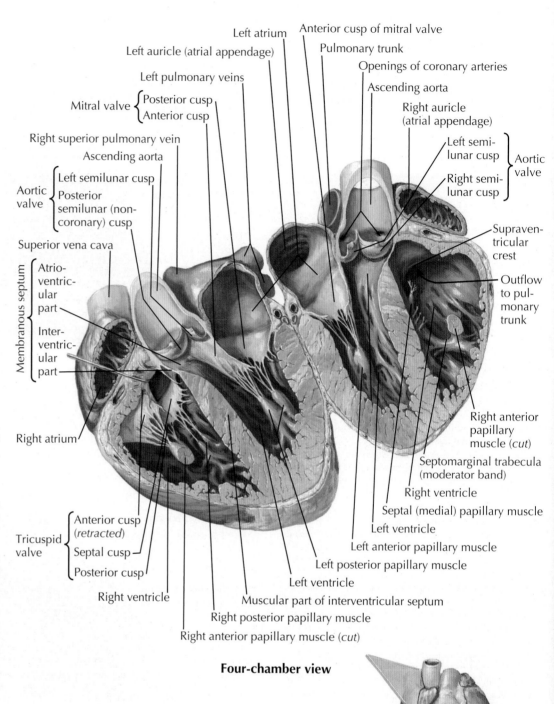

Four-chamber view

Plane of section

ATRIA AND VENTRICLES
(Continued)

shape may be long and kinked in one or more places. Its lumen contains small pectinate muscles, and there usually is a distinct waist-like narrowing proximally.

LEFT VENTRICLE

The *left ventricle* (see Plate 1.8) is egg shaped with the blunt end cut off, where the *mitral valve* and *aortic valve* are located adjacent to each other. The valves are separated only by a fibrous band giving off most of the *anterior* (aortic) *cusp of the mitral valve* and the adjacent portions of the *left* and *posterior aortic valve cusps*. The average thickness of the left ventricular (LV) wall is about three times that of the right ventricular (RV) wall. The LV trabeculae carneae are somewhat less coarse, with some just tendinous cords. As in the right ventricle, the trabeculae are much more numerous and dense in the apex of the left ventricle. The basilar third of the septum is smooth.

Usually there are two stout *papillary muscles*. The dual embryonic origin of each is often revealed by their bifid apices; each receives *chordae tendineae* from both major *mitral valve cusps*. Occasionally a third, small papillary muscle is present laterally.

Most of the *ventricular septum* is muscular. Normally it bulges into the right ventricle, showing that a transverse section of the left ventricle is almost circular. The *muscular* portion has approximately the same thickness as the parietal LV wall. The ventricular septum consists of two layers, a thin layer on the RV side and a thicker layer on the LV side. The major septal arteries tend to run between these two layers. In the human heart a variable but generally small area of the septum immediately below the *right* and *posterior aortic valve cusps* is thin and membranous.

The demarcation between the muscular and the *membranous* part of the ventricular septum is distinct and is called the *limbus marginalis*. As seen from the opened right ventricle (see Plate 1.7, bottom), the

membranous septum lies deep to the *supraventricular crest* and is divided into two parts by the origin of the *medial* (septal) *cusp* of the *tricuspid valve*. As a result, one portion of the membranous septum lies between the left ventricle and the right ventricle—the *interventricular part*—and the other between the left ventricle and the right atrium—the *atrioventricular part*.

On sectioning of the septum in an approximately transverse plane, the basilar portion of the ventricular septum, including the membranous septum, is seen to deviate to the right, so that a plane through the major portion of the septum bisects the *aortic valve*. It must be emphasized that the total cardiac septum shows a complex, longitudinal twist and does not lie in any single plane.

Plate 1.10

Anatomy

CARDIAC VALVES OPEN AND CLOSED

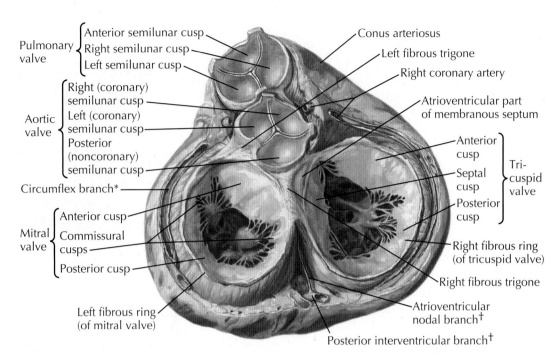

Pulmonary valve
- Anterior semilunar cusp
- Right semilunar cusp
- Left semilunar cusp

Aortic valve
- Right (coronary) semilunar cusp
- Left (coronary) semilunar cusp
- Posterior (noncoronary) semilunar cusp

Circumflex branch*

Mitral valve
- Anterior cusp
- Commissural cusps
- Posterior cusp

Left fibrous ring (of mitral valve)

Conus arteriosus

Left fibrous trigone

Right coronary artery

Atrioventricular part of membranous septum

Tricuspid valve
- Anterior cusp
- Septal cusp
- Posterior cusp

Right fibrous ring (of tricuspid valve)

Right fibrous trigone

Atrioventricular nodal branch†

Posterior interventricular branch†

Heart in diastole: viewed from base with atria removed

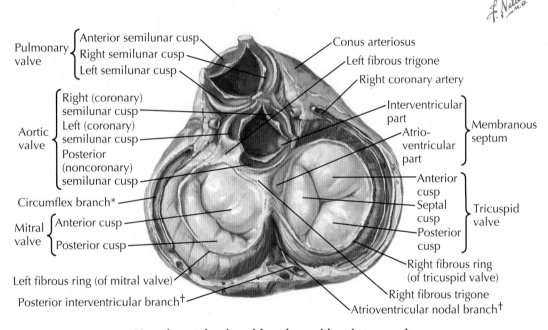

Pulmonary valve
- Anterior semilunar cusp
- Right semilunar cusp
- Left semilunar cusp

Aortic valve
- Right (coronary) semilunar cusp
- Left (coronary) semilunar cusp
- Posterior (noncoronary) semilunar cusp

Circumflex branch*

Mitral valve
- Anterior cusp
- Posterior cusp

Left fibrous ring (of mitral valve)

Posterior interventricular branch†

Conus arteriosus

Left fibrous trigone

Right coronary artery

Membranous septum
- Interventricular part
- Atrioventricular part

Tricuspid valve
- Anterior cusp
- Septal cusp
- Posterior cusp

Right fibrous ring (of tricuspid valve)

Right fibrous trigone

Atrioventricular nodal branch†

Heart in systole: viewed from base with atria removed

*Of left coronary artery
†Of right coronary artery

VALVES

Each *atrioventricular* (AV) *valve* apparatus consists of a number of cusps, chordae tendineae, and papillary muscles. The cusps are thin, yellowish white, glistening trapezoid-shaped membranes with fine, irregular edges. They originate from the *annulus fibrosus*, a poorly defined and unimpressive fibrous ring around each AV orifice. The amount of fibrous tissue increases only at the *right* and *left fibrous trigones*.

The atrial surface of the AV valve is rather smooth (except near the free edge) and not well demarcated from the atrial wall. The ventricular surface is irregular because of the insertion of the chordae tendineae and is separated from the ventricular wall by a narrow space.

The extreme edges of the cusps are thin and delicate with a sawtooth appearance from the insertion of equally fine chordae. Away from the edge, the atrial surface of the cusps is finely nodular, particularly in small children. These nodules are called the *noduli Albini*. On closure of an AV valve, the narrow border between the row of Albini's nodules and the free edge of each cusp presses against that of the next, resulting in a secure, watertight closure. The chordae tendineae may be divided into the following three groups:

- The chordae of the first order insert into the extreme edge of the valve by a large number of very

fine strands. Their function seems to be merely to prevent the opposing borders of the cusps from inverting.
- The chordae of the second order insert on the ventricular surface of the cusps, approximately at the level of Albini's nodules or even higher. These are stronger and less numerous. They function as the mainstays of the valves and are comparable to the stays of an umbrella.

- The chordae of the third order originate from the ventricular wall much nearer the origin of the cusps. These chordae often form bands or fold-like structures that may contain muscle.

The first two groups originate from or near the apices of the papillary muscles. They form a few strong, tendinous cords that subdivide into several thinner strands as they approach the valve edges. Occasionally, particularly on the left side, the chordae of the first two

Plate 1.11

Cardiovascular System: VOLUME 8

VALVES AND FIBROUS SKELETON OF HEART

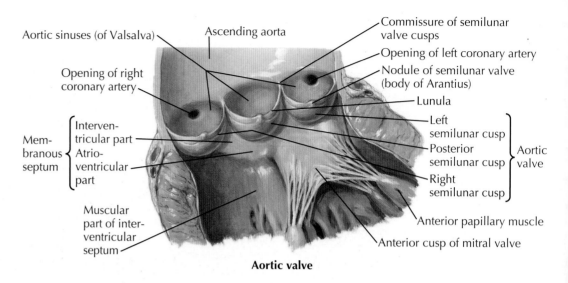

Aortic sinuses (of Valsalva)
Ascending aorta
Commissure of semilunar valve cusps
Opening of left coronary artery
Nodule of semilunar valve (body of Arantius)
Opening of right coronary artery
Lunula
Membranous septum
Interventricular part
Atrioventricular part
Left semilunar cusp
Posterior semilunar cusp
Right semilunar cusp
Aortic valve
Muscular part of interventricular septum
Anterior papillary muscle
Anterior cusp of mitral valve

Aortic valve

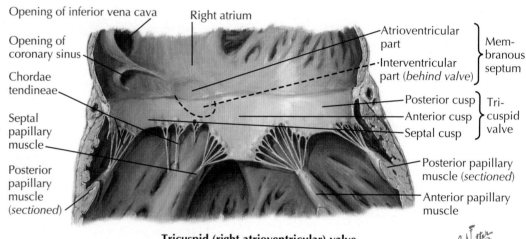

Opening of inferior vena cava
Right atrium
Atrioventricular part
Membranous septum
Opening of coronary sinus
Interventricular part (behind valve)
Chordae tendineae
Posterior cusp
Anterior cusp
Septal cusp
Tricuspid valve
Septal papillary muscle
Posterior papillary muscle (sectioned)
Posterior papillary muscle (sectioned)
Anterior papillary muscle

Tricuspid (right atrioventricular) valve

VALVES (Continued)

orders may be wholly muscular, even in normal hearts, so that the papillary muscle seems to insert directly into the cusp. This is not surprising because the *papillary muscles,* the *chordae tendineae,* and most of the *cusps* are derived from the embryonic ventricular trabeculae and therefore were all muscular at one time.

The *tricuspid valve* consists of an *anterior,* a *medial* (septal), and one or two *posterior* cusps. The depth of the *commissures* between the cusps is variable, but the commissures never reach the *annulus,* so the cusps are only incompletely separated from each other.

The *mitral* (bicuspid) *valve* actually is made up of four cusps: two large ones—the *anterior* (aortic) and *posterior* (mural) *cusps*—and two small *commissural cusps.* Here, as in the tricuspid valve, the commissures are never complete, and they should not be so constructed in the surgical treatment of mitral stenosis.

The arterial or semilunar valves differ greatly in structure from the AV valves. Each consists of three pocket-like cusps of approximately equal size. Although functionally the transition between the ventricle and the artery is abrupt and easily determined, this cannot be done anatomically in any simple manner. There is no distinct, circular ring of fibrous tissue at the base of the arteries from which these and the valve cusps arise; rather, the arterial wall expands into three dilated

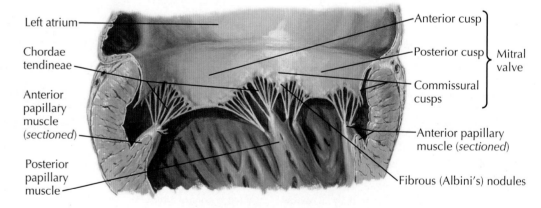

Left atrium
Anterior cusp
Chordae tendineae
Posterior cusp
Mitral valve
Anterior papillary muscle (sectioned)
Commissural cusps
Posterior papillary muscle
Anterior papillary muscle (sectioned)
Fibrous (Albini's) nodules

Mitral (left atrioventricular) valve

pouches, the sinuses of Valsalva, whose walls are much thinner than those of the aorta or pulmonary artery. The origin of the valve cusps is therefore not straight but scalloped.

The cusps of the arterial semilunar valve are largely smooth and thin. At the center of the free margin of each cusp is a small fibrous nodule called the *nodulus Arantii.* On each side of the nodules of Arantius,

along the entire free edge of the cusp, there is a thin, half-moon–shaped area called the *lunula* that has fine striations parallel to the edge. The lunulae are usually perforated near the insertion of the cusps on the aortic wall. In valve closure, because the areas of adjacent lunulae appose each other, such perforations do not cause insufficiency of the valve and are functionally of no significance.

Plate 1.12   Anatomy

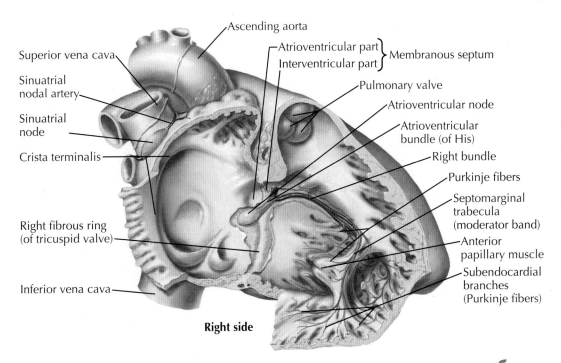

Right side

SPECIALIZED CONDUCTION SYSTEM OF HEART

The specialized heart tissues include the *sinuatrial* (SA) *node, atrioventricular* (AV) *node*, common atrioventricular bundle or bundle of His, right and left bundle branches, and peripheral ramifications of these bundle branches, which make up the subendocardial and intramyocardial Purkinje network. In addition, other fiber groups in the atria meet some of the histologic and electrophysiologic criteria for specialization. These tissues constitute Bachmann's bundle and the internodal conducting paths of the right atrium.

The body of the SA node is in the wall of the right atrium, at the junction between the atrium proper and the *superior vena cava*. At the lower end, the nodal fibers change and form the common bundle. The common bundle divides into right and left bundle branches, which extend subendocardially along both septal surfaces. The left bundle branch rapidly subdivides, forming a broad sheet of fascicles sweeping over the left interventricular septal surface. The right bundle branch extends for a distance without subdivision; one branch usually passes through the *moderator band*, and other parts extend over the endocardial surface of the ventricle. Peripherally, both bundle branches subdivide and form the subendocardial network of *Purkinje fibers*, which extend a variable distance into the ventricular walls and are in direct continuity with fibers of the ventricular muscle.

In definitive histologic studies of the human atrium, James demonstrated the existence of three discrete internodal paths and the relationship of one of these to Bachmann's bundle. The *anterior internodal tract* leaves the head of the sinus node and spreads to the left, dividing to form two branches: One extends along the dorsal aspect of the interatrial band to ramify over the left atrium. This subdivision constitutes the specialized fibers of Bachmann's bundle. The other branch curves across the interatrial septum to the region of the AV node, where it merges with fibers from other nodal tracts. The *middle internodal tract* leaves the posterodorsal margin of the sinus node and crosses the interatrial septum to merge at the AV node with other specialized atrial fibers. This tract corresponds to the

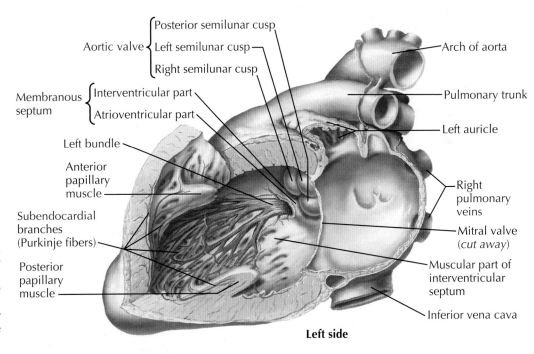

Left side

bundle described by Wenckebach. The *posterior internodal tract* extends from the tail of the sinus node along the crista terminalis, through the eustachian ridge, which is the right superior margin of the AV node. A description of the interconnections of internodal tracts with the atrium and AV node follows.

Physiologic evidence suggests that the spread of the sinus impulse to the left atrium and from the sinus node to the AV node normally depends primarily on activation of the anterior internodal tract and Bachmann's bundle. The physiologic significance of these tracts is also described here.

The only normal anatomic *communication* between the atria and ventricles of the mammalian heart is the *atrioventricular node* with the common bundle of His. On the atrial side, the AV node communicates with the atrium through the branched and interweaving fibers of the internodal tracts and perhaps through connections with ordinary atrial musculature. In addition, in studies of the canine AV node, fiber tracts appear to bypass the nodal body and connect with distal portions close to the junction of nodal fibers and the common AV bundle. Similar "bypass" fibers can be demonstrated in studies of the human AV node.

Plate 1.13

Cardiovascular System: VOLUME 8

STERNOCOSTAL AND DIAPHRAGMATIC SURFACES

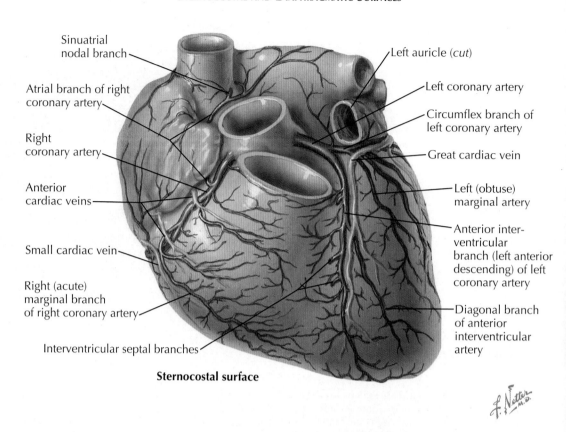

Sinuatrial nodal branch

Atrial branch of right coronary artery

Right coronary artery

Anterior cardiac veins

Small cardiac vein

Right (acute) marginal branch of right coronary artery

Interventricular septal branches

Left auricle (*cut*)

Left coronary artery

Circumflex branch of left coronary artery

Great cardiac vein

Left (obtuse) marginal artery

Anterior interventricular branch (left anterior descending) of left coronary artery

Diagonal branch of anterior interventricular artery

Sternocostal surface

CORONARY ARTERIES AND CARDIAC VEINS

The normal heart and the proximal portions of the great vessels receive their blood supply from two coronary arteries. The *left coronary artery* (LCA) originates from the left sinus of Valsalva near its upper border, at about the level of the free edge of the valve cusp. The LCA usually has a short (0.5–2 cm) common stem that bifurcates or trifurcates. One branch, the *anterior interventricular (descending) branch,* courses downward in the anterior interventricular groove (largely embedded in fat), rounds the acute margin of the heart just to the right of the apex, and ascends a short distance up the posterior interventricular groove.

The left anterior descending branch of the LCA gives off branches to the adjacent anterior RV wall (which usually anastomose with branches from the right coronary artery) and septal branches (which supply anterior two-thirds and apical portions of septum), as well as a number of branches to the anteroapical portions of the left ventricle, including the anterior papillary muscle.

One septal branch originating from the upper third of the anterior interventricular branch is usually larger than the others and supplies the mid septum, including the bundle of His and bundle branches of the conduction system. This branch also may supply the anterior papillary muscle of the right ventricle through the moderator band. The second, usually smaller *circumflex branch of the left coronary artery* runs in the left AV sulcus and gives off branches to the upper lateral left ventricular wall and the left atrium. The circumflex branch usually terminates at the obtuse margin of the heart, but it can reach the crux (junction of posterior interventricular sulcus and posterior AV groove). In this case, the circumflex branch supplies the entire left ventricle and ventricular septum with blood, with or without the right coronary artery.

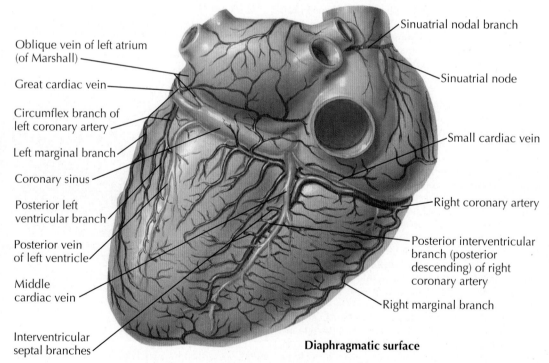

Oblique vein of left atrium (of Marshall)

Great cardiac vein

Circumflex branch of left coronary artery

Left marginal branch

Coronary sinus

Posterior left ventricular branch

Posterior vein of left ventricle

Middle cardiac vein

Interventricular septal branches

Sinuatrial nodal branch

Sinuatrial node

Small cardiac vein

Right coronary artery

Posterior interventricular branch (posterior descending) of right coronary artery

Right marginal branch

Diaphragmatic surface

In cases where the LCA trifurcates, the third branch, coming off between the anterior interventricular and the circumflex branches, is merely an LV branch that originates from the main artery.

The *right coronary artery* (RCA) arises from the right anterior sinus of Valsalva of the aorta and runs along the right AV sulcus, embedded in fat. The RCA rounds the acute margin to reach the crux in the majority of cases, and it gives off a variable number of branches to

the anterior RV wall. A usually well-developed and large branch runs along the acute margin of the heart. The *posterior interventricular* (descending) *branch* descends along the posterior interventricular groove, not quite reaching the apex, and supplies the posterior third or more of the interventricular septum. The *diaphragmatic* part of the right ventricle is largely supplied by small, parallel branches from the marginal and posterior descending arteries, not from the parent vessel

Plate 1.14   Anatomy

ARTERIOVENOUS VARIATIONS

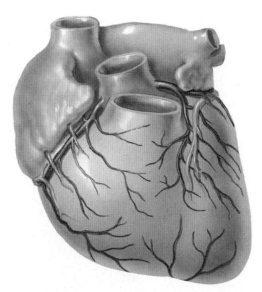

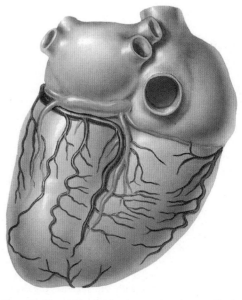

Anterior interventricular (left anterior descending) branch of left coronary artery is very short. Apical part of anterior (sternocostal) surface supplied by branches from posterior interventricular (posterior descending) branch of right coronary artery curving around apex.

Posterior interventricular (posterior descending) branch is derived from circumflex branch of left coronary artery instead of from right coronary artery.

CORONARY ARTERIES AND CARDIAC VEINS (Continued)

itself. The latter generally crosses the crux, giving off the posterior interventricular branch and a small branch to the atrioventricular node. It terminates in a number of branches to the LV wall.

The posterior papillary muscle of the left ventricle usually has a dual blood supply from both the left and the right coronary artery.

Of the *right atrial branches of the right coronary artery,* one is of great importance. This branch originates from the RCA shortly after its takeoff and ascends along the anteromedial wall of the right atrium. It enters the upper part of the atrial septum, reappears as the *superior vena cava branch* (nodal artery) posterior and to the left of the SVC ostium, rounds the ostium, and runs close to (or through) the *sinuatrial node* (see Plate 1.13), giving off branches to the crista terminalis and pectinate muscles.

Variations in the branching pattern are extremely common in the human heart. In about 67% of cases the RCA crosses the crux and supplies part of the LV wall and the ventricular septum. In 15% of cases (as in dogs and many other mammals), the LCA circumflex branch crosses the crux, giving off the posterior interventricular branch and supplying the entire left ventricle, the ventricular septum, and part of the RV wall. In about 18% of cases, both coronary arteries reach the crux. No real posterior interventricular branch may exist, but the posterior septum is penetrated at the posterior interventricular groove by many branches from the LCA, RCA, or both. In about 40% of cases the SVC branch is a continuation of a large *anterior atrial branch* of the LCA rather than of the anterior atrial branch of the RCA.

Also, the first branch of the RCA may originate independent of the right sinus of Valsalva rather than from the parent artery. Rarely, the second or even the third RCA branch arises independently.

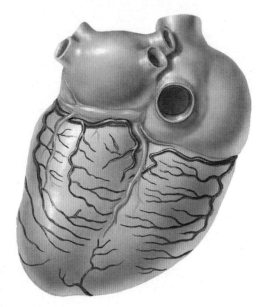

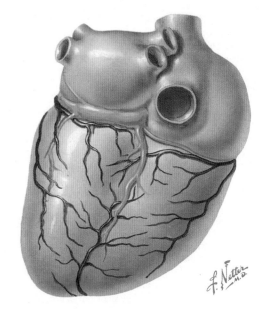

Posterior interventricular (posterior descending) branch is absent. Area supplied chiefly by small branches from circumflex branch of left coronary artery and from right coronary artery.

Posterior interventricular (posterior descending) branch is absent. Area supplied chiefly by elongated anterior interventricular (left anterior descending) branch curving around apex.

Most of the cardiac or coronary veins enter the *coronary sinus.* The three largest veins are the *great cardiac vein, middle cardiac vein,* and *posterior left ventricular vein.* The ostia of these veins may be guarded by fairly well-developed unicuspid or bicuspid valves. The *oblique vein of the left atrium* (of Marshall) enters the sinus near the orifice of the great cardiac vein, and its ostium never has a valve. The *small cardiac vein* may

enter the right atrium independently, and the *anterior cardiac veins* always do.

Small venous systems in the atrial septum (and probably in ventricular walls and septum) enter the cardiac chambers directly, called the *thebesian veins.* The existence of so-called arterioluminal and arteriosinusoidal vessels is debatable, and the evidence is inconclusive.

Plate 1.15

Cardiovascular System: VOLUME 8

INNERVATION OF HEART

The heart is supplied by sympathetic and parasympathetic nerves that arise primarily in the cervical region because the heart initially develops in the neck. Later the heart migrates downward into the thorax, along with its nerves.

The *cervical* and upper *thoracic sympathetic trunk ganglia* contribute cardiac branches, all of which pass through the *cardiac plexus,* usually without forming synapses. These ganglia are ultimately distributed to the various layers of the heart wall through the coronary plexuses. Three pairs of sympathetic cardiac nerves are derived from the cervical ganglia of the sympathetic trunks, and others arise from the upper thoracic ganglia.

The *superior cervical sympathetic cardiac nerve* originates by several rootlets from the corresponding ganglion. It often unites with the *superior vagal cardiac nerve(s),* and this *conjoined nerve* then descends behind the carotid sheath, communicating en route through slender rami with the pharyngeal, laryngeal, carotid, and thyroid nerves. On the right side, the conjoined nerve passes posterolateral to the subclavian and brachiocephalic arteries and aortic arch; on the left it curves downward across the left side of the aortic arch.

The *middle cervical sympathetic cardiac nerve* is often the largest of the cervical cardiac nerves. It is formed by filaments from the *middle* and *vertebral ganglia* of the sympathetic trunk. This cardiac nerve usually runs independent of the cardiac plexus but may unite with other cardiac nerves, and it is interconnected with tracheal, esophageal, and thyroid branches of the sympathetic trunks.

The *inferior cervical sympathetic cardiac nerves* consist of filaments arising from the *stellate* (cervicothoracic) *ganglion* and *ansa subclavia.* These cardiac nerves often combine with each other or with other cardiac nerves before reaching the cardiac plexus, and inconstant communications exist between these nerves and the *phrenic nerves.*

The *thoracic sympathetic cardiac nerves* are four or five slender branches on each side that arise from the corresponding upper thoracic sympathetic trunk ganglia. These cardiac nerves run forward and medially to the cardiac plexus. Some enter the plexus directly, whereas others are united for variable distances with filaments destined for the lungs, aorta, trachea, and esophagus.

The vagal (parasympathetic) cardiac branches vary in size, number, and arrangement but can be grouped as superior and inferior cervical and thoracic vagal cardiac nerves. The *superior cervical vagal cardiac nerve* forms from two or three filaments that leave the *vagus* in the upper part of the neck and usually unites with the corresponding sympathetic cardiac nerve. This conjoined nerve then descends to the cardiac plexus (see earlier). The *inferior cervical vagal cardiac nerve(s),* one to three in number, arise in the lower third of the neck and often join or communicate with the cardiac branches from the *middle cervical sympathetic ganglia* and the vertebral and/or stellate sympathetic ganglia. If they remain separate, these cardiac nerves lie posterolateral to the brachiocephalic artery and aortic arch on the right side and lateral to the left common carotid artery and aortic arch on the left side.

The *thoracic vagal cardiac nerves* are a series of filaments arising from the vagus nerve of each side, at or

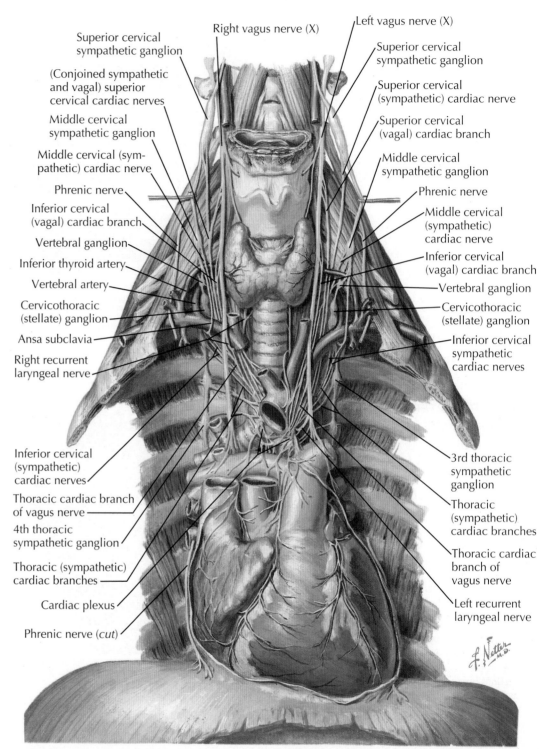

below the level of the thoracic inlet, and also from both *recurrent laryngeal nerves,* with the left contributing more filaments than the right. These often unite with other cardiac nerves in their passage to the cardiac plexus.

CARDIAC PLEXUS

All of the vagal and the sympathetic cardiac nerves converge on the cardiac plexus, and filaments from the right and left sides of the plexus surround and accompany the coronary arteries and their branches. The cardiac plexus lies between the concavity of the aortic arch and the tracheal bifurcation and is sometimes described as consisting of superficial and deep parts, although their depths vary minimally, and they are intimately interconnected. However, a superficial tenuous preaortic plexus exists over the ascending aorta.

A proportion of the vagal fibers relay in several ganglia present in the cardiac plexus. The largest, the

Plate 1.16

Anatomy

SCHEMA OF INNERVATION

INNERVATION OF HEART
(Continued)

ganglion of Wrisberg, lies below the aortic arch between the division of the pulmonary trunk and the tracheal bifurcation. Other, smaller collections of parasympathetic cells—the intrinsic cardiac ganglia—are located mainly in the atrial subendocardial tissue, along the AV sulcus and near the roots of the great vessels. Relatively few cardiac ganglia are found over the ventricles, but enough exist to question the view that the ventricular innervation is entirely or predominantly sympathetic.

The cardiac sympathetic and parasympathetic nerves carry both *afferent* and *efferent* fibers. The afferents transmit impulses to the central nervous system from discrete cardiac receptor endings and terminal networks plentiful in these reflexogenous zones, such as the endocardium around openings of the caval and pulmonary veins, over the interatrial septum, and in the AV valves. The efferents carry impulses that are modified reflexively by afferent impulses from the heart and great vessels. Efferent fibers are under the overall control of the higher centers in the brain, the hypothalamus, and the brainstem.

The more important pathways are illustrated in Plates 1.15 and 1.16. Afferents from the heart and the great vessels are shown traveling to the cord via the *sympathetic cardiac nerves*, whereas others are carried upward to nuclei in the *medulla oblongata* by the *vagus nerves*. The efferents pursue similar routes but travel in a centrifugal direction. The cell bodies of the afferent neurons are situated in the dorsal root ganglia of the upper four or five *thoracic nerves* and in the *inferior vagal* ganglia.

The *preganglionic parasympathetic* fibers are the axons of cells in the *dorsal vagal nuclei,* and these fibers relay in cardiac plexus or intrinsic cardiac ganglia. The *preganglionic sympathetic* fibers are the axons of cells located in the lateral gray columns of the upper four or five thoracic segments. These fibers enter the corresponding spinal nerves and leave them in *white rami communicantes,* which pass to adjacent ganglia in the sympathetic trunks. Some fibers relay in these ganglia, however, and the postganglionic fibers (the axons of ganglionic cells) are conveyed to the heart in the *thoracic sympathetic cardiac nerves.* Others ascend in the sympathetic trunks to form synapses with cells in the *superior, middle,* and *vertebral ganglia,* and the *postganglionic fibers* reach the heart via cardiac branches of these ganglia. Therefore the parasympathetic relays occur in ganglia near or in the heart, whereas the sympathetic relays are located in ganglia at some distance from the heart. Consequently, the parasympathetic postganglionic fibers are relatively short and circumscribed in their distribution.

Afferent and efferent fibers probably run in all the sympathetic and the parasympathetic cardiac nerves, although afferents may not be present in the *superior cervical sympathetic cardiac nerves.* Many afferent vagal fibers from the heart and great vessels are involved in reflexes depressing cardiac activity, and in some animals these fibers are aggregated in a separate "depressor nerve" and in humans may run in cardiac branches of the laryngeal nerves.

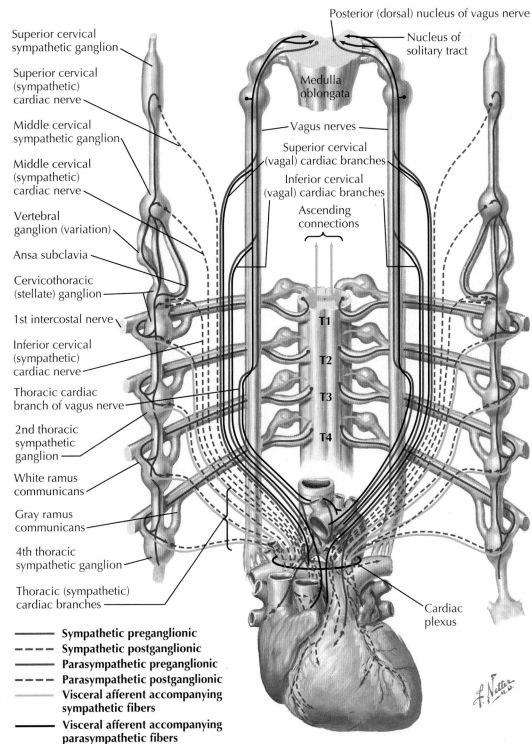

Symbols:
- —— **Sympathetic preganglionic**
- - - - **Sympathetic postganglionic**
- —— **Parasympathetic preganglionic**
- - - - **Parasympathetic postganglionic**
- —— **Visceral afferent accompanying sympathetic fibers**
- —— **Visceral afferent accompanying parasympathetic fibers**

Labels: Superior cervical sympathetic ganglion; Superior cervical (sympathetic) cardiac nerve; Middle cervical sympathetic ganglion; Middle cervical (sympathetic) cardiac nerve; Vertebral ganglion (variation); Ansa subclavia; Cervicothoracic (stellate) ganglion; 1st intercostal nerve; Inferior cervical (sympathetic) cardiac nerve; Thoracic cardiac branch of vagus nerve; 2nd thoracic sympathetic ganglion; White ramus communicans; Gray ramus communicans; 4th thoracic sympathetic ganglion; Thoracic (sympathetic) cardiac branches; Posterior (dorsal) nucleus of vagus nerve; Nucleus of solitary tract; Medulla oblongata; Vagus nerves; Superior cervical (vagal) cardiac branches; Inferior cervical (vagal) cardiac branches; Ascending connections; T1; T2; T3; T4; Cardiac plexus

Despite their insignificant size, the thoracic sympathetic cardiac nerves carry many efferent accelerator and afferent fibers to and from the heart and great vessels. Other cardiac pain afferents run in the middle and *inferior cervical sympathetic cardiac nerves,* but after entering the corresponding cervical ganglia, they descend within the sympathetic trunks to the thoracic region before passing through rami communicantes into the upper four or five thoracic nerves and then to the spinal cord. Because many cardiac pain fibers run through the preaortic plexus, some advocate excision of this plexus as a simpler, safer alternative to upper thoracic sympathetic ganglionectomy for relief of angina pectoris.

Afferent fibers from the pericardium are carried mainly in the phrenic nerves, although afferents from the visceral serous pericardium are conveyed in the coronary plexuses.

PHYSIOLOGY

Plate 2.1

Cardiovascular System: VOLUME 8

EVENTS IN THE CARDIAC CYCLE: LEFT VENTRICLE

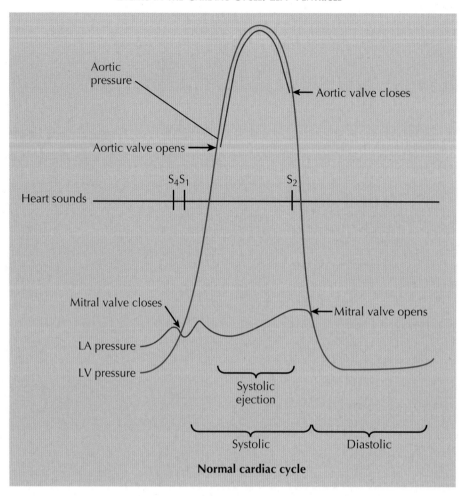

Aortic pressure

Aortic valve closes

Aortic valve opens

Heart sounds — $S_4 S_1$ — S_2

Mitral valve closes

Mitral valve opens

LA pressure

LV pressure

Systolic ejection

Systolic

Diastolic

Normal cardiac cycle

CARDIOVASCULAR EXAMINATION

EVENTS IN THE CARDIAC CYCLE: LEFT VENTRICLE

The events occurring during the cardiac cycle are driven by the left ventricular (LV) pressure. The mitral valve closes and results in the first heart sound (S_1) when LV pressure rises above left atrial (LA) pressure (Plate 2.1). The aortic valve opens when LV pressure rises above aortic diastolic pressure and is the onset of systolic ejection. The aortic valve closes and produces the second heart sound (S_2) when LV pressure falls below aortic pressure and terminates systolic ejection. The mitral valve opens when LV pressure falls below LA pressure. The fourth heart sound (S_4) occurs in late diastole following atrial contractions.

Cardiac auscultation is not the only way to examine the cardiovascular system. Peripheral vessels reflect what is occurring in the cardiovascular system; for example, carotid and femoral artery examination can reveal peripheral vascular disease. Bruits over these vessels may indicate carotid stenosis or aortofemoral stenosis. An abdominal bruit may indicate renal artery stenosis. A decrease in blood pressure in either arm suggests subclavian artery stenosis. If the ankle-brachial index (ratio of systolic pressure in the arm to systolic pressure in the ankle using Doppler technique) is less than 0.9, some peripheral artery disease may be present.

Jugular venous pulsations seen when the patient is lying with the upper body elevated to 30 degrees suggests elevated right atrial (RA) pressure of several causes.

Precordial palpation before auscultation of the heart can help the examiner make the proper cardiac diagnosis. The apical impulse can suggest LV hypertrophy (enlargement) if sustained and slow rising. Palpation along the left sternal border may reveal a parasternal lift, which suggests an elevated right ventricular (RV) pressure of about 40 mm Hg. Plate 2.2 illustrates some examples of carotid pulses and venous pulsations and cardiac apical impulses associated with specific cardiac disease states.

The basic instrument of auscultation is the human ear. Although the stethoscope has technical advantages, it often distorts, decreases, or selectively emphasizes certain vibrations. Frequently, the naked ear is superior to the stethoscope in the detection of *low-pitched* vibrations (S_3, S_4) because the ear is a larger collector of sound and fuses auditory with palpatory perception.

POSITIONS FOR CARDIAC AUSCULTATION

In auscultation, various patient positions can be used (see Plate 2.3). The patient may be sitting, supine, lying on the left side, or bent forward to increase the contact of the apex with the chest wall, as preferred for mitral or LV sounds and murmurs. The left side (left decubitus) position accentuates the rumbling murmur of mitral stenosis. The bent-forward position is preferred for

aortic diastolic murmurs, whereas the supine position is best for pulmonic and tricuspid murmurs.

AREAS OF CARDIAC AUSCULTATION

The conventional designations for areas of auscultation have been *mitral, tricuspid, aortic,* and *pulmonary.* Current understanding divides the thorax into seven areas: left ventricular, right ventricular, left atrial, RA, aortic, pulmonary, and descending thoracic aortic (see Plate 2.4).

Left Ventricular Area

The apical area ("mitral" area) is the best location for detecting not only the murmur of mitral stenosis or insufficiency but also the LV or atrial gallops and the *aortic component of the second sound* (A component of S_2). The murmurs of aortic stenosis and especially of aortic insufficiency are also often heard well at this location. However, these vibrations are detected over a larger area formed by the entire left ventricle, centering around the apical beat and extending to the fourth and fifth left interspaces medially and to the anterior axillary line laterally. In patients with ventricular enlargement, the sound shifts to either the left or the right.

Right Ventricular Area

The "tricuspid" area has been renamed the right ventricular area. In addition to the murmurs of tricuspid stenosis and insufficiency, RV and atrial gallops and the murmurs of pulmonary insufficiency and ventricular septal defect

Plate 2.2   Physiology

IMPORTANT COMPONENTS OF CARDIAC EXAMINATION

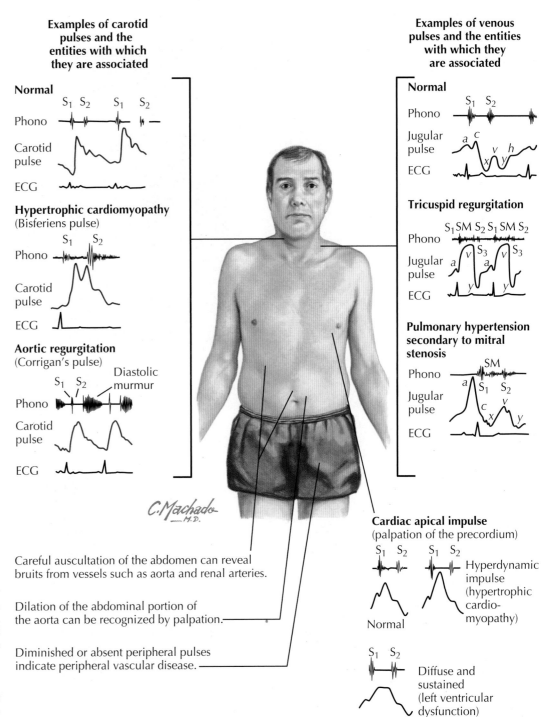

Examples of carotid pulses and the entities with which they are associated

Normal

Phono — S_1 S_2 S_1 S_2

Carotid pulse

ECG

Hypertrophic cardiomyopathy
(Bisferiens pulse)

Phono — S_1 S_2

Carotid pulse

ECG

Aortic regurgitation
(Corrigan's pulse)

S_1 S_2 Diastolic murmur

Phono

Carotid pulse

ECG

Examples of venous pulses and the entities with which they are associated

Normal

Phono — S_1 S_2

Jugular pulse — a c v h x y

ECG

Tricuspid regurgitation

Phono — S_1 SM S_2 S_1 SM S_2

Jugular pulse — v S_3 a v S_3 a y y

ECG

Pulmonary hypertension secondary to mitral stenosis

Phono — SM a S_1 S_2

Jugular pulse — c v x y

ECG

Careful auscultation of the abdomen can reveal bruits from vessels such as aorta and renal arteries.

Dilation of the abdominal portion of the aorta can be recognized by palpation.

Diminished or absent peripheral pulses indicate peripheral vascular disease.

Cardiac apical impulse
(palpation of the precordium)

S_1 S_2 S_1 S_2

Normal   Hyperdynamic impulse (hypertrophic cardio-myopathy)

S_1 S_2

Diffuse and sustained (left ventricular dysfunction)

CARDIOVASCULAR EXAMINATION (Continued)

can be well heard here. The RV area includes the lower part of the sternum and the fourth and fifth interspaces, 2 to 4 cm to the left and 2 cm to the right of the sternum. This area may extend also to the point of maximal impulse in the presence of severe RV enlargement; the "apex" in such patients is formed by the right ventricle.

Aortic Area

The aortic component of S_2 and the murmurs of aortic valve defects are often heard well at the third left interspace (Erb's area). This point is frequently more revealing than the second right interspace, except in patients with dilation of the ascending aorta, where the manubrium or the second right interspace may be more informative. The aortic area should designate both the aortic root and part of the ascending aorta. The vibrations heard best in this area include the murmurs caused by aortic stenosis, aortic insufficiency, augmented flow across the aorta or dilation of the ascending aorta, and abnormalities of the neck arteries as well as the aortic ejection click and aortic component of S_2.

Pulmonary Area

The pulmonary area should refer to the *pulmonary artery* rather than the pulmonary (pulmonic) valve. The

murmurs of pulmonary stenosis and insufficiency, the murmur caused by increased flow or dilation of the pulmonary artery, the pulmonary ejection click, the *pulmonary component of the second sound* (P component of S_2), and the murmur of patent ductus arteriosus are heard best here. The pulmonary area is formed by the second left interspace near the sternal edge and extends upward to the clavicle and downward to the third left interspace near the sternal margin. However, it may also extend posteriorly at the level of the fourth and fifth dorsal vertebrae.

MOST SIGNIFICANT AUSCULTATORY FINDINGS

Heart Sounds

The *first heart sound* (S_1) is often louder over the LV area (apex and midprecordium), whereas the *second heart sound* (S_2) is frequently louder over the aortic and pulmonary areas (base). The first sound is a long noise of *lower* tonality, whereas the second sound is shorter and sharper.

In normal adolescents or young adults, S_1 may be split. The best area for hearing this split sound is at the

Plate 2.3   Cardiovascular System: VOLUME 8

POSITIONS FOR CARDIAC AUSCULTATION

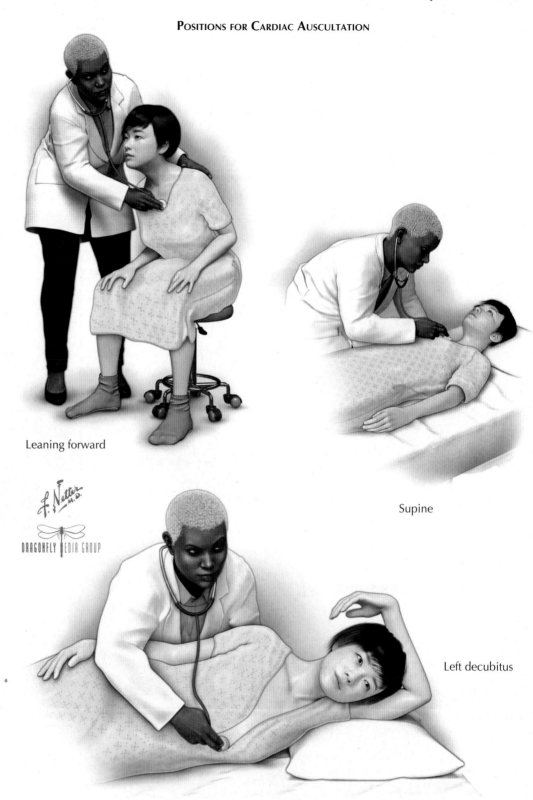

Leaning forward

Supine

Left decubitus

CARDIOVASCULAR EXAMINATION (Continued)

third left interspace. This splitting is not influenced by respiration. The loudness of S_1 is decreased in myocarditis, myocardial infarction (MI), myocardial fibrosis, hypothyroidism, mitral insufficiency (soft), aortic insufficiency, and pericarditis with effusion. S_1 is increased in mitral stenosis, systemic hypertension, and hyperthyroidism.

The second sound is frequently split during inspiration and in normal children and young adults. The best area for hearing this splitting is the third left interspace, close to the sternum (Erb's point). S_2 has an increased loudness of the aortic component in systemic hypertension, coarctation of the aorta, and aortitis. Decreased loudness of S_2 characterizes aortic stenosis. The aortic component may be so delayed as to follow the pulmonary component, a paradoxical splitting. S_2 has increased loudness of the pulmonary component in pulmonary hypertension, whereas loudness is decreased in pulmonary stenosis. The pulmonary component not only is smaller but also is delayed, causing a wider splitting. S_2 has wider, fixed splitting in conditions presenting a diastolic overload of the right side of the heart and in right bundle branch block (BBB) because of a delay in the pulmonary component. Patients with left BBB

may present with such a delay in the aortic component as to cause paradoxical splitting.

The *third heart sound* (S_3) may be normal in children, adolescents, and young athletes but may be audible over the LV or RV area in ventricular overload, myocarditis, tachycardia, or heart failure.

The *fourth heart sound* (S_4) is not heard in the normal heart. S_4 is audible over the LV area in hypertension, during myocardial ischemia, or when the ventricle

is stiff and noncompliant, as in diastolic dysfunction. S_4 can also be heard in patients with ventricular volume overload, myocarditis, tachycardia, atrial flutter, and complete or incomplete atrioventricular (AV) block or obstruction. The fourth sound is then called *atrial gallop*. A left atrial gallop is frequently heard in aortic stenosis or systemic hypertension. An RA gallop is often heard in pulmonary stenosis or pulmonary hypertension. A slightly different type is the *summation*

Plate 2.4

Physiology

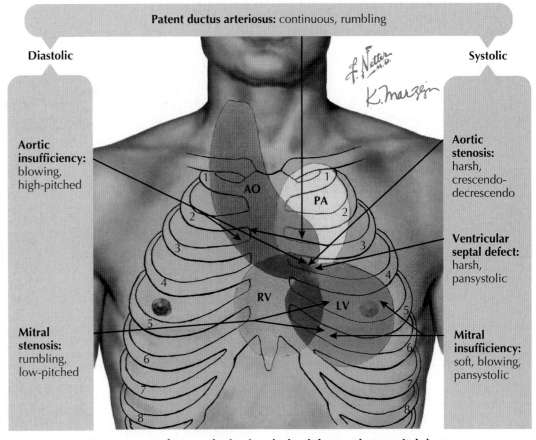

AREAS OF CARDIAC AUSCULTATION

Patent ductus arteriosus: continuous, rumbling

Diastolic

Systolic

Aortic insufficiency: blowing, high-pitched

Aortic stenosis: harsh, crescendo-decrescendo

Ventricular septal defect: harsh, pansystolic

Mitral stenosis: rumbling, low-pitched

Mitral insufficiency: soft, blowing, pansystolic

Common areas for auscultation in valvular defects and congenital shunts

AO = aortic area (murmurs of aortic stenosis and aortic insufficiency)
PA = pulmonary artery area (murmurs of pulmonary stenosis and insufficiency)
RV = right ventricular area (murmurs of tricuspid valve disease)

LV = left ventricular area (murmurs of mitral stenosis and mitral insufficiency)
3rd left interspace (most murmurs of pulmonary, aortic, and tricuspid origin, and of ventricular septal defect; splitting of 2nd sound)
Arrows point to best areas for auscultation.

CARDIOVASCULAR EXAMINATION (Continued)

gallop, caused by the summation of S_3 and S_4. This is most often seen in patients with tachycardia and grade 1 AV block.

A *systolic ejection click* can be heard over either the pulmonary area (pulmonary ejection sound) or the aortic area (aortic ejection sound). These clicks are caused by "doming" of the aortic or pulmonary valve; the aortic valve may be bicuspid. These ejection sounds occur with dilation of the aorta or pulmonary artery or narrowing of the aortic or pulmonary valve, usually with poststenotic dilation. The ejection click is a high-frequency sound due to abrupt halting of the valve opening.

A *diastolic opening snap* can be heard in the fourth left interspace, close to the sternum, over the entire LV area, or even over the entire precordium, in patients with a pliable noncalcified valve. This is the *mitral* opening snap most often heard in mitral stenosis. Occasionally it can be heard in diastolic overload of the left side of the heart (mitral insufficiency, patent ductus). A *tricuspid* opening snap is audible over the RV area in patients with tricuspid stenosis and occasionally can be heard in diastolic overload of the right ventricle (tricuspid insufficiency, atrial septal defect).

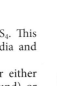

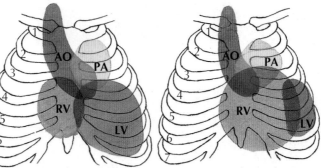

Projection of auscultatory areas in isolated left ventricular enlargement

Projection of auscultatory areas in isolated right ventricular enlargement

Usual transmission of "inflow" and "outflow" tract murmurs of left heart: AS = aortic stenosis AI = aortic insufficiency MS = mitral stenosis MI = mitral insufficiency

Murmurs

The regurgitant murmur of AV valve insufficiency is *holosystolic* and usually loud (see Plate 2.5). The murmur of mitral insufficiency is maximal over the LV area and easily audible at the left axilla, whereas the murmur of tricuspid insufficiency is maximal over the RV area and is well heard over the right precordium. Inspiration or inspiratory apnea increases the loudness of the tricuspid murmur but decreases the loudness of the mitral murmur.

The murmur of AV valve stenosis is a typical, *low-pitched rumble* that acquires higher pitch and greater loudness in presystole (presystolic accentuation) if there is sinus rhythm. It is heard best in mitral stenosis in the fourth left intercostal space, halfway between the apex and the sternal border. In tricuspid stenosis this rumble is heard best over the RV area. This murmur becomes louder in inspiration because of increased flow across the tricuspid valve during inspiration.

Plate 2.5

Cardiovascular System: VOLUME 8

MURMURS

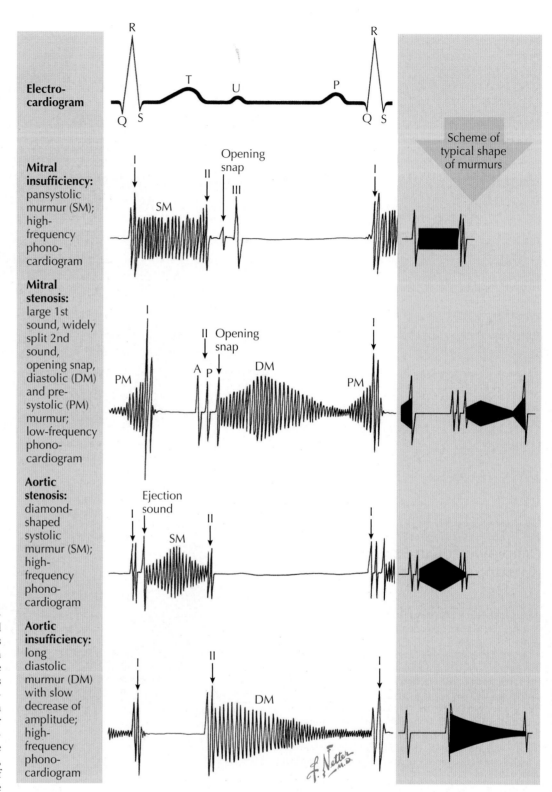

Scheme of typical shape of murmurs

Electro-cardiogram

Mitral insufficiency: pansystolic murmur (SM); high-frequency phono-cardiogram

Mitral stenosis: large 1st sound, widely split 2nd sound, opening snap, diastolic (DM) and pre-systolic (PM) murmur; low-frequency phono-cardiogram

Aortic stenosis: diamond-shaped systolic murmur (SM); high-frequency phono-cardiogram

Aortic insufficiency: long diastolic murmur (DM) with slow decrease of amplitude; high-frequency phono-cardiogram

CARDIOVASCULAR EXAMINATION (Continued)

The *regurgitant* murmur of semilunar valve insufficiency is a high-pitched, blowing, occasionally musical decrescendo. In aortic insufficiency the murmur is loudest in the third left interspace (Erb's area) and can be followed along the left sternal border toward the apex. If the ascending aorta is dilated, the murmur is louder in the second right interspace and can be followed downward along the right sternal border. In pulmonary insufficiency the murmur is loudest over the second left interspace and can be followed downward from the upper left to the lower right part of the sternum. If the patient has pulmonary hypertension, the murmur sounds similar to aortic regurgitation. If the pulmonary artery pressure is normal or low, the murmur may have a rumbling character.

The *stenotic murmur* of the semilunar valves is the loudest of all murmurs. It is harsh, starts slightly after S_1 with aortic valve opening, and is often preceded by an ejection click, especially if the valve is bicuspid and mobile. The murmur often has a crescendo-decrescendo quality and ends before or with S_2, depending on the severity of the stenosis. In aortic stenosis the murmur is maximal in the third left or second right interspace. It is readily heard over the suprasternal area and the carotid arteries and can be heard at the apex. In subvalvular

aortic stenosis, it is maximal over the LV area. In pulmonary stenosis, the murmur is best heard over the pulmonary area. It radiates moderately downward and often can be heard in the back over the lungs.

The murmur caused by a ventricular septal defect is long, harsh, and pansystolic. It is heard best over the RV area.

The murmur caused by patency of the ductus arteriosus is a continuous, machinery-like murmur because

aortic systolic and diastolic pressures are higher than pulmonary systolic and diastolic pressures. It is best heard over the first and second intercostal spaces.

Friction Rubs

Friction rubs can be heard over various areas and resemble the sound made by rubbing new leather. Friction rubs can be heard in atrial systole, ventricular systole, and ventricular diastole (i.e., three-component rub).

Plate 2.6

Physiology

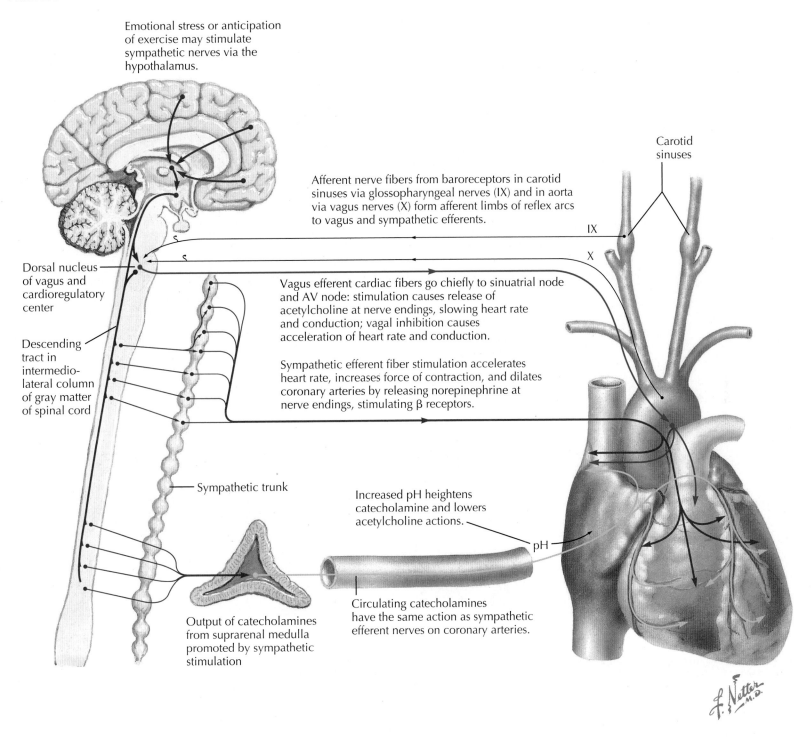

Emotional stress or anticipation of exercise may stimulate sympathetic nerves via the hypothalamus.

Afferent nerve fibers from baroreceptors in carotid sinuses via glossopharyngeal nerves (IX) and in aorta via vagus nerves (X) form afferent limbs of reflex arcs to vagus and sympathetic efferents.

Carotid sinuses

IX

X

Dorsal nucleus of vagus and cardioregulatory center

Descending tract in intermediolateral column of gray matter of spinal cord

Vagus efferent cardiac fibers go chiefly to sinuatrial node and AV node: stimulation causes release of acetylcholine at nerve endings, slowing heart rate and conduction; vagal inhibition causes acceleration of heart rate and conduction.

Sympathetic efferent fiber stimulation accelerates heart rate, increases force of contraction, and dilates coronary arteries by releasing norepinephrine at nerve endings, stimulating β receptors.

Sympathetic trunk

Increased pH heightens catecholamine and lowers acetylcholine actions.

pH

Output of catecholamines from suprarenal medulla promoted by sympathetic stimulation

Circulating catecholamines have the same action as sympathetic efferent nerves on coronary arteries.

NEURAL AND HUMORAL REGULATION OF CARDIAC FUNCTION

The efferent innervation of the heart is controlled by both the sympathetic nervous system and the parasympathetic nervous system. *Afferent fibers* accompany the *efferents* of both systems. The *sympathetic fibers* have positive chronotropic (rate-increasing) effects and positive inotropic (force-increasing) effects. The *parasympathetic fibers* have a negative chronotropic effect and may be somewhat negatively inotropic (but small and masked) in the intact circulatory system by the

increased filling that occurs when diastolic filling time is increased.

The heart is normally under the restraint of *vagal inhibition,* and thus bilateral vagotomy increases the heart rate. *Vagal stimulation* not only slows the heart but also slows conduction across the AV node. Sectioning of the cardiac sympathetics does not lower heart rate under normal circumstances.

The totally denervated heart loses some (but surprisingly little) of its capacity to respond to changes in its load. The denervated heart still responds to *humoral* influences, more slowly and less fully, but it is remarkable how well the secondary mechanisms, such as the suprarenal medullary output of catecholamines, can substitute for the primary mechanism that controls heart rate in exercise.

The nervous mechanisms controlling heart rate include the *baroreceptor reflexes,* with afferent arms from the carotid sinus, the arch of the aorta, and other pressoreceptor zones operating as negative feedback mechanisms to regulate pressure in the arteries. These reflexes affect not only heart activity but also the caliber of the resistance vessels in the vascular system.

The heart is also affected reflexively by afferent impulses via the autonomic nervous system. The response may be tachycardia or bradycardia, depending on whether the sympathetic or parasympathetic system is activated more strongly in the individual patient. Tachycardia is the common response in excitement.

Plate 2.7

Cardiovascular System: VOLUME 8

Hematologic changes in pregnancy

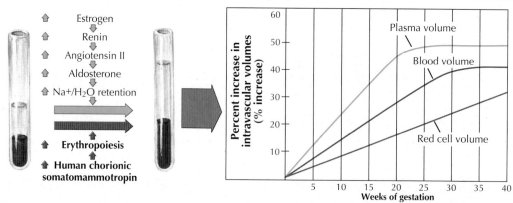

Multifactorial stimulation of fluid retention and erythropoiesis in pregnancy results in a 50% increase in plasma volume and a 30% increase in red cell volume, creating a relative "physiologic" anemia and an increased blood volume.

Changes in cardiac output

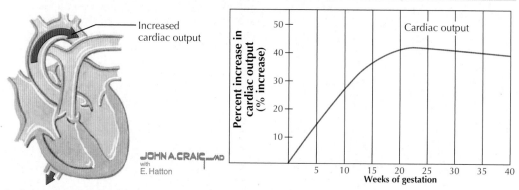

Cardiac output increases up to 50% in normal pregnancy, predominantly from increased stroke volume in first and second trimesters and increased pulse rate in third trimester.

Postural changes

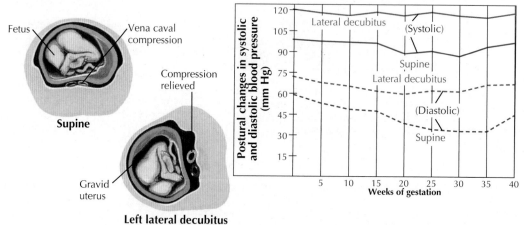

Positional changes have hemodynamically significant effects on pregnant women. Compression of the inferior vena cava by the gravid uterus in the supine position may cause hypotension and syncope. Condition is relieved by altering position from supine to lateral decubitus to relieve compression and restore venous return and cardiac output.

PHYSIOLOGIC CHANGES DURING PREGNANCY

During a normal pregnancy, the female undergoes multiple cardiovascular physiologic changes to support the increased metabolic demands of the parent and the unborn child. The changes are fairly typical in a healthy pregnant female but may vary in magnitude from patient to patient. Early in the pregnancy, the first trimester, the changes are usually mild or may not be evident. The classic changes include the following:

- Blood volume gradually increases from mild in the first trimester to moderate in the second trimester to marked in the third trimester. These volume changes often are not reflected in ventricular volume changes, and systolic function of the left ventricle usually remains normal, as determined by cardiac ultrasound.
- With the increase in blood volume, a concomitant increase in cardiac output usually occurs, possibly from the Starling mechanism. It becomes maximal in the second trimester and decreases to moderate in the third trimester.
- Stroke volume tends to increase when cardiac output increases in the second trimester but usually normalizes or decreases in the third trimester.
- Systolic blood pressure tends to decrease or remain normal throughout pregnancy, whereas pulse pressure widens because of a decrease in diastolic

pressure. This is related to a marked decrease in systemic vascular resistance, especially in the second trimester, which probably influences the marked increase in cardiac output and stroke volume.

- Heart rate gradually increases from normal or slightly increased to greatly increased in the third trimester.
- Along with the changes in heart rate, oxygen consumption gradually increases from normal or

slightly increased to greatly increased in the third trimester.

Anatomic factors related to the enlarged uterus can also influence physiologic changes, particularly in the third trimester. Inferior vena cava compression can increase femoral venous pressure and can elevate the diaphragm, which in turn can shift the axis of the heart and alter the axis of the electrocardiogram (ECG) toward the left.

Plate 2.8

Physiology

VASCULAR ACCESS

Points of measuring pressure

Right heart catheterization

Catheter can be introduced into basilic vein, travels via axillary, subclavian, brachiocephalic veins, and superior vena cava to right heart

Catheter may be introduced via jugular or saphenous vein

Superior vena cava

Wedged in small branch of pulmonary artery

Pulmonary trunk

Right ventricle

Right atrium

Inferior vena cava

Left heart catheter access

Guidewire in the left coronary artery

Guide catheter

Brachial artery

Radial artery

Femoral artery

CARDIAC CATHETERIZATION

VASCULAR ACCESS AND RIGHT-SIDED HEART CATHETERIZATION

Cardiac catheterization, first attempted by Forssmann on himself in 1928, was developed by Cournand, Richards, and their colleagues and is now a common procedure in both clinical and research laboratories.

Technique

The primary goal of right-sided heart catheterization is to access the conditions existing in the chambers and great vessels of the right side of the heart. In these procedures, a radiopaque flexible catheter of various designs, including balloon tipped, is introduced percutaneously into a vein, usually the femoral or jugular, with the patient under local anesthesia. After introduction into the vein, the catheter is manipulated under fluoroscopic control and constant electrocardiographic monitoring downstream through the venous system to the right atrium and eventually into the right ventricle and pulmonary artery. The catheter is often *wedged* and is advanced into the most peripheral branch of the pulmonary artery that will accept the catheter tip or occlusion by a balloon-tipped catheter. A pressure recorded from the wedge position has essentially the same mean pressure as the left atrium and the same but delayed phasic features. If there is no mitral stenosis, the pulmonary capillary wedge pressure (PCWP) reflects the left ventricular end-diastolic pressure.

Diagnostic Procedures

The position of the catheter in the fluoroscopic image may indicate some departure from the intracardiac course normally taken by a catheter. Examples include passage into a persistent left superior vena cava through the coronary sinus from the right atrium, passage through a patent ductus arteriosus, and traversal of an interatrial or interventricular septal defect.

Blood can be sampled for oxygen or other analysis, and pressures can be measured through the catheter from any point reached. Oxygen samples can be used to determine the site of entry into the right side of the heart and the size of a left-to-right intracardiac shunt at atrial, ventricular, or pulmonary artery levels in patients with congenital heart disease. Oxygen values from the pulmonary artery are used with other data to calculate the pulmonary blood flow with thermodilution and balloon-tipped catheters. Measurement of pressures through the catheter using external pressure transducers allows determination of the phasic form of the pressure in any location. Pressures recorded as the catheter traverses a valve permit an evaluation of the site and degree of valvular stenosis.

Special sensors at the tip of a catheter have been designed for the detection and recording of intracardiac ECGs and pressures.

Complications

Brief arrhythmias, vasovagal episodes, and minor phlebitis may be observed in patients undergoing catheterization. More serious complications are rare.

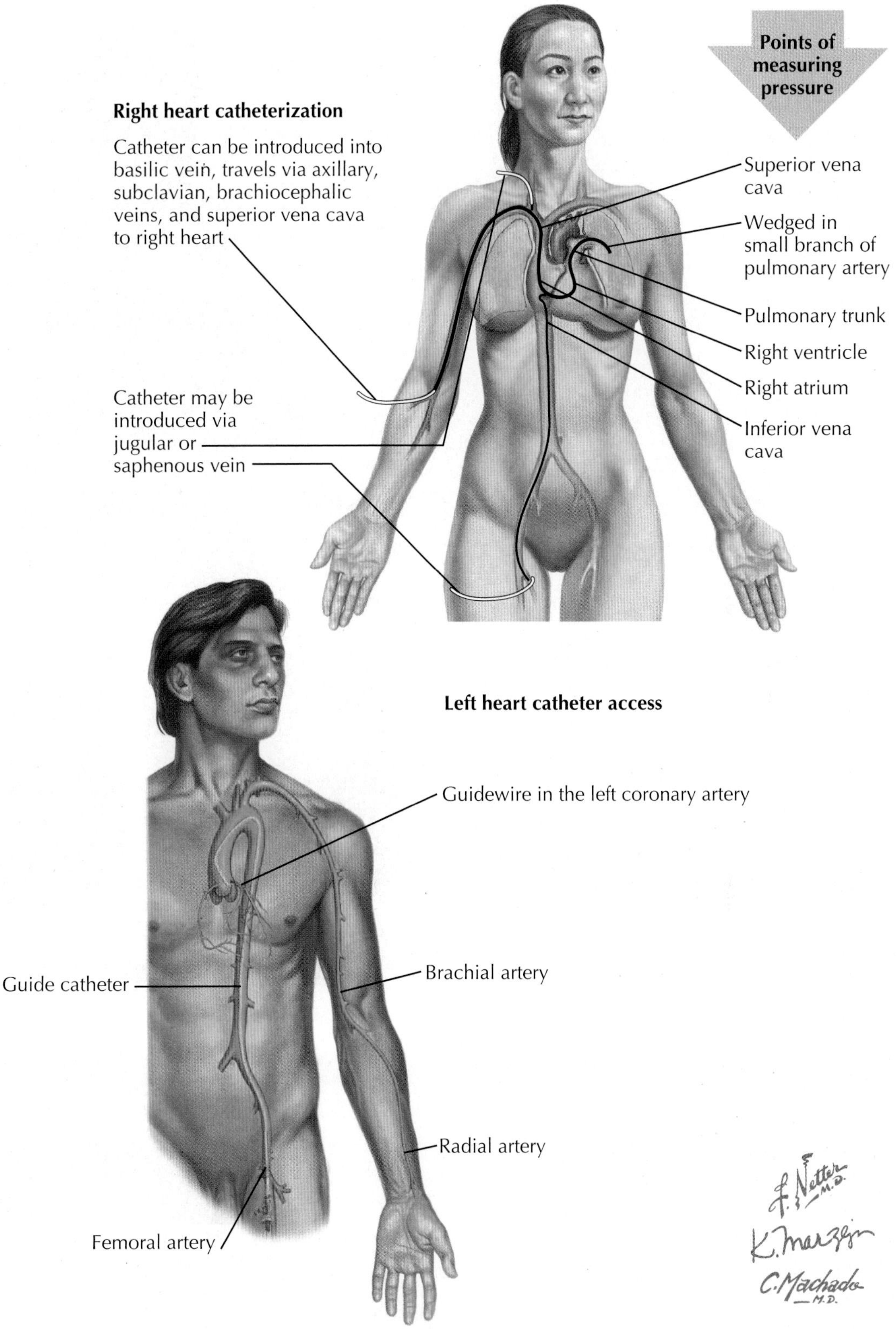

Plate 2.9

Cardiovascular System: VOLUME 8

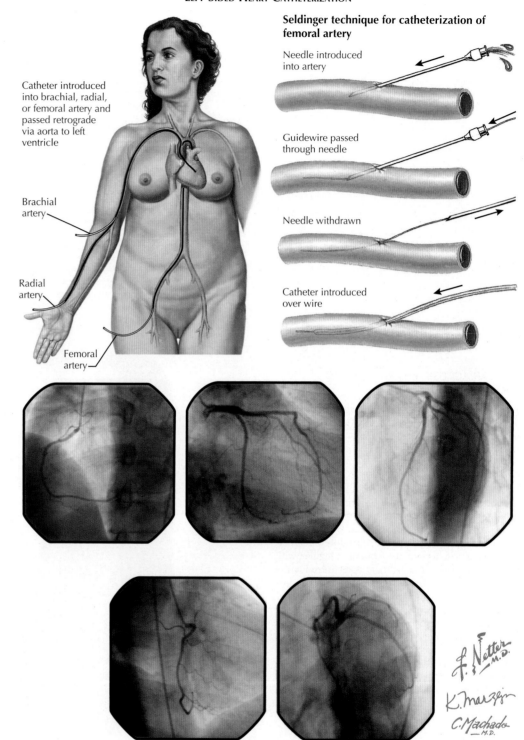

LEFT-SIDED HEART CATHETERIZATION

Seldinger technique for catheterization of femoral artery

Needle introduced into artery

Guidewire passed through needle

Needle withdrawn

Catheter introduced over wire

Catheter introduced into brachial, radial, or femoral artery and passed retrograde via aorta to left ventricle

Brachial artery

Radial artery

Femoral artery

CARDIAC CATHETERIZATION (Continued)

LEFT-SIDED HEART CATHETERIZATION

Technique

The aim of *left-sided heart catheterization* is to study the conditions in the chambers and vessels of the left side of the heart. In congenital heart disease, the catheter may reach the left side of the heart from a right-sided heart chamber, passing through an atrial septal defect or a patent ductus arteriosus.

More often the left side of the heart is approached by *retrograde passage* of the catheter from its point of insertion into a peripheral *artery,* most commonly by percutaneous technique. This technique was designed by Seldinger (Plate 2.9).

The catheter is manipulated under fluoroscopic control in a retrograde direction using the Seldinger technique through the artery to the aorta and frequently across the aortic valve into the left ventricle. Entry into the left atrium retrograde through the mitral valve is possible but not typically used. Approach to the left atrium can also be accomplished using a transseptal technique by passage of the transseptal catheter and transseptal needle from a right femoral vein to the right atrium and across the atrial septum at the level of the fossa ovalis. The catheter can then be advanced into the left ventricle. Direct percutaneous needle puncture of the LV apex may be done to reach the left ventricle in special circumstances, such as LV pressure measurement in patients with mechanical aortic and mitral valves.

Diagnostic Procedures

Sampling and pressure measurements for left-sided heart catheterization do not differ from right-sided procedures. Valvular abnormalities can be estimated using simultaneous pressure measurements on both sides of the valve.

Complications

Arrhythmias, the most common complication of left-sided catheterization, usually respond to simple catheter withdrawal, although they rarely may require therapy. Other complications include arterial spasm and the rare dissection or occlusion of the artery. Perforations

of the walls of an artery or the aorta, a heart chamber, or a coronary artery also can occur rarely. Fluid should never be forced through a catheter from which blood cannot be withdrawn, particularly if the catheter is in the ascending aorta; a clot can be expressed and embolize peripherally to the brain.

CARDIAC OUTPUT: THERMODILUTION TECHNIQUE

A balloon-tipped pulmonary artery catheter (Swan-Ganz catheter) with a thermistor at the tip (introduced in 1970) floats into the pulmonary artery from the right

ventricle as an embolus when the balloon is inflated. The balloon occludes the distal pulmonary branches, and a pressure similar to the PCWP can be measured. When deflated, the catheter measures pulmonary artery pressure, and the thermistor measures a *thermodilution curve* after injection of 10 mL of cold saline or glucose into the right atrium. The *cardiac output* can be calculated from the measured thermodilution curve. When the cardiac output is low, the temperature change from right to distal pulmonary artery changes little. When the cardiac output is high, the temperature change is large. Thus the degree of change in temperature is directly proportional to the cardiac output.

Plate 2.10

Physiology

NORMAL SATURATIONS (O$_2$) AND PRESSURE

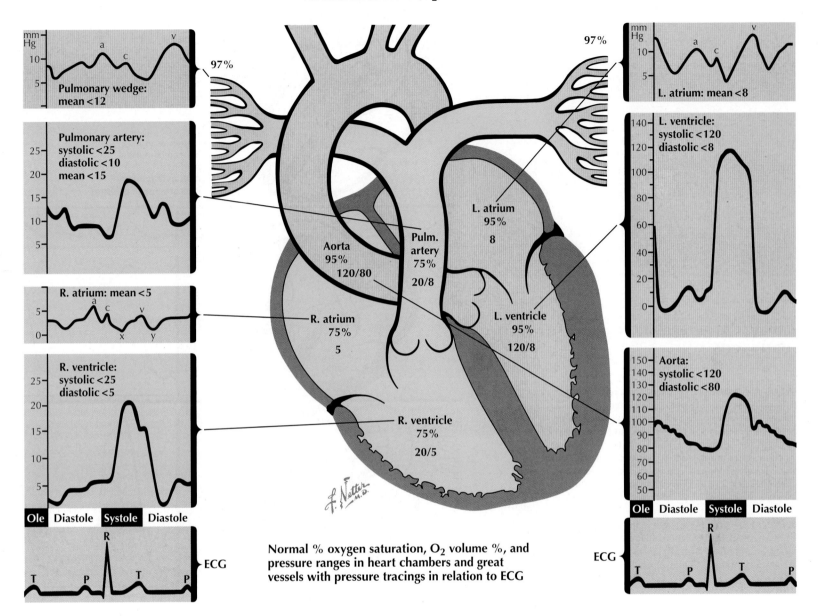

Normal % oxygen saturation, O$_2$ volume %, and pressure ranges in heart chambers and great vessels with pressure tracings in relation to ECG

CARDIAC CATHETERIZATION (Continued)

NORMAL OXYGEN SATURATIONS AND PRESSURE

In the venae cavae, right atrium, right ventricle, and pulmonary arteries, *oxygen saturation* (SO$_2$) is normally close to 75% (Plate 2.10). Small, phasic variations in SO$_2$ of blood sampled from the right-sided heart chambers can be measured. The variation is maximal in the right atrium, where contributions of blood from the renal veins (with a relatively high So$_2$), from the hepatic veins (with relatively low So$_2$), from the coronary sinus (with very low So$_2$), and from the lower inferior vena cava and superior vena cava (with intermediate So$_2$) meet and start mixing. The mixing is probably complete by the time the blood reaches the pulmonary artery. In the *pulmonary wedge* position, 97% to 99% saturated blood can be withdrawn through the wedged catheter, approximating the values of pulmonary venous blood. Blood leaving the pulmonary capillary bed is at least

97% saturated. Blood entering the *left atrium* is slightly less saturated because of its admixture with blood passing through pulmonary arteriovenous and other small shunts.

NORMAL INTRACARDIAC PRESSURES

Atrial and Wedge Pressures

The phasic pressures in the right atrium, the left atrium, and the pulmonary artery wedge position (essentially a slightly delayed left atrial pressure) share the same characteristics, with small differences in the amplitude and timing of the phasic features. In normal sinus rhythm, the pressure pulse in these chambers is characterized by an *a* wave produced by the atrial contraction that begins with completion of the atrial P wave in the ECG. After a brief delay, the P wave is followed by the QRS signaling the depolarization of the ventricular myocardium. Immediately after depolarization, ventricular contraction begins. The AV valves close, and the *c* waves in the atrial pressure curves are produced by changes in the dimensions of the atria and by bulging of the valves into the atria secondary to ventricular contraction. After the

c wave, pressure decreases to a low value (the *x* descent) in response to further atrial volume changes during continued ventricular contraction. During the remainder of *systole*, continuous venous inflow produces an increase in pressure, the *v* wave). The peaks of the *v* waves coincide with the opening of the mitral and tricuspid valves. A pressure decrease in the atria (the *y* descent) accompanies the transfer of blood from the atria into the ventricles.

Ventricular Pressures

Except for the peak systolic pressure in the left ventricle being approximately five times greater than that in the right, the phasic pressures in the left and right ventricles are similar in contour. The ventricles begin to contract approximately 60 milliseconds after the QRS in the ECG, with the right preceding the left. This action is associated with closure of the AV valves, resulting in elevated ventricular pressures. During the subsequent period of sequential myocardial contraction, lasting 10 milliseconds and 40 milliseconds for the right and left ventricles, respectively, there are no volume changes; this is considered the period of *isovolumic contraction*.

Plate 2.11

Cardiovascular System: VOLUME 8

Examples of O₂ and Pressure Findings and Pressure Tracings in Heart Diseases

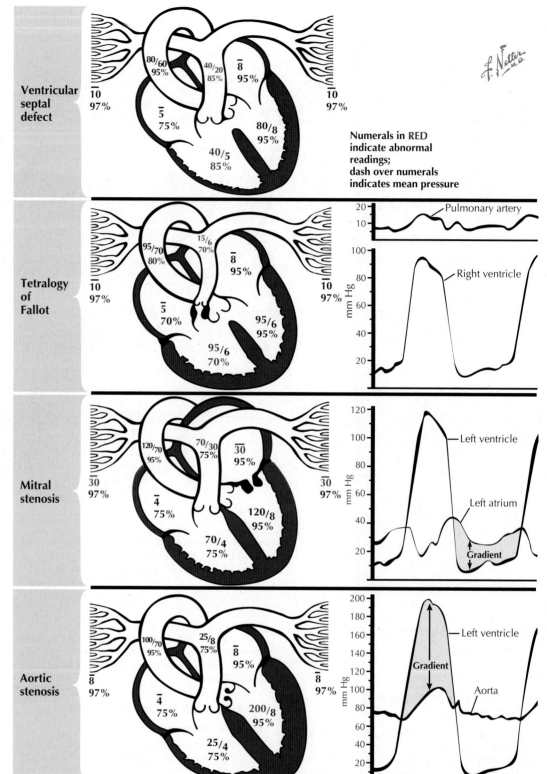

Ventricular septal defect

Numerals in RED indicate abnormal readings; dash over numerals indicates mean pressure

Tetralogy of Fallot

Pulmonary artery

Right ventricle

mm Hg

Mitral stenosis

Left ventricle

Left atrium

Gradient

mm Hg

Aortic stenosis

Left ventricle

Gradient

Aorta

mm Hg

CARDIAC CATHETERIZATION (Continued)

When the ventricular pressures exceed the end-diastolic pressures in the pulmonary artery and aorta, the semilunar valves open and ejection begins. During the ejection period, the right ventricle and pulmonary artery and the left ventricle and aorta have the same phasic pressures until, systole being completed, the semilunar valves close and the pressures begin to drop in the ventricles. This is followed by the brief period of *isovolumic relaxation*.

As soon as the ventricular pressures fall below the pressures in the atria, the AV valves open, and diastole starts and proceeds with venous filling of the common ventricular and atrial chambers, leading to superposable pressures in the atria and ventricles.

Aortic and Pulmonary Artery Pressures

During ejection, the ventricular pressures and the pressures in the aorta or pulmonary artery are identical and are characterized by a smooth rise to a peak and then a steady fall to the dicrotic notch, signaling the closure of the aortic and pulmonary valves. This is followed by a steady decrease in pressure as a "runoff" of blood from the arterial system into the venous system occurs through the capillary beds. This is abruptly terminated by the next ejection.

ABNORMAL OXYGEN AND PRESSURE FINDINGS

Ventricular Septal Defect

In ventricular septal defect, a shunt of 95% saturated blood is ejected during systole by the left ventricle through the defect into the right ventricle, under the influence of the normally occurring pressure difference between the two ventricles (Plate 2.11). There the shunted blood contaminates the less-saturated mixed venous blood. Thus an increased volume of blood with a greater than normal So_2 (85%) flows into the pulmonary artery. In the majority of cases the volume of blood shunted depends on the systolic pressure difference between the two ventricles and on size of the defect. The increased So_2 of the blood in the pulmonary artery is in direct proportion to the volume of the

shunt. The pressures in the pulmonary artery and right ventricle are usually elevated because of the increased pulmonary vascular resistance, which is secondary to the failure of neonatal involution to take place in the normal prenatal medial hypertrophy of the small arteries. The pressures may be greatly elevated by subsequent intimal and other pathologic changes. Eventually, after development of very high RV pressures, the shunt may be reversed, and desaturated blood may flow from the right to the left ventricle and the systemic arteries.

Tetralogy of Fallot

The basic abnormalities in tetralogy of Fallot are pulmonary stenosis (valvular or infundibular) interventricular septal defect, disproportion in the diameter between and usually some displacement of the aorta and pulmonary artery, with secondary RV hypertrophy (Plate 2.11). Because of the pulmonary stenosis, which significantly increases normal outflow resistance, RV hypertension may reach systemic levels. This results in a shunt of unsaturated blood through the defect, with a

Plate 2.12

Physiology

NORMAL CARDIAC BLOOD FLOW DURING INSPIRATION AND EXPIRATION

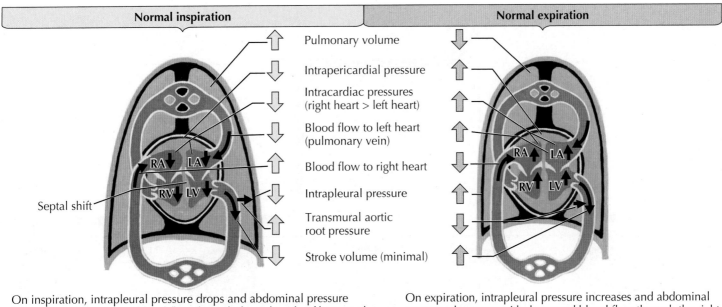

| Normal inspiration | Normal expiration |

Pulmonary volume

Intrapericardial pressure

Intracardiac pressures
(right heart > left heart)

Blood flow to left heart
(pulmonary vein)

Blood flow to right heart

Intrapleural pressure

Transmural aortic
root pressure

Stroke volume (minimal)

Septal shift

On inspiration, intrapleural pressure drops and abdominal pressure increases with increased blood flow through the right side of heart and slight decrease in flow to left side of heart. Increased aortic root transmural pressure adds a minor amount of LV afterload.

On expiration, intrapleural pressure increases and abdominal pressure decreases with decreased blood flow through the right side of heart and increase in flow to left side of heart.

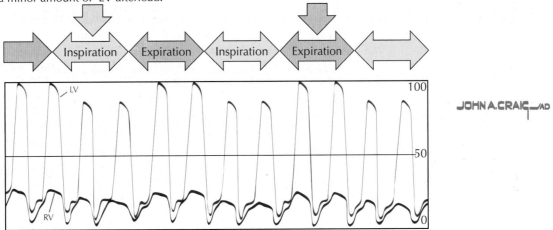

Inspiration — Expiration — Inspiration — Expiration

JOHN A. CRAIG—AD

Simultaneous measurement of RV and LV systolic pressure reveals a concordant decrease in pressure in both chambers during inspiration, with a similar concordant increase in pressure in both ventricles during expiration. Pressure changes are exaggerated for emphasis.

CARDIAC CATHETERIZATION (Continued)

mild reduction in So$_2$ in the left ventricle and a greater reduction in the aorta and systemic arteries. The latter causes the cyanosis characteristic of these patients. The greatly reduced pulmonary blood flow reaches full saturation in the lungs. Systolic pressure in the right ventricle reaches the level of the aortic pressure. Distal to the pulmonary stenosis, however, the pressures are lower than normal, and the pressure contour is often distorted.

Mitral Stenosis

The resistance to diastolic flow from left atrium to left ventricle after narrowing of the mitral valve increases LA pressures and eventually reduces LV flow (Plate 2.11). A pressure gradient across the mitral valve throughout diastole can be demonstrated by simultaneous PCWP measurements or direct LA and LV pressure measurements. This gradient is inversely proportional

to the square of the cross-sectional area of the valve orifice and is directly proportional to the square of the volume flow. The gradient is greater with increases in the degree of stenosis and during exercise. The LA hypertension is accompanied by pulmonary venous hypertension, which results in pulmonary hypertension and RV hypertension, increased RV work, and hypertrophy. Diastolic pressures in the pulmonary artery and left atrium are identical until pulmonary vascular resistance is increased because of pathologic changes in the vascular bed, resulting in a gradient between the two pressures. Acute bouts of LA hypertension lead to pulmonary edema, whereas chronic pulmonary artery hypertension may eventually cause RV failure.

Aortic Stenosis

In aortic stenosis, obstruction to the ejection of blood from the ventricle into the aorta, caused by subvalvular, valvular, or supravalvular stenosis, results in abnormally high pressure in the left ventricle and abnormally low pressure in the aorta and thus a systolic pressure gradient across the valve. Progressive obstruction to LV

outflow magnifies these effects and leads to LV hypertrophy and eventually acute or chronic LV systolic and diastolic failure (Plate 2.11).

EFFECTS OF INSPIRATION AND EXPIRATION ON INTRACARDIAC PRESSURES AND FLOW

During inspiration, systolic blood pressure decreases and pulse rate increases slightly because the intrathoracic pressure becomes more negative relative to atmospheric pressure. Systemic venous return increases, more blood flows into the right side of the heart, and pulmonary vasculature compliance increases (see Plate 2.12). This results in pooling of blood in the lungs and a decrease in pulmonary venous return, reducing flow to the left side of the heart. The reduced left-sided heart filling leads to a decreased stroke volume and systolic blood pressure. The decrease in systolic blood pressure leads to a faster heart rate because of the baroreceptor reflex, which stimulates sympathetic outflow to the heart. These changes are reversed with expiration.

Plate 2.13

Cardiovascular System: VOLUME 8

PHYSIOLOGY OF SPECIALIZED CONDUCTION SYSTEM

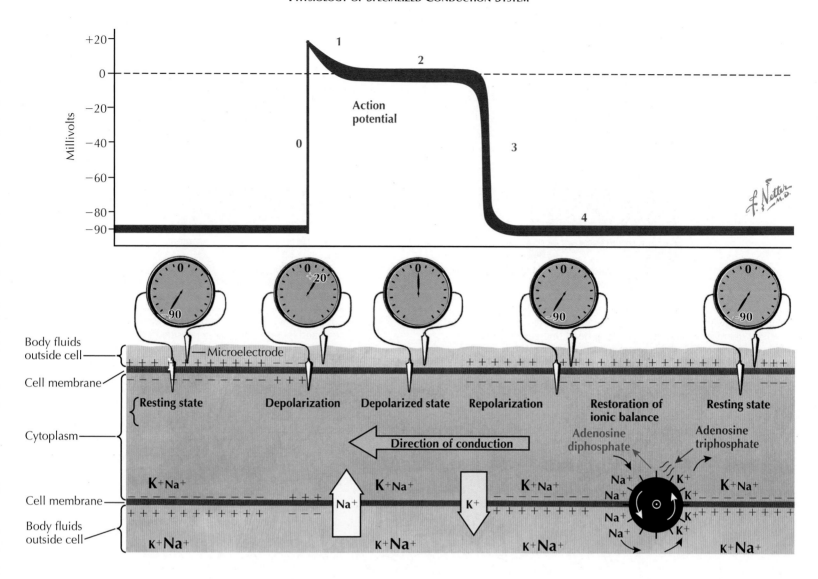

SPECIALIZED CONDUCTION SYSTEM

PHYSIOLOGY OF SPECIALIZED CONDUCTION SYSTEM

Under normal conditions, heart activation results from an impulse originating in a cell or cell group (the pacemaker) and from the propagation of this impulse to all fibers of the atria and ventricles. Arrival of the electrical signal at the contractile fibers of the heart initiates contraction. Regular rhythmic activity requires the presence of specialized automatic fibers. Coordinated contraction of the atria and ventricles requires a system that distributes the electrical impulse to the muscle fibers of these chambers in the proper sequence and at the proper time. Both of these functions are performed by specialized groups of cardiac fibers.

The automaticity that underlies pacemaker activity is a unique property not only of the fibers in the sinuatrial (SA) node but also of other groups of specialized atrial fibers and cells of the His-Purkinje system. The conduction system is composed of the fibers of the internodal tracts, Bachmann's bundle, the atrioventricular node, the bundle of His, the bundle branches, and the peripheral Purkinje fibers. The cells of the conduction system, in addition to having a characteristic histologic appearance, possess unique electrical properties. These properties, and the basis for electrical activity of all cardiac fibers, can best be understood by recording the transmembrane potentials through intracellular microelectrodes.

Basis for Transmembrane Potentials

As with other excitable mammalian tissues, cardiac cells have an intracellular ionic composition that differs from that found in the extracellular fluids (Plate 2.13). For our consideration, the most important ions are sodium (Na^+) and potassium (K^+). The relative magnitude of the concentration of these ions is indicated by the sizes of the symbols in the illustration. Intracellular K^+ concentration is approximately 30 times greater than the extracellular concentration, whereas intracellular Na^+ concentration is approximately 30 times less. Because of this difference, and because the resting membrane is more permeable to K^+ than to Na^+, the membrane of the resting fiber is polarized. The magnitude of this polarization, the *transmembrane resting potential,* can be measured by inserting a microelectrode inside the cell and measuring the potential difference across the membrane. This is shown schematically both as

the recorded voltage (-90 mV) and as an oscilloscopic tracing.

With the onset of excitation, there is a change in the permeability of the membrane that permits sodium ions, carrying a positive charge, to move rapidly down their electrochemical gradient, across the membrane, and inside the fiber. This sudden influx of positive charge carried by Na^+ actually *reverses* the transmembrane potential, and the inside becomes 20 to 30 mV more positive than the outside. The inward Na^+ current is represented by the large arrow in Plate 2.13; the resulting change in transmembrane potential is shown as the upstroke (phase 0) of the oscilloscopic tracing. After excitation there is a period of variable duration (phases 1 and 2) when the membrane potential remains close to zero. This period, often described as the *plateau* of the transmembrane action potential, results from a decrease in Na^+ and K^+ permeability. Subsequently, *repolarization,* or restoration of the normal resting potential, takes place because of an increase in K^+ permeability and an efflux of K^+ from the cells. The phase of rapid repolarization (phase 3) is followed by a period of stable resting potential (phase 4) until the arrival of the next wave of excitation. To maintain the normal concentration gradients for the sodium and potassium ions, an active transport system, often referred to as a

Plate 2.14   Physiology

ELECTRICAL ACTIVITY OF THE HEART

SPECIALIZED CONDUCTION SYSTEM (Continued)

"pump," must extrude the sodium that has entered and pump in an equivalent amount of potassium. The pump is represented by the wheel with gates.

Plate 2.13 is a representation of a longitudinal section of a single fiber during propagation of the impulse. The activity, *conduction,* spreads from right to left. At the extreme left of the tracing, the resting potential has not yet been changed by the coming wave of excitation. At the right, repolarization is complete, and the resting potential has been restored. In the middle of the figure, the current flow associated with excitation is shown under the upstroke (phase 0) of the action potential; the currents associated with repolarization appear under phase 3. The relative magnitude and polarity of the transmembrane potential are suggested by the plus and minus signs inside and outside the membrane. *Propagation,* or the spread of the impulse, occurs because a change in transmembrane potential at one point, during phase 0, causes a local longitudinal potential difference. This produces a flow of current across the membrane in advance of the action potential upstroke, resulting in excitation of the next adjacent segment of the fiber. During propagation these processes are continuous, and thus activity spreads from its point of origin throughout all excitable fibers.

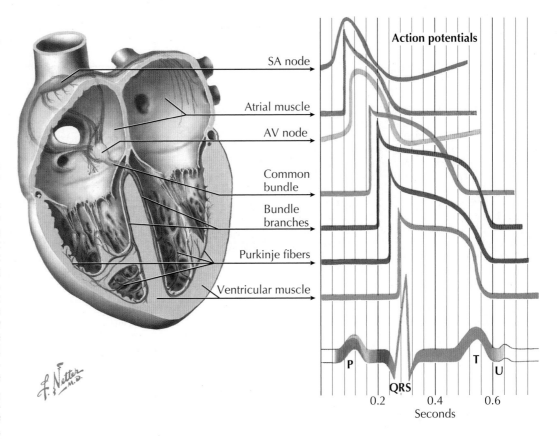

ELECTRICAL ACTIVITY OF THE HEART

The previous description applies in general to all cardiac fibers. However, records of transmembrane action potentials recorded from cells in different parts of the heart show special characteristics in the initiation and spread of the normal cardiac impulse (Plate 2.14).

Sinuatrial Node and Atrium

This trace is recorded from a single automatic fiber in the SA node. There is no steady resting potential; instead, after repolarization the transmembrane potential decreases spontaneously. This slow, spontaneous *depolarization* during phase 4 causes the automatic activity of sinus fibers. A similar cause of automaticity has been recorded from all the specialized cardiac fibers capable of normal pacemaker activity. Further, the rate of rise of the upstroke of the action potential is slow, causing slow conduction of the impulse within the node. The action potential recorded from an ordinary atrial muscle fiber is shown below that from the SA node. Here the upstroke is rapid and the resting potential steady.

Atrioventricular Node

Action potentials recorded from fibers of the AV node resemble those shown for sinus fibers. The extremely slow spread of the impulse through the AV node results largely from the slow rate of rise of the action potential. The phase 4 depolarization shown probably causes automatic activity only in fibers of the lower node in proximity to the common bundle.

His-Purkinje System

The action potentials recorded from the fibers of this part of the specialized conduction system (Purkinje fibers) have the following important characteristics:

1. The rate of rise of the action potential is fast, and thus conduction is rapid.
2. The duration of the action potential is great, and thus the refractory period is long.
3. Under appropriate conditions, each of these fiber groups (not shown) may develop spontaneous phase 4 depolarization and become an automatic pacemaker.

The bottom trace in Plate 2.14, recorded from an ordinary muscle fiber of the ventricle, is included to contrast the time of excitation and action potential duration with the other records.

SEQUENCE OF EXCITATION AND THE ELECTROCARDIOGRAM

The seven tracings of transmembrane action potentials indicate the normal sequence of heart activation in relation to the schematic ECG shown below them. The coloring of the ECG trace suggests the temporal relationship of each type of action potential to the normal ECG, as well as the contribution of electrical activity in each type of cell to the ECG recorded from the body surface.

Activity of pacemaker fibers in the SA node precedes the first indication of activity in the ECG (the P wave) and cannot be demonstrated in the body surface leads. Depolarization of atrial muscle fibers, in a sequence largely determined by the specialized atrial paths shown, causes the P wave. Repolarization of atrial fibers ordinarily is not seen in the surface ECG. Activity reaches the upper part of the AV node early during the P wave. Propagation through the node is slow, and excitation of fibers in the His bundle does not occur until the middle of the PR interval. The spread of activity through the common bundle, the bundle branches, and parts of the Purkinje system precedes the earliest excitation of ventricular muscle. There is no indication in the surface ECG of excitation of the fibers of the His-Purkinje system. The QRS complex results from activation of the muscle fibers of the ventricles. The isoelectric ST segment corresponds to the plateau of the ventricular action potential, and the T wave results from repolarization of ventricular fibers. The U wave corresponds in time with repolarization of the specialized fibers of the bundle branches and Purkinje system and may reflect this event as recorded at the body surface.

Although the normal sequence of heart activation results from the anatomic distribution and unique electrical properties of specialized cardiac cells, no signal recorded in the ECG corresponds to these events. Thus the sequence of excitation of the specialized tissues can be determined only by implication when noting the temporal characteristics of the P wave and QRS complexes and their interrelationships. Further, because excitation and the resulting depolarization cause contraction of the myocardial fibers, the coordinated mechanical activity of the heart depends on the specialized cardiac fibers.

Plate 2.15

Cardiovascular System: VOLUME 8

ELECTROCARDIOGRAM

An ECG is a graphic representation of voltage variations plotted against time. The variations result from the depolarization and repolarization of the cardiac muscle, which produces electric fields that reach the surface of the body where electrodes are located. An ECG machine is a galvanometer that records voltage variations, usually on paper tape. The first such machine was developed by Wilhelm Einthoven in 1906. It consisted of a silver-plated quartz string situated in a fixed magnetic field. Voltage variations from the body passed through the string, and the interaction of the electric fields between the magnet and the string resulted in the string's movement, which was photographed. The modern ECG machine is similar to these early models, but microelectronics and computer interfaces have been incorporated, making them more useful and powerful. Although more convenient to use, these newer machines are no more accurate than the original ECG built by Einthoven.

Since the development of a practical method of recording the ECG, much has been learned about the electrophysiology of the heart. In the major contribution, Nobel Prize winner Einthoven described the *vector* concept and stated that the action current of the heart, often called the "accession" or "regression" wave, can be represented by a vector that has magnitude, direction, and sense. The magnitude of the voltage of the accession wave is the length of the *arrow shaft*, the direction is determined with respect to a *line of reference*, and the sense is indicated by the presence of an *arrowhead* on the shaft. In its simplest concept, the vector represents the magnitude of a single *dipole* (i.e., a paired electric charge, minus and plus). Likewise, the electrical effect of a group of dipoles can be represented by a vector.

NORMAL ELECTROCARDIOGRAM

The ECG is a record of voltage variations plotted against time. The paper on which the ECG is recorded is ruled in 1-mm-spaced lines, horizontally and vertically. When the tracing is properly standardized (1-mV change produces 10-mm stylus deflection), each vertical space represents a voltage change of 0.1 mV, and each horizontal space an interval of 40 milliseconds. Each fifth line, horizontal and vertical, is heavy. The time between the heavy lines is 0.2 seconds. The voltage change between two heavy lines is 0.5 mV.

A P wave is the result of atrial depolarization and should not exceed 2.5 mm (0.25 mV) in height in lead II or longer than 0.12 seconds. The PR interval, which includes the P wave plus the PR segment, is a measure of the interval from the beginning of atrial depolarization to the beginning of ventricular depolarization. This interval should not be greater than 0.2 seconds for rates greater than 60 beats/min. The Q wave is the first downward deflection of the QRS complex and represents septal depolarization. The R wave is the *first positive,* or upward, *deflection* of the QRS complex, normally caused by apical LV depolarization. The S wave is the *first negative deflection* after the R wave, caused by depolarization of the posterior basal region of the left ventricle. The voltage of the R wave in the precordial

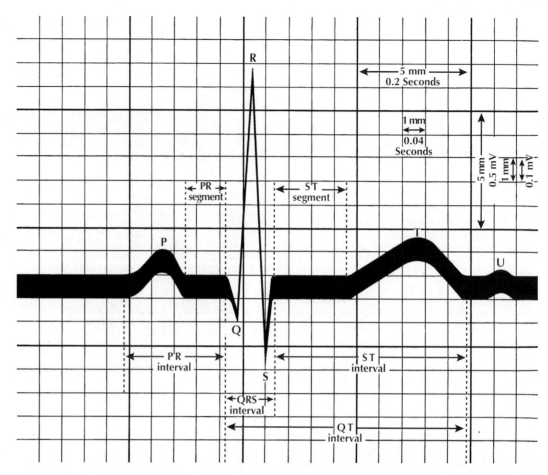

		PR interval	QRS interval	Rate	QT interval	ST segment
Normal ranges	Adults	180 to 200 msec	70 to 100 msec	60	330 to 430 msec	140 to 160 msec
	Children	150 to 180 msec		70	310 to 410 msec	130 to 150 msec
				80	290 to 380 msec	120 to 140 msec
				90	280 to 360 msec	110 to 130 msec
				100	270 to 350 msec	100 to 110 msec
				120	250 to 320 msec	60 to 70 msec

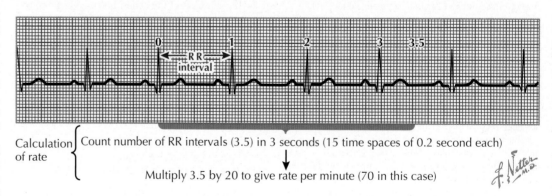

Calculation of rate { Count number of RR intervals (3.5) in 3 seconds (15 time spaces of 0.2 second each)

Multiply 3.5 by 20 to give rate per minute (70 in this case)

leads should not exceed 27 mm. The QT interval is measured from the beginning of the QRS complex to the end of the T wave, including the QRS complex, ST segment, and T wave intervals, the latter two constituting the ST interval. The QT interval varies with the cardiac rate and should not be greater than 0.43 seconds for rates greater than 60 beats/min. The total QRS interval should not exceed 0.1 seconds.

The *cardiac rate* may be determined by counting the number of RR intervals within 16 heavy vertical time

lines (15 time spaces) and multiplying by 20. The first interval counted is coincident with the zero time line (Plate 2.15).

ELECTROCARDIOGRAPHIC LEADS AND REFERENCE LINES

The conventional electrical connections used for recording the ECG are the limb leads, augmented limb leads, and precordial leads.

Plate 2.16

Physiology

ELECTROCARDIOGRAM
(Continued)

Limb Leads

The bipolar limb leads detect electrical variations at two points and display the difference. Lead I is the connection between the electrodes on the left arm and right arm; the galvanometer is between these points of contact (Plate 2.16). When the left arm is in a positive field of force with respect to the right arm, an upward (positive) deflection is written in lead I. Lead II is the connection between the left leg and right arm electrodes. When the left leg is in a positive field of force with respect to the right arm, an upward deflection is written in lead II. Lead III is the connection between the left leg and left arm. When the left leg is in a positive field of force with respect to the left arm, a positive deflection is written in lead III.

Augmented Limb Leads

The unipolar augmented limb leads register the electrical variations in potential at one point (right arm, left arm, or left leg) with respect to a point that does not vary significantly in electrical activity during cardiac contraction (Plate 2.16). The lead is augmented by virtue of the type of electrical connection, which results in a trace of increased amplitude, versus the older Wilson unipolar lead connections. Lead aV_R inscribes the electrical potentials of the right arm with respect to a null point, which is made by uniting the wires from the left arm and left leg. Lead aV_L records the potentials at the left arm in relation to a connection made by the union of wires from the right arm and left foot. Lead aV_F reveals the potentials at the left foot in reference to a junction made by the union of wires from the left and right arms.

Precordial Leads

The unipolar precordial leads are recorded in chest positions 1 through 6 (Plate 2.16). The V designation indicates that the movable electrode registers the electric potential under the electrode with respect to a V, or central terminal, connection, which is made by connecting wires from the right arm, left arm, and left leg. The electric potential of the central terminal connection does not vary significantly throughout the cardiac cycle; therefore the recordings made with the V connection show the electrical variations occurring under the movable precordial electrode. Position V_1 is at the fourth intercostal space to the right of the sternum, V_2 is at the fourth intercostal space to the left of the sternum, V_4 is at the left midclavicular line in the fifth intercostal space, V_3 is halfway between V_2 and V_4, V_5 is at the fifth intercostal space in the anterior axillary line, and V_6 is at the fifth intercostal space in the left midaxillary line.

At times, other precordial lead placements are helpful, including those elevated 2 inches (5 cm) above the usual positions (EV_1, EV_2, etc.), which may help detect MIs. Precordial leads are also placed 2 inches below the usual positions (LV_1, LV_2, etc.) when the heart is unusually low in the thorax, as in patients with pulmonary emphysema. Leads to the right of V_1 (V_3R, V_4R, etc.) are used to differentiate right BBB and right ventricular

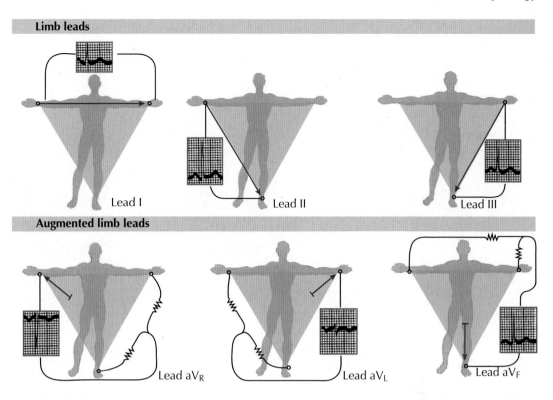

Limb leads

Lead I   Lead II   Lead III

Augmented limb leads

Lead aV_R Lead aV_L Lead aV_F

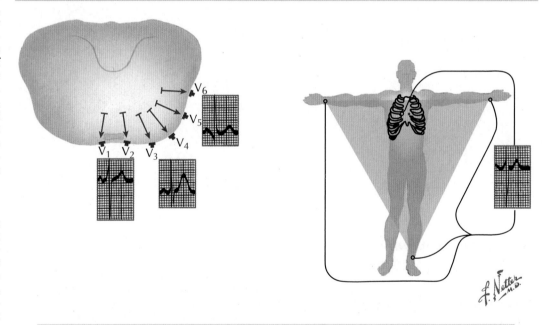

Precordial leads

V_6
V_5
V_1 V_2 V_3 V_4

When current flows toward red arrowheads, upward deflection occurs in ECG.

When current flows away from red arrowheads, downward deflection occurs in ECG.

When current flows perpendicular to red arrows, no deflection or biphasic deflection occurs.

hypertrophy from the normal condition. Leads farther to the left (V_7, V_8, etc.) are used to explore the left ventricle when it is directed posteriorly.

Reference Lines

For the various leads, the reference lines of Einthoven are shown in Plate 2.16 as red arrows. For example, the line of reference for lead I connects the left and right arm electrodes. An accession wave (vector) directed toward the arrowhead of any of the red arrows results in an upward (positive) deflection in the ECG. If the electrical activity, or accession wave, is directed toward the tail of the reference arrow, a downward (negative) deflection is written, but if this wave is perpendicular to the line (90 degrees), no deflection (or a small biphasic one) will be written. The height of the ECG wave is proportional to the magnitude of the projection of the accession wave vector on a reference line.

Plate 2.17

Cardiovascular System: VOLUME 8

PROGRESSION OF DEPOLARIZATION

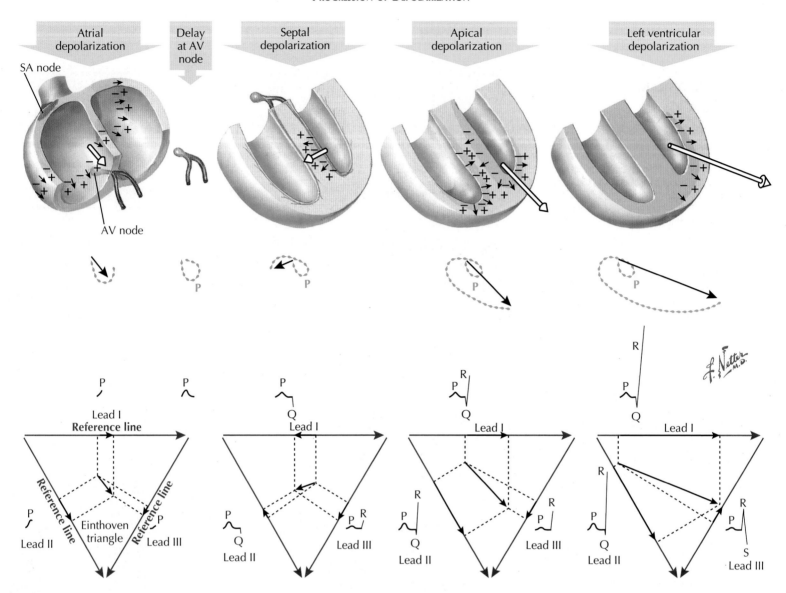

CARDIAC DEPOLARIZATION AND REPOLARIZATION AND MEAN INSTANTANEOUS VECTORS

PROGRESSION OF DEPOLARIZATION

Atrial Depolarization and Mean Vectors

The cardiac impulse originates in the sinus node and starts the process of atrial depolarization by lowering the resistance of the cell membrane, allowing neutralization or reversal of certain dipoles. This leaves an electric wave front, an accession wave, which is preceded by positive forces and followed by negative ones. Normally, this wave is initiated at the *SA node* (Plate 2.17). Early during atrial depolarization, however, the wave spreads toward the foot and AV node. Toward the end of atrial depolarization, the accession wave is directed toward the left atrium and left arm. The early atrial depolarization wave may be represented as a vector, the length of which indicates the magnitude (strength) of the voltage generated by the accession wave. The late atrial depolarization voltage is represented by a second vector, the length of which is a measure of the voltage generated at this time. If the heads of these vectors are connected

with their points of origin, a loop is formed; this is the P loop of the *vectorcardiogram* (VCG). The P loop is seen in the frontal plane.

A mean P vector can be determined from the instantaneous vectors 1 and 2 by using the *parallelogram law*. To derive the mean vector from two instantaneous vectors, a parallelogram is drawn. The instantaneous vectors are drawn as originating from a common point of origin E. The parallelogram is completed by drawing a line from each arrowhead, parallel to the opposite vector. The *mean vector* is an arrow connecting E with the opposite angle of the parallelogram. The mean vector indicates the average direction taken by the atrial accession wave, and its magnitude as the wave travels over the atria.

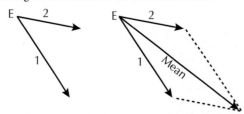

The mean atrial depolarization vector can be analyzed against the *Einthoven triangle* reference frame to

predict the type of P waves that will appear in leads I, II, and III. Projecting the mean vector against the reference line of lead I creates a projected vector, the length of which is proportional to the amplitude of the P wave in that lead. The direction of the wave (up or down) is determined by the direction of the projected atrial vector with respect to the polarity of the reference line. The direction of the P wave will be upward (positive) when the projected vector points in the same direction as the reference arrow for that lead and downward (negative) when the opposite relationship exists.

Just before atrial depolarization is complete, depolarization of the AV node begins. However, the nodal depolarization process is of such low magnitude that the ECG instrument is unable to detect these changes, and it is not until the interventricular septum is invaded that a QRS complex begins. Normally, there is a time interval from the end of the P wave to the beginning of the QRS complex (PR segment), which is usually opposite in direction to the P wave and is a result of atrial repolarization.

Septal Depolarization

The first important electric movement in *septal depolarization* normally begins at the left side of the septum, moves to the right, and results from the entry of bundle

Plate 2.18

Physiology

END OF DEPOLARIZATON FOLLOWED BY REPOLARIZATION

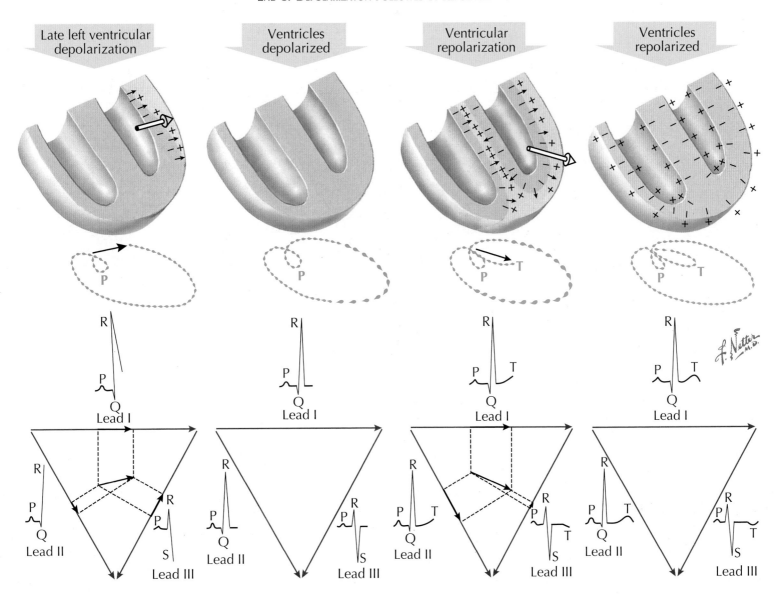

CARDIAC DEPOLARIZATION AND REPOLARIZATION AND MEAN INSTANTANEOUS VECTORS (Continued)

of His branches into the septum at a higher level on the left than the right. The septal left-to-right movement is important because it writes the normal septal Q wave in leads I, aV_L, and V_6. If the first electric movement is analyzed (using Einthoven reference frame), it is evident that a Q wave will initiate the QRS complex in leads I and II and an R wave in lead III.

Apical Depolarization

The second electric movement of significance is apical depolarization, which follows the early depolarization of the right ventricle. Projection of the second instantaneous vector onto the Einthoven triangle indicates that leads I, II, and III will develop R waves at this time.

Left Ventricular Depolarization

Depolarization of the right ventricle occurs quickly and is completed early because of the thinness of

this structure compared with that of the left ventricle. The *third* significant electric movement is toward the lateral wall of the left ventricle. At this time the amplitude of the R waves is increased in leads I and II, and S waves appear in lead III. The forces at this time are strong because there are no counterforces from the right ventricle and the LV muscle mass is thick.

END OF DEPOLARIZATION FOLLOWED BY REPOLARIZATION

Late Left Ventricular Depolarization

The fourth, or late, instantaneous vector (electric movement) exists toward the base of the left ventricle and occurs just before the end of the ventricular depolarization process. This force results in a deepening of the S waves in lead III and an accentuation of the amplitude of the R waves in leads I and II.

Ventricles Depolarized

When the dipoles are removed or reversed, with no potential differences on the body as a result of electric changes affecting the heart, the heart is in the

depolarized state. The myocardium is in a refractory condition during this period, and a myocardial stimulus will fail to elicit a contraction. Because there are no voltage differences, the ECG trace returns to the baseline in all leads; the ST segment is written during this time.

Ventricular Repolarization

Repolarization of the ventricles is a complex process in which a vector appears opposite the wave of depolarization. As a result, development of positive (upward) T waves is shown in the standard leads I and II. The normal direction of T waves in lead III is variable.

Ventricles Repolarized

Finally, each cell of the myocardium becomes repolarized, with a preponderance of negative charges inside the cell and positive charges outside. The heart is now ready for its next stimulation and contraction. The heart muscle is thus in a *receptive state,* and a stimulus will elicit a contraction. Now the trace is *isoelectric* because there are no net potential differences on the body surface.

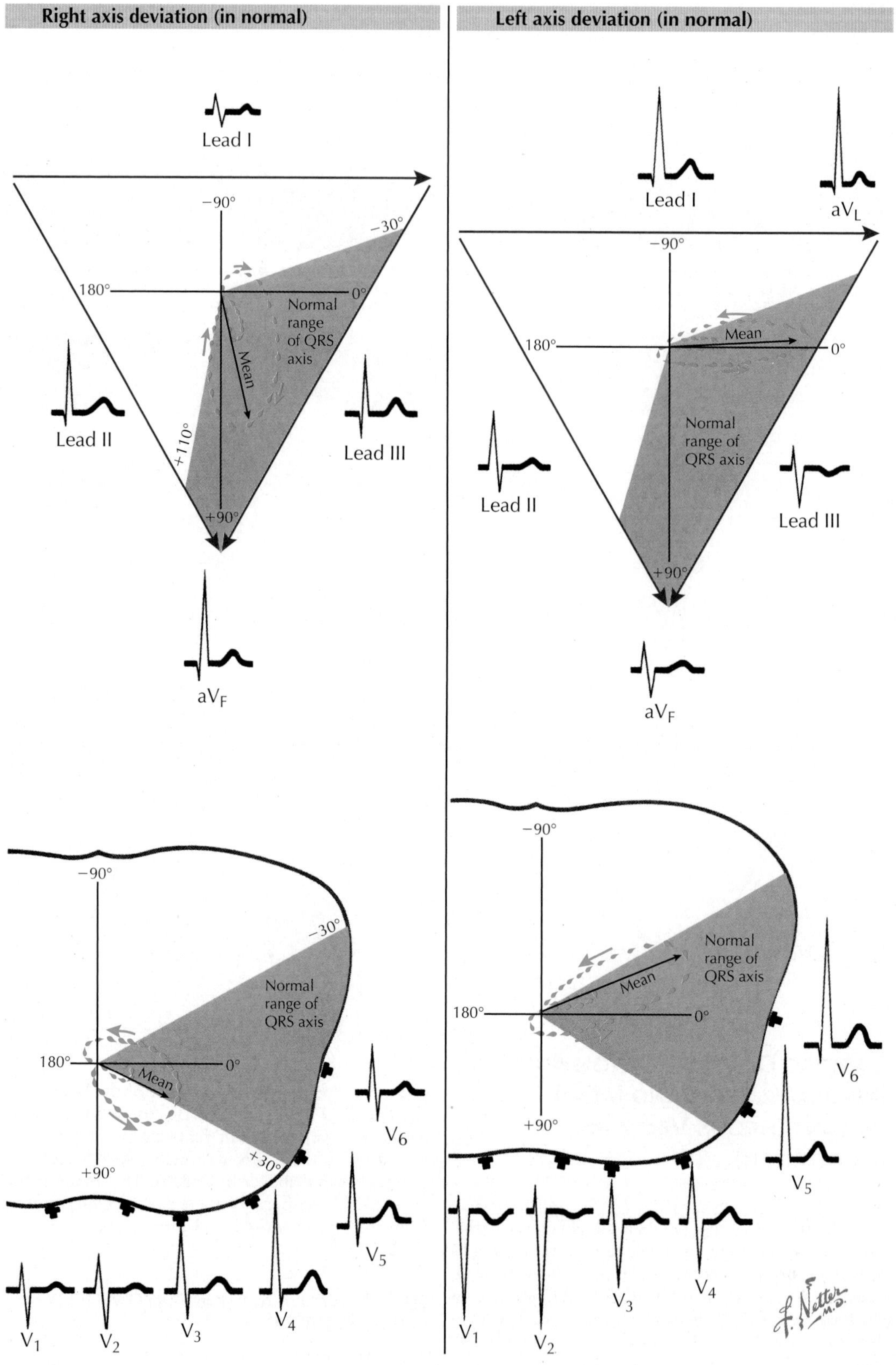

Plate 2.19

Cardiovascular System: VOLUME 8

Right axis deviation (in normal)

Left axis deviation (in normal)

AXIS DEVIATION IN NORMAL ELECTROCARDIOGRAM

In the normal individual, the *mean* electric axis of the P wave, QRS complex, and T wave often reflects the anatomic position of the heart in the chest; an abnormal axis can result from heart disease. Plate 2.19 illustrates normal variations in the vectorcardiographic loop. The QRS and T loops in the frontal plane vary between −30 and +110 degrees and in the horizontal plane between +30 and −30 degrees, measured from the left arm.

In *right axis deviation* in the frontal plane, the P and QRS loops are directed toward the right, often to +90 degrees. Electrocardiographically, there are tall R waves in leads II, III, aV_F, V_2, and V_3.

Left axis deviation is characterized by a QRS loop that points toward the left shoulder blade (left, up, and back). The mean electric axis is often close to −30 degrees in the frontal plane and approaches −30 degrees in the horizontal plane (toward the back). The S waves are deep in leads V_1 and V_2, and the R waves are tall in leads I, aV_L, V_5, and V_6.

It is important to understand the relationship between the position of the heart in the chest and the ECG because the heart's position has a profound influence on the tracing. The concept is complex; the heart can rotate around an anteroposterior axis, a transverse axis, and an anatomic axis that runs from the base to the apex of the heart. Actually, the heart can rotate from front to back, side to side, and around the anatomic axis, all simultaneously. The rotation around the anatomic axis is the most difficult to visualize. Rotation here consists of turning around an axis that runs from the valvular base of the heart through the septum, finally emerging from the apex. An observer at the left of a patient would see the emerging axis at the apex of the heart. Then visualizing a clock at the base of the heart, the observer could also visualize any rotational change around the axis and could designate the direction of rotation as clockwise or counterclockwise.

In a patient with an intermediately placed heart, the right ventricle is in front, to the right, and superior to the left ventricle. The left ventricle is in back, below, and to the left of the right ventricle. If an electrode were placed directly on the right ventricle, a "right ventricular complex" (small R, large S, inverted T) would be recorded. If an electrode were placed directly on the left ventricle, a "left ventricular complex" (small Q, large R, upward T) would be recorded. An electrode on the body or on a limb, facing one ventricle or the other, will record in the lead the type of complex that is typical of that ventricle. In the intermediate heart position, neither the right nor the left ventricle directly faces the aV_L or aV_F electrode; thus these leads have small complexes that do not look exactly as do the right or left ventricular complexes. With inspiration and the descent of the diaphragm, or in a patient with an asthenic body build, the heart rotates clockwise, causing the left ventricle to face the foot and the right ventricle to face the left arm. Thus typical complexes of a left ventricular type will be recorded from lead aV_F, whereas aV_L will record complexes of a right ventricular type. In an obese or pregnant subject, or during expiration with a high diaphragm, the heart rotates counterclockwise, and LV (predominantly positive) complexes are recorded in lead aV_L and RV (predominantly negative) complexes in lead aV_F (Plate 2.19).

Plate 2.20

Physiology

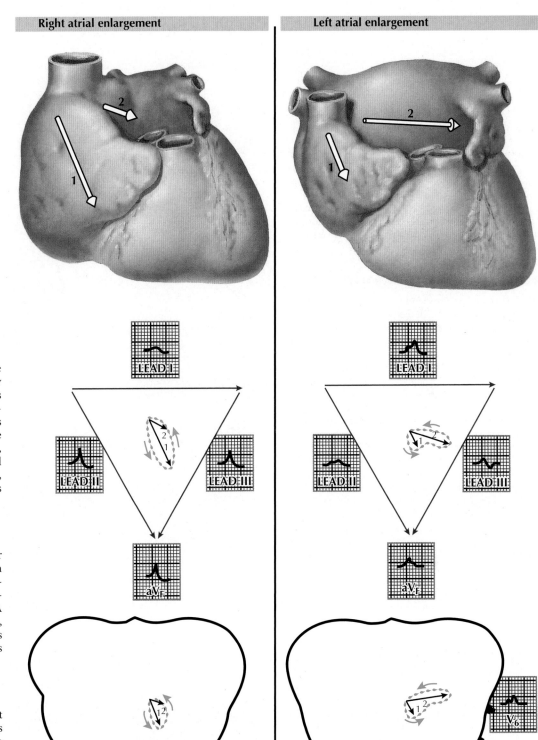

Right atrial enlargement

Left atrial enlargement

ATRIAL ENLARGEMENT

Enlargement of the right atrium, compared with the left, occurs in patients with cor pulmonale, pulmonary hypertension, and tricuspid or pulmonary stenosis. As a result, the first atrial electric movement predominates, and the electric axis of the P wave generally is toward the foot and to the front. As a consequence, the P waves are small in lead I but are tall in leads II, III, and aV_F, often exceeding the upper limit of normal (2.5 mm) for lead II. The vector loop is down, forward, and large. Moderately tall P waves are present in leads V_1 and V_2.

RIGHT ATRIAL ENLARGEMENT

RA enlargement is found when there is a pressure or flow overload in the right atrium compared with the left (Plate 2.20). The pressure is increased characteristically in the right atrium in patients with tricuspid stenosis, and the "P pulmonale" picture of RA enlargement occurs. Here, the P waves are tall, peaked, narrow, and unnotched (easily seen in leads II, III, and aV_F), with a tendency toward right axis deviation.

LEFT ATRIAL ENLARGEMENT

In contrast to the right atrium, left atrial enlargement causes the ECG picture of "P mitrale." This usually is caused by mitral stenosis or regurgitation incident to rheumatic heart disease. The P waves are notched and wide in lead II, with a tendency to left axis deviation, but typically are normal in height. There is enlargement of the left atrium compared with the right; therefore the electric forces are directed toward the left axilla. Characteristically, the P waves in lead II are wide (≥ 0.12 seconds). The loop of the P wave is unusually large and shows a left axis deviation. Wide, notched P waves also are seen in lead V_6. With left atrial enlargement, the late P vectors are large compared with the early vectors (Plate 2.20).

ENLARGEMENT OF BOTH ATRIA

When both right and left atria are enlarged, the P waves are tall—more than 2.5 mm in lead II—and wide (≥ 0.12 seconds). Notching is present. This condition occurs when mitral valve disease prevails in the presence of an interatrial septal defect or when multiple valvular defects are present. The atrial T waves or the repolarization waves of the atria are normally small, often being undetectable or lost in the QRS complexes. Normally, the T wave is discordant with the P wave, in that a positive P wave is usually followed by a very small, negative T wave. Generally, the area under the atrial T wave is slightly smaller than the area under the P wave.

With enlargement of the P waves, in either "P mitrale" or "P pulmonale," the atrial T waves enlarge in proportion to the increased size of the P waves, with resultant depression of the PR segments. Large atrial T waves often call attention to atrial abnormalities and are helpful diagnostically.

Plate 2.21

Cardiovascular System: VOLUME 8

VENTRICULAR HYPERTROPHY

Various terms have been used to describe the ECG picture of ventricular hypertrophy, including *ventricular preponderance, strain, systolic* or *diastolic overload,* and *enlargement*. Some of these describe a functional state of overwork of one ventricle versus the other or refer to an anatomic condition with increased muscle of one ventricle compared with the other. Ventricular preponderance is an all-inclusive term that broadly includes most conditions, and enlargement covers both hypertrophy and dilation.

RIGHT VENTRICULAR HYPERTROPHY

The QRS forces are directed to the right because of the thick right ventricle, which distorts the horizontal loop to the right and forward, and is associated with tall R waves relative to normal in leads V_1 and V_2 and deep S waves in leads V_4 and V_5 (Plate 2.21). The R/S amplitude ratio in lead V_1 is abnormal, indicating a tall R wave with respect to the depth of the S wave. Normally, this ratio should be less than 1. Characteristically, the ST segments and T waves are opposite in direction to that portion of the QRS complex of greatest area (usually the R wave), and the T loop is opposite to the QRS loop. Thus the R wave is up and the T wave is down in leads V_1 and V_2, but in leads V_5 and V_6, the S wave is always down and the T wave is up.

Right ventricular hypertrophy may be caused by congenital or acquired heart disease, and the hypertrophy may result from a pressure or volume overload. As a result, the RV muscle thickens with respect to the LV, and a RV preponderance develops. The *net* electric change of the whole heart writes the ECG and VCG, and thus the QRS electric forces are directed in general from the left to the right of the heart and of the body. The direction of the electric forces will usually be from the smaller muscle mass toward the larger mass; that is, from the normal toward the hypertrophied ventricle.

LEFT VENTRICULAR HYPERTROPHY

The large muscle mass of the left hypertrophied ventricle compared with the right distorts the QRS loop toward the left scapula. This results in small R waves and deep S waves in leads V_1 and V_2, with high R waves and small or no S waves in leads V_5 and V_6 (Plate 2.21). Again, the ST segments and T waves are opposite in direction to the major deflection of the QRS complex, which means that in lead V_1 the deep S wave is associated with a *positive* ST segment and T wave, whereas in lead V_6 the tall R wave is associated with a *negative* ST segment and T wave. In the horizontal loop the early forces in the patient are from left to right and to the front, later toward the left scapula, and finally returning to the zero point. When the shifts of the ST segments are characteristic of LV enlargement, there is an open QRST loop in the VCG (i.e., beginning and end of a QRS complex are at different levels), and usually a T wave follows that is 180 degrees discordant with the major portion of the QRS loop. The frontal loop is displaced toward the left shoulder, with discordant QRS and T-wave relationships. An open loop may be seen here as well.

The *J point* is the junction between the end of the QRS complex and the beginning of the T wave in

the ECG. The point just in front of the J point, which is the end of the PR interval and the beginning of the QRS complex, is called the *I point*. The open loop in the VCG is found when the I and J points in the ECG are at different horizontal levels. In a normal person the I and J points usually are on the same level, often on the isoelectric line. With severe LV hypertrophy, the J point shifts below the I point in lead V_5, and in severe RV hypertrophy, J is below I in lead V_1. The

I-J relationships are also changed by digitalis, hypokalemia, MI, myocardial ischemia, pericarditis, and BBB.

RIGHT AND LEFT VENTRICULAR HYPERTROPHY

When both RV and LV hypertrophy exist, the muscle with the greater degree of enlargement will dominate the electrical picture.

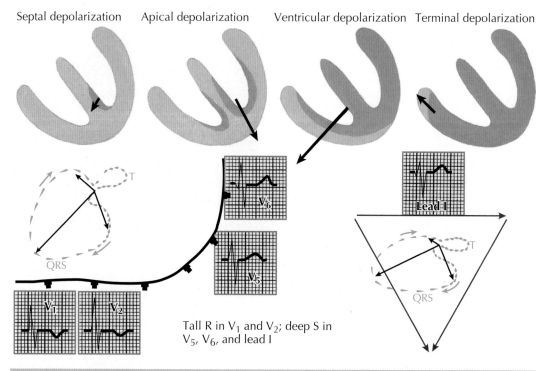

Right ventricular hypertrophy

Septal depolarization   Apical depolarization   Ventricular depolarization   Terminal depolarization

Tall R in V_1 and V_2; deep S in V_5, V_6, and lead I

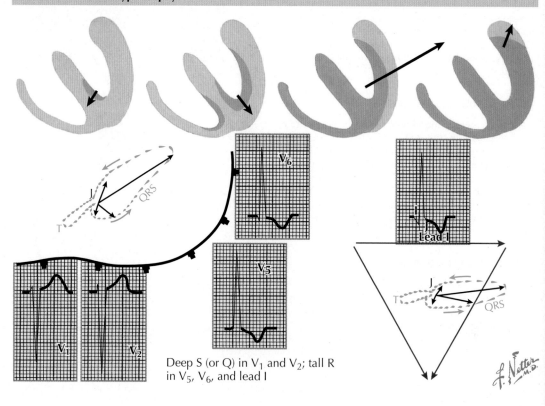

Left ventricular hypertrophy

Deep S (or Q) in V_1 and V_2; tall R in V_5, V_6, and lead I

Plate 2.22

Physiology

BUNDLE BRANCH BLOCK

The term *bundle branch block* (BBB) indicates disease in, or altered transmission through, certain branches of the conduction system of the heart. Blocks may occur in the left or right ventricle or in both. A characteristic change is widening of the QRS complex greater than 0.1 seconds. When the duration of this complex ranges from 0.1 to 0.12 seconds, the block is *incomplete*; if greater than 0.12 seconds, a *complete* BBB exists. With a complete right BBB, the first 0.04 seconds of the QRS complex is normal in configuration but the last portion is abnormal (Plate 2.22). With a left BBB the total duration of the wave is written by an abnormal depolarization wave, and the tracing is abnormal.

BBBs may be typical or atypical. A *typical* BBB has a lesion only in the bundle of His or one of its branches, and there is no associated lesion. An *atypical* BBB, in addition to the block, has some other lesion (e.g., MI). A typical block has T waves in the opposite direction as the wave of greatest duration in the QRS complex (i.e., T is opposite S in right BBB in V_6, but T is opposite R in lead V_1). An atypical block does not necessarily follow this rule.

RIGHT BUNDLE BRANCH BLOCK

A small defect in the distal His bundle or right bundle branch itself is sufficient to cause right BBB. In right BBB, the first electric activation is normal from the left side of the septum to the right; this writes the usual septal Q wave in leads V_5 and V_6. The next movement is through the left ventricle from the endocardium to the epicardium, which writes a normal R wave in leads V_5 and V_6. Finally, there is a slow progression of the activation wave through the septum and the Purkinje system on the right and through the right ventricle, which requires more time. As a result, there is a wide S wave in leads V_5 and V_6, and the duration of the S wave is usually greater than that of the R wave in the QRS complex. This order of depolarization—right, then left, then right—registers an R, an S, and an R' wave in lead V_1; here the duration of the R' wave is greater than that of the R wave. The VCG shows the electromotive forces going first to the right, then to the left, and then back to the right again. Writing of the VCG slows (dots closer together) during late ventricular depolarization because the activation of the right ventricle is slow. The horizontal-plane VCG is to the right, then to the left, and then to the right front, whereas the frontal-plane VCG is right, then left, then right, and often up. Recall that in a right BBB the first part of the QRS loop is normal but the last part is abnormal.

Right BBB often is caused by arteriosclerosis or prolonged strain on the right ventricle, as in pulmonary hypertension or pulmonary stenosis.

LEFT BUNDLE BRANCH BLOCK

A block in the left bundle of His alters the entire ventricular depolarization pathway. Ventricular depolarization starts from the right side of the septum and

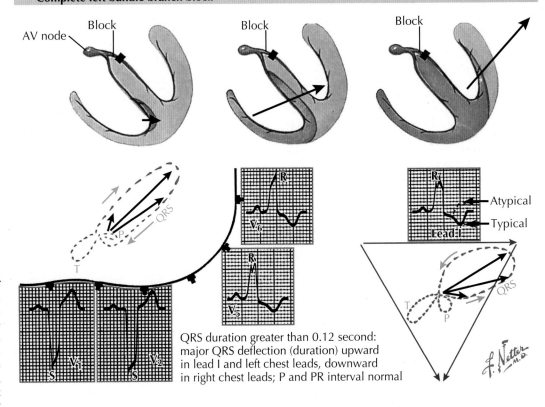

Complete right bundle branch block

AV node
Block
Block
Block

QRS duration greater than 0.12 second: major QRS deflection (duration) downward in lead I and left chest leads, upward in right chest leads; P and PR interval normal

Complete left bundle branch block

AV node
Block
Block
Block

QRS duration greater than 0.12 second: major QRS deflection (duration) upward in lead I and left chest leads, downward in right chest leads; P and PR interval normal

progresses toward the left front, writing small R waves in leads V_1 and V_2. The voltage next swings toward the left near the cardiac apex, then toward the left base, writing tall R waves in leads I, V_5, and V_6 and S waves in leads V_1 and V_2. The electric movement is generally toward the left scapula, and characteristically the ST segments and T waves are *opposite* in direction to the major deflection of the QRS complex. When this QRS complex–T wave relationship occurs, the tracing is characteristic of *typical* left BBB. When the QRS complex and the T wave are not opposite or are concordant, the tracing is referred to as *atypical*, and another lesion (e.g., MI) probably is present as well as the block.

Left BBB is caused by arteriosclerosis, MI, cardiac failure, or severe strain on the left ventricle, as in hypertension.

Plate 2.23

Cardiovascular System: VOLUME 8

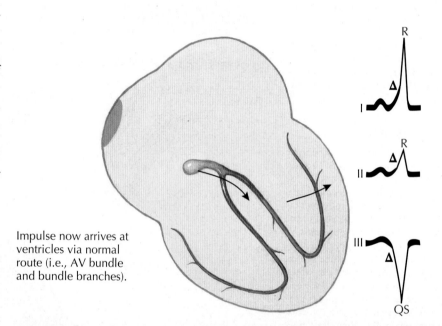

Impulse originates at SA node, passes through atrium, is delayed at AV node, but passes rapidly through accessory bundle of Kent.

P wave is normal, but almost immediately thereafter Δ wave appears due to arrival of impulses at ventricles via abnormal route, resulting in short or absent PR segment.

WOLFF-PARKINSON-WHITE SYNDROME

Wolff-Parkinson-White (WPW) syndrome is caused by the presence of an accessory pathway. About 20% of patients with an accessory pathway have organic heart disease, and 80% have the ECG abnormality only. The accessory pathway connects the atria to the ventricles, over which depolarization occurs rapidly from atria to ventricles, resulting in ventricular preexcitation. The syndrome related to preexcitation is most often seen in young subjects who may have frequent paroxysms of supraventricular tachycardia. Between episodes of rapid heartbeat, the QRS complexes consist of a short PR interval (usually <0.11 seconds), a QRS complex widened by a Δ *wave*, and usually a QRS complex with a duration of 0.11 to 0.14 seconds. The PR interval is decreased by the amount the QRS complex is increased, so that the P-J interval remains quite normal (Plate 2.23). The P-J interval is from the beginning of the P wave to the end of the QRS. "J" stands for the junction between the QRS and ST segment on the ECG.

The upstroke of the R wave in lead I in a patient with a right-sided accessory pathway is usually "slurred" because of the Δ wave at the beginning of the QRS complex. If the accessory pathway connects left atrium to left ventricle, depolarization will be from left to right, which will produce QRS complexes in lead I that are primarily negative. Most often, however, the accessory pathway is on the right, with the accession wave going from right to left and a Δ wave appearing at the beginning of the QRS complex in lead I. The accessory pathway could be posterior or anterior, and different ECG configurations result. The precise location of the accessory pathway is determined at electrophysiologic study before an ablation procedure.

Impulses from the sinus node travel more rapidly through the accessory pathway than through the AV node and bundle of His. The widening of the QRS complex and the slurring of the upstroke of the R wave in lead I are explained by the depolarization wave entering the right ventricle early and without delay, through the abnormal connection between the atria and the ventricles. Because the depolarization process through the ventricles is longer than normal due to its abnormal direction, the QRS complex is exceptionally wide. After the early depolarization of the ventricle from the accessory pathway has begun, the normal atrial impulses, which were delayed at the AV node, enter the ventricle by the normal pathway, and the depolarization of the ventricles is completed in a normal fashion. Thus the terminal portions of the QRS complexes are normal.

Impulse now arrives at ventricles via normal route (i.e., AV bundle and bundle branches).

The QRS complex is completed, but total result is a short PR interval and a long, slurred QRS complex.

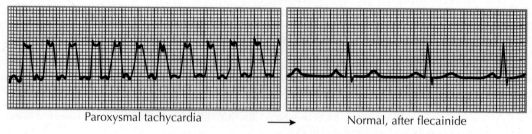

Paroxysmal tachycardia → Normal, after flecainide

The accessory pathway predisposes the patient to *paroxysmal reentrant tachycardia* by facilitating retrograde conduction into the atria with the initiation of circus movements or antegrade conduction in the pathway with retrograde conduction in the His-Purkinje system. Therefore all young patients reporting attacks of tachycardia should have an ECG during a period of normal heart rate to determine whether a WPW pattern exists.

Antiarrhythmic drugs such as flecainide may be used successfully to block preexcitation. Digitalis is usually ineffective and may be dangerous if given alone because of 1:1 conduction to the ventricle in certain atrial arrhythmias (e.g., atrial fibrillation or flutter), which may result in ventricular fibrillation. Other drugs that block conduction through the AV node can enhance conduction through the accessory pathway as well (e.g., calcium blockers, adenosine).

Plate 2.24

Physiology

Representation of dual-pathway physiology

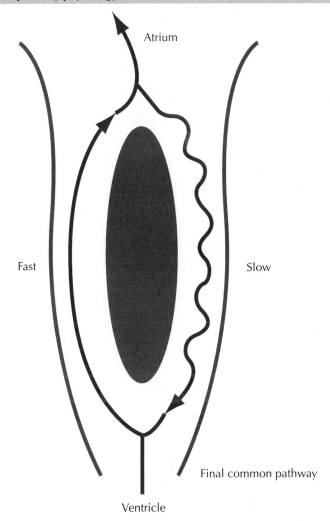

Atrium

Fast

Slow

Final common pathway

Ventricle

Typical ECG recordings and anatomic representation of the common supraventricular tachycardias

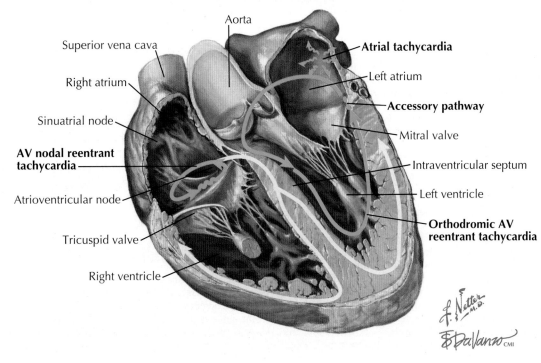

Aorta

Superior vena cava

Right atrium

Sinuatrial node

AV nodal reentrant tachycardia

Atrioventricular node

Tricuspid valve

Right ventricle

Atrial tachycardia

Left atrium

Accessory pathway

Mitral valve

Intraventricular septum

Left ventricle

Orthodromic AV reentrant tachycardia

ATRIOVENTRICULAR NODAL REENTRANT TACHYCARDIA

The other common reentrant arrhythmia is atrioventricular nodal reentrant tachycardia. This arrhythmia is characterized by the presence of two distinct pathways within the AV node, the "fast" and "slow" pathways. The pathways allow reentrant tachycardia to occur within the AV node, using a final common pathway to exit the AV node and travel to the ventricle through the bundle of His. This arrhythmia can be treated with AV nodal blockers, antiarrhythmic drugs such as flecainide, and ablation.

Plate 2.25   Cardiovascular System: VOLUME 8

SINUS AND ATRIAL ARRHYTHMIAS

Certain arrhythmias are caused by a disturbance at the sinus node, including sinus bradycardia, sinus tachycardia, sinus arrhythmia, and wandering pacemaker. The sinus node is under the control of the parasympathetic and sympathetic nerves, and altered function of these nerves may influence cardiac activity. The SA node is depressed by parasympathetic *(vagus)* functions or stimulated by sympathetic activity.

SINUS BRADYCARDIA

In sinus bradycardia the sinus node originates impulses at a slow rate, less than 60 beats/min (Plate 2.25). Sinus bradycardia is common in patients with high vagal tone, hypothyroidism, and increased intracranial tension; during athletic training; and during treatment with digitalis and/or reserpine. Usually the slow rate is caused, at least in part, by vagal inhibition of the sinus node.

SINUS TACHYCARDIA

Sympathetic nerve stimulation or the blocking of vagus nerves can produce sinus tachycardia. The sinus node originates impulses at a rate greater than 100 beats/min, and close inspection of these curves shows some variation in the RR interval (Plate 2.25). It is important to observe this variation to differentiate sinus tachycardia from *atrial tachycardia,* in which there is no significant variation between the RR intervals. Sinus tachycardia is found in patients after exercise or smoking; in hyperthyroidism, anxiety, toxic states, fever, anemia, and diseases involving the heart or lungs; and from other causes. Sinus tachycardia is characterized by a slowing of the pulse rate during carotid sinus pressure, followed by the gradual return of the rate to its basic level on release of pressure. This is in contrast to the reaction to carotid pressure in atrial tachycardia, which may cause the rhythm to change abruptly to a sinus rhythm.

SINUS ARRHYTHMIA

Sinus arrhythmia is a variation in cardiac rate during breathing or sometimes with other organ function, such as contraction of the spleen. The arrhythmia is typically found in children or in patients with Cheyne-Stokes respiration. Usually, afferent impulses from the lungs travel to the cardiac center, with efferent impulses traveling over the vagus nerve to the sinus node. The pacemaker activity at the node varies reflexively with respiration. Generally, there are about five cardiac beats to each respiratory cycle. With expiration, the cardiac rate is slow; with inspiration, it is more rapid (Plate 2.25).

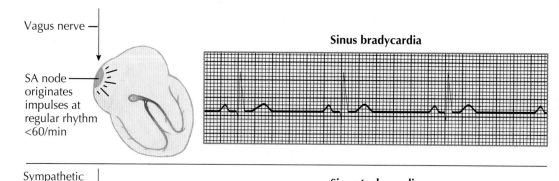

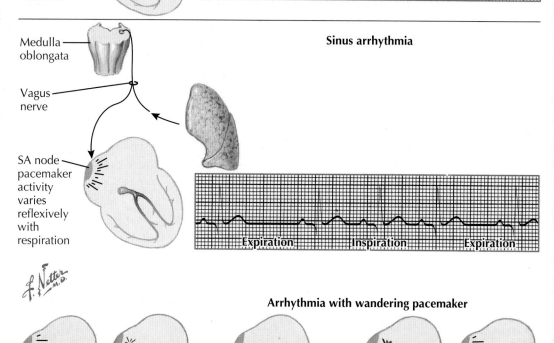

WANDERING PACEMAKER

A wandering pacemaker is present when, with each beat, the pacemaker changes its position in the atrium, often traveling down to and into the AV node and back to the sinus node again. This occurs when there is a variation in the vagal tone at the sinus node or there are changes in sympathetic stimulation. In the ECG the PR interval becomes progressively shorter, and the P waves often disappear within the QRS complexes or may even appear *after* the QRS complexes. In lead II, the P waves may at times be *inverted* because the atria are depolarized from the AV node to the sinus node instead of in the usual direction. A wandering pacemaker is not a serious irregularity; it is often transient and may be stopped by anticholinergic agents such as atropine (Plate 2.25).

Plate 2.26

Physiology

PREMATURE CONTRACTION

Three common terms used to describe certain abnormal cardiac contractions are *premature contractions* (beats occurring early in time), *ectopic beats* (beats with sites of origin outside the sinus node), and *extrasystoles* (added beats). Only extrasystoles are truly added or additional beats, often interpolated or added between two normal beats without interfering with the basic rhythm.

ATRIAL PREMATURE CONTRACTIONS

Premature atrial contractions are caused by an irritability of the atria, with early contractions emanating from an impulse in the atria outside the SA node. Atrial is differentiated from ventricular premature contractions by measurement of the compensatory pause. With atrial contractions the compensatory pause is incomplete, whereas with ventricular premature contractions the pause is complete (Plate 2.26). Measurement of the compensatory pause for atrial premature beats follows:

1. Select the atrial premature beat (P wave) that appears different from the P waves of the basic mechanism and is premature in time; this is the atrial premature contraction.
2. Measure the interval from the premature P wave to the P wave immediately in front.
3. Add this measured interval to the time between the premature P wave and the P wave immediately following (<2×).

This total duration is shorter than the time between two normal PP intervals that do not include a premature contraction (2×).

NODAL PREMATURE CONTRACTIONS

Nodal premature contractions result from stimulation of the AV node. Usually there is retrograde conduction starting at the AV node, with an accession wave moving over the atria from the AV node to the SA node, and P waves of an abnormal form are written. At times there is no retrograde conduction, and P waves and atrial contraction do not occur. The stimulus at the AV node often is vagal or is caused by disease (Plate 2.26).

High Atrioventricular Nodal Rhythm

High AV nodal rhythm prevails when the *head* of the AV node becomes the pacemaker, and atrial depolarization occurs in a retrograde fashion from the AV node to the SA node. With nodal premature contractions, *inverted* P waves are written in leads II, III, and aV$_F$ because of retrograde auricular depolarization. The PR interval is short, P waves precede the QRS complexes, and the QRS and T waves are of normal configuration.

Middle Nodal Rhythm

When the junctional tissue is stimulated below the AV node near its *center*, atrial and ventricular depolarizations occur simultaneously. Here the P waves fall within the QRS complexes, and the summation complexes (QRS + P) are slightly different in appearance from the normal QRS complexes of the basic mechanism.

Low Nodal Impulse

If the pacemaker is *low* in the junctional tissues, the ventricles are depolarized before the atria, the QRS complexes are written first, and *inverted* P waves in leads II, III, and aV$_F$ are written later.

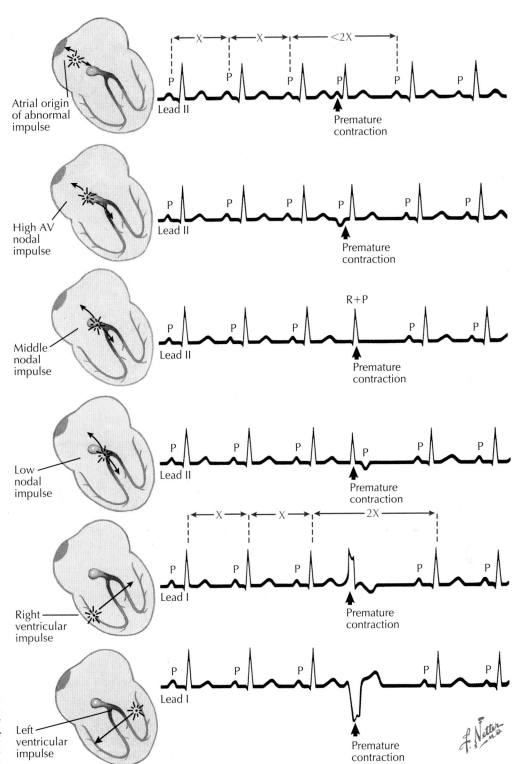

RIGHT VENTRICULAR IMPULSE

The P wave rhythm is not disturbed. The ventricles contract early from a stimulus in the region of the right ventricle. The accession wave travels from right to left and, moving in this direction, produces *upright* QRS deflections in lead I. The duration of this complex is long because of the abnormally long pathway and is longer than 0.10 seconds, followed by ST segments and T waves in the opposite direction as the major deflections of the QRS complexes. The compensatory pause is complete; that is, the interval between two normal QRS complexes that do not contain an ectopic beat is the same as the time from a QRS complex before the ectopic QRS beat to the QRS complex that follows this beat (Plate 2.26).

LEFT VENTRICULAR IMPULSE

A pacemaker in the LV wall produces an accession wave that travels from left to right in lead I, resulting in negative (*inverted*) wide QRS complexes with positive (*upward*) ST segments and T waves and complete compensatory pauses.

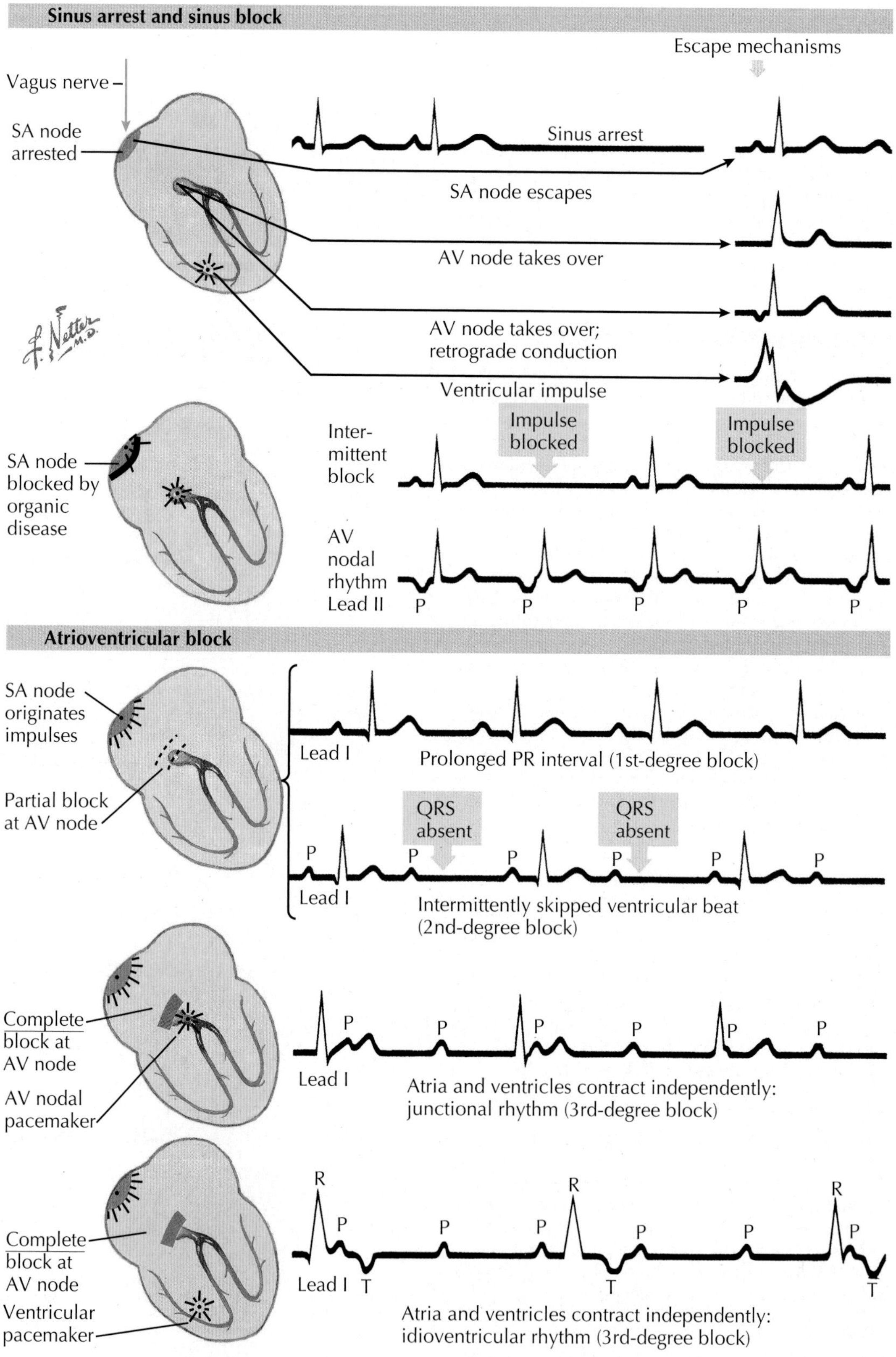

Plate 2.27

Cardiovascular System: VOLUME 8

SINUS ARREST, SINUS BLOCK, AND ATRIOVENTRICULAR BLOCK

SINUS ARREST

Sinus arrest is usually a functional condition in which the sinus node fails to send impulses to the atria, resulting in a period of cardiac asystole. Eventually, recovery occurs. The first beat after the asystole may be a normal sinus beat (known as a *sinus escape* beat), or the AV node may take over for the first beat, originating from a pacemaker in the AV node, called a *nodal escape* beat (Plate 2.27). Here, the P wave may be detectable when there is *retrograde atrial conduction*. In this case, *inverted* P waves either precede or follow the QRS complexes in leads II, III, and aV$_F$, or there may be no retrograde conduction and hence no P waves. A ventricular escape beat has all the characteristics of a ventricular ectopic beat. Escape beats of these various types may precede sinus rhythm, sinus bradycardia, sinus tachycardia, nodal rhythm, ventricular tachycardia, or other cardiac rhythms or arrhythmias.

SINUATRIAL BLOCK

In SA block the sinus node is blocked organically or chemically (Plate 2.27). The block may occur intermittently, in which case every other beat may fail to appear. The sinus node recovers slowly after depolarization, and the refractory period is such that only every other beat is written. Periodically, in some cases more than one beat is skipped. In other cases, the SA node is more severely diseased, and repolarization of the P wave occurs slowly. An AV nodal rhythm develops and takes over the role of pacemaker, and the P waves are *inverted* in leads II, III, and aV$_F$.

ATRIOVENTRICULAR BLOCK

Atrioventricular block often is classified as a first-, second-, or third-degree AV block (Plate 2.27). A *first-degree* AV block has a prolonged PR interval. A *second-degree* AV block is characterized by the occasional dropping of a QRS complex. A *third-degree* AV block shows a complete dissociation between atrial and ventricular contractions. With a first-degree AV block, the PR interval is long, exceeding 0.2 seconds for rates above 60 beats/min. With a second-degree AV block, an occasional P wave is not followed by a QRS complex. Normally there is one P wave for every QRS complex, but with a second-degree block there may be seven P waves for every six QRS complexes (or some other ratio of P to QRS). This degree of block would be designated 7:6. A complete AV block may be of two types: (1) the pacemaker may be in the AV nodal tissue, with QRS complexes essentially normal in appearance and not

wide, or (2) the pacemaker may be in the His-Purkinje system, and the QRS complexes will be wide and abnormal in shape. In either case, there will be a complete dissociation between the beating of the atria and the ventricles. There also will be two different frequencies: one frequency of about 76 beats/min, which represents the atrial depolarization rate, and the other of 30 beats/min, which is the ventricular depolarization rate.

These arrhythmias are important clinically because a slow rate from any cause greatly decreases cerebral, coronary, and other organ circulation, which results in tissue damage and often death. Every medical or surgical effort should be made to maintain a normal rate. Stopping drugs such as beta blockers and calcium antagonists or initiating pacemaker therapy may be of great benefit.

Sinus arrest and sinus block

Vagus nerve

SA node arrested

Escape mechanisms

Sinus arrest

SA node escapes

AV node takes over

AV node takes over; retrograde conduction

Ventricular impulse

SA node blocked by organic disease

Impulse blocked

Impulse blocked

Inter-mittent block

AV nodal rhythm Lead II

Atrioventricular block

SA node originates impulses

Partial block at AV node

Lead I — Prolonged PR interval (1st-degree block)

QRS absent

QRS absent

Lead I — Intermittently skipped ventricular beat (2nd-degree block)

Complete block at AV node

AV nodal pacemaker

Lead I — Atria and ventricles contract independently: junctional rhythm (3rd-degree block)

Complete block at AV node

Ventricular pacemaker

Lead I — Atria and ventricles contract independently: idioventricular rhythm (3rd-degree block)

Plate 2.28

Physiology

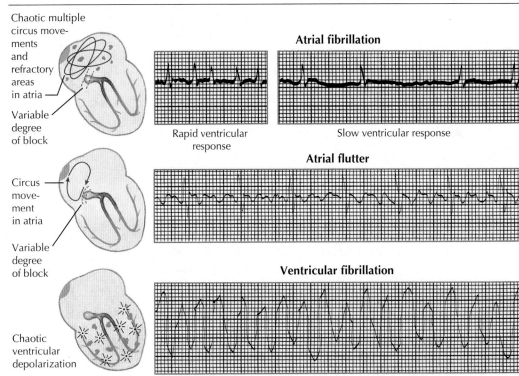

TACHYCARDIA, FIBRILLATION, AND ATRIAL FLUTTER

PAROXYSMAL TACHYCARDIA

Paroxysmal Atrial Tachycardia

Paroxysmal atrial tachycardia (PAT) is caused by a pacemaker in the atria that gives rise to rapid regular impulses at a rate above 100 beats/min, often as much as 180 beats/min (Plate 2.28). P waves can usually be identified, although in some cases the P and T waves fall on each other. The RR intervals are regular. PAT is characterized by an abrupt beginning and ending. The onset and end often occur within the course of a single beat. Carotid sinus pressure may cause a sudden reversion to sinus rhythm, which is diagnostic of PAT.

Paroxysmal Atrial Tachycardia with Block

It is important to recognize PAT with block because it may be caused by digitalis intoxication, in which case the digitalis should be withdrawn. This condition is the same as PAT.

Paroxysmal Nodal Tachycardia

This disturbance is characterized by inverted P waves in leads II, III, and aV$_F$ because of retrograde atrial conduction. The P waves fall before, within, or after the QRS complexes. Retrograde conduction may occur. Paroxysmal nodal tachycardia often is caused by disease of the AV node.

Ventricular Tachycardia

Ventricular tachycardia is caused by rapid impulse formation in a ventricle. The arrhythmia is serious and often associated with the toxic effects of digitalis and many antiarrhythmics (e.g., sotalol), or it may be caused by serious organic cardiac disease. The ventricular rate is more rapid than the atrial rate, and close inspection of the tracing allows identification of occasional P waves occurring at the basic atrial rate. The ventricular contractions are

generally more than 150 beats/min and may be greater than 200 beats/min. The QRS complexes are wide, with T waves that are discordant with the QRS complexes, and the PR intervals are not identical.

ATRIAL FIBRILLATION

Atrial fibrillation (AF) is the most common arrhythmia on hospital admission in older patients. AF is caused by the presence of multiple islands of abnormal myocardium in various states of *refractoriness*, so that the atrial depolarization wave must wind its way in and out of these islands of tissue, resulting in electric potentials of low voltage with variable directions. Only some of these impulses are transmitted through the AV node; thus all of the RR intervals are different because of the irregularity of conduction (Plate 2.28).

Plate 2.29   Cardiovascular System: VOLUME 8

Sudden Cardiac Death (SCD)

Structural congenital abnormalities

Hypertrophic cardiomyopathy (HCM)

Ventricular tachycardia (VT) is common in patients with HCM and asymmetric septal hypertrophy.

HCM is usually inherited as an autosomal dominant trait with incomplete penetrance. Patients with family history of syncope or sudden cardiac death are at particularly high risk.

HCM is one of most common causes of SCD in young athletes.

JOHN A.CRAIG—AD
with E. Hatton

Channelopathies

Long QT syndrome

Autosomal dominant (Romano-Ward syndrome)

Autosomal recessive (Jervell syndrome) (Lange-Nielsen syndrome)

Congenital deafness

Acquired form (drugs, ischemia, metabolic abnormalities)

Brugada syndrome

Autosomal dominant

Patients have structurally normal hearts on echocardiography but exhibit ST elevations in V_1–V_3 characterized by accentuated J wave often followed by inverted T wave. Administration of Na^+ channel blockers or other drugs may initiate polymorphic VT resembling VF.

Na^+

K^+

Rate = 71/min   QT 0.42 s

ECG demonstrating prolonged QT interval

Adrenergic stimulation   (Exercise, fear, startle)

ECG of polymorphic VT (Torsades de pointes)

Long QT syndrome may result from genetic or acquired factors that affect number and function of ion channels, resulting in prolonged QT interval and increased risk of developing fatal arrhythmias.

Na^+

V_1 V_2 V_3

Resting ECG findings in Brugada syndrome

Na^+ channel blocker

Na^+

Polymorphic VT pattern after administration of Na^+ channel blocker

Tachycardia, Fibrillation, and Atrial Flutter (Continued)

Rheumatic heart disease, hyperthyroidism, and arteriosclerotic heart disease are common causes of AF. There are no consistently identifiable P waves in the tracing with AF. The ventricular rate may be rapid or slow, depending on the degree of conduction through the AV node and the presence of heart failure or digitalis and other drugs that slow or accelerate conduction. If the ventricular rate is rapid and heart failure is present, the rate can be slowed greatly by beta blockers, calcium antagonists, and digitalis. Sinus rhythm can be achieved by electrical or chemical cardioversion and antiarrhythmics as well as by catheter-based ablation of atrial tissue in the pulmonary vein or other sites of origin of the arrhythmia. The antiarrhythmic drugs commonly used include flecainide, propafenone, sotalol, dofetilide, amiodarone, and dronedarone. Additionally, ibutilide may be used for chemical rather than electrical cardioversion.

ATRIAL FLUTTER

Atrial flutter is caused by a circus movement or a low atrial pacemaker that fires regularly at a rapid rate, usually about 220 beats/min (see Plate 2.28). Often there is a *variable block* at the AV node, and only every other beat, or every third or fourth beat, is transmitted to the ventricles. A clinical clue to the diagnosis of atrial flutter is a ventricular rate of 150 beats/min. This usually means atrial flutter with 2:1 block. In leads II, III, and aV_F, *inverted* P waves are usually followed by atrial T waves, or continuous atrial activity results from the circus movement. These waves have a sawtooth appearance.

Arteriosclerotic heart disease, hyperthyroidism, and rheumatic heart disease are common causes of atrial flutter. This is a macro–reentrant arrhythmia and can be ablated with radiofrequency energy applied in the right atrium (see Plate 2.24).

VENTRICULAR FIBRILLATION

Multiple periodic ventricular pacemakers result in erratic depolarization of the ventricles, producing an ECG that resembles distorted sine waves irregular in amplitude and duration. The waves may be of high or low voltage. With ventricular fibrillation there is no effective pumping of the heart. Severe organic cardiac disease or the toxic effects of digitalis or antiarrhythmics that prolong the QT interval can produce a similar condition. Other causes of ventricular arrhythmias include hypertrophic cardiomyopathy and channelopathies such as the long QT syndrome and Brugada syndrome (Plate 2.29). The treatment of choice is immediate electrical defibrillation (see Plate 2.28).

Plate 2.30

Physiology

EFFECT OF DIGITALIS AND CALCIUM/POTASSIUM LEVELS ON ELECTROCARDIOGRAM

DRUG EFFECTS: DIGITALIS

The effect of common drugs such as digitalis and other antiarrhythmic agents on the ECG depends on the dose, the rate of excretion, responsiveness of the patient, and previous ECG abnormalities. Small doses of digitalis produce a mild digitalis effect with sagging depression of the ST segment, negative J shifts, and lowering of the T waves (Plate 2.30, *A*). The QT interval may be shortened slightly because of increases in the rate of ventricular repolarization. Digitalis usually slows the cardiac rate and AV conduction because of vagal depression of the SA and AV nodes. With large doses a further depression of J occurs, with sagging of the ST segments and a distinct decrease in the QT intervals, which fall outside of normal limits (Plate 2.30, *B*). With *toxic* doses there is a depression of the AV conduction tissue with prolonged PR intervals, and a state of ventricular irritability with *ventricular ectopic beats*, which may be single or multiple and multifocal (Plate 2.30, *C*). *Coupling* is common, and atrial fibrillation or flutter, with paroxysmal atrial tachycardia, and block or variable degrees of *AV block* may occur.

Drugs such as procainamide and lidocaine tend to depress the electric activity of the atria and ventricles. Characteristically, the P waves increase in duration, with a slight increase in amplitude. Drugs such as ibutilide often cardiovert the AF to sinus rhythm, but the patient should receive intravenous magnesium sulfate before treatment to prevent torsades de pointes. Intravenous amiodarone also prolongs the QT interval and frequently will cardiovert the patient to sinus rhythm.

CALCIUM AND POTASSIUM LEVELS

Hypercalcemia may be encountered in patients with hyperparathyroidism. The ECG is characterized by shortening of the QT intervals, often with increased amplitudes of the T waves (Plate 2.30, *D*). The T waves begin immediately after the ending of the QRS complexes, so the QRS complexes and T waves appear compressed.

Hypocalcemia increases the duration of the ST and QT intervals (Plate 2.30, *F*). The QRS complexes and T waves merely appear to be widely separated from each other by long ST segments, which often are isoelectric.

Hyperkalemia depresses the atria, the AV node, and the ventricles but has less effect on the sinus node. Consequently, increases in potassium concentration produce prolonged PR intervals (Plate 2.30, *H*), high

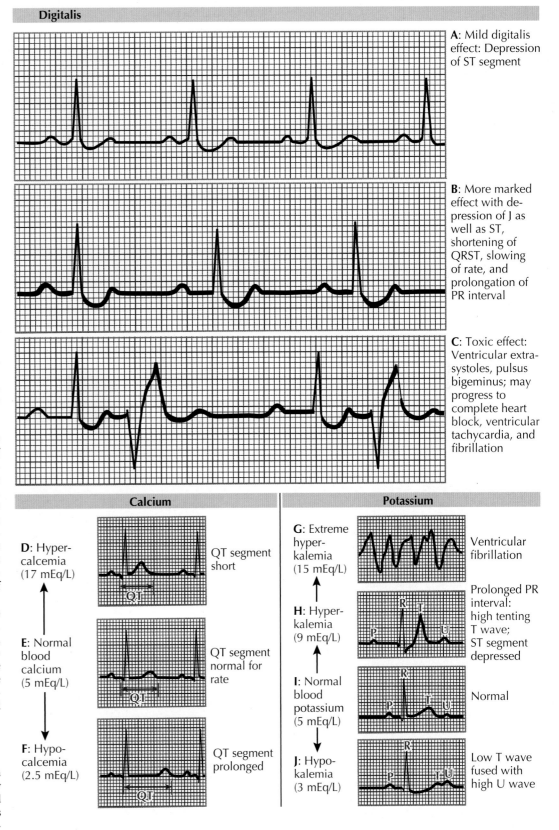

Digitalis

A: Mild digitalis effect: Depression of ST segment

B: More marked effect with depression of J as well as ST, shortening of QRST, slowing of rate, and prolongation of PR interval

C: Toxic effect: Ventricular extra-systoles, pulsus bigeminus; may progress to complete heart block, ventricular tachycardia, and fibrillation

Calcium

D: Hypercalcemia (17 mEq/L) — QT segment short

E: Normal blood calcium (5 mEq/L) — QT segment normal for rate

F: Hypocalcemia (2.5 mEq/L) — QT segment prolonged

Potassium

G: Extreme hyperkalemia (15 mEq/L) — Ventricular fibrillation

H: Hyperkalemia (9 mEq/L) — Prolonged PR interval: high tenting T wave; ST segment depressed

I: Normal blood potassium (5 mEq/L) — Normal

J: Hypokalemia (3 mEq/L) — Low T wave fused with high U wave

T waves, SA block with small or absent mechanical contractions of the atria, tenting of the T waves (tall and narrow at base), intraventricular block with widening of QRS complexes, abnormal shifts of the ST segment, and ventricular standstill or ventricular fibrillation (Plate 2.30, *G*).

Hypokalemia frequently results from administration of diuretics or cortisone or from vomiting, diarrhea, surgical suction, or low intake of potassium.

Hypokalemia causes an amplitude loss in the T waves (Plate 2.30, *J*) and a prominence of the U waves, with easily measured Q-U intervals. T and U waves are clearly separated in some leads but may *fuse* in others, causing a T-U complex. Deviations of the ST segment (depression or elevation) may occur. It is difficult to recognize hypokalemia associated with other abnormal states, such as myocardial ischemia or infarction, or with cardiac drugs.

Plate 2.31

Cardiovascular System: VOLUME 8

A. Dual-chamber pacing

The endocardial leads are usually introduced via the subclavian or the cephalic vein (left or right side), then positioned and tested.

A pocket for the pulse generator is commonly made below the mid-clavicle adjacent to the venous access for the pacing leads. The incision is parallel to the inferior clavicular border, approximately 1 inch below it.

The pulse generator is placed either into the deep subcutaneous tissue just above the prepectoralis fascia, or into the submuscular region of the pectoralis major muscle.

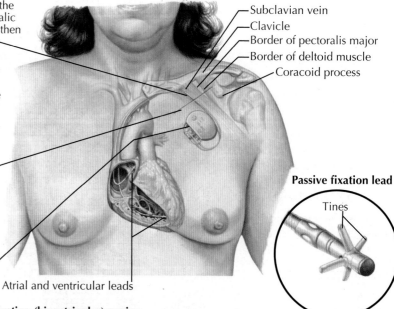

Subclavian vein
Clavicle
Border of pectoralis major
Border of deltoid muscle
Coracoid process

Atrial and ventricular leads

Passive fixation lead

Tines

B. Cardiac resynchronization (biventricular) pacing

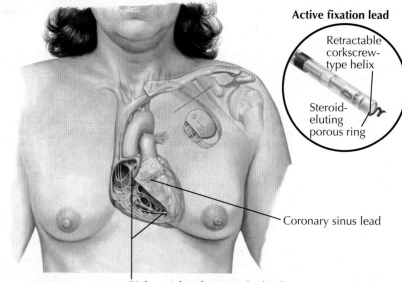

Active fixation lead

Retractable corkscrew-type helix

Steroid-eluting porous ring

Coronary sinus lead

Right atrial and ventricular leads

CARDIAC PACING

When patients have symptomatic bradycardia (e.g., syncope, dizziness, lethargy), a cardiac pacemaker can effectively decrease or eliminate symptoms because it treats the pathophysiologic problem: slow heart rate, which can result from sinus node dysfunction or AV block. Some devices pace only the atrium, some only the right ventricle, and some pace both the atrium and the ventricle sequentially. Some pacemakers also are combined with an implantable cardioverter-defibrillator (ICD), and others can improve cardiac synchronization (e.g., biventricular [BiV] pacemakers).

CURRENT TRANSVENOUS PACEMAKERS

A modern pacemaker generator (usually a lithium battery) is placed subcutaneously under the clavicle. This generator is sealed to avoid imbibing body fluids and can deliver electrical impulses to the electrode leads within the RA appendage and right ventricle and to the left ventricle by way of a coronary sinus electrode lead (BiV pacing). The pacemaker generator is immunologically inert.

Permanent Pacing

The pacemaker implant procedure is performed under fluoroscopy, usually by a trained cardiologist or cardiac surgeon. Most often, percutaneous access to the left subclavian vein is used to pass the electrode leads into the heart, but the right subclavian vein can be used when the left is not available. Fluoroscopy confirms the positioning of the pacing leads in the RA or right ventricular chambers and of the left ventricular epicardial lead when BiV pacing is used.

The leads connecting the pulse generator to the endocardium can be different types: unipolar or bipolar and of active fixation or passive fixation. The unipolar system has a single electrode (cathode, negative pole) in contact with the endocardium, and the anode is the pulse generator itself. The bipolar system lead has both a cathode and an anode at the tip of the same lead. Passive fixation leads have tines, or barbs, that anchor the lead to the endocardial trabecular muscle of the chamber in which it is implanted. Active fixation leads have a corkscrew-type device or helix that is placed into the myocardium. Both types irritate the myocardium, causing an inflammatory reaction and cellular growth around the lead. To minimize the inflammatory reaction, most leads have steroid-eluting tips. The coronary sinus lead allows for "resynchronization" of disorganized ventricular contraction in selected patients with impaired cardiac function and conduction block.

Pacemaker Types

Pacemakers can be of three types and are used to pace a single chamber or multiple chambers of the heart. A *single-chamber pacemaker* involves the placement of a single lead into an atrium or ventricle, which then can sense and pace either the atrium or the ventricle. The most common reason for pacing only the atrium is dysfunction of the sinus node, such as sick sinus syndrome. The most frequent reason for pacing only the right ventricle is atrial fibrillation.

In contrast, a *dual-chamber pacemaker* consists of two leads inserted into the heart (Plate 2.31). One lead can be inserted into the RA appendage and fixated in that position, pacing the atrium. Another pacing lead can be inserted into the right ventricle and fixated in that position. When activated and functioning, these two pacing leads pace the atrium and ventricle sequentially, closely simulating the natural conduction system of the heart. This type of pacing is the most common type currently used.

Plate 2.32

Physiology

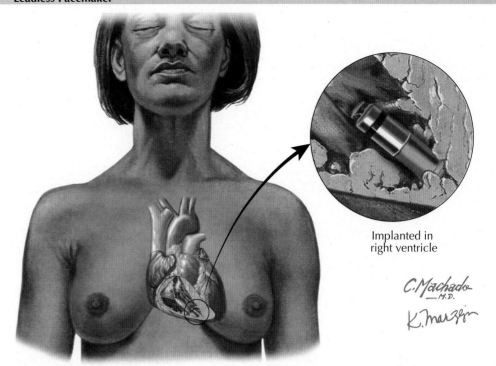

Leadless Pacemaker

Implanted in right ventricle

C. Machado M.D.

K. Marzejon

Subcutaneous Implantable Cardioverter Defibrillator (S-ICD)

Electrode in heart

Intermuscular implantation of S-ICD showing concealment of the device

Implanted device (generator)

CARDIAC PACING (Continued)

A *rate-responsive pacemaker* is usually a dual-chamber pacemaker (can be single chamber) that responds to increased demand for an increased heart rate. The patient's increased physical activity (exercise) activates a sensor contained in the pacemaker, most commonly an accelerometer or a sensor that responds to minute ventilation. Once the sensor is activated, the pacemaker increases the rate of electrical impulses and increases heart rate to meet the patient's physiologic demands for increased cardiac output. Rate-responsive pacemakers are often used for patients with symptomatic bradycardia.

Biventricular Pacing

In contrast to standard two-lead AV sequential pacing, BiV pacing consists of three leads: RA appendage lead, RV lead, and a lead introduced into the coronary sinus and advanced to a lateral vein on the epicardial surface of the LV free wall. The position of the epicardial lead corresponds to the position of an obtuse marginal artery. This lead system, in addition to AV pacing, enables pacing of the LV free wall (see Plate 2.31).

Cardiac resynchronization therapy (CRT) uses BiV pacing because the lead system paces both the septal LV wall and the lateral LV wall. When viable tissue is present in these areas, the left ventricle resynchronizes the contraction of a heart whose opposing walls do not contract in synchrony. *Dyssynchrony* frequently occurs in patients with systolic heart failure, many with QRS duration longer than 120 milliseconds, which qualifies a patient for CRT. These patients are at high risk for sudden cardiac death because many have an LV ejection fraction of 35% or less. The BiV lead system can be combined with an ICD to prevent sudden cardiac death

from ventricular tachycardia or ventricular fibrillation, a common companion to severe heart failure.

Leadless Technology

Leadless pacing offers an innovative approach for cardiac pacing and defibrillation. Although not appropriate for all patients, leadless pacing and defibrillation offers the advantage of no transvenous access. This is particularly useful in patients with complex anatomy and no option of endovascular lead implantation (Plate 2.32).

SUBCUTANEOUS IMPLANTABLE CARDIOVERTER DEFIBRILLATORS

Subcutaneous ICD systems are an established therapy for prevention of sudden cardiac death and an alternative to a transvenous ICD system in selected patients. These systems offer the advantage of no transvenous access. One major limitation is that they provide no pacing option, thus not allowing programming of painless antitachycardia pacing for ventricular arrhythmias (Plate 2.32).

IMAGING

Plate 3.1

Cardiovascular System: VOLUME 8

RADIOLOGY AND CATHETER-BASED ANGIOCARDIOGRAPHY

RADIOLOGY

Radiologic examination is an essential part of the evaluation of cardiac disease. The size of the heart and identification of chamber enlargement and pericardial, cardiac, and coronary calcification, as well as information on heart function and hemodynamics, can be determined from chest radiography, fluoroscopic examination, and angiocardiographic observations.

The myocardium, valves, and other heart structures have similar radiodensity and therefore cannot be distinguished radiologically unless calcified. Similarly, the walls of the cardiac chambers cannot be visually separated from the blood within unless the opacity of the blood is increased by the injection of a contrast material. The outer borders of the heart can be seen because the relatively homogeneous cardiac silhouette is contrasted against the lucent, air-containing lungs.

The shadow of the heart seen on standard radiographs or by fluoroscopy is magnified and somewhat distorted. At the target-to-film or screen distances customarily used, the x-ray beam diverges as it passes through the patient. The structures farther from the film are more magnified than those closer. The distortion can be largely eliminated if the x-ray beam is composed of parallel rather than divergent rays. For most purposes, heart size can be adequately estimated from the standard 6-ft chest film by comparing the apparent cardiac size with that of the thorax. Allowances must be made for the degree of inspiration—the higher the diaphragm, the larger the apparent size of the heart—and the age of the patient. An infant's heart is relatively large compared with the chest, whereas an older patient's chest is often small in relation to the heart.

Because the heart is a three-dimensional (3D) structure and only two borders are seen in any one view, radiographs need to be secured in several projections to bring the various chambers and great vessels into profile. Plain films of the chest also allow an evaluation of the pulmonary vasculature and the lung changes that may be associated with heart disease. Increased size and tortuosity of the pulmonary arteries and veins usually indicate a left-to-right shunt, whereas decreased prominence of these vessels is associated with a right-to-left shunt. When the pulmonary artery flow is greatly decreased, as in severe tetralogy of Fallot, the vascular pattern in the lungs often is reticular and nondirectional rather than an orderly radiation of vessels from the lung hilum. This indicates the presence of a significant collateral flow through the bronchial arteries.

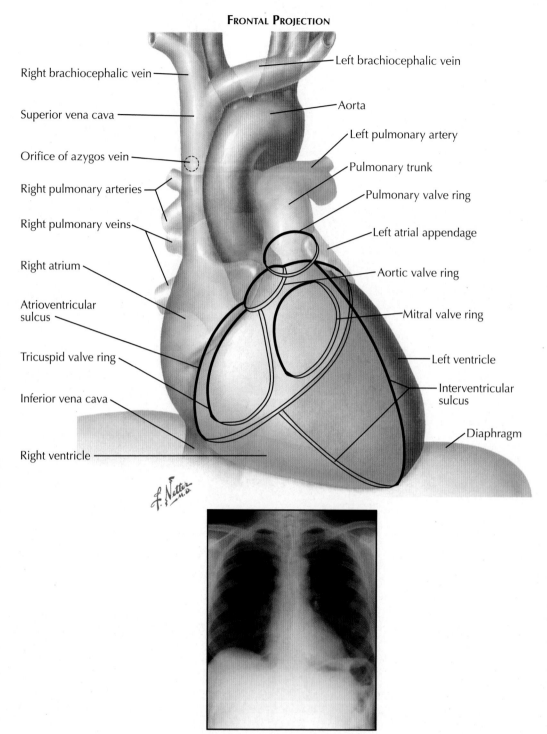

FRONTAL PROJECTION

Right brachiocephalic vein — Left brachiocephalic vein

Superior vena cava — Aorta

Orifice of azygos vein — Left pulmonary artery

Right pulmonary arteries — Pulmonary trunk

Right pulmonary veins — Pulmonary valve ring

Right atrium — Left atrial appendage

Atrioventricular sulcus — Aortic valve ring

Tricuspid valve ring — Mitral valve ring

Inferior vena cava — Left ventricle

Right ventricle — Interventricular sulcus

Diaphragm

F. Netter M.D.

In congestive failure or obstruction on the left side of the heart, as in mitral stenosis, the pulmonary veins become engorged. If this progresses to pulmonary hypertension, the veins, together with the peripheral pulmonary arteries, become quite small while the central pulmonary arteries dilate and become bulbous.

Frontal Projection

Most chest films are made in the frontal projection, so this is the view of the heart usually seen, often providing the first suggestion of cardiac disease. Frontal is the most easily reproducible projection, and thus heart size generally is evaluated in this view (Plate 3.1). Enlargement of the left atrium and left ventricle, as well as the

right atrium, generally can be recognized in the frontal projection. The right ventricle, although it forms no borders, can produce characteristic changes in the cardiac contour.

The upper half of the right contour of the cardiac silhouette is formed by the superior vena cava (SVC) and the lower half by the lateral wall of the right atrium. The margin of the SVC is straight, but that of the right atrium bulges outward. The angle between these two contours represents the superior aspect of the right atrium. If the patient takes a deep inspiration, an indentation on the right border of the heart can be seen just above the diaphragm, identifying the junction of the inferior vena cava (IVC) and right atrium.

Plate 3.2

Imaging

RADIOLOGY AND CATHETER-BASED ANGIOCARDIOGRAPHY (Continued)

On the left side, the uppermost part of the cardiovascular silhouette is formed by the distal arch of the aorta as it curves posteriorly and inferiorly to become the *descending thoracic aorta*. This is seen as a localized bulge extending from the left side of the mediastinum above the right tracheobronchial angle. This bulge usually produces a localized indentation on the left side of the esophagus. In the presence of a right aortic arch, the bulge will be on the right side and will displace the esophagus to the left. Immediately below the aortic bulge, the main pulmonary trunk and left main pulmonary artery are border forming. A small segment of the left cardiac silhouette below the pulmonary artery is formed by the *left atrial appendage*. This segment normally is flat or slightly convex and is continuous with the curve of the left ventricle, which forms the largest part of the left border of the cardiac contour. The point of transition between the normal left atrial appendage and the left ventricle usually cannot be identified on radiographs.

The *apex* of the heart is formed by the left ventricle. In the frontal projection, the right ventricle is completely hidden within the cardiac silhouette. Occasionally on deep inspiration, a part of the diaphragmatic surface of the heart near the cardiac apex is disclosed. An indentation in this region marks the *interventricular sulcus* between the two ventricles.

Enlargement of the right atrium causes outward bowing and increased curvature of the border of the right side of the heart. When the right ventricle increases in size, the heart enlarges to the left, the apex is usually lifted, and the groove of the interventricular sulcus appears higher on the apex of the heart than normal. As it enlarges, the right ventricle elongates as well as widens, resulting in elevation of the main pulmonary artery. As the left ventricle enlarges, the cardiac apex is displaced downward and to the left. Often the entire left cardiac border is displaced to the left, becoming increasingly convex.

Left atrial enlargement is detected in the frontal view primarily by dilation of the left atrial appendage, which produces a localized bulge of the left contour below the pulmonary artery segment. In addition, the enlarged left atrium often increases the density of the central part of the cardiac silhouette and, when sufficiently large, may elevate the left main bronchus. With increasing dilation, the right border of the left atrium may be seen within the cardiac silhouette to the right of the spine, producing a second curved contour medial to the right atrial margin. With further enlargement, the left atrium may project behind and beyond the right atrium so that

the left atrium will form the right border of the cardiac shadow. The border of the right atrium will then be seen within the shadow of the left atrium.

Calcification of the cardiac valves is most often caused by rheumatic valvulitis, calcific aortic stenosis, or bacterial endocarditis and involves the mitral and aortic valves. In the frontal projection the *mitral valve* lies to the left of the spine, and as the heart beats, calcifications on this valve will describe a flat, elliptical trajectory extending downward and to the left. The *aortic valve* is usually projected over the left side of the spine and moves in a relatively straight line upward and slightly to the right. Because of the overlapping shadows of the vertebral bodies, small calcific deposits on the aortic valve may be difficult to detect in the frontal view but

are readily seen in the lateral projection. The *pulmonic (pulmonary) valve* is projected to the left of the spine, higher than the aortic and mitral valves, and moves vertically with the cardiac pulsation. The *tricuspid valve* lies over the spine and moves in a horizontal plane.

Right Anterior Oblique Projection

The right anterior oblique (RAO) view is used mainly to evaluate left atrial enlargement and abnormalities of the right ventricular outflow (outlet) tract (Plate 3.2). RAO is also the best projection in which to study calcification of the mitral valve. During selective left ventricular angiocardiography, the RAO view is used to evaluate mitral stenosis or insufficiency because the mitral valve is seen tangentially, and the left atrium is projected

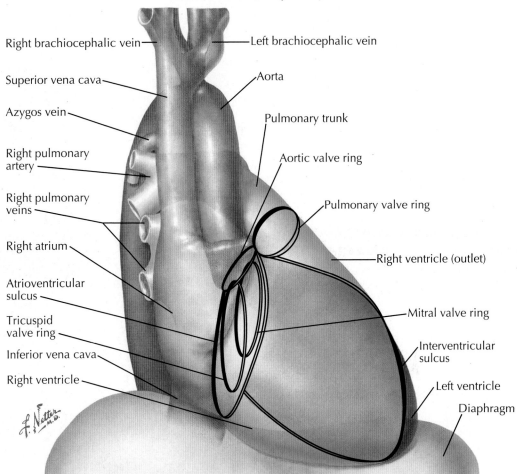

RIGHT ANTERIOR OBLIQUE PROJECTION

Right brachiocephalic vein — Left brachiocephalic vein
Superior vena cava — Aorta
Azygos vein — Pulmonary trunk
Right pulmonary artery — Aortic valve ring
Right pulmonary veins — Pulmonary valve ring
Right atrium — Right ventricle (outlet)
Atrioventricular sulcus — Mitral valve ring
Tricuspid valve ring — Interventricular sulcus
Inferior vena cava — Left ventricle
Right ventricle — Diaphragm

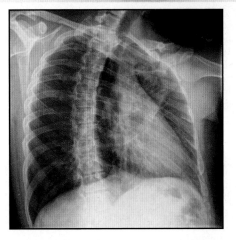

Plate 3.3

Cardiovascular System: VOLUME 8

LEFT ANTERIOR OBLIQUE PROJECTION

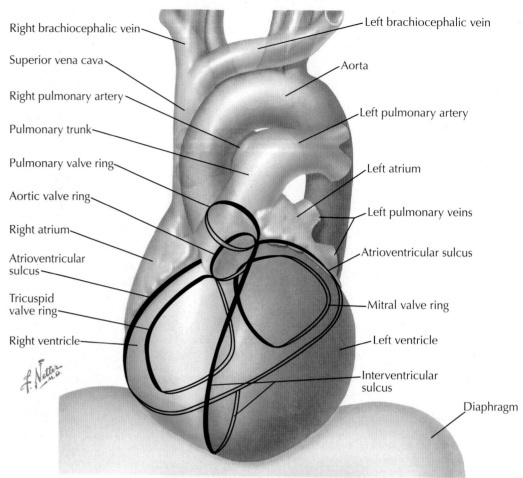

Right brachiocephalic vein
Superior vena cava
Right pulmonary artery
Pulmonary trunk
Pulmonary valve ring
Aortic valve ring
Right atrium
Atrioventricular sulcus
Tricuspid valve ring
Right ventricle

Left brachiocephalic vein
Aorta
Left pulmonary artery
Left atrium
Left pulmonary veins
Atrioventricular sulcus
Mitral valve ring
Left ventricle
Interventricular sulcus
Diaphragm

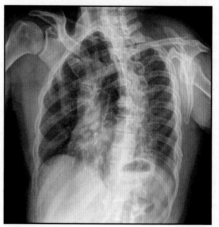

RADIOLOGY AND CATHETER-BASED ANGIOCARDIOGRAPHY (Continued)

entirely behind the left ventricle. RAO is the only view in which these two chambers do not overlap.

In a properly positioned RAO view, the shadow of the spine lies to the left of the cardiac silhouette, and a thin vertical band of air-containing lung separates the two structures. The aortic arch is foreshortened in this view, and the descending aorta partially overlaps the vertebral column.

The right border of the heart is formed by the right posterior aspect of the left atrium above and the posterior border of the right atrium below. As the obliquity of the projection is increased, more of the left atrium comes into profile.

The uppermost part of the left border of the cardiovascular silhouette is almost vertical and represents the *ascending aorta*. Just below this segment, the cardiac contour slopes downward and to the left in a gentle curve and is formed by the outflow tract (outlet) of the right ventricle and pulmonary trunk. The inferior continuation of this curve is formed by the anterior wall of the left ventricle. As in the frontal view, the body of the right ventricle is in contact with the diaphragm and cannot be visualized.

The mitral valve is seen almost tangentially and is projected over the midpart of the cardiac silhouette. Because confusing overlapping shadows are absent and the direction of mitral valve motion is perpendicular to the x-ray beam, calcification of the mitral valve is best detected fluoroscopically in RAO projection. The elliptical orbit of the valve is mainly directed horizontally. The aortic valve is thrown clear of the spine, and although in contact with the upper border of the mitral valve, calcification of the aortic valve can be recognized as it moves mostly in an up-and-down direction. This projection also provides the greatest separation of the aortic and pulmonic valves. The pulmonary valve lies at a level higher than the aortic valve and to its left, touching the left border of the cardiac silhouette. The line of motion of the pulmonic valve is directed upward and to the right. The tricuspid valve is seen almost tangentially and slightly behind the mitral valve. The tricuspid valve moves horizontally with the cardiac pulsation, and in the rare case of tricuspid calcification, the valve is easily mistaken for a calcified mitral valve.

Left Anterior Oblique Projection

Although no longer used for plain chest radiographs, the left anterior oblique (LAO) view is useful in evaluating the size of the left atrium and left ventricle during

angiography (Plate 3.3). The *aortic arch* is seen clearly because it is oriented approximately parallel to the film and is projected with minimal foreshortening. A selective left ventricular angiocardiogram in the left oblique projection is useful in the detection of a ventricular septal defect because most of the muscular interventricular septum and a part of the membranous septum are seen tangentially.

The right border of the cardiac contour is formed by the right atrium above and the right ventricle below. As the degree of obliquity is increased, more of the right ventricle becomes border forming. Enlargement of the right atrium increases the convexity of the upper right cardiac border, whereas enlargement of the right ventricle

usually results in a more generalized increase in curvature of the upper right border.

The left cardiac contour is formed mostly by the left ventricle, except for the upper quarter, which is contributed by the left posterior aspect of the left atrium, directly beneath the left main bronchus. In a proper 45-degree oblique view, the shadow of a normal left ventricle will not usually extend to the left of the shadow of the spine; extension of this shadow indicates an enlarged left ventricle. However, this sign must be evaluated cautiously because with lesser degrees of obliquity, or if the film is not made in full inspiration, a normal left ventricle may not clear the spine. If the stomach is distended with air,

Plate 3.4   Imaging

LATERAL PROJECTION

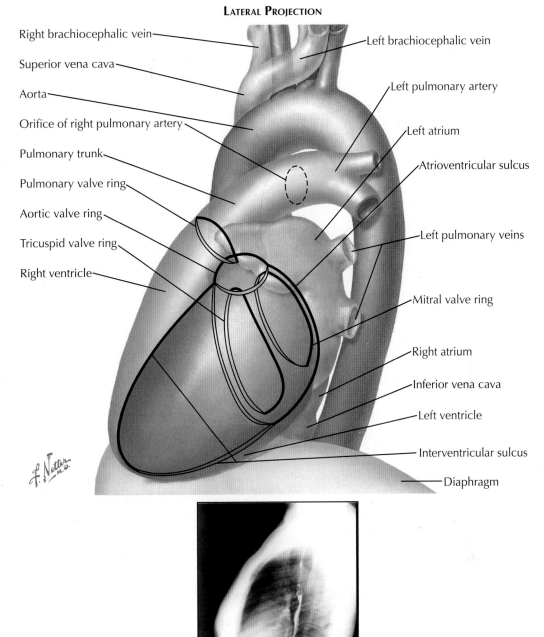

Right brachiocephalic vein
Superior vena cava
Aorta
Orifice of right pulmonary artery
Pulmonary trunk
Pulmonary valve ring
Aortic valve ring
Tricuspid valve ring
Right ventricle

Left brachiocephalic vein
Left pulmonary artery
Left atrium
Atrioventricular sulcus
Left pulmonary veins
Mitral valve ring
Right atrium
Inferior vena cava
Left ventricle
Interventricular sulcus
Diaphragm

RADIOLOGY AND CATHETER-BASED ANGIOCARDIOGRAPHY (Continued)

the diaphragmatic surface of the left ventricle can also be evaluated.

The left atrial part of the cardiac contour is usually straight or minimally convex. An outward bulging in this region denotes left atrial enlargement, probably its most sensitive radiographic sign. The esophagus is projected directly over the left atrial segment; therefore barium must not be given until after the LAO film has been made because significant degrees of left atrial enlargement could be obscured. With greater degrees of enlargement, the dilated left atrium will push the left main bronchus upward and horizontally. The dilated atrium will also encroach on the clear space below the aortic arch.

The greatest length of the aortic arch is seen in the LAO view, and the origins of the great vessels are maximally separated. Thus LAO is the best projection for identifying aneurysms of the aortic arch and for opacification studies of the aorta and great vessels.

The mitral valve is seen almost directly en face. As a result, calcific deposits on the cusps may be difficult to see because these move on an axis perpendicular to the fluoroscopic screen, with minimal horizontal excursion. In addition, the mitral valve may be hidden partially by the shadow of the spine. Calcification of the tricuspid valve can be differentiated from that of the mitral valve by the complete separation of the two valves in the LAO projection, with the tricuspid valve lying in the right half of the cardiac silhouette. The LAO view is well suited for identifying calcification of the aortic valve, which lies in the upper part of the cardiac silhouette, clear of the spine, and moves along an axis directed upward and to the right. The pulmonic valve is situated slightly higher than the aortic valve and moves upward and toward the left.

Lateral Projection

In plain radiographs the lateral view is used primarily for evaluating the presence of right ventricular (RV) enlargement, left atrial enlargement, and combined enlargement of the left atrium and left ventricle. Lateral is also the best view for distinguishing between calcification of the aortic and mitral valves. A selective RV angiocardiogram in the lateral projection provides the best visualization of the outflow part of the right ventricle and the pulmonic valve (Plate 3.4).

In the lateral view, the heart is projected clear of the confusing shadows of the sternum and spine. The anterior margin of the cardiac silhouette is formed by the apex and the RV outflow tract. Normally, this abuts on the lower quarter or third of the anterior chest wall. The upper two-thirds of the anterior cardiac contour is formed by two convex arcs, slanting upward and posteriorly. The lower, more oblique arc is formed by the RV outflow tract, and the upper arc is formed by the ascending aorta. The radiolucent lung is interposed between these two arcs and the sternum. As it enlarges, the right ventricle bulges forward and progressively obliterates the retrosternal space. Similarly, dilation and tortuosity, or an aneurysm of the ascending aorta, will encroach on the upper retrosternal space. The upper margin of the aortic arch distal to the origin of the great vessels can usually be identified in the lateral view.

The posterior border of the heart is formed mostly by the posterior wall of the left atrium. Just above the diaphragm, small parts of the right atrium and IVC come into profile. When enlarged, however, the left ventricle may extend farther posteriorly than the right atrium, forming the lower part of the posterior heart border as well. The esophagus lies immediately behind the left atrium and left ventricle, and an enlargement of these chambers will indent the anterior wall of the esophagus and displace it posteriorly. If only the left atrium is enlarged, the indentation on the esophagus is localized at the level of the upper half of the cardiac silhouette; the lower part of the esophagus is in its normal position. When the left ventricle is enlarged as well, it also

Plate 3.5

Cardiovascular System: VOLUME 8

ANTEROPOSTERIOR PROJECTION OF RIGHT-SIDED HEART STRUCTURES

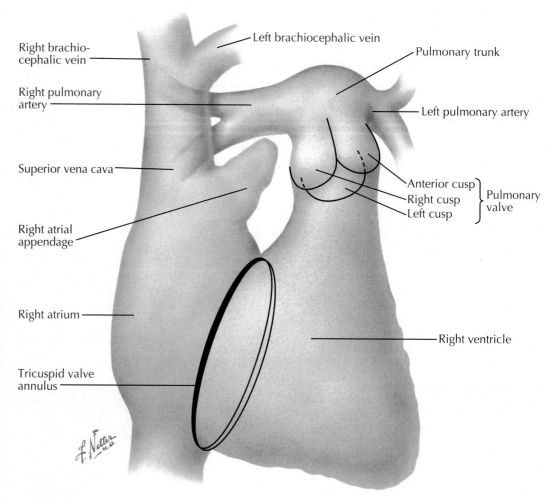

Right brachio-
cephalic vein

Right pulmonary
artery

Superior vena cava

Right atrial
appendage

Right atrium

Tricuspid valve
annulus

Left brachiocephalic vein

Pulmonary trunk

Left pulmonary artery

Anterior cusp
Right cusp — Pulmonary valve
Left cusp

Right ventricle

RADIOLOGY AND CATHETER-BASED ANGIOCARDIOGRAPHY (Continued)

pushes the esophagus posteriorly, and the backward curve of the displaced esophagus is then continuous over the entire length of the cardiac silhouette to the diaphragm.

Identifying localization of a calcific deposit in the mitral or aortic valve may be difficult. This problem can be resolved in the lateral view. If a line is drawn from the anterior costophrenic sulcus to the point of bifurcation of the trachea, the aortic valve will lie above and in front of this line, whereas the mitral valve will be below and posterior. The mitral valve moves more or less horizontally in the lateral view, and the aortic valve moves on a vertical axis that is tilted slightly anteriorly and upward. The pulmonic valve is located above the aortic valve and more anteriorly, extending to the anterior border of the cardiac shadow.

ANGIOCARDIOGRAPHY

Chest radiography and fluoroscopy demonstrate only the outer borders of the heart and great vessels. Considerably more information is obtained when the blood is opacified by introducing a radiopaque contrast medium into the vascular system to visualize the inner borders of the cardiac chambers and vessels during catheter-based angiography. The structure and motion of the cardiac valves can be studied, as well as cardiac and pulmonary hemodynamics.

The basic requirements for successful catheter-based angiocardiography are (1) rapid injection of the radiopaque contrast material so that it flows as a bolus and (2) cineangiography of the heart to follow the course of the contrast material. The iodinated contrast medium can be injected into a peripheral vein, where it is carried to the heart through the SVC or IVC, or it can be injected through a catheter directly into a specific cardiac chamber, great vessel, or coronary artery. The latter technique, *selective angiocardiography*, provides greater anatomic detail because the contrast material reaches the chamber as a denser, more compact bolus and is not diluted in the right atrium by nonopaque blood.

A catheter can be placed in the right atrium, right ventricle, or pulmonary trunk by introducing the catheter into a peripheral vein and then advancing it through the SVC or IVC. In children the left atrium can usually be entered by manipulating a catheter in the right atrium, across the foramen ovale. In adults a similar route is used; the atrial septum is punctured by

a transseptal needle and a catheter advanced over the needle into the left atrium. The left ventricle is reached by inserting a catheter into a peripheral artery and passing it retrograde through the aortic valve into the ventricle. If the catheter has the proper curve, it can be manipulated backward through the mitral valve into the left atrium. The left ventricle can also be reached by a transseptal catheter passed from the right atrium into the left atrium and advanced through the mitral valve. The left ventricle can be punctured directly through the anterior chest wall, however, and angiocardiography by this route carries substantial risk and is no longer used.

Frontal Projection of Right Side of Heart

The right side of the heart usually can be well visualized by venous angiocardiography as well as selective injection (Plate 3.5). In the frontal, or anteroposterior (AP), projection, the SVC and IVC lie in a straight line to the right of the spine, entering opposite ends of the right atrium. The free wall of the right atrium is thin and is represented by the space between the right border of the contrast-filled atrium and the right border of the cardiac silhouette. Normally, this space is 2 to 3 mm in diameter; increased width of this space indicates a pericardial effusion separating the wall of the right atrium from the pericardium.

The right atrial appendage extends medially and upward from the upper part of the right atrium. The

tricuspid valve lies in an oblique plane relative to the AP projection, and the line of attachment of its cusps is often seen as an ellipse overlying the spine. The inferior margin of the *tricuspid annulus* lies adjacent to the entrance of the IVC into the right atrium. The opening of the coronary sinus lies in the same region. Clinicians must keep this in mind when catheterizing the right ventricle because a catheter that has entered the coronary sinus and has advanced into the great cardiac vein will follow almost the identical course in the frontal projection as a catheter that has crossed the tricuspid valve and lies within the RV outflow tract. The left border of the tricuspid valve ring forms the left border of the atrium and corresponds to the posterior margin of the tricuspid valve. The right ventricle is in front of the atrium and extends to the right (or anterior) border of the tricuspid valve. Therefore, within the elliptical projection of the tricuspid valve, the atrium and ventricle overlie each other.

The right ventricle is a triangular-shaped chamber that can be divided into two parts: a large, trabeculated inflow part and a smooth, narrow outflow tract. In the frontal view these two parts can be separated by a line drawn from the uppermost margin of the tricuspid valve downward and to the left, toward the apex of the ventricle. This line approximates the course of the septal and moderator bands. The RV inflow tract lies below

Plate 3.6

Imaging

LATERAL PROJECTION OF RIGHT-SIDED HEART STRUCTURES

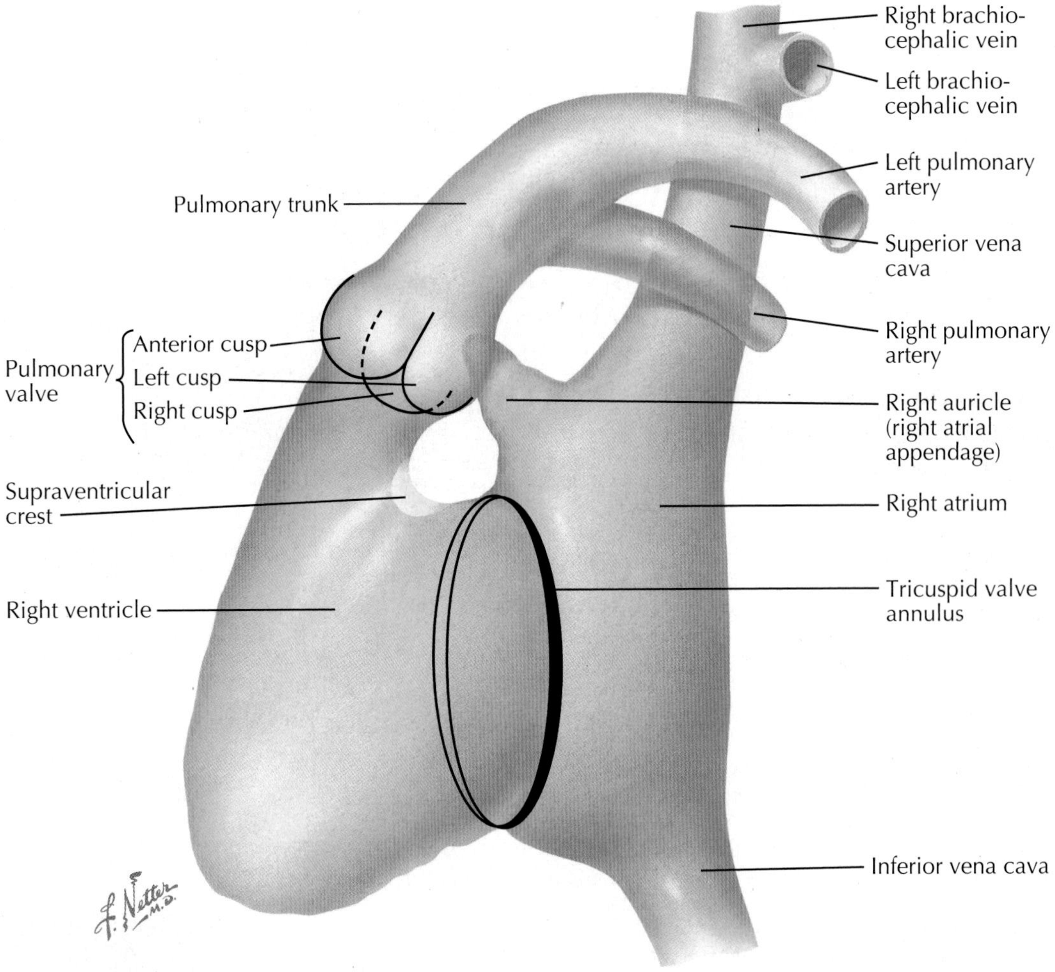

Labels on illustration:
- Right brachio-cephalic vein
- Left brachio-cephalic vein
- Left pulmonary artery
- Superior vena cava
- Right pulmonary artery
- Right auricle (right atrial appendage)
- Right atrium
- Tricuspid valve annulus
- Inferior vena cava
- Pulmonary trunk
- Pulmonary valve { Anterior cusp / Left cusp / Right cusp }
- Supraventricular crest
- Right ventricle

RADIOLOGY AND CATHETER-BASED ANGIOCARDIOGRAPHY (Continued)

the line, and the RV outflow tract lies above the line, extending to the pulmonic valve. The right border of the inflow part is formed by the tricuspid valve and the left border by the interventricular septum. The diaphragmatic RV surface is a free wall. The right border of the RV outflow tract is also a free wall, formed by a sheet of muscle extending from tricuspid to pulmonic valve and lying in front of the aortic root. A localized prominence in this sheet of muscle, the crista supraventricularis, is projected en face in this view and cannot be identified. The line of attachment of the tricuspid valve can often be seen during diastole on a selective RV angiocardiogram because contrast material is trapped between the open valve cusps and the walls of the ventricle and the orifice of the valve is filled by nonopaque blood entering from the atrium.

The pulmonic valve is projected partially en face and is not well visualized in the frontal view. The pulmonary trunk is usually seen well, but its root may be obscured in part by the RV outflow tract. The right pulmonary artery courses almost directly to the right, and its greatest length can be seen in the AP projection, whereas the left pulmonary artery is directed posteriorly and is foreshortened. A steep LAO or left lateral view is best for the study of the left pulmonary artery. On a venous angiocardiogram, a part of the right pulmonary artery is often obscured by contrast material in the SVC or right atrium, especially if this chamber is enlarged.

Lateral Projection of Right Side of Heart

In the lateral view the right atrium is projected almost entirely behind the right ventricle (Plate 3.6). The posterior border of the atrium is a free wall. The interatrial septum lies in an oblique plane and cannot be visualized in either the frontal or the lateral projection. The septum is seen tangentially only in a steep right posterior oblique view. The anterior margin of the right atrium is formed by the tricuspid valve. The atrial appendage arises at a level higher than the valve and extends anteriorly and superiorly. The appendage is triangular shaped, its base continuous with the atrial cavity. The border of the atrial appendage cavity is irregular because of the pectinate muscles.

The ostium of the coronary sinus lies in the inferior part of the atrium just in front of the entrance of the IVC, and the great cardiac vein extends along the posterior aspect of the heart. Therefore a catheter passed through the SVC that has entered the great cardiac vein will curve posteriorly in the lateral view rather than anteriorly, as occurs when the catheter traverses the tricuspid valve to enter the right ventricle.

The right ventricle is best studied by selective angiocardiography because in the lateral view the opacified right atrial appendage, especially if large, often extends far enough anteriorly to obscure part of the RV outflow tract or the pulmonic valve. On a selective study the tricuspid valve can usually be identified as an oblique ring on the posterior aspect of the ventricle. The anterior border of this ring corresponds to the right margin of the tricuspid valve. The main body of the right ventricle, the inflow part, lies directly in front of the tricuspid valve. Just above the upper level of the tricuspid valve, the ventricle becomes narrowed because of the intrusion of a soft tissue mass on the posterior aspect. This represents the crista supraventricularis and marks the level of the entrance to the infundibulum, the RV outflow tract. The anterior border of the RV cavity forms a continuous curve to the pulmonary valve.

The pulmonic valve and its cusps are easily identified in the lateral view, which is an ideal projection for the study of pulmonic valvular stenosis. The lateral view not only can show the limitation in the opening of the valve cusps but also allows study of the infundibular region and evaluation of associated infundibular stenosis. The pulmonary trunk courses upward and backward, continuing the curve of the anterior RV wall. The left pulmonary artery is well seen in the lateral view because it courses posteriorly, whereas the right pulmonary artery is foreshortened.

Frontal Projection of Left Side of Heart

The left atrium lies partly above and to the right of the left ventricle (see Plate 3.7). The upper border of the atrial cavity in the frontal (AP) view is straight, slanting upward and to the left. The lower margin is bowed downward. The part of the lower atrial margin that crosses the left ventricular (LV) chamber is formed by the inferior margin of the mitral valve. The two superior pulmonary veins enter the uppermost part of the atrium, and the inferior pulmonary veins enter at a slightly lower level. The left atrial appendage often has a hook-like contour in the AP view, extends to the left border of the heart, and overlies the left superior pulmonary vein. It may be difficult to distinguish fluoroscopically whether a catheter in the left atrium has entered the atrial appendage or the left superior pulmonary vein. This can be resolved by viewing the patient in an oblique or lateral projection, because the pulmonary vein extends posteriorly while the appendage lies anteriorly, or by injecting a small quantity of contrast material and outlining the structure.

The left ventricle differs basically from the right ventricle in that the inflow (mitral) valve and the outflow (aortic) valve lie adjacent to each other. Indeed, the

Plate 3.7

Cardiovascular System: VOLUME 8

RADIOLOGY AND CATHETER-BASED ANGIOCARDIOGRAPHY (Continued)

anterior cusp of the mitral valve arises from a common annulus with part of the aortic valve. The LV body lies below the two valves, rather than interposed as in the right ventricle. The left ventricle is oval shaped, with its apex pointing downward and to the left. The trabeculation of the LV body is finer than the RV trabeculation. On a selective LV injection, the inferior part of the mitral valve ring can usually be identified as a curvilinear interface between the contrast material trapped under the posterior mitral cusp and the nonopaque blood entering from the left atrium above. The superior margin of the mitral ring is continuous with the aortic ring and usually is not well seen in the frontal view. During ventricular systole, the mitral cusps bulge toward the left atrium, the valve orifice is obscured by the contrast material in the ventricle, and the line of attachment of the cusps can no longer be observed. Finger-like indentations arising from the left and right margins of the ventricle are often seen during systole intruding into the ventricular lumen, representing the papillary muscles.

The location of the membranous part of the interventricular septum can be determined in relation to the aortic valve by ventriculography. It lies beneath the anterior part of the posterior (noncoronary) cusp and a small part of the adjacent *right (coronary) cusp* and the commissure between the two. In the AP projection the right cusp is seen en face, the left cusp forms the left border of the aortic valve, and the noncoronary cusp forms the right border. The membranous septum thus forms a segment of the right LV border immediately beneath the aortic valve.

The right coronary artery arises from the midpart of the aortic valve in the AP view and extends slightly to the right and downward, running in the sulcus between the right atrium and ventricle. The left coronary artery originates from the left border of the aortic valve. The anterior descending branch courses downward in the interventricular sulcus overlying the left part of the left ventricle. The circumflex branch curves to the right, paralleling the inferior attachment of the mitral valve as it runs in the sulcus between the left atrium and ventricle on the posterior aspect of the heart.

The relationships of the structures on the right and left sides of the heart can be appreciated when the drawings of the two ventricles and their great vessels are superimposed. The ventricles, for the most part, are projected on top of one another. The RV outflow tract is directed upward and toward the left, whereas blood in

the left ventricle reaches the aorta by passing upward and to the right. Thus the outflow tracts cross each other, the left passing behind the right. Almost the entire right border of the left ventricle is formed by the interventricular septum, with the uppermost part membranous and the remainder muscular. In addition, a segment of the upper left LV border also represents the interventricular septum. This is the basal part of the muscular septum, which lies in the lower part of the infundibulum just above the septal band on the right side. The uppermost margin of the tricuspid valve attachment reaches almost to the aortic valve, and the origin of the septal cusp of the tricuspid valve actually crosses the membranous septum. Thus the membranous

septum on the left side lies completely within the left ventricle, whereas on the right side the anterior part lies in the right ventricle (interventricular septum), and the posterior part lies behind the tricuspid valve in the right atrium (atrioventricular septum).

The upper outflow tract of the right ventricle lies above the left ventricle at the level of the aortic sinuses of Valsalva. The pulmonic valve is at a level higher than the aortic valve, and the two valves touch only near the commissures between right and left cusps.

Lateral Projection of Left Side of Heart

In the lateral view the left atrium is projected almost completely behind the left ventricle (see Plate 3.8). The

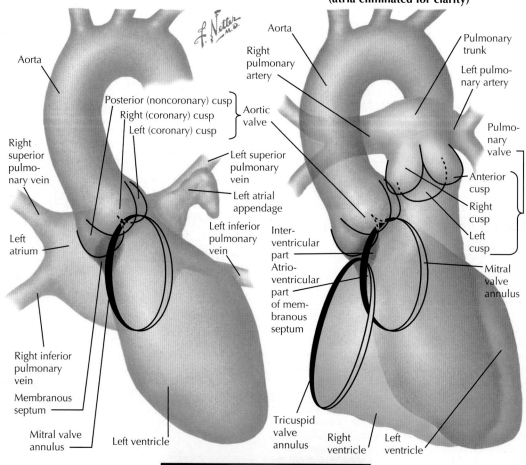

ANTEROPOSTERIOR PROJECTION OF LEFT-SIDED HEART STRUCTURES
Left and right sides of heart superimposed (atria eliminated for clarity)

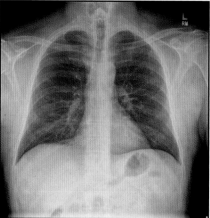

Plate 3.8   Imaging

RADIOLOGY AND CATHETER-BASED ANGIOCARDIOGRAPHY (Continued)

anteroinferior margin of the atrium is formed by the mitral valve. The left atrial appendage (auricle) arises somewhat above the mitral valve and extends anteriorly, crossing the aorta just above the sinuses of Valsalva. If the atrial appendage is sufficiently large, its tip may overlie the pulmonic valve. The posterior border of the atrial cavity is formed by the free wall of the atrium, and the pulmonary veins enter its upper and middle parts.

On a selective LV angiocardiogram the line of insertion of the mitral cusps can usually be seen during diastole as an opaque ring surrounding the radiolucent blood within the valve orifice. The mitral valve forms the posterior boundary of the ventricle. The upper margin of the mitral valve reaches the aortic valve in the region of the commissure between the left (coronary) and posterior (noncoronary) cusps. The LV body extends forward and downward from the mitral valve. The posteroinferior border of the LV body is formed by the free ventricular wall, and the entire anterior border is bounded by the interventricular septum. The papillary muscles may sometimes be seen as radiolucent defects arising from the midpart of the lower border of the ventricle and directed toward the mitral valve.

In the lateral view the right coronary cusp of the aortic valve is seen tangentially, forming the valve's anterior border. The left and posterior cusps are projected obliquely and lie posteriorly, with the posterior (noncoronary) cusp always the lower of the two. The membranous part of the interventricular septum directly below the commissure between right and noncoronary cusps is not border forming. The superior part of the muscular septum is directly in front of the membranous septum and forms the anterior subvalvular border of the left ventricle.

The right coronary artery arises from the upper part of the right sinus of Valsalva and courses anteriorly a short distance before curving almost directly downward. The main trunk of the left coronary artery is parallel to the x-ray beam and is foreshortened in this view. Its circumflex branch parallels the posterior aspect of the mitral ring. The left anterior or descending branch extends anteriorly and downward, overlying the aortic root, and then courses over the right sinus of Valsalva slightly below the origin of the right coronary artery and crosses this artery, so that the lower part of the anterior descending branch is the most anterior of the major coronary vessels.

When the right ventricle is enlarged, the sulcus between the ventricle and the right atrium is displaced anteriorly. The right coronary artery lies within this sulcus and in the lateral view is seen completely in front of the left anterior descending branch. In this way, RV enlargement can be recognized on a selective LV angiocardiogram.

When lateral views of the right and left ventricles are superimposed, the tricuspid valve lies anterior to the mitral valve. The upper margin of the tricuspid valve marks the anterior extent of the atrioventricular septum, and the mitral valve marks the posterior extent.

The interventricular portion of the membranous septum lies anterior to the insertion of the tricuspid valve. The *supraventricular crest* is directly in front of the right sinus of Valsalva, and most of the RV outflow tract thus is at a higher level than the left ventricle. Actually, a small part of the LV outflow tract immediately below the commissure between right and left aortic cusps does reach the same level as the subpulmonic region of the right ventricle. The RV and LV outflow tracts are separated in this area by the ventricular septum, and a defect in this region will produce a subpulmonic ventricular septal defect.

LATERAL PROJECTION OF LEFT-SIDED HEART STRUCTURES

Left and right sides of heart superimposed (atria eliminated for clarity)

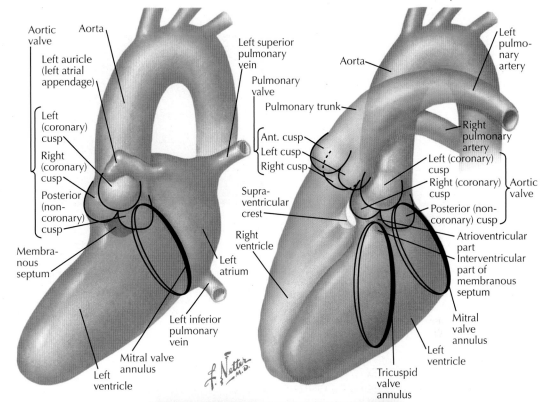

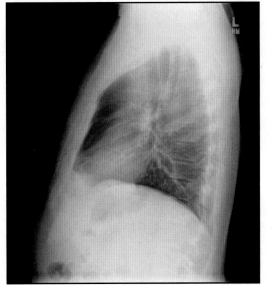

Plate 3.9

Cardiovascular System: VOLUME 8

RIGHT CORONARY ARTERY: ARTERIOGRAPHIC VIEWS

Right coronary artery: left anterior oblique view

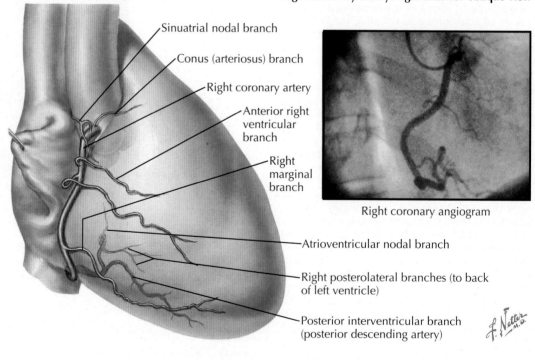

Right coronary angiogram

Sinuatrial nodal branch

Right coronary artery

Anterior right ventricular branches

Atrioventricular nodal branch

Right marginal branch

Posterior interventricular branch (posterior descending artery)

Branches to back of left ventricle

CATHETER-BASED CORONARY ANGIOGRAPHY

Until recently, diagnosis of human coronary atherosclerosis depended primarily on the physician's ability to interpret the significance of chest pain described by patients who experience infinitely variable subjective responses to stress. Objective confirmation hinged on the recognition of transient or persistent electrocardiographic changes, which usually indicate the presence of myocardial ischemia, necrosis, or scar tissue replacement of functioning myocardium. Therefore the presence of coronary atherosclerosis could be recognized in a patient only after the disease process had progressed to a point where arterial obstructions were so severe as to cause transient or permanent secondary changes in the myocardium (ischemia or infarction).

Selective cine coronary arteriography provides a clinically useful approach to the precise demonstration of the morphologic characteristics of the lumen of the human coronary artery when used in combination with intravascular ultrasound (see Plate 3.11).

TECHNIQUE

Sones Technique

With the patient under local anesthesia, the right brachial artery is usually mobilized in the right antecubital fossa immediately above its bifurcation. After heparinizing the distal brachial artery and occluding flow, an 8-Fr woven catheter 80 cm long, with a special tip that tapers to a 5-Fr diameter in its distal 2 inches (5 cm), is passed *retrograde* from the right brachial artery directly into the ascending aorta. The catheter tip is introduced directly into one coronary orifice and then the other under direct vision using an image intensifier equipped with a closed-circuit television unit to provide direct visualization during the procedure. Pressure measurements from the catheter tip are recorded constantly to permit immediate recognition of arterial occlusion by the catheter tip. The electrocardiogram (ECG) also is monitored constantly.

Multiple small doses of radiopaque contrast are injected directly into the orifice of each coronary artery, with the patient positioned in varying right and left anterior oblique projections. Individual projections for each patient are selected based on direct fluoroscopic visualization, to photograph all segments of each vessel in a plane perpendicular to that of the x-ray beam. Usually, four to six arteriograms of each artery are made in varying

Right coronary artery: right anterior oblique view

Sinuatrial nodal branch

Conus (arteriosus) branch

Right coronary artery

Anterior right ventricular branch

Right marginal branch

Right coronary angiogram

Atrioventricular nodal branch

Right posterolateral branches (to back of left ventricle)

Posterior interventricular branch (posterior descending artery)

RAO and LAO projections. On average, 4 to 6 mL of radiopaque contrast material is injected manually with a 10-mL syringe for adequate opacification of individual coronary vessels. Positioning the heart in multiple RAO and LAO projections is facilitated greatly by the use of a movable camera. The passage of the contrast medium through all branches of the coronary artery is digitally recorded (Plates 3.9 and 3.10).

After each coronary artery has been opacified effectively in the appropriate projections, the catheter tip is passed across the aortic valve into the left ventricle. Pressure measurements are recorded in the left ventricle. The LV cavity then is opacified selectively with 20 to 30 mL of radiopaque contrast. Left ventriculography is performed routinely in the RAO projection, clearly showing localized LV aneurysms or areas of impaired

Plate 3.10

LEFT CORONARY ARTERY: ARTERIOGRAPHIC VIEWS

Left coronary artery: left anterior oblique view

Left coronary angiogram

- Left coronary artery
- Circumflex branch
- Anterior interventricular branch (left anterior descending)
- Diagonal branches of anterior interventricular branch
- Atrioventricular branch of circumflex branch
- Left (obtuse) marginal branch
- Posterolateral branches
- (Perforating) interventricular septal branches

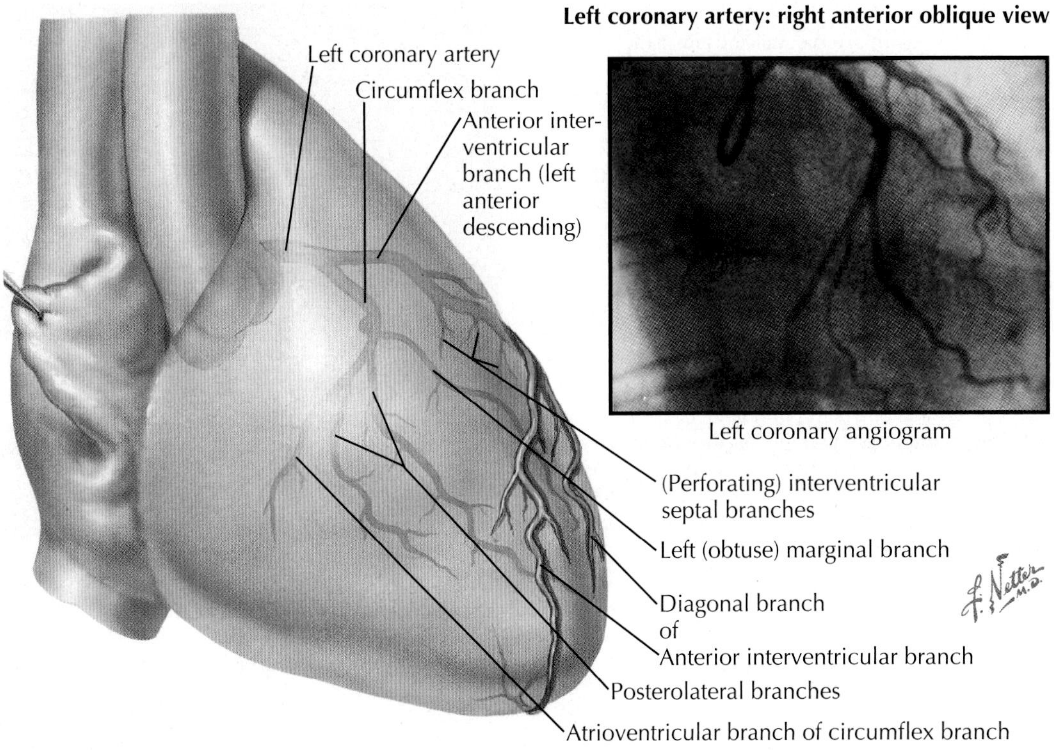

CATHETER-BASED CORONARY ANGIOGRAPHY (Continued)

contractility in the ventricular myocardium caused by interstitial scar tissue replacement or grossly impaired myocardial perfusion. Left ventriculography also permits the ready identification of associated mitral or aortic valve lesions or severely impaired LV function caused by generalized preexisting myocardial injury. The LAO ventriculogram visualizes the ventricular septum and lateral LV wall.

On completion of the procedure, the catheter is withdrawn and the brachial arteriotomy closed by direct suture.

The Sones technique is rarely used now in catheterization laboratories.

Judkins Technique

In contrast to the Sones technique, the Judkins technique is done percutaneously with preformed catheters from the femoral artery. Three catheters are required to perform ventriculography and right and left coronary injections. Ventriculography is usually performed with a "pigtail" catheter before selective coronary angiography. As with the Sones technique, multiple projections are used to identify coronary stenoses. Other catheters (e.g., multipurpose, Amplatz) are introduced percutaneously and often are used if the coronary arteries cannot be engaged by the Judkins catheters.

Radial Artery Technique

Small catheters can be used percutaneously for diagnostic coronary angiography, as well as percutaneous coronary intervention (PCI), if blood flow to the hand is adequate in the radial and ulnar arteries.

CLINICAL APPLICATIONS

Coronary angiography can demonstrate distal vessels of the coronary artery as small as 100 to 200 μm in lumen diameter. Segmental variations in lumen diameter of the major branches caused by atherosclerosis result in up to a 10% reduction in diameter (minimal irregularities). More advanced stenotic lesions can limit myocardial perfusion and are visualized easily. Selective opacification of the vessels allows precise delineation of the presence, sites of origin, and distribution of effective intercoronary collateral channels, which compensate for severe stenotic or occlusive lesions. In patients with angiographically normal vessels, coronary atherosclerosis may still be present,

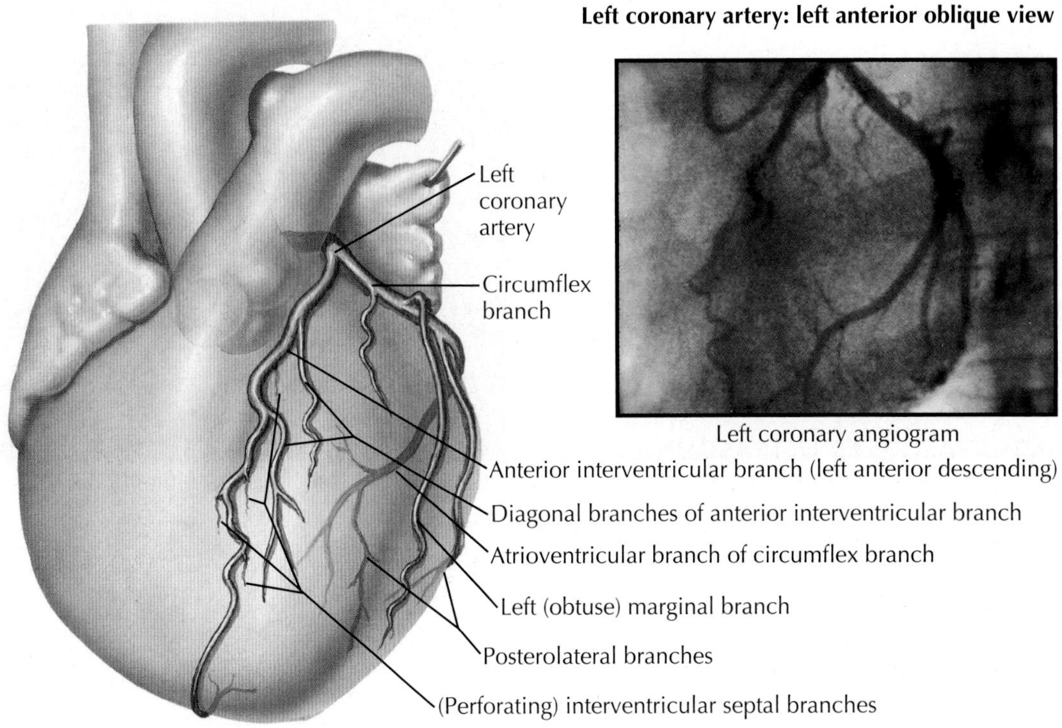

Left coronary artery: right anterior oblique view

Left coronary angiogram

- Left coronary artery
- Circumflex branch
- Anterior interventricular branch (left anterior descending)
- (Perforating) interventricular septal branches
- Left (obtuse) marginal branch
- Diagonal branch of Anterior interventricular branch
- Posterolateral branches
- Atrioventricular branch of circumflex branch

but myocardial ischemia caused by epicardial vessel stenosis can be ruled out.

Coronary arteriography is essential in selecting patients with coronary atherosclerosis who may benefit from revascularization procedures to improve myocardial perfusion, as well as objectively assessing results. Severe localized obstructions in major proximal arteries are now removed by direct angioplasty/stent or coronary artery bypass. More diffuse obstructive lesions provide an objective basis for planning optimal medical therapy.

After angioplasty or stent placement or postoperatively, repeated coronary arteriograms and selective conduit angiograms permit long-term assessment of the effectiveness of such revascularization procedures, as well as the evolving disease process in the individual patient.

Plate 3.11

Cardiovascular System: VOLUME 8

INTRAVASCULAR ULTRASOUND

Intravascular ultrasound (IVUS) uses high-frequency sound waves to acquire 3D images to determine the extent and composition of the atherosclerotic lesions in the coronary arteries. IVUS is an invasive technique used in the catheterization laboratory to complement catheter-based coronary angiography and thus requires cardiac catheterization.

A small wire is inserted into a coronary artery, and an echocardiographic transducer is passed over the guidewire into the coronary artery by way of the cardiac catheter (Plate 3.11). High-frequency sound waves produce pictures of the arterial wall and any pathology seen in the wall, such as a clot, cholesterol, calcium, or disruption of the endothelium. Both IVUS and angiography can evaluate the length and severity of stenosis, but IVUS adds assessment of the vascular wall, including plaque morphology and cross-sectional area of the stenosis and layers of the vessel wall. IVUS is useful for clinical decision making on whether a patient needs an intracoronary interventional procedure when catheter-based assessment of stenotic severity is equivocal (Plate 3.11). It is also frequently used to optimize an interventional coronary procedure.

IVUS combined with angiography, fractional flow, and coronary flow reserve provides a complete assessment of the anatomy and physiology of the blood vessel. The cardiologist uses all of this information in management of the patient, including diagnosis of disease and its severity and potential clinical implications, and for guidance and optimization of a coronary interventional procedure.

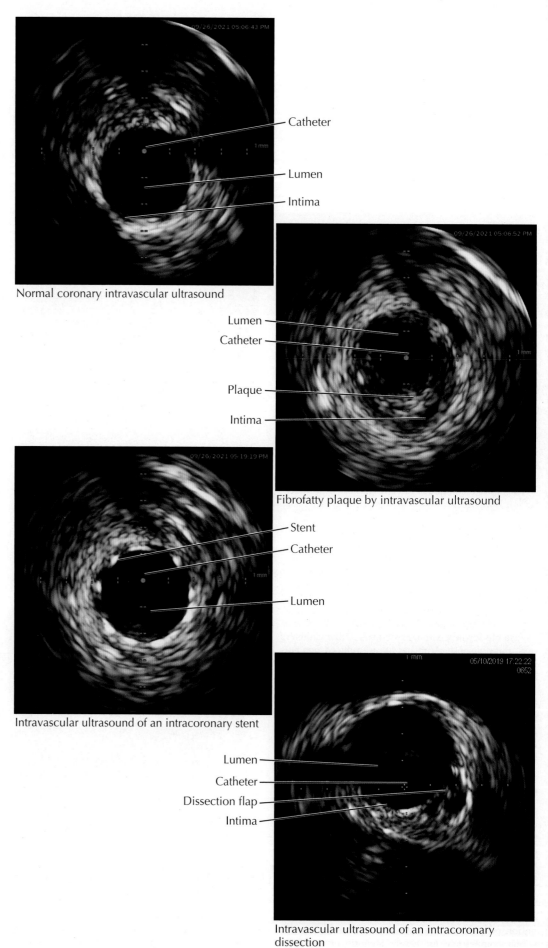

Normal coronary intravascular ultrasound

Fibrofatty plaque by intravascular ultrasound

Intravascular ultrasound of an intracoronary stent

Intravascular ultrasound of an intracoronary dissection

Images courtesy R. David Anderson, MD, MS, FACC, FSCAI

Plate 3.12

Imaging

TRANSDUCER POSITIONS IN ECHOCARDIOGRAPHIC EXAMINATION

Parasternal position

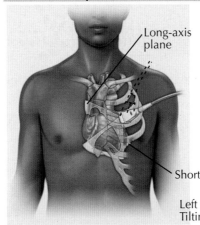

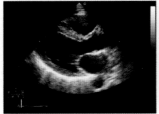

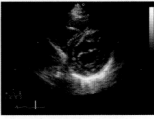

Long-axis plane

Short-axis plane

Normal long-axis view during systole

Normal short-axis view at mitral valve level

Left parasternal position allows views in long- and short-axis planes. Tilting the transducer allows multiple sections.

TRANSTHORACIC CARDIAC ULTRASOUND

Understanding cardiac ultrasound (US) requires knowledge of cardiac anatomy and physiology. In addition, performing echocardiography requires considerable experience to develop the necessary technical skills. Cardiac US records reflected sound waves from blood tissue interfaces within the heart and great vessels, thus visualizing the complex cardiac anatomy and providing a remarkably detailed image of heart motion and structure during all phases of the cardiac cycle (Plate 3.12). Transthoracic cardiac US is one of the most useful diagnostic tests available.

The most common echocardiogram is a two-dimensional (2D) image of cardiac anatomy in different planes, similar to angiography. The 2D echocardiogram provides a detailed picture of spatial relations of the cardiac chambers and valves. One weakness is that the image is somewhat difficult to quantitate. A major limitation is too much lung between the transducer and the heart, making it difficult to obtain good images in patients with chronic obstructive pulmonary disease. Parameters that can be measured with US include the following:

1. Ventricular chamber size and wall thickness
2. Ventricular function
3. Mitral valve: motion, valve thickness, prolapse, calcification, vegetations
4. Aortic valve: thickness, extent of motion, calcification, vegetations, number of cusps, aortic root size
5. Left atrium: size, presence of clots, tumors
6. Pericardial effusion
7. Congenital cardiac malformations

Apical position

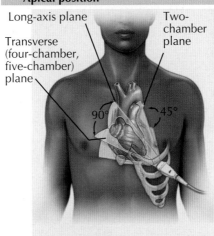

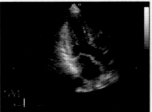

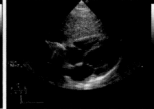

Long-axis plane

Transverse (four-chamber, five-chamber) plane

Two-chamber plane

90° 45°

Normal apical long-axis view

Normal apical four-chamber view

Apical studies imaged from point of maximal impulse toward base. Four-chamber plane passes through atrioventricular valves; upward tilt gives five-chamber plane. Counterclockwise rotation of 45 degrees gives two-chamber plane. 90-Degree rotation gives long-axis plane.

Subcostal position

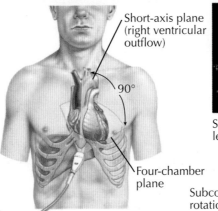

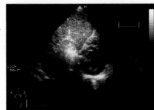

Short-axis plane (right ventricular outflow)

90°

Four-chamber plane

Subcostal short-axis view of left ventricle

Subcostal four-chamber view

Subcostal position allows multiple short-axis views; 90-degree rotation provides four-chamber view.

Suprasternal position

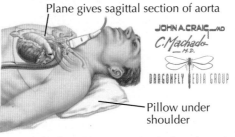

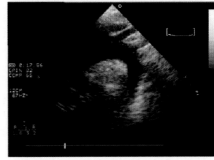

Plane gives sagittal section of aorta

JOHN A. CRAIG—MD
C. Machado—M.D.
DRAGONFLY MEDIA GROUP

Pillow under shoulder

Suprasternal view of aortic arch and origins of left common carotid and left subclavian

Suprasternal position uses plane of aortic arch to provide views of aorta and mediastinum.

Plate 3.13

Cardiovascular System: VOLUME 8

Principles of Doppler Echocardiography

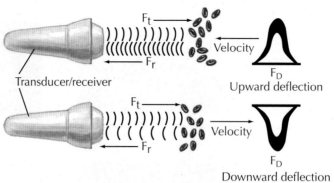

Doppler shift

$$F_D = F_r - F_t$$

(Doppler frequency) (reflected frequency) (transmitted frequency)

Doppler shift (F_D) based on principle that transmitted ultrasonic frequency (F_t) is reflected at greater frequency (F_r) by target moving toward transducer and at decreased frequency (F_r) by target moving away from transducer

$$F_D = 2F_t \frac{V \cos \cdot \theta}{C}$$

$$V = \frac{F_D}{2F_t} \frac{C}{(\cos \cdot \theta)}$$

Doppler frequency (F_D) can be used to determine flow velocity (V) if angle of insonation (θ) and velocity of sound (C) are known.

Doppler Echocardiography

Echocardiography with Doppler US is based on the principle of estimating velocity and direction of blood flow by using moving red blood cells as a target (Plate 3.13). There are two types of Doppler US: continuous wave and pulse wave. With the *continuous wave* technique, the transducer can be aimed along the long axis of the ventricle of the aorta and can record all flow patterns encountered. The *pulse wave* technique allows simultaneous recording of the Doppler and 2D echocardiography. The pulsed technique allows the localization of a Doppler sample in the area of interest (e.g., mitral and aortic valves). Using these Doppler techniques, a transvalvular gradient across the aortic or mitral valves can be derived in addition to estimation of the pressure and severity of mitral, aortic, and tricuspid valve regurgitations.

Doppler color flow imaging techniques allow noninvasive imaging of blood flow through the heart and the display of flow data on the 2D echocardiogram. Color flow imaging can provide the approximate size and direction of any abnormal flow velocity within the heart, including mitral or aortic insufficiency and ventricular septal defect. Doppler echocardiography is extremely sensitive and will detect even the slightest amount of tricuspid regurgitation, even in patients with no evidence of cardiac disease.

The accepted indications of cardiac US include the following:

- Valvular heart disease (native cardiac valve, prosthetic cardiac valve), suspected or proven infective endocarditis
- Ischemic heart disease (i.e., myocardial infarction), when the physician asks a specific question that can be answered by cardiac US
- Heart muscle disease, to establish the morphologic diagnosis and hemodynamic assessment of patients with cardiomyopathy, systemic illness associated with cardiac involvement and clinical symptoms, and exposure to cardiotoxic agents
- Pericardial disease, to evaluate clinical manifestations or suspicion of pericardial disease
- Cardiac masses, to evaluate patients with suspected cardiac masses
- Cardiac murmurs, to evaluate an organic murmur in a patient with cardiorespiratory symptoms or a murmur in an asymptomatic patient if clinical features indicate at least moderate probability that the murmur is organic

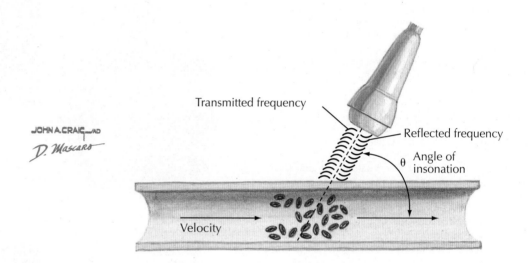

JOHN A. CRAIG—AD
D. Mascaro

Doppler signal processing (waveform spectral analysis)

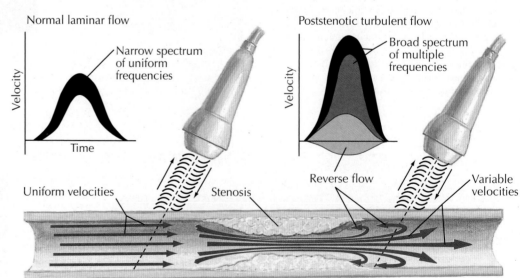

Laminar flow consists of zones of unidirectional flow of fairly uniform velocities, resulting in narrow Doppler spectral waveform of similar frequencies.

Turbulent flow made up of widely different velocities and reverse flow, creating waveform made up of broad spectrum of frequencies (spectral broadening)

Plate 3.14

Imaging

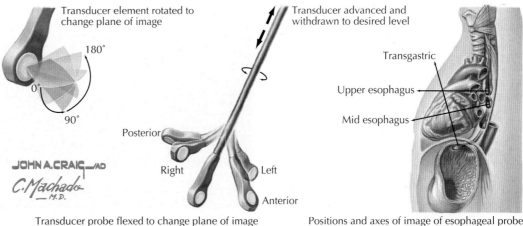

Transducer element rotated to change plane of image

180°

0°

90°

Transducer probe flexed to change plane of image

JOHN A. CRAIG—MD
C. Machado —M.D.

Transducer advanced and withdrawn to desired level

Posterior

Right   Left

Anterior

Transgastric

Upper esophagus

Mid esophagus

Positions and axes of image of esophageal probe

TRANSESOPHAGEAL ECHOCARDIOGRAPHY

Transesophageal echocardiography (TEE) requires an ultrasound transducer at the tip of a probe that can be passed into the patient's esophagus, which lies directly behind the left atrium, as well as into the gastric area (Plate 3.14). Sedation is required, and TEE should be performed only by a certified physician (e.g., cardiologist, cardiac anesthesiologist), not echo technologists. TEE does not replace transthoracic echocardiography but does provide clearer images, especially images that are more difficult to view with transthoracic US, such as the left atrial appendage. This feature is extremely important before cardioversion of patients in atrial fibrillation with uncertain onset. If the atrial appendage is free of clots, the patient is considered at very low risk for emboli to the brain.

The structures evaluated best in adults with TEE are the aorta, pulmonary artery, cardiac valves, both atria and ventricular septum, left atrial appendage, and coronary arteries. However, TEE is rarely used as a diagnostic tool to detect coronary abnormalities in the adult. As with any invasive technique, there is some risk with anesthesia, esophageal perforation, and drug side effects.

In patients undergoing valve surgery, particularly reconstruction (e.g., mitral valve repair), anesthesiologists trained in TEE provide important information to the surgeon on ventricular function and valve status after repair.

Upper esophageal position

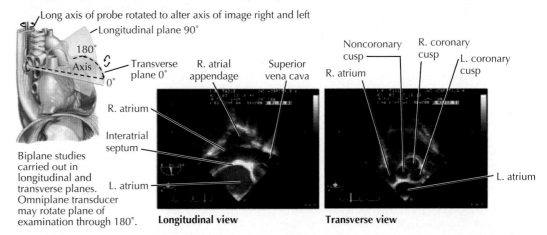

Long axis of probe rotated to alter axis of image right and left

Longitudinal plane 90°

180°

Axis

Transverse plane 0°

0°

Biplane studies carried out in longitudinal and transverse planes. Omniplane transducer may rotate plane of examination through 180°.

R. atrial appendage

Superior vena cava

R. atrium

Interatrial septum

L. atrium

Longitudinal view

Noncoronary cusp

R. coronary cusp

L. coronary cusp

R. atrium

L. atrium

Transverse view

Mid esophagus position

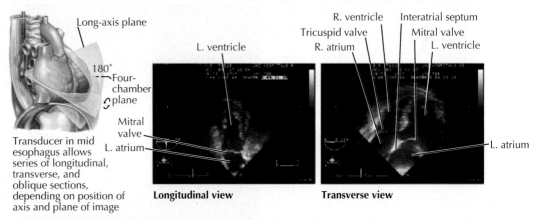

Long-axis plane

180°

Four-chamber plane

Mitral valve

L. atrium

Transducer in mid esophagus allows series of longitudinal, transverse, and oblique sections, depending on position of axis and plane of image

L. ventricle

Mitral valve

Longitudinal view

R. ventricle

Tricuspid valve

R. atrium

Interatrial septum

Mitral valve

L. ventricle

L. atrium

Transverse view

Transgastric position

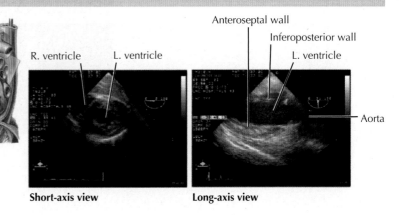

Longitudinal plane (long-axis view)

Short-axis plane

0°   180°

90°

Anteflexion alters axis of image up and down

Transducer head in proximal stomach for short-axis and long-axis planes

R. ventricle   L. ventricle

Short-axis view

Anteroseptal wall

Inferoposterior wall

L. ventricle

Aorta

Long-axis view

Plate 3.15

Cardiovascular System: VOLUME 8

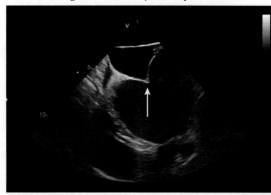

Tenting of foramen by transeptal needle

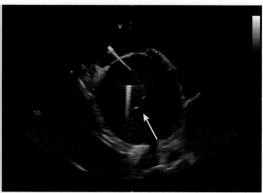

Ablation catheter curled in LA

Left atrial access via transseptal puncture utilizing intracardiac echo (ICE) guidance. The ICE catheter is introduced from the femoral vein and positioned in the mid-right atrium. ***Left,*** The membranous foramen ovale is "tented" toward the left atrium by forward pressure from a sheath/needle assembly introduced into the right atrium via the femoral vein. The needle itself is not visualized in this frame because it is out of plane with the 2D echo slice. ***Right,*** After transseptal puncture has been accomplished, ICE demonstrates the ablation catheter crossing the foramen ovale and curled in the left atrium (LA). Tenting of the foramen is no longer evident.

INTRACARDIAC ECHOCARDIOGRAPHY

Intracardiac echocardiography is a type of cardiovascular ultrasound that provides high-resolution, real-time visualization of intracardiac structures. As opposed to traditional echocardiography, these transducers are placed inside the heart via a transfemoral approach. It is commonly used for accurate visualization of intracardiac structures during interventional procedures such as ablations and structural heart interventions.

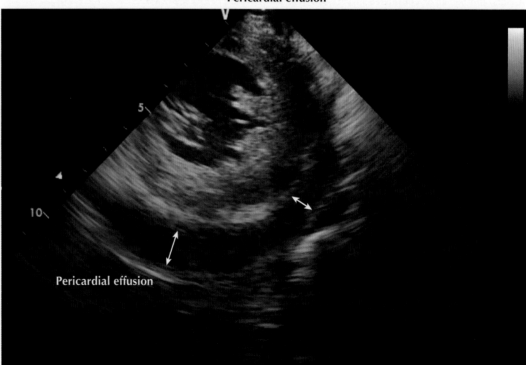

Pericardial effusion

Pericardial effusion

Demonstration of a pericardial effusion by intracardiac echo (ICE) during an electrophysiology procedure. The ICE catheter is introduced via the femoral vein and advanced to the mid-right ventricle. In addition to the effusion, the left ventricular cavity, wall muscle, papillary muscle, and chordae can be identified. If pericardiocentesis is necessary, needle entry into the pericardial space can be verified on ICE by injection of agitated saline, and ICE provides real-time monitoring of effective pericardial drainage.

Images courtesy William Murrell Miles, MD, FACC

Plate 3.16

Imaging

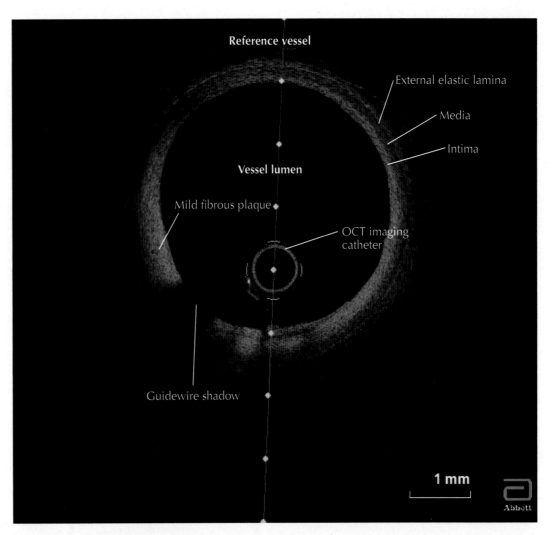

OPTICAL COHERENCE TOMOGRAPHY

Optical coherence tomography (OCT) is an intravascular imaging tool that uses near-infrared light to capture high temporal and spatial resolution images of a coronary artery. This technology is used in addition to coronary angiography and requires cardiac catheterization because the imaging catheter is advanced through a guide catheter over a wire into the coronary artery being studied. Contrast is then injected to clear the vessel of blood, allowing the infrared light to reflect off the vessel. This creates the image, which can be analyzed in different planes, both longitudinal and cross-sectional. OCT prior to PCI can be used to identify culprit lesions, degree of stenosis, amount of calcium burden, plaque burden, and morphology. The software allows for angiographic coregistration leading to accurate measurement of vessel diameter and length, which is then applied to optimize stent selection and deployment. After a coronary stent is deployed, OCT can be performed again to assess the quality of stent deployment with attention to stent apposition and expansion, as well as stent edge assessment for potential dissection. OCT-guided PCI allows the operator to plan a more precise treatment of the vessel with regards to lesion preparation (predilation, atherectomy, etc.) and stent optimization (adequate landing zones and appropriate balloon sizes for dilation). This can help improve outcomes by reducing the risk of stent thrombosis and in stent restenosis.

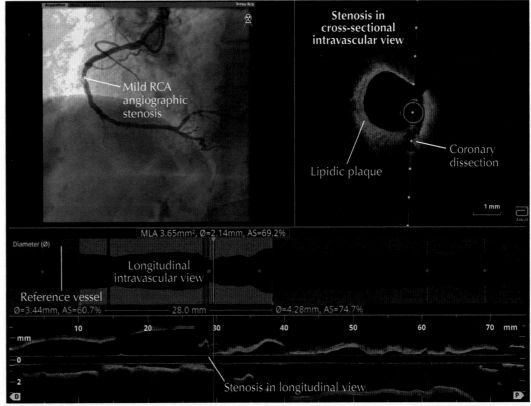

Images courtesy Michael R. Massoomi, MD

Plate 3.17

Cardiovascular System: VOLUME 8

EXERCISE AND CONTRAST ECHOCARDIOGRAPHY

EXERCISE ECHOCARDIOGRAPHY

This type of stress test generally involves walking on a treadmill after a baseline echocardiogram is obtained (Plate 3.17). During treadmill exercise, the heart rate increases; if myocardial ischemia occurs, wall motion abnormalities can be detected, which return to baseline at rest or after nitroglycerin. This is highly suggestive of a high-grade stenosis of a coronary artery; identification of the specific artery depends on the distribution of the wall motion abnormality. For example, if the ventricular septum contracts normally at rest but with exercise barely moves, this suggests disease in the anterior descending coronary artery. In contrast, a similar situation with the inferior wall suggests disease of the vessel supplying the posterior descending coronary artery.

If the patient reaches 85% to 90% of predicted maximum heart rate with no transient wall motion changes on the echocardiogram, high-grade coronary stenosis can be excluded in the majority of cases (i.e., excellent negative predictive value).

CONTRAST ECHOCARDIOGRAPHY

Early attempts at contrast echocardiography involved intravenous injection of agitated saline, which did not cross the pulmonary vascular bed and thus was seen only in the right atrium and right ventricle. Right-to-left shunts could be detected by bubbles in the left atrium or left ventricle. Left-to-right shunts at the atrial or ventricular level could be detected as negative images. Other contrast agents were developed later that allowed passage through the lung after bolus injection in a peripheral vein. These contrast agents consisted of microspheres and were helpful in defining intracardiac structures, demonstrating intracardiac shunts, and enhancing Doppler velocity signals through heart valves. Probably the most important use of these agents is to clearly identify the borders of the left ventricle, which allows an easier and better assessment of left ventricular function than when these agents are not used (Plate 3.17).

Exercise echocardiography

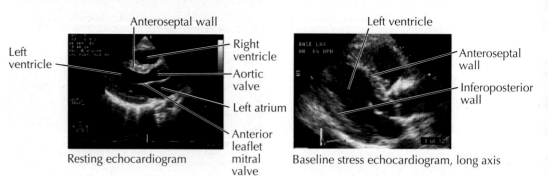

Resting echocardiogram

Left ventricle — Anteroseptal wall — Right ventricle — Aortic valve — Left atrium — Anterior leaflet mitral valve

Baseline stress echocardiogram, long axis

Left ventricle — Anteroseptal wall — Inferoposterior wall

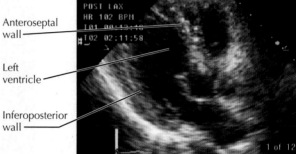

Diastolic postexercise echocardiogram, long axis

Anteroseptal wall — Left ventricle — Inferoposterior wall

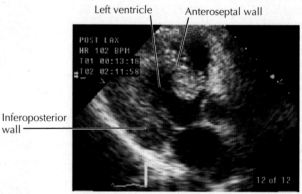

Systolic postexercise echocardiogram, long axis

Left ventricle — Anteroseptal wall — Inferoposterior wall

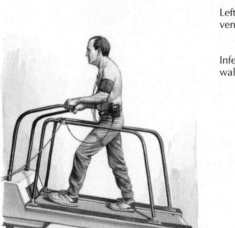

Exercise performed to elicit ischemic signs and postexercise echocardiogram used to evaluate ventricular function, wall motion, and thickness. Often correlated with stress echocardiography

JOHN A. CRAIG ___ MD
C. Machado ___ M.D.

Contrast echocardiography

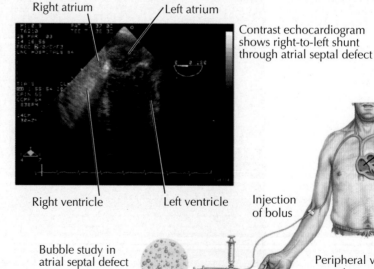

Right atrium — Left atrium

Right ventricle — Left ventricle

Bubble study in atrial septal defect

Microbubble solution

Injection of bolus

Contrast echocardiogram shows right-to-left shunt through atrial septal defect

Peripheral venous contrast agent confined to right side of heart in normal patient

Peripheral venous injection of solution contains acoustically dense microbubbles, affording contrast agent that delineates intracardiac structures and identifies shunts.

Plate 3.18

Imaging

MYOCARDIAL PERFUSION IMAGING

Use of myocardial perfusion imaging (MPI) is preferable to stress nuclear imaging, but both terms are used interchangeably. In general, images at peak stress and at rest reflect changes in the distribution of the radiopharmaceutical if ischemia is present (Plate 3.18; *SPECT*, single-photon emission computed tomography [CT]). Indications for MPI are as follows:

1. To detect and provide semiquantitative information about ischemia, especially when the ECG may not be useful during exercise (e.g., patients with left bundle branch block).

2. To distinguish a false-positive ECG response for patients who are asymptomatic during exercise but have striking ECG alteration (e.g., ST-segment depression); normal radionuclide uptake in these patients is highly suggestive of a false-positive ECG response to exercise.

3. To assess previous or new myocardial infarction and to provide some semiquantitative information about the size of the infarction.

4. To provide information on the functional significance of a specific coronary artery stenosis found at angiography (e.g., patient with 50%–60% stenosis of left anterior descending coronary artery and 90% stenosis of a right coronary artery undergoes an exercise radionuclide test to detect regional abnormality in distribution of descending and right coronary arteries).

Unfortunately, a false-positive test for ischemia can occur, especially in patients who have any type of infiltrative disease within the myocardium, such as myocarditis or tumors. False-negative results are also found, especially when the ischemic area of the myocardium is too small to be detected by this technique.

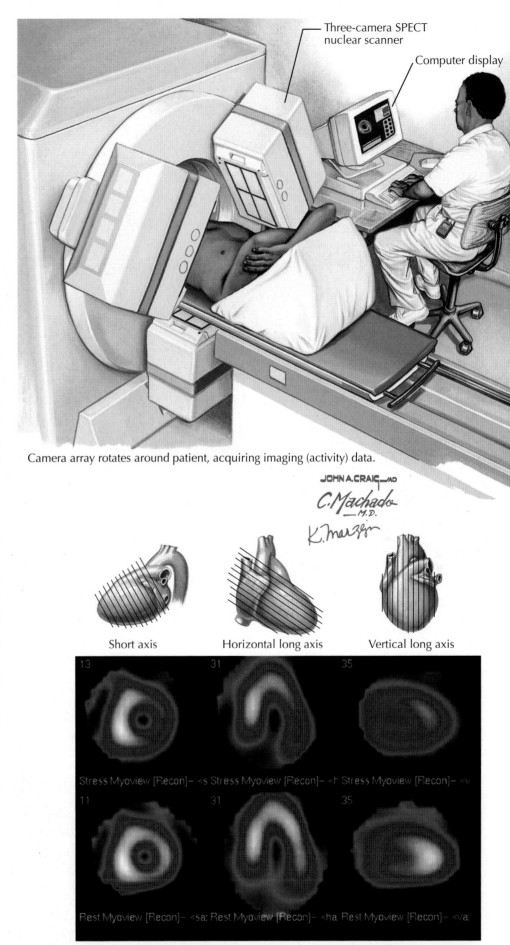

Camera array rotates around patient, acquiring imaging (activity) data.

Short axis Horizontal long axis Vertical long axis

Computer reconstructs acquired image data into a series of tomographic slices displayed in three standard views: short axis, horizontal long axis, and vertical long axis.

Plate 3.19

Cardiovascular System: VOLUME 8

VENTRICULOGRAPHY

In ventriculography, a catheter (usually pigtail) is introduced into the ventricle and radiopaque contrast material is injected (Plate 3.19). The ventricle is then visualized by fluoroscopy/cine as it contracts and relaxes, to assess ventricular wall motion and calculate ejection fraction (EF; normal $\geq$55%). Ejection fraction is calculated by the formula EF = SV/EDV, where *SV* is stroke volume and *EDV* is end-diastolic volume.

Hemodynamic study for ischemic heart disease is incomplete without assessment of ventricular function. Catheter-based ventriculography enables identification of areas of akinesis or hypokinesis and allows measurement of global EF if an LAO view is obtained. This information complements coronary angiography; for example, areas of hypokinesis corresponding to the distribution of the coronary arteries with stenotic lesions may provide information that encourages the physician to perform PCI or cardiac surgery to improve contraction of that part of the ventricle.

Ventriculography can be performed in both RAO and LAO projections. In the RAO view, the anterior, apical, and inferior walls are visualized. In the LAO projection, the septum, apex, and lateral wall are assessed (Plate 3.19).

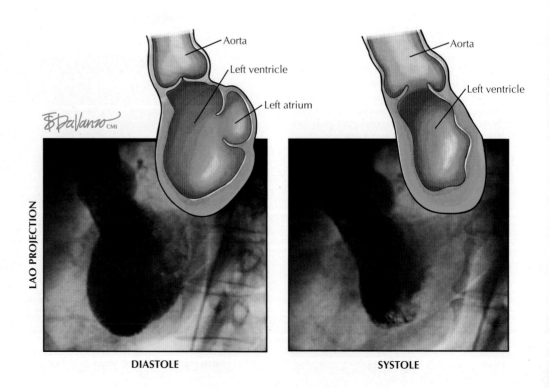

Plate 3.20

Imaging

COMPUTED TOMOGRAPHIC ANGIOGRAPHY

Computed tomographic angiography (CTA) is a 3D image reconstructed from multiple slices of tomographic images of a particular body part (e.g., brain, chest, blood vessels, abdomen, pelvis, joints). CTA of the heart includes the coronary arteries. Because CT studies are created by computer processing, the images can be seen in multiple planes, and ventricles, atria, veins, and arteries can be easily delineated. Pulmonary CTA can reveal emboli in both right and left pulmonary arteries and some subdivisions, as well as in the main pulmonary artery (see Plate 3.21).

CARDIAC CYCLE AND CALCIUM CONTRAST STUDIES

High resolution and high speed allow imaging of the coronary arteries as well as all chambers of the heart and the great vessels. When imaging the coronary arteries, ionizing radiation is usually confined to diastole because the majority of blood flow in the coronary arteries occurs during that time in the cardiac cycle (Plate 3.20). Coronary artery calcium deposits can be quantitated. CTA is especially useful in identifying the course of anomalous coronary arteries (between, posterior/anterior to great vessels).

The radiation dose using CT coronary angiography initially once was quite high, 10 to 15 millisieverts (mSv) per study. The dose is now considerably reduced, particularly when imaging the coronary arteries, which can be imaged in diastole, thus decreasing the amount of radiation exposure as much as 1 to 3 mSv. However, many studies still require greater exposure. Importantly, patients' exposure to radiation has greatly increased over the last several years; 49% results from CT-related ionizing radiation, although CT makes up only 12% of medical radiation procedures. All healthcare personnel should be aware of patient exposure to radiation.

Because CTA studies require administration of intravenous contrast agents, similar to catheter-based coronary angiography, patient risks include allergic reaction and contrast nephropathy.

ADVANCES AND INTERPRETATION

As systems improve, many new clinical CTA investigations will become possible. CT can help assess the coronary artery calcium score and evaluate the cardiac chambers and valves, congenital heart disease, aortic and pulmonary disease, and extracardiac structures and abnormalities (see Plate 3.21). Techniques are now being developed to assess not only the anatomic pathology of the coronary arteries but also the physiopathology of a specific lesion that may need a revascularization procedure (i.e., PCI or coronary artery bypass surgery). Preliminary results are encouraging compared with catheter-based coronary angiography and fractional flow reserve, the current reference standard for the physiologic significance of a specific coronary artery stenosis.

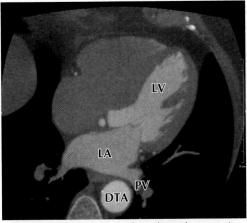

CT of the heart taken in systole. Iodinated contrast is visible in the left ventricle; the right side of the heart is free of contrast agent. Just anterior and left (of the patient, right of the image) of the spine, the descending thoracic aorta is visible. Anterior to the aorta is the left atrium with two pulmonary veins visible entering from either side.

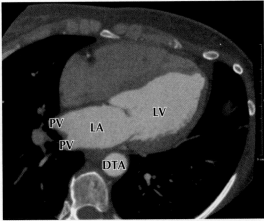

CT of the heart taken in diastole. Iodinated contrast is visible in the left ventricle; the right side of the heart is free of contrast agent. Just anterior (up) and left (of the patient, right of the image) of the spine, the descending thoracic aorta is visible. Anterior to the aorta is the left atrium with two right pulmonary veins visible entering from the left side of the image.

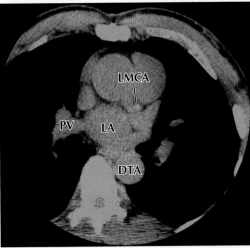

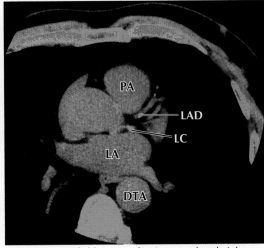

Coronary artery calcium study. All structures that are more than 150 Hounsfield units in density are colored pink: the spine, sternum, and ribs. This cutoff is used to identify calcium in the arteries. **Left CT,** In the middle of the chest, there is a small area of calcified plaque in the distal portion of the left main coronary artery. At this level of the chest, few other cardiac structures are readily identifiable. **Right CT,** Several small areas of pink in the middle of the image represent calcified plaque of the left anterior descending artery and left circumflex. More calcium appears to be in the wall of the ascending aorta, and a small amount of calcium is also seen in the medial wall of the descending thoracic aorta.

KEY	
LV = Left ventricle	LMCA = Left main coronary artery
DTA = Descending thoracic aorta	LAD = Left anterior descending artery
LA = Left atrium	LC = Left circumflex
PV = Pulmonary veins	

Plate 3.21

Cardiovascular System: VOLUME 8

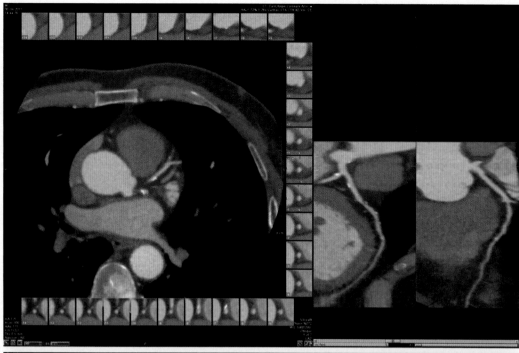

CT coronary angiogram. Several methods of interpreting images are seen. The large image at left is an axial image, as would be seen in a routine CT of the chest. Starting at the top left corner and proceeding clockwise, the small images around the main image are sequential cross-sectional images from the left main and left anterior descending arteries starting at the origin in the aorta and proceeding distally. Minor, nonobstructive calcified lesions are seen throughout the vessel. On the right, a multiplanar reconstruction of the vessel is displayed. Using the slider bar at the bottom of this display, the vessel can be "rolled" about its central lumen to assess the severity of disease from any angle.

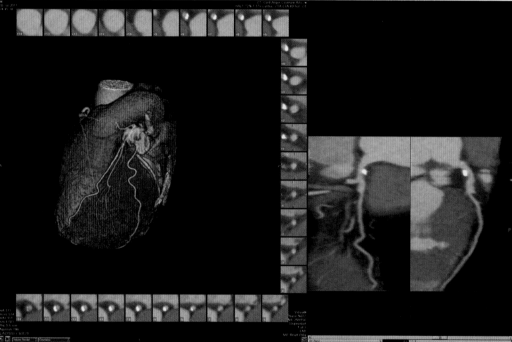

CT coronary angiogram. Several methods of interpreting images are seen. The color image at the left is a 3D representation of the heart generated from axial data acquired during the scan. Starting at the top left corner and proceeding clockwise, the small images around the 3D image are sequential cross-sectional images from the left main and left anterior descending coronary arteries starting at the origin in the aorta and proceeding distally. The bottom images show the calcified lesion (white) resulting in moderate to severe stenosis of the vessel lumen. On the right, a multiplanar reconstruction of the vessel is displayed. Using the slider bar at the bottom of this display, the vessel can be "rolled" about its central lumen to assess the severity of disease from any angle.

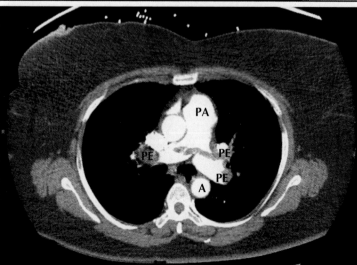

CT, axial view. Iodinated contrast has opacified the pulmonary arterial circuit to assess for emboli in this patient who presented acutely with severe dyspnea. Several dark areas in the pulmonary arteries demonstrate massive saddle emboli affecting each of the main and segmental pulmonary arteries.

KEY	PA = Pulmonary artery
	PE = Pulmonary emboli
	A = Aorta

Plate 3.22

Imaging

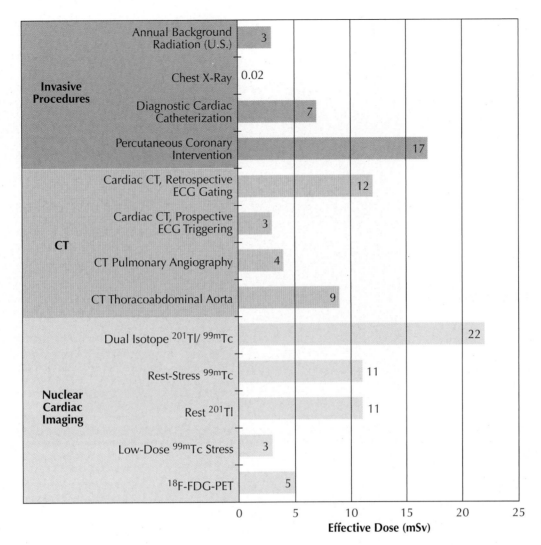

Reused with permission from Meinel FG. Radiation risk from cardiovascular imaging tests. Circulation. 130(5):442–445.

RADIATION DOSE CONCERNS

It is not easy to quantify radiation doses with precision because there is considerable variability in radiation dose reported for each diagnostic procedure performed. What is available must be considered as an average radiation dose of the different imaging modalities.

It is estimated that ionizing radiation exposure has increased approximately 600% from 1980 to 2021. Although CT studies make up only 12% of the medical radiation procedures, almost half of the radiation dose exposure in the United States is related to these procedures.

In radiation-producing procedures, weight, heart rate, and specified protocols may make a difference in the radiation dose. A millisievert is commonly used to measure the dose equivalent in diagnostic medical procedures (i.e., chest radiographs, nuclear studies, CT, and cardiac catheterization). One Sievert is the equivalent of about 50,000 chest radiographs. An acute full-body equivalent dose of 1 Sv causes slight blood

changes; 2 to 5 Sv cause nausea, hair loss, hemorrhage, and death in many cases.

CT CORONARY ANGIOGRAPHY

In 2008, Choi and his investigator colleagues reported that they could not recommend CT-based coronary angiography as a screening tool with the rationale that CT-based coronary angiography can produce false-positive results, turning subjects into patients. False-positive results may also trigger anxiety, further diagnostic procedures, and possibly unnecessary treatment. As technology improves, these concerns have lessened, although they remain valid and worthy of consideration prior to exposing patients to additional radiation.

WHAT NEEDS TO BE DONE?

Decision making between pharmacologic treatment, PCI, and coronary artery bypass grafting based solely on noninvasive imagining will become a reality, according

to Patrick Serruys. Nonobstructive coronary artery disease diagnosed by noninvasive CT imaging can be used to encourage lifestyle modification with or without aggressive pharmacologic therapy. Whatever is found with noninvasive CT angiography should be correlated with functional significance before any revascularization procedure is attempted in patients with stable angina.

Noninvasive plaque imaging can provide information previously obtained only by invasive intravascular cardiac catheterization. CTA-derived physiologic assessment of epicardial conductance and myocardial resistance is a surrogate for catheter-based coronary pressure and velocity measurements and can be used in decision making and management for both primary and secondary cardiovascular prevention.

In the near future, CTA may replace invasive procedures for the assessment of anatomy, functionality, and plaque composition. Complete CTA assessment could provide a one-stop shop for diagnosis, decision making, and risk management for treatment of coronary artery disease.

Plate 3.23

Cardiovascular System: VOLUME 8

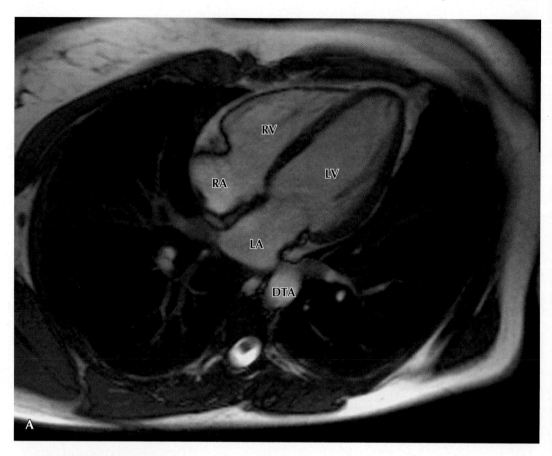

CARDIAC MAGNETIC RESONANCE IMAGING

Cardiac magnetic resonance imaging (MRI) does not use radiation and is based on fundamental principles related to the presence of water in all tissues. Because two protons are contained in a water molecule, when put in a magnetic field, they can be aligned. If the magnetic field is turned off, the protons can return to their original position and generate a radio signal that can be detected and quantitated for an image. The images obtained can help assess ventricular function, aortic disease, ischemic heart disease, cardiomyopathies, pericardial disease, valvular heart disease, cardiac masses, congenital heart disease, pulmonary vascular disease, and coronary artery bypass grafting. In the near future, electrophysiologists will be using cardiac MRI to evaluate atrial morphology before atrial fibrillation ablation therapy (Plates 3.23 and 3.24).

Most cardiac MR images are obtained using gadolinium as a contrast agent. Although gadolinium is generally benign, some patients have developed devastating problems, including nephrogenic systemic fibrosis, a serious, occasionally fatal condition.

At this time, most radiologists will not perform cardiac MRI in patients who have implantable devices such as pacemakers or defibrillators. However, some device companies are producing MR-compatible devices, and all devices will probably be MR compatible in the future.

KEY

A = Arch of aorta
AA = Ascending aorta
AV = Aortic valves
DTA = Descending thoracic aorta
LA = Left atrium
LV = Left ventricle
PA = Pulmonary artery
RA = Right atrium
RV = Right ventricle
S = Stomach

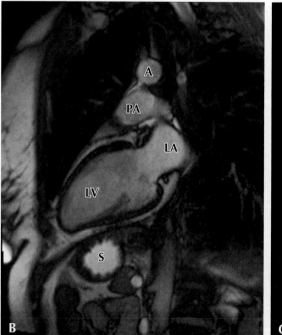

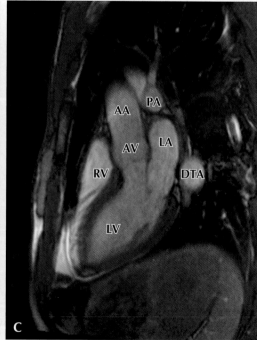

MRI allows for high-resolution images of the heart in any desired imaging plane. Standard four-chamber (**A**), two-chamber (**B**), and three-chamber (**C**) imaging planes are shown.

Plate 3.24

Imaging

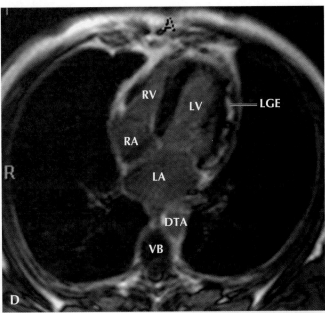

Abnormal white enhancement on images acquired late after gadolinium injection occurs in tissues with increased water content. Abnormal enhancement in the mid-wall of the left ventricle is shown in a young male with rheumatic carditis.

KEY

A = Arch of aorta
AA = Ascending aorta
DTA = Descending thoracic aorta
LA = Left atrium
LGE = Late gadolinium enhancement
LV = Left ventricle
PV = Pulmonary vein
RA = Right atrium
RV = Right ventricle
VB = Vertebral body

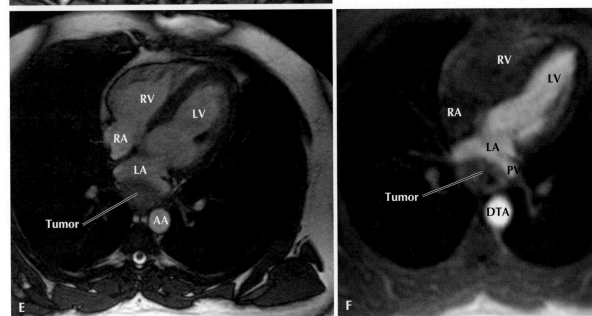

Cardiac MRI allows for characterization of thoracic masses. **E,** Mass posterior to the left atrium. **F,** Gadolinium contrast is seen within the mass, suggesting that the mass is highly vascular. Also, there are areas void of contrast, suggesting a necrotic core. This mass was excised and found to be a moderately differentiated extra-adrenal pheochromocytoma.

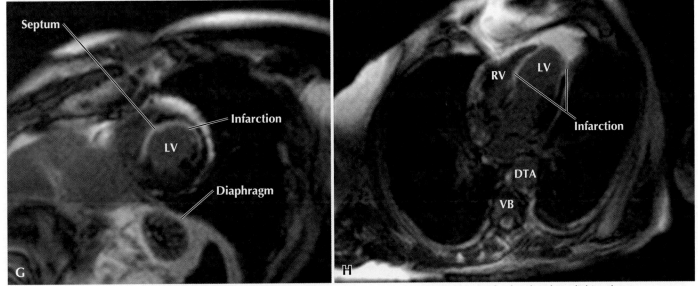

Myocardial infarction is shown in short axis (**G**) and long axis (**H**). Infarction is transmural in certain areas and only subendocardial in others.

EMBRYOLOGY

Plate 4.1

Cardiovascular System: VOLUME 8

EARLY EMBRYONIC DEVELOPMENT

In humans, as in most other primates, fertilization takes place in the distal part of the uterine tube, near its fimbriated end, about 12 to 24 hours after ovulation. The fertilized ovum, or *zygote,* is transported to the uterus by rhythmic contractions of the tube, aided by the action of the cilia of the epithelium. During this passage down the uterine tube, which takes about 4 days, the zygote executes a number of cell divisions and, on reaching the uterus, consists of a clump of blastomeres, the *morula,* which has not increased appreciably in size from the zygote.

After entering the uterus, a *blastocyst* is formed as a fluid-filled cavity develops in the enlarging morula. The wall of the blastocyst consists of a single layer of flattened cells, the *trophoblast,* and an eccentrically placed mass of cells, the inner cell mass or *embryoblast.* The trophoblast of the blastocyst attaches to the uterine epithelium to begin the process of implantation into the endometrium during the second week. Its cells soon differentiate into an inner *cytotrophoblast* and an outer *syncytiotrophoblast* (syntrophoblast) and will eventually form the outer embryonic membrane (the *chorion*) and the fetal portion of the placenta. The embryo develops from the inner cell mass, which also contributes to the formation of the amnion and umbilical vesicle.

Soon after implantation, the cells of the inner mass differentiate into two layers: an inner *hypoblast* (future endoderm) and an outer *epiblast* (future ectoderm). Together, these two layers form the embryonic disc. At the same time, a space appears within the inner cell mass, the *primitive amniotic cavity,* lined by the cells that are continuous with the epiblast cells of the embryonic disc. The cavity of the blastocyst becomes lined by hypoblast cells from the embryonic disc migrating along the trophoblast to form the *primitive umbilical vesicle* (yolk sac). Cells of the primitive umbilical vesicle also give rise to *extraembryonic mesoderm,* loose connective tissue that separates the umbilical vesicle from the trophoblast. The embryo proper now is a disc made of two layers of cells and from which all the intraembryonic tissues will be derived: the *ectoderm,* consisting of a simple columnar epithelium that is also the floor of the amnion, and the *cuboidal endodermal cells* that form the roof of the yolk sac. Small cavities appear in the extraembryonic mesoderm and coalesce to form the *extraembryonic coelom* (chorionic cavity), except for a mesodermal stalk that connects the amnion to the trophoblast. This remaining mesodermal stalk later forms the *connecting stalk* (future umbilical cord).

With the formation of the extraembryonic coelom, the extraembryonic mesoderm separates into two thin layers, completing formation of the three extraembryonic membranes. The trophoblast, with its inner coating of extraembryonic mesoderm, is now called the *chorion.* The primitive amnion with its outer coating of extraembryonic mesoderm is the amnion proper, and the primitive umbilical vesicle (yolk sac) becomes the umbilical vesicle proper with its outer coating of mesoderm.

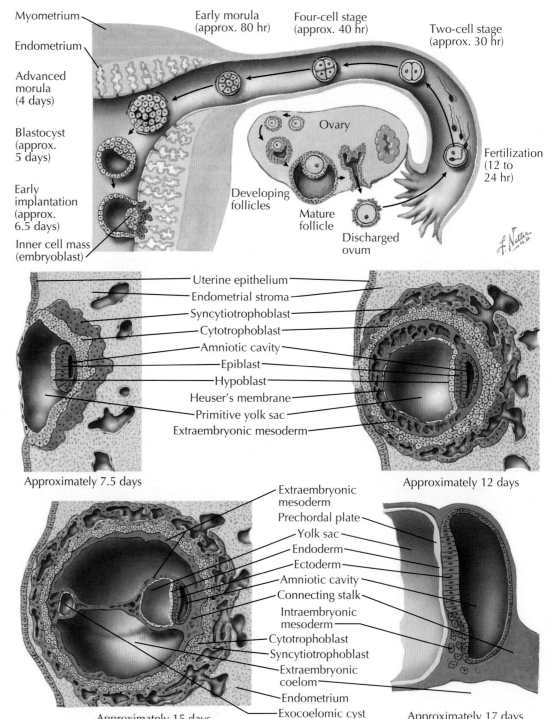

Approximately 7.5 days

Approximately 12 days

Approximately 15 days

Approximately 17 days

At the future caudal end of the embryonic disc, ectodermal cells form in the midline a thickened ectodermal *primitive streak* with a *primitive node* at the cephalic end of the streak. The primitive streak and node give rise to a third germ layer, the *intraembryonic mesoderm,* situated between the ectoderm and endoderm. This creation of intraembryonic mesoderm is through the process of *gastrulation,* occurring during the third week. The mesodermal cells migrate laterally and cranially until ectoderm and endoderm are separated from each other by intraembryonic mesoderm, except at the cephalic *oropharyngeal membrane* and the caudal *cloacal membrane,* where ectoderm remains in contact with endoderm. The primitive streak mesoderm cranial to the oropharyngeal membrane in the midline is the

cardiogenic mesoderm. Laterally, all along the margin of the embryonic disc, the intraembryonic mesoderm is continuous with the extraembryonic mesoderm. The embryo, now trilaminar, becomes more elongated and pear shaped when viewed from its dorsal (ectodermal) or ventral (endodermal) side. The embryo is attached at its narrow caudal end to the chorion by the connecting stalk.

The ovulation age of the embryo at this stage of development is about 20 days, and its length is almost 1.5 mm. The time is now rapidly approaching when simple diffusion of oxygen and nutrients cannot adequately provide for the greatly increasing metabolic needs of the embryo, and a functional circulatory system becomes necessary.

Plate 4.2

Embryology

Presomite stage (1.5-mm embryo) at approximately 20 days

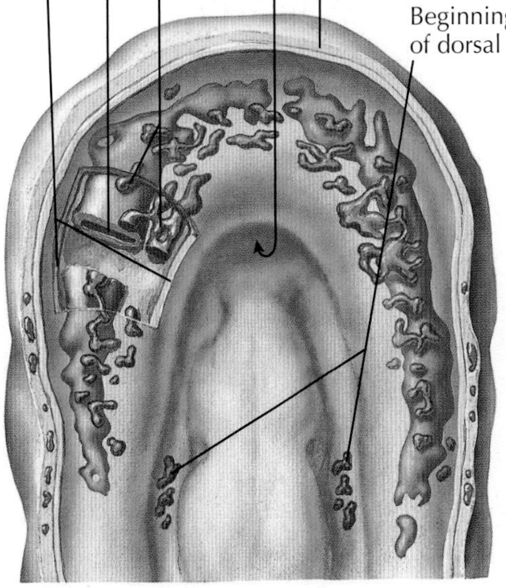

Window cut in endoderm

Intraembryonic coelom

Blood islands (of cardiogenic plate)

Foregut

Amnion

Beginnings of dorsal aortae

Yolk sac

Blood island

Intraembryonic coelom

Foregut

Oropharyngeal membrane

Neural plate

Amniotic cavity

Ventral dissection

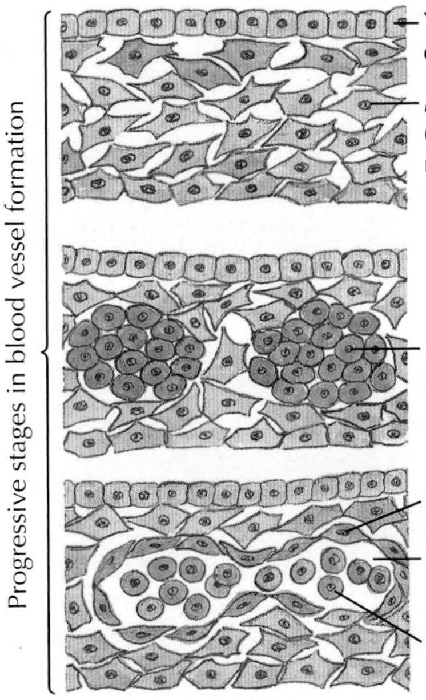

EARLY INTRAEMBRYONIC VASCULOGENESIS

PRESOMITE STAGE

Although not the first organ system to make its appearance in the embryo, the cardiovascular system reaches a functional state long before the other systems, while still in a relatively primitive state of development. The vascular system grows from a simple, bilaterally symmetric plexus into an asymmetric, complex system of arteries, veins, and capillaries—a necessarily dynamic process involving the formation of new vessels and temporary detours, rerouting of the bloodstream, and the disappearance of previously dominant channels or even of entire vascular subsystems. The vascular system needs to enlarge as the embryo grows, adapting to marked changes in embryonic shape and developmental changes in other organ systems. While hard at work, the heart also must grow and differentiate from a simple tube into a complex, four-chambered organ with sets of valves. Finally, because the very young embryo is tiny compared with the mass of extraembryonic (placental) tissue, which the young heart also supplies with blood, this heart is relatively enormous compared with its relative size in the adult.

Describing the development of the cardiovascular system first requires review of the *intraembryonic coelom* ("body cavity") formed by the confluence of small, initially isolated spaces that appear in the lateral mesoderm and cardiogenic mesoderm. The spaces fuse together and form the single, horseshoe-shaped intraembryonic coelom that extends the length of the embryo in the lateral mesoderm on each side, communicating across the midline cranially in the cardiogenic mesoderm. Later in development, a communication develops on each side between the caudal ends of the intraembryonic coelom and the extraembryonic coelom.

The formation of the coelom separates the lateral mesoderm into two layers: the *parietal* layer in contact with the ectoderm and the *visceral* layer in contact with the endoderm. The ectoderm with its parietal layer of lateral plate mesoderm is called *somatopleure;* endoderm with its visceral mesodermal layer is called *splanchnopleure.*

In the late *presomite* embryo, scattered masses of angiogenic cells differentiate in the cardiogenic mesoderm and the splanchnopleure mesoderm ventral to the entire extent of the horseshoe-shaped coelom. These cells also appear earlier in the wall of the umbilical vesicle (yolk sac). The angiogenic cell clusters, called *blood islands,* rapidly increase in number and size, acquire a lumen surrounded by a simple squamous endothelium, and unite to form a plexus of vessels. The angiogenic clusters can also form angioblastic cords that canalize to form vessels. In the cardiogenic

Progressive stages in blood vessel formation

Yolk sac endoderm

Mesenchyme cells (splanchnopleuric mesoderm)

Blood island

Endothelium

Lumen of primitive vessel

Primitive blood cell

Endoderm

Connecting stalk

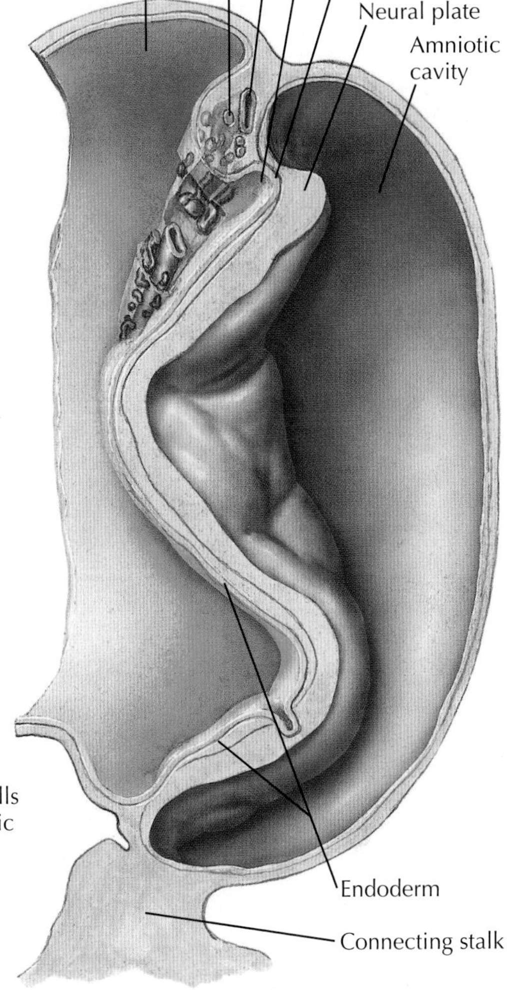

Sagittal dissection (paramedian)

mesoderm, paired endothelial heart tubes develop from paired angioblastic cords. The tubes are ventral to the central part of the U-shaped coelom that will form the pericardial cavity. The paired heart tubes begin to beat by day 21 or 22 and fuse into a single heart tube a few days later.

Another pair of angioblastic cords appear bilaterally, parallel and rather close to the midline of the embryo. These cords also acquire a lumen and form a pair of

longitudinal vessels, the *dorsal aortae* (aortas). These vessels connect with the dorsocranial aspect of the endothelial (endocardial) heart tubes to establish the arterial pole of the developing heart. The caudal ends of the endothelial heart tubes make contact with vessels arising in the yolk sac mesoderm (vitelline veins) and later with the developing umbilical veins and common cardinal veins. Thus the venous pole of the heart, still paired, is determined.

Plate 4.3

Cardiovascular System: VOLUME 8

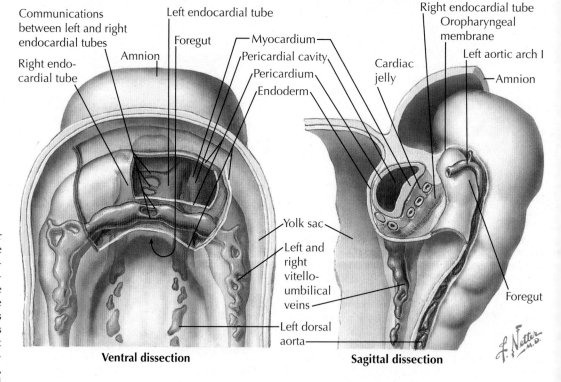

One-somite stage (1.5 mm) at approximately 20 days

Intraembryonic coelom (pericardial cavity)
Right endocardial tube
Foregut
Amnion
Left endocardial tube
Yolk sac
Left dorsal aorta

Ventral dissection

Right endocardial tube
Myocardium
Intraembryonic coelom (pericardial cavity)
Foregut
Left aortic arch I
Forebrain
Amnion

Sagittal dissection

Two-somite stage (1.8 mm) at approximately 21 days

Communications between left and right endocardial tubes
Right endo-cardial tube
Amnion
Left endocardial tube
Foregut
Myocardium
Pericardial cavity
Pericardium
Endoderm
Yolk sac
Left and right vitello-umbilical veins
Left dorsal aorta

Ventral dissection

Right endocardial tube
Oropharyngeal membrane
Left aortic arch I
Amnion
Cardiac jelly
Foregut

Sagittal dissection

FORMATION OF THE HEART TUBE

ONE-SOMITE AND TWO-SOMITE STAGES

As the primitive, bilaterally symmetric cardiovascular system appears, shaping of the embryo during the fourth week profoundly influences the relative position of the cardiac portion of this system. The trilaminar embryonic disc folds into a cylinder, and the amnion tucks around the embryo on each side. The amnion also envelops the head end of the embryo as the ectodermal tube of the forebrain rapidly increases in size in a cranial and ventral direction. The result is a 180-degree sagittal plane rotation of the cardiogenic mesoderm and oropharyngeal membrane, which were originally cranial to the neural plate and the developing neural tube. The heart is now caudal to the oropharyngeal membrane rather than cranial, and the heart locates dorsal to the developing pericardial cavity (Plate 4.3).

The folding of the gastrula also results in (1) formation of an endodermal gut tube consisting of a foregut, midgut, and hindgut and (2) each dorsal aorta leaving the cranial end of the endocardial tubes and curving dorsally around the foregut. Thus the first pair of *aortic arches,* or pharyngeal (branchial) arch arteries, appear.

With the folding of the trilaminar embryonic disc, the endoderm is shaped into a tube within the embryo. The *midgut* is continuous with the umbilical vesicle (yolk sac) that extends ventrally from the embryo. The *foregut* is an extension into the head region of the embryo, and the *hindgut* is a caudal extension. The umbilical vesicle is pressed against the connecting stalk, and the intraembryonic part becomes a narrow duct connected to the midgut. With the rotation of the cardiogenic mesoderm and oropharyngeal membrane from growth of the forebrain, the developing heart swings to a position ventral to the foregut, a relationship retained in the adult. The dorsal aortae are dorsal to the foregut, and pairs of pharyngeal (branchial) arch arteries flank the foregut to connect the heart tubes with the aortae.

Plate 4.4

Embryology

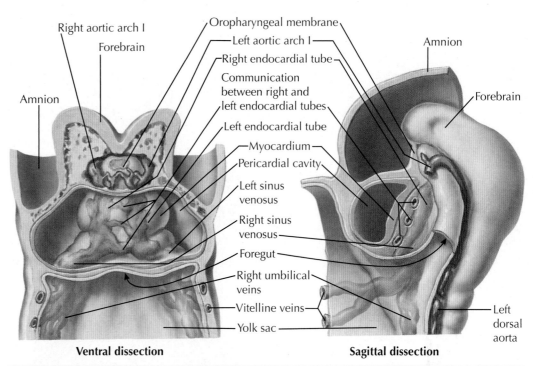

Four-somite stage (2.0 mm) at approximately 22 days

Right aortic arch I
Forebrain
Amnion
Oropharyngeal membrane
Left aortic arch I
Right endocardial tube
Communication between right and left endocardial tubes
Left endocardial tube
Myocardium
Pericardial cavity
Left sinus venosus
Right sinus venosus
Foregut
Right umbilical veins
Vitelline veins
Yolk sac
Amnion
Forebrain
Left dorsal aorta

Ventral dissection

Sagittal dissection

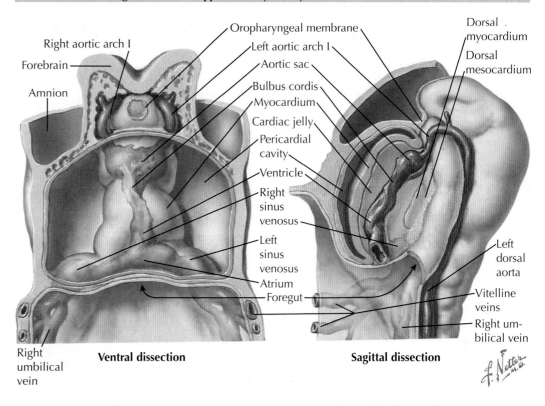

Seven-somite stage (2.2 mm) at approximately 23 days

Right aortic arch I
Forebrain
Amnion
Oropharyngeal membrane
Left aortic arch I
Aortic sac
Bulbus cordis
Myocardium
Cardiac jelly
Pericardial cavity
Ventricle
Right sinus venosus
Left sinus venosus
Atrium
Foregut
Right umbilical vein
Dorsal myocardium
Dorsal mesocardium
Left dorsal aorta
Vitelline veins
Right umbilical vein

Ventral dissection

Sagittal dissection

FORMATION OF THE HEART TUBE (Continued)

As a result of all of these changes, the endothelial heart (endocardial) tubes lie closer and parallel to each other. They quickly fuse into a single tube in a craniocaudal direction.

FOUR-SOMITE AND SEVEN-SOMITE STAGES

As indicated earlier, the heart tube is dorsal to the developing pericardial cavity. As the tube enlarges and bends, it bulges into the underlying coelom. As the heart tube comes to rest entirely within the pericardial cavity, it is suspended by the two opposing epithelial layers of the pericardial sac, the *dorsal mesocardium*. A ventral mesocardium never develops.

The mesodermal tissue surrounding the *endothelial heart* (endocardial) *tube,* meanwhile, has differentiated into three layers. The inner layer immediately around the endothelium is initially thick, gelatinous connective tissue called the *cardiac jelly.* The next layer is the cellular *primitive myocardium.* The third (outer) layer consists of flat mesothelial cells that also line the remaining pericardial cavity.

The cardiac jelly disappears. The endocardial tubes persist as the inner lining of the heart chambers, the *endocardium.* The primitive myocardium elaborates and matures to become the muscular wall of the heart, the myocardium. The simple squamous *epicardium,* although continuous with the rest of the pericardial sac, derives from cells overlying the sinus venosus of the heart tube that migrate over the heart (Plate 4.4).

The embryo now has seven somites, is about 2.2 mm long, and is approximately 23 days old. About 3 days have elapsed between the appearance of intraembryonic vasculogenesis and the formation of the endocardial tube. About this time, or slightly earlier, the heart begins to beat. No known cardiac anomaly can be attributed to the developmental phases described thus far, except the rare cases of acardia seen infrequently in twins with a common placental circulation.

Plate 4.5

Cardiovascular System: VOLUME 8

10-Somite stage (2.5 mm) at approximately 23 days

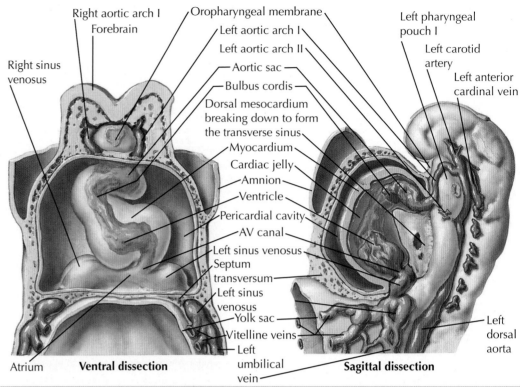

Right aortic arch I
Forebrain
Oropharyngeal membrane
Left aortic arch I
Left aortic arch II
Aortic sac
Bulbus cordis
Dorsal mesocardium breaking down to form the transverse sinus
Myocardium
Cardiac jelly
Amnion
Ventricle
Pericardial cavity
AV canal
Left sinus venosus
Septum transversum
Left sinus venosus
Yolk sac
Vitelline veins
Left umbilical vein
Right sinus venosus
Atrium
Ventral dissection
Left pharyngeal pouch I
Left carotid artery
Left anterior cardinal vein
Left dorsal aorta
Sagittal dissection

14-Somite stage (3.0 mm) at approximately 24 days

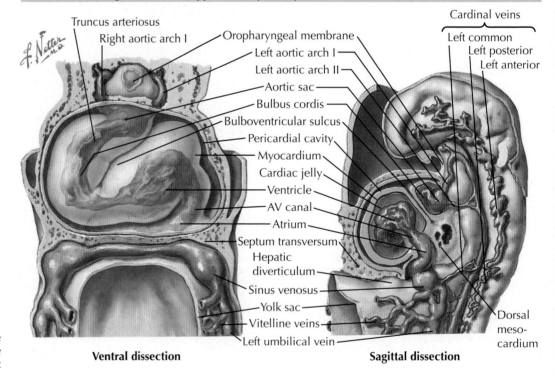

Truncus arteriosus
Right aortic arch I
Oropharyngeal membrane
Left aortic arch I
Left aortic arch II
Aortic sac
Bulbus cordis
Bulboventricular sulcus
Pericardial cavity
Myocardium
Cardiac jelly
Ventricle
AV canal
Atrium
Septum transversum
Hepatic diverticulum
Sinus venosus
Yolk sac
Vitelline veins
Left umbilical vein
Ventral dissection
Cardinal veins
Left common
Left posterior
Left anterior
Dorsal mesocardium
Sagittal dissection

FORMATION OF THE HEART LOOP

At the beginning of the next phase of development, the heart, as described earlier, is essentially a straight tube with a caudal venosus end and cranial arterial end. It lies within the *pericardial cavity* and is attached posteriorly only by the *dorsal mesocardium*.

10-SOMITE AND 14-SOMITE STAGES

A series of chambers forms in sequence within the tube. At the venous end the *sinus venosus* develops left and right horns and receives blood from the common cardinal veins, vitelline veins, and umbilical veins (two initially, one later). These veins return blood from the embryo, umbilical vesicle (yolk sac), and placenta, respectively (Plate 4.5). From the sinus venosus, blood flows into a *primordial atrium,* a *primordial ventricle,* a chamber called the *bulbus cordis,* and then out the arterial end of the heart tube through the *truncus arteriosus*. Blood from the truncus arteriosus flows into a dilated *aortic sac* ventral to the foregut. The first pair of pharyngeal (branchial) arch arteries (aortic arches) connects the aortic sac to the dorsal aortae. The ventricle and bulbus cordis grow faster than the other parts of the heart tube. Because its two ends are fixed, the heart tube is forced to bend to adapt to the available pericardial space. The bend is between the ventricle and bulbus cordis, forming a *bulboventricular loop* that extends ventrally and to the right. A result of the bend is the more cranial and dorsal position of the atrium and sinus venosus behind the truncus arteriosus outflow tract of the heart

Plate 4.6

Embryology

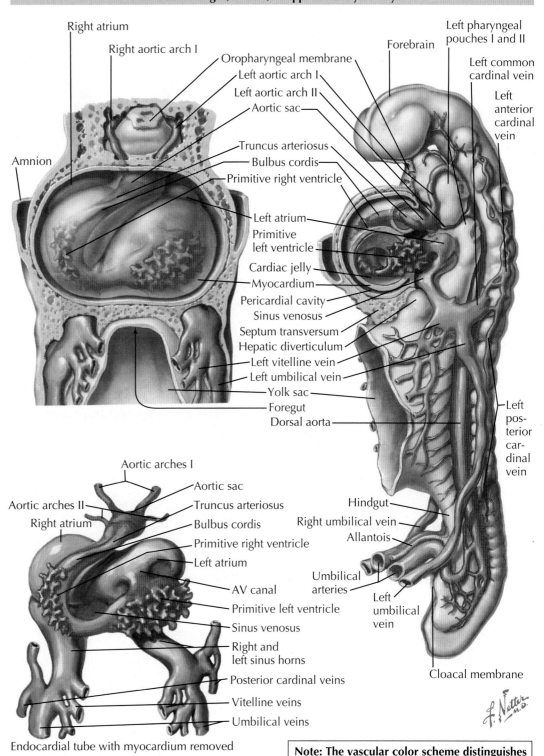

20-Somite stage (3.2 mm) at approximately 25 days

Right atrium
Right aortic arch I
Oropharyngeal membrane
Left aortic arch I
Left aortic arch II
Aortic sac
Amnion
Truncus arteriosus
Bulbus cordis
Primitive right ventricle
Left atrium
Primitive left ventricle
Cardiac jelly
Myocardium
Pericardial cavity
Sinus venosus
Septum transversum
Hepatic diverticulum
Left vitelline vein
Left umbilical vein
Yolk sac
Foregut
Dorsal aorta

Forebrain
Left pharyngeal pouches I and II
Left common cardinal vein
Left anterior cardinal vein
Left posterior cardinal vein

Aortic arches I
Aortic sac
Aortic arches II
Truncus arteriosus
Right atrium
Bulbus cordis
Primitive right ventricle
Left atrium
AV canal
Primitive left ventricle
Sinus venosus
Right and left sinus horns
Posterior cardinal veins
Vitelline veins
Umbilical veins

Hindgut
Right umbilical vein
Allantois
Umbilical arteries
Left umbilical vein
Cloacal membrane

Endocardial tube with myocardium removed

Note: The vascular color scheme distinguishes veins from arteries. It does not reflect blood oxygenation levels.

FORMATION OF THE HEART LOOP (Continued)

tube. At the same time, perforations appear in the dorsal mesocardium, leading to its disappearance as the openings increase in size. The result is the formation of the *transverse pericardial sinus,* the space between the arteries and veins at the top of the adult heart that connects the left and right aspects of the pericardial cavity.

20-SOMITE STAGE

At the close of this phase of development, numerous *diverticula* appear in the ventral aspect of the early ventricle and in the proximal third of the bulbus cordis.

These diverticula project initially into the cardiac jelly and later into the myocardium, expanding the capacity of the heart sections involved and becoming the mechanism of formation of the trabecular muscle of the ventricular walls. At this point, although bending and local elaborations have changed its appearance, the heart still consists of essentially a single tube. A small, *interventricular septum* appears, marking the start of

left and right ventricles and an *interventricular canal,* but these are still in sequence with regard to blood flow. Although still a tube, the heart's external appearance already strongly suggests its future four-chambered structure. The elaboration of septa will further define the atria and ventricles. The embryo is now about 3.2 mm long and approximately 25 days old, and it possesses 20 somites (Plate 4.6).

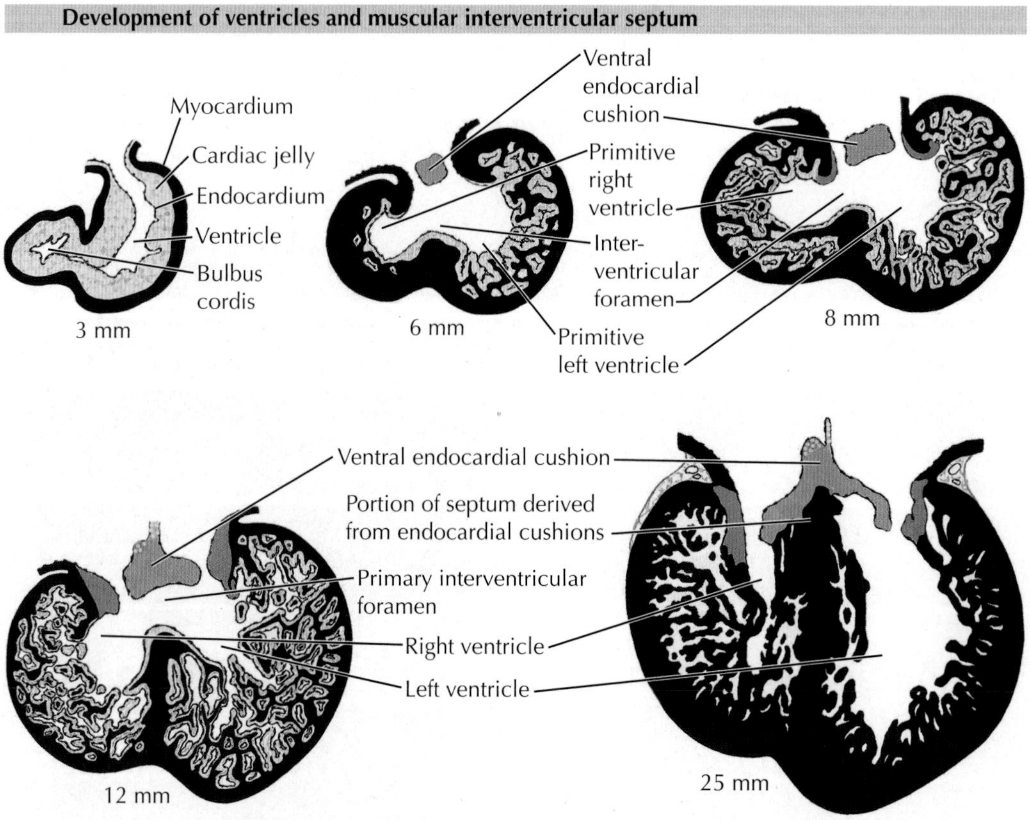

Plate 4.7

Cardiovascular System: VOLUME 8

Development of ventricles and muscular interventricular septum

Myocardium
Cardiac jelly
Endocardium
Ventricle
Bulbus cordis

3 mm

Ventral endocardial cushion
Primitive right ventricle
Inter-ventricular foramen
Primitive left ventricle

6 mm

8 mm

Ventral endocardial cushion
Portion of septum derived from endocardial cushions
Primary interventricular foramen
Right ventricle
Left ventricle

12 mm

25 mm

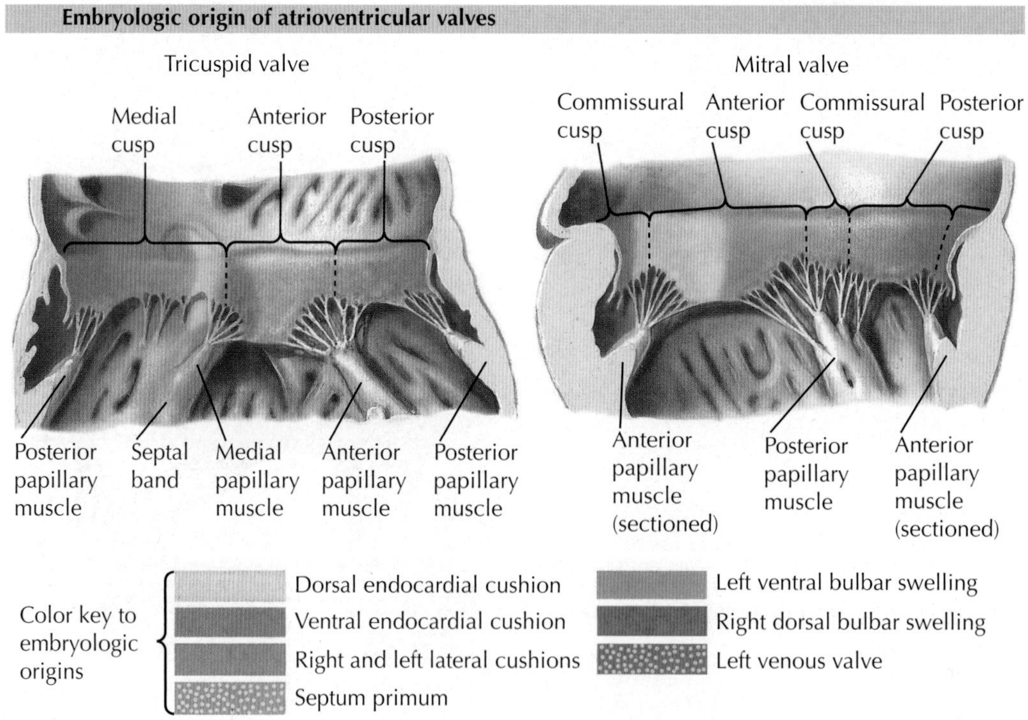

Embryologic origin of atrioventricular valves

Tricuspid valve

Medial cusp
Anterior cusp
Posterior cusp

Posterior papillary muscle
Septal band
Medial papillary muscle
Anterior papillary muscle
Posterior papillary muscle

Mitral valve

Commissural cusp
Anterior cusp
Commissural cusp
Posterior cusp

Anterior papillary muscle (sectioned)
Posterior papillary muscle
Anterior papillary muscle (sectioned)

Color key to embryologic origins

Dorsal endocardial cushion
Ventral endocardial cushion
Right and left lateral cushions
Septum primum

Left ventral bulbar swelling
Right dorsal bulbar swelling
Left venous valve

FORMATION OF CARDIAC SEPTA

At the close of the preceding phase of development, the heart completely occupies the pericardial cavity. Blood flows in a single path through the sinus venosus and atrium, through an atrioventricular canal into the left ventricle, though an interventricular canal above the free edge of the *primordial interventricular septum* into the right ventricle, and then out the bulbus cordis and truncus arteriosus. The stage is now set for the septation of the heart, which lasts about 10 days. No major changes occur in the external appearance of the heart. The formation of the various cardiac septa occurs more or less simultaneously; for descriptive purposes, however, it is necessary to consider their development separately.

ATRIOVENTRICULAR CANAL

Blood flow through the heart is first separated into left and right sides by dorsal and ventral *endocardial cushions* that appear about day 24. Endocardial cushions are swellings of mesenchymal tissue that grow toward each other and then fuse to divide the *atrioventricular* (AV) *canal* into left and right AV canals (Plate 4.7). The primordial atrium begins to shape into a left atrium and a right atrium, although at this early stage the atria are in wide communication with each other. With the appearance of the endocardial cushions and primordial interventricular septum, the four chambers can be identified, but blood from the sinus venosus still enters the

heart in one location, the right atrium, and it exits the heart in one location, the right ventricle. Half the blood in the right atrium passes through the right AV canal into the right ventricle and then out through the bulbus cordis and truncus arteriosus. The other half of the blood in the right atrium passes into the left atrium, through the left AV canal into the left ventricle, and then to the right ventricle and the same exit path through bulbus cordis and truncus arteriosus.

ATRIA, ATRIAL SEPTUM, AND PULMONARY VEINS

The atria are divided by two adjacent septa that function as a valve permitting blood to flow from primitive right atrium to left atrium but not in the other direction. This plays a crucial role in having blood bypass the nonfunctioning prenatal lungs and in converting the prenatal circulatory pattern to the postnatal configuration soon after the first breath of the newborn.

Plate 4.8

Embryology

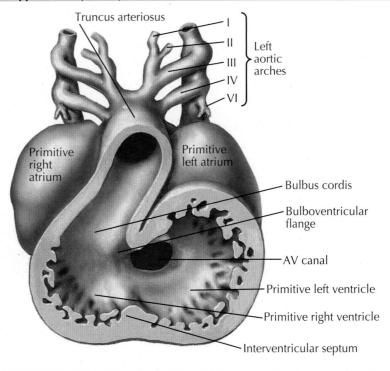

4 to 5 mm (approximately 27 days)

Truncus arteriosus

I
II
III
IV
VI

Left aortic arches

Primitive right atrium

Primitive left atrium

Bulbus cordis

Bulboventricular flange

AV canal

Primitive left ventricle

Primitive right ventricle

Interventricular septum

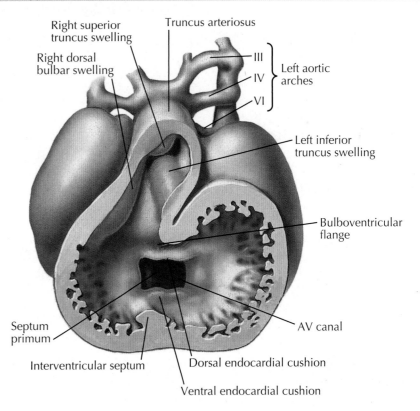

6 to 7 mm (approximately 29 days)

Right superior truncus swelling

Truncus arteriosus

Right dorsal bulbar swelling

III
IV
VI

Left aortic arches

Left inferior truncus swelling

Bulboventricular flange

AV canal

Septum primum

Interventricular septum

Dorsal endocardial cushion

Ventral endocardial cushion

FORMATION OF CARDIAC SEPTA (Continued)

The truncus arteriosus forms a depression on the external surface of the common atrium that corresponds on the inside to a crescent-shaped ridge, the *septum primum* (see Plate 4.7). It grows inferiorly toward the fused endocardial cushions. The transient interatrial passage inferior to it is the *foramen primum,* which disappears as the septum primum fuses with the endocardial cushions. Before this happens, holes appear high up on the septum primum and coalesce to form a *foramen secundum* in the septum primum. On the right atrium side of the septum primum, a thick, muscular *septum secundum* grows inferiorly toward the endocardial cushions. It also has a crescent shape that, with continued growth, will circumscribe an oval foramen in the septum secundum, the *foramen ovale.* The foramen secundum is at a higher level than the foramen ovale. Oxygen-rich blood in the fetal inferior vena cava is directed at the foramen ovale. It pushes the septum primum away from the septum secundum to allow blood to pass through the foramen secundum into the left atrium. With increased blood pressure in the left atrium at birth from increased pulmonary blood flow, however, the septum primum is pressed against the relatively stiff septum secundum, effectively closing the foramen ovale. After fusion of septum primum with septum secundum, the foramen ovale becomes the *fossa ovalis* of the right atrium. Growth of

the septum secundum occurs during the fifth and sixth weeks.

A single embryonic *pulmonary vein,* present in a 5- to 6-mm embryo, develops as an outgrowth of the posterior left atrial wall. It connects with the splanchnic plexus of veins in the region of the developing lung buds. Later in development, the vein itself and parts of its first four branches (two from the left lung and two from the right) expand tremendously and become incorporated into the left atrium to form the larger,

smooth, posterior part of the adult atrium. In the fully developed heart, the original embryonic left atrium is represented by little more than the trabeculated atrial appendage (auricle). The intrapulmonary part of the splanchnic venous plexus ultimately loses its connections with the systemic veins and drains exclusively by way of the pulmonary veins.

On the right side, the right sinus horn is similarly incorporated into the right atrium; it enlarges mainly in its vertical diameter, and the relative distance

Plate 4.9

Cardiovascular System: VOLUME 8

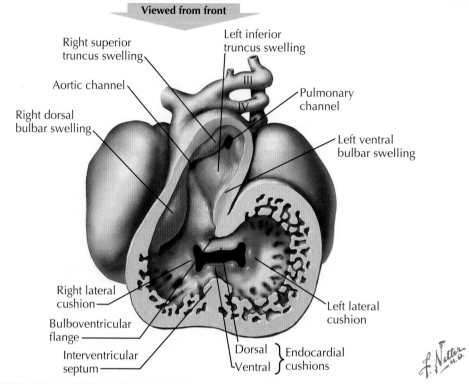

8 to 9 mm (approximately 31 days)

Viewed from front

Right superior truncus swelling

Left inferior truncus swelling

Aortic channel

Pulmonary channel

Right dorsal bulbar swelling

Left ventral bulbar swelling

Right lateral cushion

Left lateral cushion

Bulboventricular flange

Dorsal
Ventral } Endocardial cushions

Interventricular septum

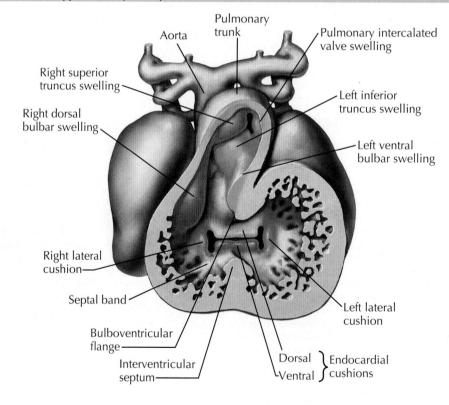

9 to 10 mm (approximately 33 days)

Pulmonary trunk

Aorta

Pulmonary intercalated valve swelling

Right superior truncus swelling

Left inferior truncus swelling

Right dorsal bulbar swelling

Left ventral bulbar swelling

Right lateral cushion

Septal band

Left lateral cushion

Bulboventricular flange

Dorsal
Ventral } Endocardial cushions

Interventricular septum

FORMATION OF CARDIAC SEPTA (Continued)

between the common cardinal vein (proximal *superior vena cava* [SVC]) and the *inferior vena cava* (from the right vitelline vein) increases. The original embryonic right atrium becomes the *right atrial appendage* (auricle), containing the earliest-appearing pectinate muscles. A lateral wall with pectinate muscle will grow to become the largest component of the right atrial wall. Thus the primitive right atrium becomes the right atrial appendage with its pectinate muscle, the right horn of the sinus venosus becomes the smooth back wall of the right atrium, and new pectinate muscle develops into the lateral wall.

DEVELOPMENT OF THE VENTRICLES

The primordial right and left ventricles are little more than sequential local widening of the original cardiac tube, and they are connected to each other by a smooth-walled, relatively narrow channel, the *primary interventricular foramen*. As the heart tube folds, the interventricular foramen is bounded inferiorly by the developing *interventricular septum* (see Plate 4.8). Completion of the ventricular separation is intimately related to division of the outflow tract of the primitive heart tube: the bulbus cordis and truncus arteriosus.

In an embryo of about 4 to 5 mm, the AV canal still leads into the primitive left ventricle, and blood can

reach the primitive right ventricle only by way of the primary interventricular foramen. After division of the AV canal by the endocardial cushions into left and right AV canals, blood still must pass from the left ventricle to the right ventricle before exiting the heart. If the interventricular septum simply grew to fuse with the endocardial cushions, there would be no exit of blood from the left ventricle.

Enlargement of the ventricles is accomplished by centrifugal growth of the myocardium, always closely followed by increasing diverticulation and formation of trabeculae internally; this prevents the compact outer layer of the myocardium from becoming too thick and solid. Typically, the ventricles of the embryonic heart consist of a tremendous mass of trabeculae enclosed by a rather thin outer layer of compact myocardium. Most

Plate 4.10

Embryology

16 mm (approximately 37 days)

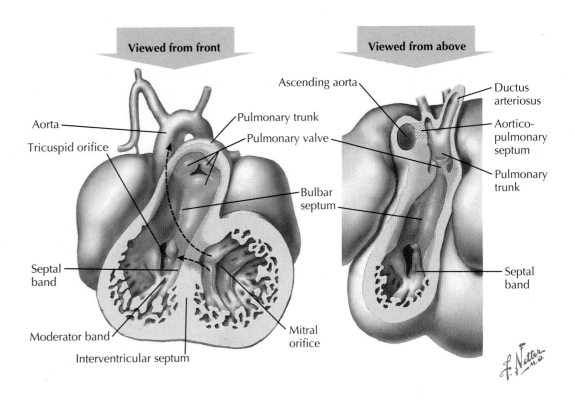

Viewed from front

Viewed from above

Ascending aorta

Ductus arteriosus

Aorta

Pulmonary trunk

Aortico-pulmonary septum

Tricuspid orifice

Pulmonary valve

Bulbar septum

Pulmonary trunk

Septal band

Septal band

Moderator band

Mitral orifice

Interventricular septum

40 mm (approximately 55 days)

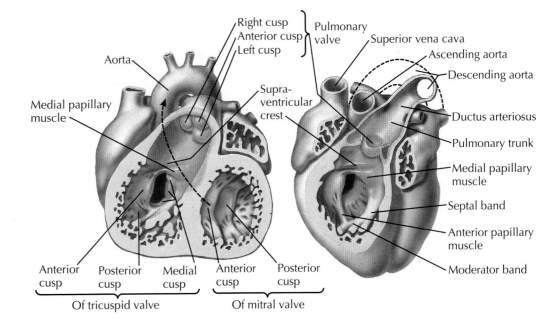

Right cusp

Anterior cusp

Pulmonary valve

Left cusp

Superior vena cava

Ascending aorta

Aorta

Descending aorta

Medial papillary muscle

Supraventricular crest

Ductus arteriosus

Pulmonary trunk

Medial papillary muscle

Septal band

Anterior cusp

Posterior cusp

Medial cusp

Anterior cusp

Posterior cusp

Anterior papillary muscle

Moderator band

Of tricuspid valve

Of mitral valve

FORMATION OF CARDIAC SEPTA (Continued)

of the trabeculae eventually disappear. Of the remaining trabeculae, some coalesce to form larger structures such as *papillary muscles* and the *moderator band;* others are reduced to thin, fibrous strands (e.g., *chordae tendineae*) that connect the papillary muscles to the atrioventricular valve cusps (see Plate 4.7).

The primary interventricular septum is thick and gives rise to the inferior, muscular part of the adult septum. Again, it does not continue to grow to fuse with the endocardial cushions. Instead, it will fuse with a septum that divides the bulbus cordis and truncus arteriosus. The *primary interventricular foramen* never closes but actually enlarges and, in the fully developed heart, gives access to the *aortic vestibule,* the smooth upper part of the left ventricle that leads to the aortic valve.

TRUNCUS ARTERIOSUS AND BULBUS CORDIS

Distal to the ventricles in the outflow part of the heart tube is a dilation, the *bulbus cordis,* followed by a tapering *truncus arteriosus* (see Plate 4.8). Potentially confusing terms have been used to describe these structures; some consider these two outflow chambers to be a single structure, sometimes referred to as the bulbus cordis, sometimes as the truncus arteriosus. Another term used for the interface between the two is the "conus

cordis." Word combinations are also used, such as "truncoconal" to describe septal swellings (see Plate 4.9). This section uses more recent and common terms, the bulbus cordis leading to the truncus arteriosus.

The bulbus cordis and truncus arteriosus are divided lengthwise by a *spiral septum,* also called the *aorticopulmonary septum,* named after the ascending aorta and pulmonary trunk that are derived from the truncus arteriosus ("arterial trunk"). Two streams of blood spiral

through this part of the heart tube, and longitudinal septa form in the path of least resistance between the two streams (Plate 4.10).

The process begins in the 6-mm embryo at the end of the fourth week and is completed near the end of the sixth week (14- to 15-mm embryo). It proceeds in a distal-to-proximal direction; the truncus arteriosus is divided first, followed by the bulbus cordis. The two opposing ridges dividing the bulbus cordis are called *left*

Plate 4.11

Cardiovascular System: VOLUME 8

HEART TUBE DERIVATIVES
Heart tube primordia

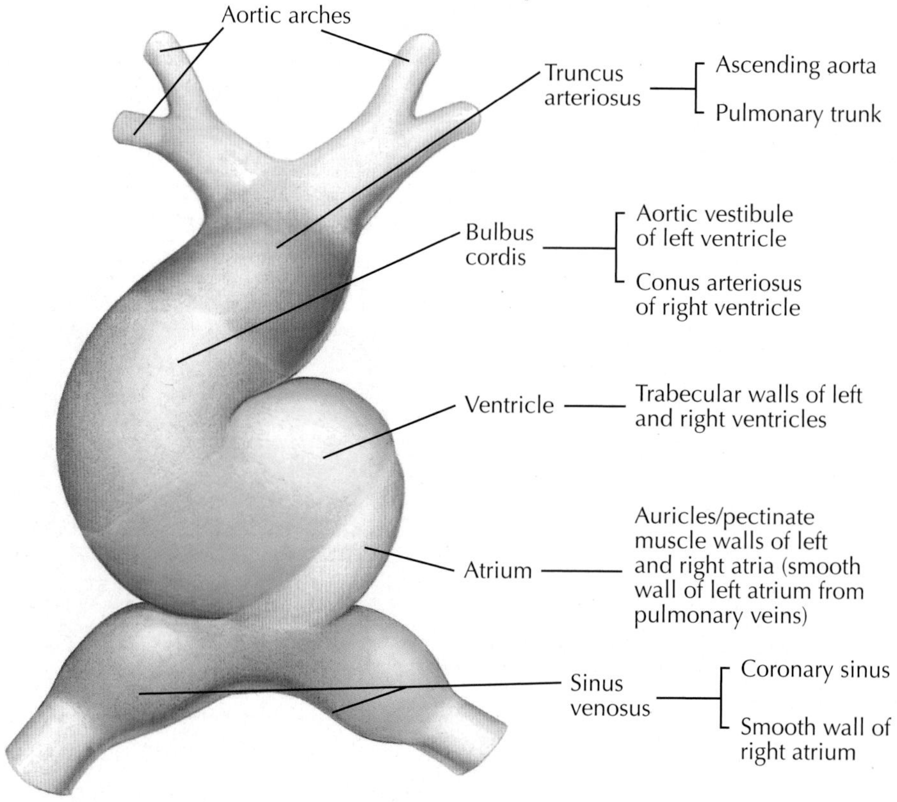

Aortic arches

Truncus arteriosus — Ascending aorta / Pulmonary trunk

Bulbus cordis — Aortic vestibule of left ventricle / Conus arteriosus of right ventricle

Ventricle — Trabecular walls of left and right ventricles

Atrium — Auricles/pectinate muscle walls of left and right atria (smooth wall of left atrium from pulmonary veins)

Sinus venosus — Coronary sinus / Smooth wall of right atrium

Heart tube derivatives

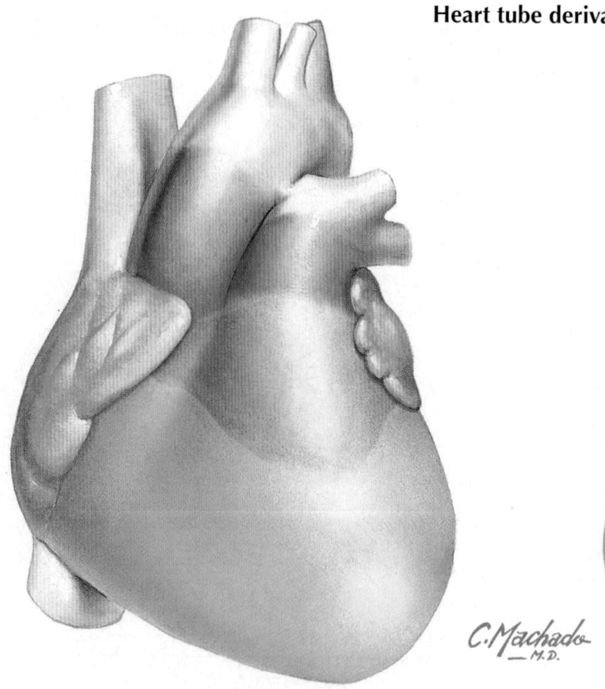

Adult heart, anterior view

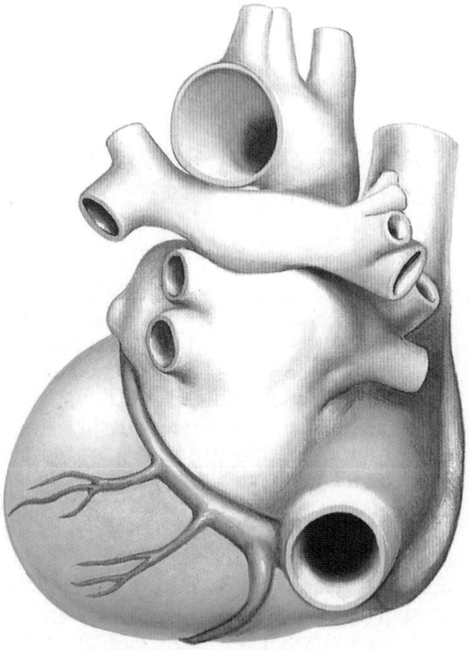

C. Machado M.D.

Adult heart, posterior view

FORMATION OF CARDIAC SEPTA (Continued)

and right bulbar ridges, which are the proximal parts of the developing spiral septum. The ridges are continuous with the attached edges of the *muscular* interventricular septum. The fusion of these ridges with each other, with the interventricular septum, and with the endocardial cushions completes division of the ventricles and creates an outflow path for each chamber. The thin upper *membranous* interventricular septum derives from an extension of tissue on the right side of the endocardial cushions. It fuses with the muscular interventricular septum and bulbar ridges of the spiral septum. Membranous septal defects are the most common heart defect (25% of all congenital heart defects), partly because three basic primordia (interventricular septum, spiral septum, endocardial cushions) are required to fuse in an area of very dynamic blood flow. There is considerable opportunity for a failure of fusion of these elements at the location of the membranous interventricular septum.

The spiral septum is a suitable synonym for the aorticopulmonary septum because of its orientation in the outflow part of the embryonic heart tube and the resulting relationship of the adult arterial derivatives of the chambers it divides. The ascending aorta arises posterior to the pulmonary trunk in the adult heart, spirals up to the right of the pulmonary trunk, and continues anteriorly to form the aortic arch that passes over the bifurcation of the trunk into left and right pulmonary arteries.

The bulbus cordis is incorporated into the ventricles, forming the upper smooth-walled outflow part of each ventricle: the *conus arteriosus* in the right ventricle, just below the pulmonic semilunar valve, and the *aortic vestibule* of the left ventricle, leading to the aortic semilunar valve (Plate 4.11). The inferior trabeculated part of each ventricle derives from the primitive ventricle. Because of the oblique orientation of the bulbar (spiral septum) ridges, part of the primitive right ventricle is captured by the left ventricle when the ridges fuse to the interventricular septum. As a result, the embryonic interventricular foramen above the primary interventricular septum is retained as the interface between the aortic vestibule and trabecular part of the left ventricle.

SINUS VENOSUS

The cardiovascular system in the early embryo is paired and symmetric. At about day 23, the seven-somite stage, the paired endothelial heart tubes fuse, beginning in

Plate 4.12

Embryology

PARTITIONING OF THE HEART TUBE: ATRIAL SEPTATION

After fusion of the endocardial cushions and the establishment of a left and right flow of blood, the heart still has one primary site of entry for blood (right atrium) and one primary site of exit (right ventricle). Blood must be able to pass between the atria and between the ventricles.

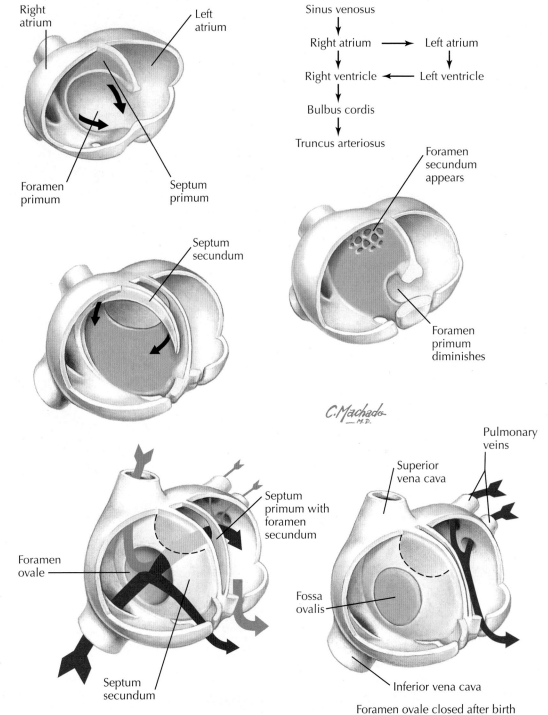

Right atrium

Left atrium

Sinus venosus → Right atrium → Left atrium
Right ventricle ← Left ventricle
Bulbus cordis
Truncus arteriosus

Foramen primum

Septum primum

Foramen secundum appears

Septum secundum

Foramen primum diminishes

C. Machado —M.D.

Pulmonary veins

Superior vena cava

Septum primum with foramen secundum

Foramen ovale

Fossa ovalis

Septum secundum

Inferior vena cava

Foramen ovale closed after birth with increased pulmonary flow

FORMATION OF CARDIAC SEPTA (Continued)

the bulboventricular region and progressing toward the venous pole of the heart. The sinus venosus maintains its paired condition. Early in the fourth week, a central unpaired part of the sinus venosus opens into the primitive atrium and right and left sinus horns.

At this stage the sinus venosus receives three pairs of veins. Most medially, at the junction of the sinus horns and the central portion, the *vitelline veins* enter the floor of the sinus. Lateral to the vitelline veins, the *umbilical veins* enter the sinus horns from below, with the *common cardinal veins* coming from above. The proximal parts of the umbilical veins soon disappear (and the distal segment of the left umbilical vein connects with the developing inferior vena cava). Because anastomotic channels develop between the right and left systemic veins (e.g., future left brachiocephalic vein) and blood flow is preferential to the right side of the embryo, the right horn of the sinus venosus and the right proximal cardinal and vitelline veins become more important, whereas their left counterparts are greatly reduced in size. Thus the right sinus horn becomes larger, more vertical, and incorporated into the part of the primitive atrium that will become the right atrium. The right horn will form the smooth posterior wall of the right atrium, the *sinus venarum,* named after its sinus venosus origin. The communication between the sinus venosus and the developing right atrium is now limited to the right sinus horn. The

left horn of the sinus venosus becomes the *coronary sinus.* The left common cardinal vein usually disappears.

The *sinuatrial orifice* is tall and narrow, and the folds on either side constitute the *valve of the sinus venosus*, with the right fold larger than the left fold. The vertical dimension increases until a constriction in the middle creates separate openings for the developing superior and inferior venae cavae. The left fold of the valve fuses with the septum secundum to become part of the interatrial septum. The cranial part of the right valve fold becomes a

thick, vertical ridge of muscle, the *crista terminalis,* that marks the boundary between the two primordia (sinus venosus and primitive atrium) that contribute to the right atrial wall. Posterior to the crista terminalis is the smooth-walled sinus venarum; anterior to the crista terminalis is the wall of the right atrium lined with pectinate muscle, including the right atrial appendage (auricle). The inferior part of the right fold of the valve of the sinus venosus becomes the valve of the inferior vena cava and the smaller valve of the coronary sinus.

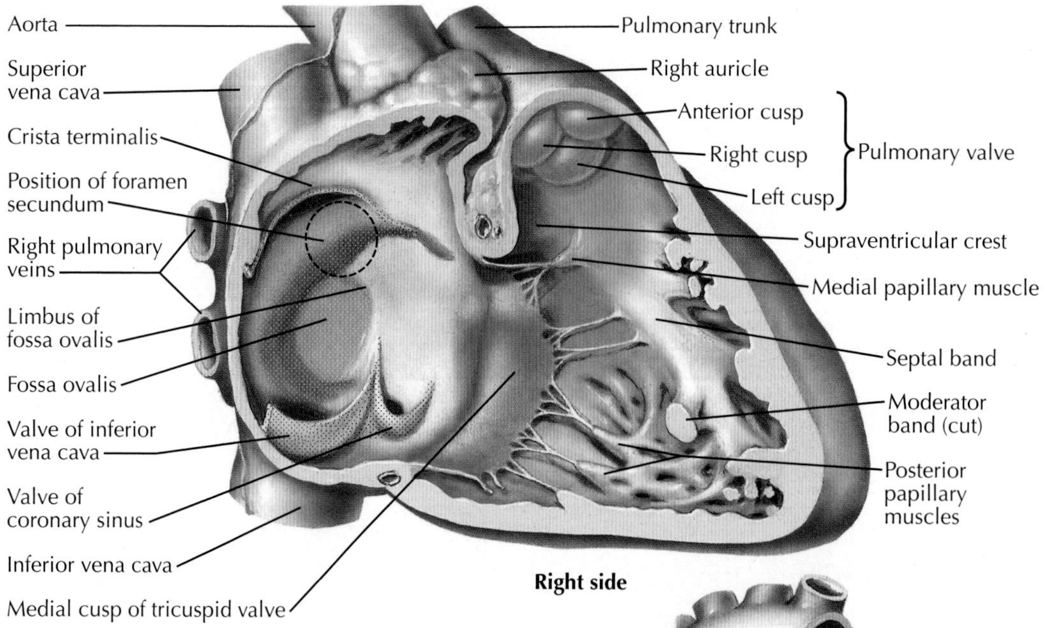

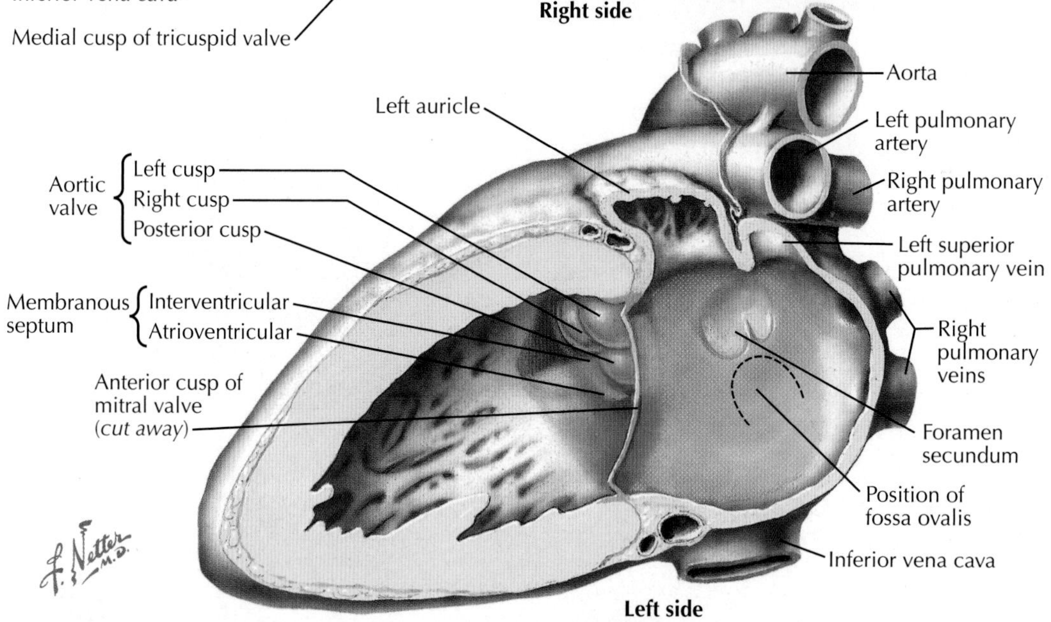

Plate 4.13

Cardiovascular System: VOLUME 8

Aorta — Pulmonary trunk

Superior vena cava — Right auricle

Crista terminalis — Anterior cusp

Position of foramen secundum — Right cusp ⎱ Pulmonary valve

Left cusp ⎰

Right pulmonary veins — Supraventricular crest

Limbus of fossa ovalis — Medial papillary muscle

Fossa ovalis — Septal band

Valve of inferior vena cava — Moderator band (cut)

Valve of coronary sinus — Posterior papillary muscles

Inferior vena cava

Medial cusp of tricuspid valve

Right side

Left auricle — Aorta

Left pulmonary artery

Aortic valve ⎰ Left cusp
Right cusp
Posterior cusp ⎱ — Right pulmonary artery

Left superior pulmonary vein

Membranous septum ⎰ Interventricular
Atrioventricular ⎱

Anterior cusp of mitral valve (cut away) — Right pulmonary veins

Foramen secundum

Position of fossa ovalis

Inferior vena cava

Left side

Color key to embryologic origins

Right sinuatrial valve flap

Left sinuatrial valve flap

Septum spurium

Septum primum

Superior endocardial cushion

Inferior endocardial cushion

Right and left lateral cushions

Right dorsal bulbar swelling

Left ventral bulbar swelling

Right superior truncus swelling

Left inferior truncus swelling

Intercalated valve swellings

FORMATION OF CARDIAC SEPTA (Continued)

Plate 4.11 summarizes the primitive heart tube chambers and their adult derivatives.

ATRIOVENTRICULAR AND SEMILUNAR VALVES

The *atrioventricular valve* cusps form from extensions of mesenchyme and ventricular muscle surrounding the AV canals (see Plate 4.7). The cusps are initially thick and fleshly, becoming thin and fibrous later. The left, bicuspid *mitral valve* initially has four cusps of equal size. The left and right cusps diminish in size and are usually identifiable in the adult valve as very small left and right *commissural cusps*. The remaining two cusps are the *anterior (aortic) cusp* and *posterior cusp*. The right *tricuspid valve* develops similarly, except three cusps develop instead of the original four (becoming two) in the mitral valve. The lateral cusp and part of the anterior cusp develop first. The medial cusp overlying the membranous interventricular septum develops later. The papillary muscles and their chordae tendineae develop from trabecular muscle. Initially thick and fleshly, the chordae tendineae become thin and fibrous as their muscular component disappears. Development of the basic structure of the mitral valve is completed by the end of the sixth week; the tricuspid valve is completed soon after (Plates 4.12 and 4.13).

The primordia of the aortic and pulmonar semilunar valves appear near the end of partitioning of the truncus arteriosus by the truncal component of the spiral septum. Four swellings of mesenchyme surround the lumen of the truncus arteriosus (see Plate 4.9). Left and right swellings are divided by the aorticopulmonary septum to form left and right valve cusps in both the ascending aorta and pulmonary trunk. The anterior swelling forms the anterior cusp in the pulmonary valve, and the posterior swelling in the truncus arteriosus forms the posterior cusp of the aortic valve. Excavation of the superior surfaces of the swellings and later thinning result in the semilunar shape of each cusp. Dilation of the proximal origins of the ascending aorta and pulmonary trunk gives rise to the pulmonary and aortic sinuses, the expanded space between each cusp and the walls of the arteries. The left and right coronary arteries arise from the left and right aortic sinuses (of Valsalva), respectively.

Plate 4.14

Embryology

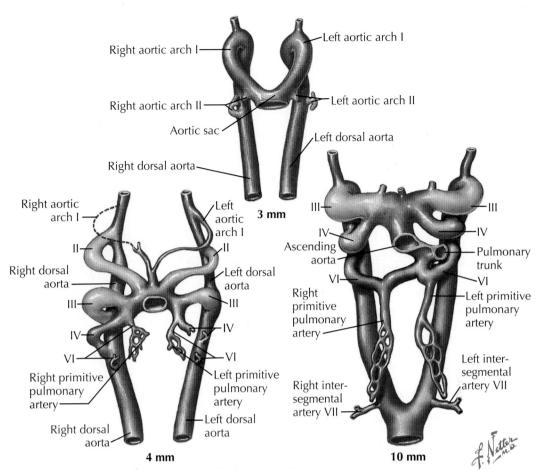

Right aortic arch I — Left aortic arch I

Right aortic arch II — Left aortic arch II

Aortic sac

Right dorsal aorta — Left dorsal aorta

3 mm

Right aortic arch I — Left aortic arch I

Right dorsal aorta — II — Left dorsal aorta

III — III

IV — IV

VI — VI

Right primitive pulmonary artery — Left primitive pulmonary artery

Right dorsal aorta — Left dorsal aorta

4 mm

III — III

IV — IV

Ascending aorta — Pulmonary trunk

VI — VI

Right primitive pulmonary artery — Left primitive pulmonary artery

Right inter-segmental artery VII — Left inter-segmental artery VII

10 mm

Development of Major Blood Vessels

The early embryonic vascular system is plexiform (intercalating). Preferential flow related to the development of organ systems, however, leads to enlargement of certain channels in the plexus. This expansion is brought about in part by the fusion and confluence of adjacent smaller vessels and by the enlargement of individual capillaries. Thus a number of vascular systems develop. As the embryo grows, new organs appear; others are transient and disappear. The various vascular systems are also continuously modified to satisfy changing needs.

Initially, the arteries and veins consist simply of endothelial tubes and cannot be distinguished from each other histologically. In later development, typical vessel walls are differentiated from the surrounding mesenchyme. The final pattern of the vascular system is genetically determined and varies with the animal species. Variations are, however, extremely common in both arterial and venous patterns, and local modifications occur in cases of abnormal development of organs.

AORTIC ARCH SYSTEM

The major arteries in an early embryo are represented by a pair of vessels, the dorsal aortae, which run with the long axis of the embryo and form the continuation of the endocardial heart tubes. Because of the changing position of the cardiogenic mesoderm containing the heart tubes, the cranial portion of each dorsal aorta comes to describe an arc on both sides of the foregut, thus establishing the first pair of aortic arch arteries, termed *aortic arches* (Plate 4.14).

In primitive vertebrates, six pairs of aortic arches appear in conjunction with the development of the corresponding pharyngeal ("branchial") arches, which are transverse swellings of mesenchyme flanking the foregut ventrally and laterally. The pharyngeal arches and their blood supply initially evolved in part to form the gills (branchiae) of aquatic vertebrates; thus their original designation as "branchial arches." In humans and other lung-breathing vertebrates, five of the six pharyngeal arches are present (the *fifth* pair of arches and arteries are rudimentary) only in early embryonic life; they become greatly modified in development as their mesenchyme differentiates into the facial skeleton and many other structures and tissues of the head and neck. As part of this process, certain aortic arches (pharyngeal arch arteries) are retained and modified to form the large arteries of the neck and thorax.

Derivatives of the aortic arch arteries and related vessels

1. Truncus arteriosus:	Proximal portions of *ascending aorta* and *pulmonary trunk*.
2. Aortic sac:	Distal portion of *ascending aorta, brachiocephalic trunk*, and aortic arch up to origin of left common carotid artery.
3. First arches:	Parts persist as components of *maxillary arteries*.
4. Second arches:	Parts persist as *stapedial arteries*.
5. Third arches:	*Common carotid arteries* and proximal segment of *internal carotid arteries*.
6. Fourth arches:	Right: Most proximal segment of *right subclavian artery*. Left: Aortic arch segment between *left common carotid* and *left subclavian arteries*.
7. Fifth arches:	No known derivations. Transient and never well developed.
8. Sixth arches:	Right: Proximal part becomes proximal segment of *right pulmonary artery*; distal part disappears early. Left: Proximal part becomes proximal segment of *left pulmonary artery*; distal part persists, until birth, as ductus arteriosus.
9. Right dorsal aorta:	Cranial portion becomes part of *right subclavian artery*; remainder disappears.
10. Left dorsal aorta:	Distal aortic arch.
11. Right seventh intersegmental artery:	Part of right *subclavian artery*.
12. Left seventh intersegmental artery:	*Left subclavian artery*.

Near the end of the third week (3-mm embryo), the first pair of arches is large; the second pair is just forming. The junction of the truncus arteriosus and the first pair of arches is somewhat dilated and is called the *aortic sac*. From this aortic sac, subsequent aortic arches originate, and new arches are added as the heart and aortic sac undergo relatively caudal displacement. Distally, the dorsal aortae fuse to form a single artery; this fusion progresses in a cranial direction, in both an absolute sense and a relative sense.

Two days later (4-mm embryo), the first arch has largely disappeared, but part of it persists as a portion of the maxillary artery. The *second arch* also regresses; all that remains of it is the tiny stapedial artery in the middle ear. The *third arch* is well developed and large. The *fourth* and *sixth arches* form as ventral and dorsal sprouts from the aortic sac and dorsal aortae, respectively, fuse with each other. The ventral portions of the sixth arches already have their major branches, the proximal portions of the left and right *primitive*

Plate 4.15

Cardiovascular System: VOLUME 8

DEVELOPMENT OF MAJOR BLOOD VESSELS (Continued)

pulmonary arteries, even though the arch itself has not yet been completed (see Plate 4.14).

Soon after the end of the fifth week (10-mm embryo), the first two aortic arches have disappeared as such; the third, fourth, and sixth arches are large. The truncus arteriosus and proximal aortic sac have divided into the ascending aorta and pulmonary trunk. The trunk is aligned with the left side of the sixth arch, which becomes the *ductus arteriosus,* a shunt from the pulmonary trunk into the aorta. The sixth aortic arch on the right disappears, and the left and right pulmonary arteries remain connected to the pulmonary trunk. *Intersegmental arteries* form between the somites; the seventh cervical pair will play an important role in the formation of the subclavian arteries and is located at about the level where the dorsal aortae join each other.

By now, the aortic arch system has largely lost its original symmetric pattern (Plate 4.15). The dorsal aortae between the third and fourth arches have disappeared on each side, and the third arches begin to elongate as the heart descends farther. The aortic sac becomes the arch of the aorta and brachiocephalic trunk, and the third arches extending from these become the left and right common carotid arteries, respectively. The fourth arch on the left becomes the short, descending part of the aortic arch between the left common carotid artery and the slightly more distal connection with the ductus arteriosus. On the right, the fourth arch becomes the proximal portion of the right subclavian artery. The rest of this artery derives from a segment of the right dorsal aorta and right seventh intersegmental artery. The right dorsal aorta disappears between the developing right subclavian artery and the site where the right dorsal aorta joins the left. If this segment persists as an abnormal origin of the right subclavian artery, it will form a "vascular sling" behind the foregut.

In summary, it may be helpful to think of the aortic arch derivatives from a purely topographic perspective. The pharyngeal (and aortic) arch territories in the embryo extend from the jaws to the thorax. Aortic arches I and II largely disappear, but arch I contributes to the maxillary arteries in the head, and arch VI gives rise to the pulmonary arteries and ductus arteriosus in the mediastinum. The common carotid arteries span the halfway point of the territory of the arches, so it makes sense that these arteries come from arch III in the middle of the sequence. Arch V is not functional, leaving arch IV to contribute to the arteries between the common carotid and pulmonary vessels: the arch of

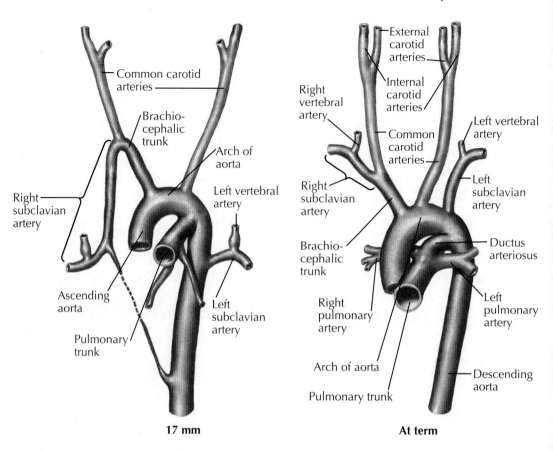

17 mm

At term

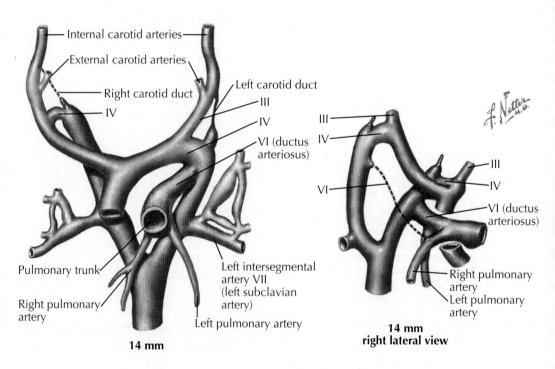

14 mm

**14 mm
right lateral view**

the aorta and the proximal part of the right subclavian artery (Plates 4.14 and 4.15).

MAJOR SYSTEMIC VEINS

The development of the great systemic veins is a complex process of clinical importance. Few organ systems in the body are so subject to variations and anomalies in their final, fully developed state. Although generally of little functional significance to the individual, the many venous variations and anomalies can cause confusion in diagnostic angiocardiographic studies and potentially disastrous accidents when surgical correction of cardiac anomalies is attempted.

In the early embryo, the major veins develop from an initially plexiform network, and a number of channels run mainly in a longitudinal direction. Three main pairs of veins connect to the sinus venosus. The *vitelline veins* carry the blood from the umbilical vesicle (yolk sac), the first site of the production of embryonic blood cells.

Plate 4.16

Embryology

DEVELOPMENT OF MAJOR BLOOD VESSELS (Continued)

The *umbilical veins,* initially paired, bring blood from the chorionic villi (developing placenta) into the embryo, entering the sinus venosus lateral to the vitelline veins. The *cardinal venous system* is entirely intraembryonic. The paired *anterior cardinal veins* drain the cranial region of the embryo. The *posterior cardinal veins* arise somewhat later; they drain the body of the embryo, including the large *mesonephric kidneys,* the first functioning embryonic/fetal kidneys. The anterior and posterior cardinal veins join to form the short *common cardinal veins* that enter the right and left horns of the sinus venosus just lateral to the umbilical veins.

Soon after the posterior cardinal veins have been established, a new venous system develops as a pair of veins, the *subcardinal veins,* appear medially to the posterior cardinal veins (Plate 4.16). Their main function is to drain the urogenital system of the developing embryo: first the mesonephric kidneys and gonads and then the *metanephric kidneys* (future adult kidneys), gonads, and suprarenal glands. Cranially, the subcardinal veins empty into the posterior cardinal veins.

In the 5-week embryo (8 to 10 mm), the cardinal venous system is symmetric and equally developed bilaterally, but this will rapidly change. The vitelline veins—in the region of the *septum transversum,* the developing liver, and around the duodenum—have broken into an anastomosing plexus that will give rise to hepatic veins and the proximal portion of the hepatic portal system of veins. The original left and right vitelline veins connecting this plexus with the sinus venosus are now called *hepatocardiac channels.* The left vitelline disappears, but the right vein becomes greatly enlarged and persists as the terminal, posthepatic part of the inferior vena cava (IVC). The SVC derives from the right common cardinal vein. The right umbilical vein disappears, and the left umbilical vein connects with the vitelline venous plexus, after which its proximal portion connecting to the sinus venosus also disappears. All of the umbilical venous blood now enters the vitelline venous (liver) plexus. A direct route, the *ductus venosus,* is created between the left umbilical vein and the right hepatocardiac channel (future IVC), allowing most of the umbilical venous blood to enter the right atrium through the IVC.

The subcardinal veins have gained importance, and numerous anastomoses with the posterior cardinal veins have been established. The growing mesonephric kidneys have brought the left and right *subcardinal veins* closer together, and an anastomosing plexus of veins has developed between them, the *intersubcardinal*

anastomosis. The right subcardinal vein connects to the right hepatocardiac channel to form the hepatic segment of the IVC.

A new venous system appears bilaterally in the caudal region of the embryo, although some view this system as originating from the posterior cardinal veins. It consists of *sacrocardinal veins* that empty into posterior cardinal veins. Two smaller caudal veins, the *sacrocardinal vein* and *caudal vein,* form the iliac

system of veins (common, internal, external branches) and veins of the pelvis.

As the subcardinal veins enlarge, the *left posterior cardinal vein* decreases in size, and the left horn of the sinus venosus, the future *coronary sinus,* becomes attenuated. Venous return is shifting to the right side of the embryo. Most of the left and right posterior cardinal veins soon disappear as the subcardinal system continues to develop.

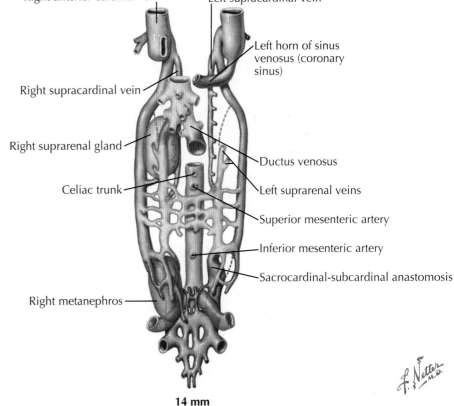

4 mm

10 mm

14 mm

Plate 4.17

DEVELOPMENT OF MAJOR BLOOD VESSELS (Continued)

The right subcardinal vein and its anastomosis with the right hepatocardiac channel (from the right vitelline vein) rapidly become the principal venous channel to the heart. The anastomosis becomes the intrahepatic component of the IVC, and the right subcardinal vein becomes an infrahepatic segment of the IVC. The subcardinal veins lose their cranial connections with the posterior cardinal veins; remaining branches become the renal and suprarenal veins as well as the gonadal veins.

Yet another new venous system appears in the form of two longitudinal channels, the *supracardinal veins* (see Plate 4.16). Cranially, the veins empty into the terminal part of the posterior cardinal veins, and caudally, anastomose with the subcardinal veins. The supracardinal veins form the azygos system of veins that drain the thoracic body wall by way of *the intercostal veins,* taking over this function from the posterior cardinal veins. The cranial part of the left supracardinal vein degenerates; the caudal thoracic portion forms the *hemiazygos vein* that connects over the midline with the right supracardinal vein (developing azygos vein). The azygos vein forms an arch that drains the azygos system into the SVC. The azygos develops from the terminal portion of the right supracardinal vein and right posterior cardinal vein. Recall that the right common cardinal vein forms the SVC. The right supracardinal vein below its connection to the subcardinal vein enlarges to become the inferior segment of the IVC. The left supracardinal vein disappears. If the terminal part of the IVC fails to develop from the right vitelline vein, blood from the lower part of the body will enter the right atrium through a greatly enlarged azygos vein.

The upper limbs and head and neck are drained by veins that empty into the left and right *anterior cardinal veins* (Plate 4.17). An anastomosis between them forms the left brachiocephalic vein, which brings superior venous return to the right side of the embryo, the same shift that occurs in venous return below the heart. The right anterior cardinal vein becomes the right brachiocephalic vein that continues into the SVC (from right common cardinal vein). The left horn of the sinus venosus has attenuated further. The left anterior and common cardinal veins become the ligament of the left SVC (ligament of Marshall), which is continuous with the coronary sinus (from the left horn of sinus venosus). The most common anomaly of the anterior cardinal veins is a persistent left SVC. An oblique vein of the left atrium may also persist.

The only functioning remnant of the left anterior cardinal vein is the small, left superior intercostal vein.

The inferior vena cava derives from more primordia than any other vessel and thus merits a summary. The contributions are as follows.

1. Terminal part, right vitelline vein: posthepatic segment
2. Subcardinohepatic anastomosis: hepatic segment
3. Part of right subcardinal vein: renal segment
4. Right supracardinal vein: prerenal segment

Of the original six connections to the sinus venosus—paired vitelline, umbilical, and common cardinal veins—only two remain: derivatives of the right common cardinal vein (SVC) and right vitelline vein (IVC). The terminal part of the right vitelline vein is also the hepatocardiac channel.

With three vascular systems in the early embryo and three sequential systems of cardinal veins, it is not surprising that variations and anomalies are extremely common.

17 mm

Left anterior cardinal vein
Left common cardinal vein
Left posterior cardinal vein
Coronary sinus (left horn of sinus venosus)
Left suprarenal veins
Left umbilical artery

24 mm

Left brachiocephalic vein
Right suprarenal gland
Right kidney (right metanephros)
Right umbilical artery
Right external iliac artery
Left suprarenal vein
Left renal vein
Gonadal veins
Left umbilical artery
Left external iliac artery

At term

Right internal jugular vein
Left brachiocephalic (left innominate) vein
Left superior intercostal vein
Ligament of left superior vena cava (Marshall)
Right subclavian vein
Right brachiocephalic (right innominate) vein
Superior vena cava
Right superior intercostal vein
Azygos vein
Accessory hemiazygos vein
Coronary sinus
Hemiazygos vein
Hepatic veins
Ductus venosus
Portal vein
Umbilical vein
Left suprarenal vein
Inferior vena cava
Left renal vein
Gonadal (testicular or ovarian) veins
Middle sacral artery and vein
Right internal iliac vein and artery
Left common iliac artery and vein
Right external iliac artery and vein
Right umbilical artery

Plate 4.18   Embryology

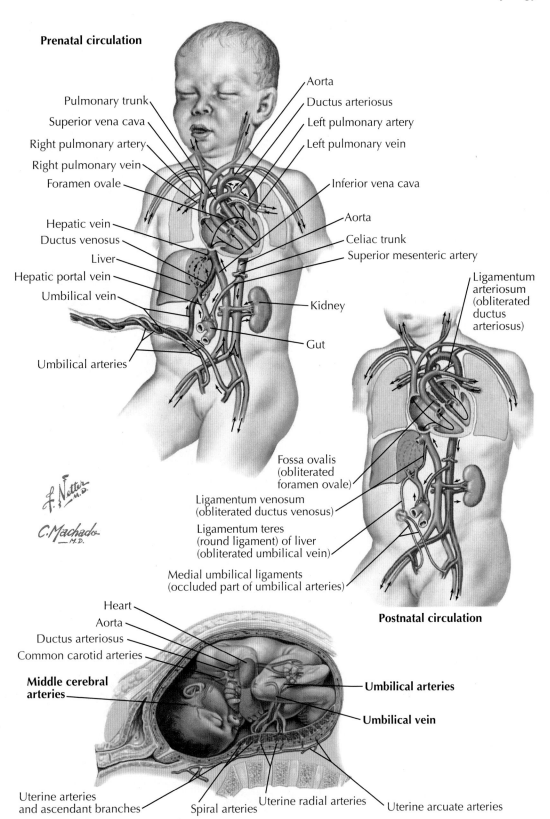

Prenatal circulation

Pulmonary trunk
Superior vena cava
Right pulmonary artery
Right pulmonary vein
Foramen ovale

Aorta
Ductus arteriosus
Left pulmonary artery
Left pulmonary vein

Inferior vena cava

Hepatic vein
Ductus venosus
Liver
Hepatic portal vein
Umbilical vein

Aorta
Celiac trunk
Superior mesenteric artery

Kidney

Umbilical arteries

Gut

Ligamentum arteriosum (obliterated ductus arteriosus)

Fossa ovalis (obliterated foramen ovale)
Ligamentum venosum (obliterated ductus venosus)
Ligamentum teres (round ligament) of liver (obliterated umbilical vein)
Medial umbilical ligaments (occluded part of umbilical arteries)

Postnatal circulation

Heart
Aorta
Ductus arteriosus
Common carotid arteries
Middle cerebral arteries

Umbilical arteries

Umbilical vein

Uterine arteries and ascendant branches
Spiral arteries
Uterine radial arteries
Uterine arcuate arteries

FETAL CIRCULATION AND CHANGES AT BIRTH

The primary vascular concept of prenatal circulation is the requirement that the intraembryonic circulation of blood bypasses the nonfunctioning lungs and liver (Plate 4.18). The placenta (villous chorion) serves the role of these organs with gas and metabolic exchange between maternal and fetal blood. The airway in the lungs is filled with amniotic fluid, and pulmonary vascular resistance is high. The lungs only receive enough blood to nourish the tissues, and pulmonary venous blood flow into the left atrium is minimal. The plan for the prenatal circulation also requires that it convert to the postnatal pattern soon after the first breath of the newborn. Two lung shunts (and a liver shunt) and the design of the interatrial septum serve these needs.

The original placental circulation consists of paired umbilical arteries that pass from the internal iliac arteries to the placenta through the umbilical cord and paired umbilical veins that bring highly oxygenated blood into the embryo to connect with the sinus venosus of the developing heart tube (Plate 4.19). The right

umbilical vein disappears, and the left proximal umbilical vein also disappears as the remaining intraembryonic segment connects with the developing IVC under the liver. As with the lungs, blood flow in the liver is also minimal. Most of the blood in the umbilical vein bypasses the liver through the *ductus venosus,* a straight continuation of the umbilical vein into the IVC.

After partitioning of the heart tube, the IVC is in line with the foramen ovale in the right atrium. Its stream of

blood pushes the septum primum away from the septum secundum, and much of this oxygenated blood passes from the right atrium to the left. This is the first lung shunt. From the left atrium, the blood will pass into the left ventricle and out the ascending aorta.

Venous blood from the SVC is directed at the right atrioventricular valve. Although some mixing of blood occurs from superior and inferior venae cavae, the streams of the blood pass each other to a degree, and

Plate 4.19

Cardiovascular System: VOLUME 8

THREE EARLY VASCULAR SYSTEMS

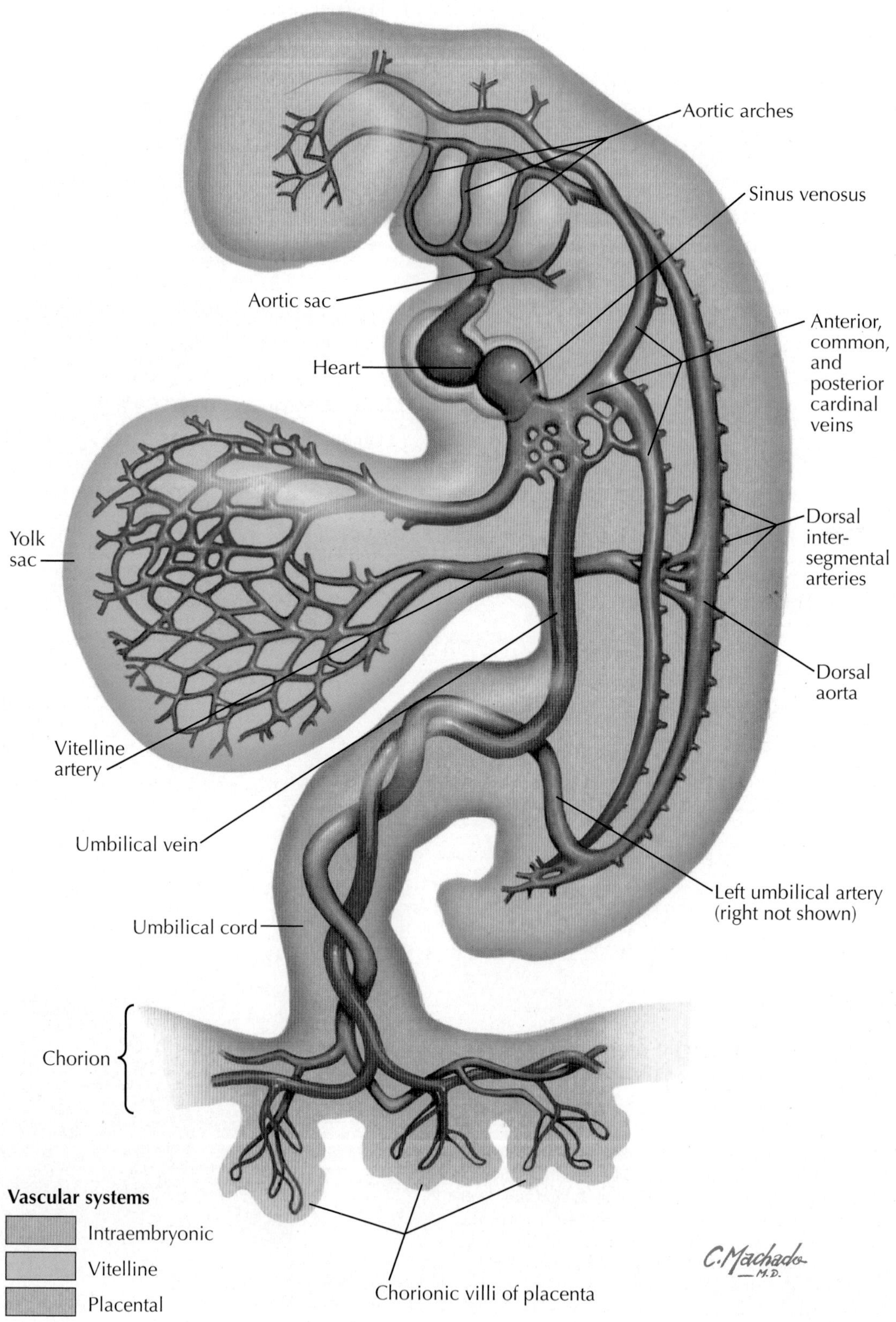

Aortic arches

Sinus venosus

Aortic sac

Heart

Anterior, common, and posterior cardinal veins

Dorsal inter-segmental arteries

Dorsal aorta

Yolk sac

Vitelline artery

Umbilical vein

Left umbilical artery (right not shown)

Umbilical cord

Chorion

Vascular systems
- Intraembryonic
- Vitelline
- Placental

Chorionic villi of placenta

FETAL CIRCULATION AND CHANGES AT BIRTH (Continued)

the most highly oxygenated blood in the fetal heart ends up on the left side. The blood in the right ventricle passes into the pulmonary trunk and continues into the arch of the aorta via the ductus arteriosus (from the sixth aortic arch). This is the second lung shunt based on simple pressure differences between the pulmonary and systemic circulations. Again, vascular resistance in the lungs is high. Pressure is much lower in the aorta, and most of the right ventricle blood flows to the descending aorta. The ductus arteriosus connects with the aortic arch just past the origin of the great arteries. The result is that the brain (and head in general) and upper extremities receive the most highly oxygenated blood in the fetus. There is a mixing of blood from the ductus arteriosus and ascending aorta, but its oxygen content is still higher than that of typical venous blood, and it is obviously sufficient to address the metabolic needs of the growing lower half of the fetus.

The conversion to the postnatal/adult configuration is triggered by the first breath. Amniotic fluid comes

out of the airway, vascular beds open in the lungs, and blood now rushes from the ductus arteriosus into the lungs rather than the aortic arch. Blood flow from the lungs to the left atrium increases rapidly, and the septum primum is pressed against the septum secundum to effectively close the foramen ovale. Over the next few weeks, the ductus arteriosus will begin to form a fibrous cord, the *ligamentum arteriosum*, and the two inter-atrial septa will permanently fuse.

Blood in the umbilical arteries now has a higher oxygen content, which causes the arteries to spasm. Eventually the umbilical arteries will form fibrous cords, the *medial umbilical ligaments*, converging on the umbilicus on the internal surface of the abdominal wall. The umbilical vein collapses from lack of blood and eventually becomes the fibrous *round ligament of the liver* (ligamentum teres). The ductus venosus becomes the ligamentum venosum.

CONGENITAL HEART DISEASE

Plate 5.1

Cardiovascular System: VOLUME 8

Ehlers-Danlos syndrome

Hyperextensibility of thumbs and fingers

Hyperextensibility of elbows

Easy splitting of the skin (so-called cigarette paper scars) over bony prominences, hyperelastic auricles

Hyperelasticity of skin

Marfan syndrome

Upper body segment

Lower body segment

Walker-Murdoch wrist sign. Because of long fingers and thin forearm, thumb and little finger overlap when patient grasps wrist.

Down syndrome
Typical facies seen in Down syndrome

Upward-slanting eyes contrasting with ethnic group

Small mouth with protruding tongue

Short, broad hands, with simian crease and clinodactyly of fifth digit

Clinodactyly

Simian crease (one elongated palmar crease)

Wide gap between the first and second toes

PHYSICAL EXAMINATION

Although many forms are not seen in adult patients, cardiologists often do see simple clues to the diagnosis of certain forms of congenital heart disease (CHD), usually acyanotic or cyanotic and postoperative. Any child with confirmed or suspected CHD should be seen by a pediatric cardiologist at an institution with interventional pediatric cardiologists and cardiac surgeons. Adult patients with CHD should be seen and advised by a pediatric cardiologist or adult cardiologist (preferably both) at a surgical center with experts in congenital heart surgery and percutaneous procedures. Many adult patients present with arrhythmias, heart failure, or failure of the original childhood surgery. Occasionally, older patients or patients with anomalous coronary artery disease present with ischemic heart disease symptoms.

Although the history generally does not provide major clues to the diagnosis, a family history of CHD raises awareness that the offspring of these patients may also have a congenital abnormality. Diagnostic clues in the adolescent or adult patient are based on simple physical examination and electrocardiographic (ECG) and chest radiographic findings characteristic of CHD (Plate 5.1).

SIMPLE DIAGNOSTIC CLUES TO CONGENITAL HEART DISEASE	
Phenotypes	(Inspection) Ehlers-Danlos syndrome, Marfan syndrome, and Down syndrome
Blood pressure measurement	**Hypertension and diminished or absent femoral pulses:** coarctation of the aorta
Inspection	**Jugular venous "A-wave":** Possible pulmonary stenosis, primary pulmonary hypertension, Ebstein's anomaly
Palpation	**Carotid bruit:** Aortic stenosis. **Left parasternal lift:** Primary pulmonary hypertension, atrial septal defect
Auscultation	**Diminished pulmonary second sound:** Pulmonic stenosis **Loud pulmonary second sound:** Primary pulmonary hypertension, atrial septal defect **Fixed split pulmonary second sound:** Secundum atrial septal defect, ostium primum atrial septal defect **Ejection click:** Pulmonic or aortic stenosis, bicuspid aortic valve with coarctation of aorta **Nonejection click and loud systolic murmur:** Mitral and tricuspid prolapse **Ejection systolic murmur:** Bicuspid aortic valve, aortic stenosis **Holosystolic murmur** (tricuspid or mitral regurgitation): Ebstein's malformation, mitral or tricuspid valve prolapse **Decrescendo diastolic murmur:** Bicuspid aortic valve with or without coarctation of aorta **Diastolic rumble** (tricuspid valve): Atrial septal defect **Continuous murmur:** Patent ductus arteriosus **Pansystolic murmur:** Ventricular septal defect
Electrocardiogram	**Normal ECG:** Can be seen in patients with a patent ductus arteriosus, ventricular septal defect, or any mild congenital defect **RSR prime in lead V$_1$** (RVH or incomplete right bundle branch block): Ostium secundum, atrial septal defect **Left axis deviation and RSR prime in lead V$_1$:** Ostium primum atrial septal defect **Right ventricular hypertrophy:** Pulmonic stenosis, atrial septal defect, primary pulmonary hypertension **Left ventricular hypertrophy:** Aortic stenosis, subaortic stenosis, hypertrophic cardiomyopathy, coarctation of aorta **PR interval prolongation and Wolff-Parkinson-White abnormality:** Ebstein's anomaly
Chest radiograph	**Normal pulmonary vascularity:** Any trivial left-to-right shunt, pulmonic stenosis, or left-sided valve disease **Increased pulmonary vascularity:** Any left-to-right shunt with increased pulmonary blood flow (e.g., atrial septal defect, ventricular septal defect, patent ductus arteriosus) **Prominent main pulmonary artery:** Idiopathic dilation of the pulmonary artery, atrial septal defect, pulmonic stenosis, ventricular septal defect, primary pulmonary hypertension **Rib notching and a "three sign":** Coarctation of aorta **Right atrial enlargement:** Ebstein's anomaly

Plate 5.2   Congenital Heart Disease

ANOMALIES OF THE GREAT SYSTEMIC VEINS

Anomalies can involve the large systemic venous trunks because of the complex embryogenesis and tremendous variability of the venous system in general. Abnormal channels almost always empty into other systemic veins and rarely cause functional changes disturbing to the patient; they are usually discovered incidentally at post-mortem examination or during cardiovascular diagnostic or surgical procedures. Venous trunk anomalies may occur as isolated malformations but more often are associated with other cardiovascular anomalies. The presence of an anomaly, if unsuspected, may lead to troublesome or even dangerous situations when total cardiopulmonary bypass techniques are used.

LEFT SUPERIOR VENA CAVA

By far the most common clinically significant anomaly of the great systemic veins is persistence of the left superior vena cava (SVC). This vein, after being formed by the confluence of the left jugular and subclavian veins, descends into the chest parallel to the right superior vena cava and anterior to the left lung hilus, usually entering the greatly dilated coronary sinus along a course normally occupied by the ligament and vein of Marshall. This topographic position is expected because, embryologically, a persistent left SVC represents retention of the left anterior and common cardinal veins and the left sinus horn. Anatomically, the hemiazygos vein resembles the normal right-side azygos vein and may approximate it in size (Plate 5.2).

The right SVC is usually present as well but may be absent. The two venae cavae may be equal in size, or one (generally the left) may be smaller than its counterpart. The left innominate vein, if present, is smaller than normal or may be more or less plexiform.

The coronary sinus ostium (coronary os) is very large because of the increased blood flow through it and is detected easily by cardiac ultrasound. Occasionally, a defect is present in the wall between the sinus and left atrium (*unroofed* coronary sinus). In general such a defect results in a left-to-right shunt; that is, left atrial blood enters the coronary sinus and is carried to the right atrium. Hemodynamically, the anomaly therefore resembles an atrial septal defect. If the defect is extremely large, particularly if the coronary os is small or atretic, the left SVC is said to "enter the left atrium."

Patients with persistent left SVC present a typical clinical picture consisting of moderate central cyanosis without other symptoms. There is no murmur, and the heart is normal in size. The ECG generally shows signs of left ventricular (LV) hypertrophy. Similar but more pronounced findings have been described in the rare cases of isolated drainage of the inferior vena cava into the left atrium.

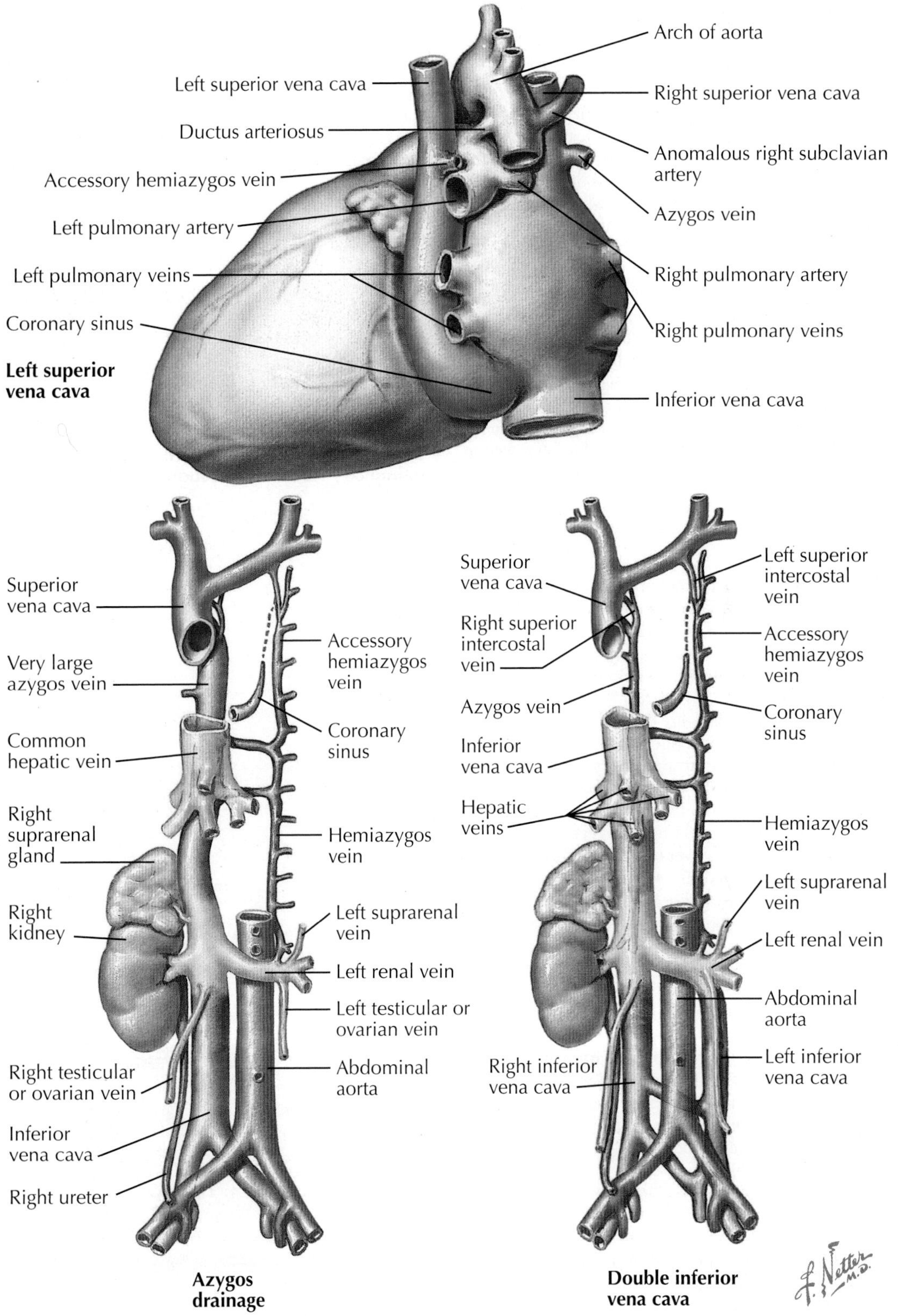

AZYGOS DRAINAGE OF INFERIOR VENA CAVA

Absence of the hepatic segment of the inferior vena cava (IVC) is an uncommon anomaly in which the prehepatic portion of the IVC drains into the right atrium by way of an enormously enlarged azygos vein. The hepatic veins empty into the right atrium by way of a short common stem that normally forms the most proximal part of the IVC (Plate 5.2). Although azygos drainage of the IVC occurs rarely as an isolated lesion,

usually it is associated with other serious cardiac anomalies (e.g., asplenia or polysplenia syndrome).

DOUBLE INFERIOR VENA CAVA

Other systemic venous anomalies, including double inferior vena cava (Plate 5.2), generally involve the IVC bed and are of more importance to general surgeons and urologists than cardiologists and cardiac surgeons.

Patients with significant cardiac anomalies associated with various types of partial inversion of the thoracic or abdominal viscera are particularly prone to harboring anomalies of the great systemic venous trunks. Because such anomalies may cause difficulties at surgery, their presence or absence should be clearly established as part of the diagnostic workup, most easily through angiocardiography, computed tomography (CT), or magnetic resonance imaging (MRI).

CARDIAC VEIN ANOMALIES

Left superior vena cava

Azygos drainage

Double inferior vena cava

Plate 5.3

Cardiovascular System: VOLUME 8

ANOMALOUS PULMONARY VENOUS CONNECTION

In patients with *anomalous pulmonary venous connection* (APVC), all or some of the pulmonary veins fail to communicate with the left atrium, instead discharging blood into major systemic veins or directly into the right atrium. This discussion only considers the isolated forms of APVC. When these occur with other cardiac malformations, the clinical and hemodynamic features are usually modified or are chiefly determined by the complicating defect.

In *partial anomalous pulmonary venous connection,* one or more pulmonary veins empty into the proximal SVC close to the right atrium or into the sinus portion or the right atrium itself. The involved veins almost always drain all or part of the right lung; the others empty normally into the left atrium. An atrial septal defect (ASD) is generally present, especially the *sinus venosus* type. The clinical picture closely resembles that seen in other forms of ASD and is not discussed here.

TOTAL ANOMALOUS PULMONARY VENOUS CONNECTION

In total anomalous pulmonary venous connection (TAPVC), all of the pulmonary venous blood enters the systemic venous system or the right atrium. An ASD or patent foramen ovale is always present. Types of TAPVC are distinguished by how the pulmonary venous blood enters the systemic circuit (Plate 5.3). Embryologically, the intrapulmonary veins are derived from the venous plexus around the foregut and anastomose freely with the systemic veins early in the embryo. After the embryonic main pulmonary vein has appeared as an outgrowth of the primitive left atrium and established connections with the pulmonary venous plexus, the systemic and pulmonary venous anastomotic channels typically are obliterated. If the embryonic pulmonary vein does not develop at all or is obliterated secondarily, some of the anastomotic channels are retained, resulting in TAPVC.

TAPVC to Left Superior Vena Cava

By far the most common form of TAPVC is that *to a persistent left superior vena cava,* illustrated as seen from behind in Plate 5.3. The right pulmonary veins converge to form a single vessel, which runs behind the small left atrium to join the left pulmonary veins. From the junction of the pulmonary veins, a large single vessel representing a persistence of the distal left SVC carries the pulmonary venous blood by way of a dilated left brachiocephalic (innominate) vein and the right SVC to the right atrium. An ASD, or more frequently a widely patent foramen ovale, allows part of the right atrial blood to enter the left atrium. Tremendous right atrial and right ventricular (RV) enlargement develops early and rapidly.

Symptoms of persistent left SVC generally appear shortly after birth: initially rapid respirations followed by dyspnea, feeding difficulties, failure to thrive, and frequent respiratory infections. As a rule the patient has no obvious cyanosis, at least at first, reflecting the mixing of a large amount of oxygenated pulmonary venous blood with a much smaller amount of systemic venous blood. Cyanosis becomes more pronounced if bronchopneumonia or congestive heart failure is present. Failure almost always appears within the first 6 months of life, and the great majority of these infants die during their first year. For unknown reasons, a small number of patients improve, a few of whom may reach adulthood.

Total anomalous pulmonary venous connection to left innominate vein

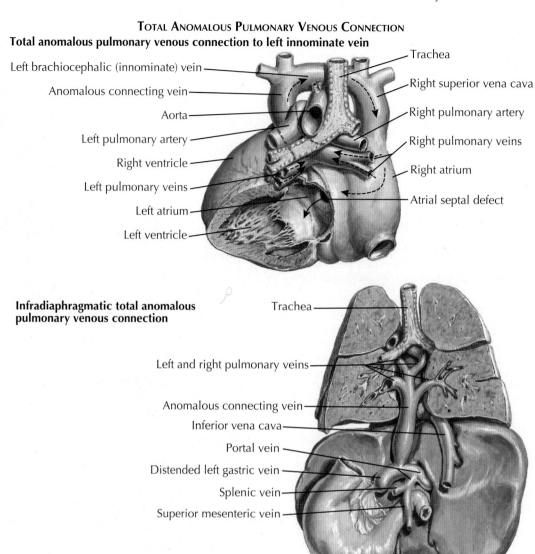

Left brachiocephalic (innominate) vein
Anomalous connecting vein
Aorta
Left pulmonary artery
Right ventricle
Left pulmonary veins
Left atrium
Left ventricle
Trachea
Right superior vena cava
Right pulmonary artery
Right pulmonary veins
Right atrium
Atrial septal defect

Infradiaphragmatic total anomalous pulmonary venous connection

Trachea
Left and right pulmonary veins
Anomalous connecting vein
Inferior vena cava
Portal vein
Distended left gastric vein
Splenic vein
Superior mesenteric vein

Total anomalous pulmonary venous connection to coronary sinus

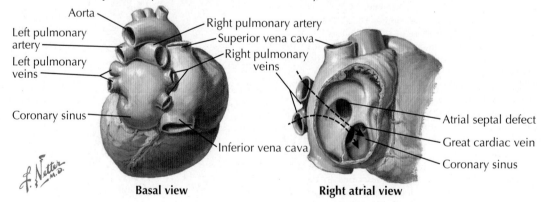

Aorta
Left pulmonary artery
Left pulmonary veins
Coronary sinus
Right pulmonary artery
Superior vena cava
Right pulmonary veins
Inferior vena cava
Atrial septal defect
Great cardiac vein
Coronary sinus

Basal view

Right atrial view

Cyanosis and clubbing of the digits are common only in older children and adults with TAPVC. The heart is enlarged. Generally there is no thrill, but a lower left parasternal "heave" is usually present. A systolic murmur of mild to moderate intensity is present at the left upper sternal border or sometimes lower. The pulmonic second sound is usually loud and often split. A diastolic tricuspid flow murmur may be present along the right lower sternal border or over the xiphoid process.

The chest radiograph features of persistent left SVC in older children and adults are characteristic. The dilated left and right superior venae cavae cause a rounded shadow in the upper mediastinum. Together with the rounded and enlarged heart shadow, a typical figure-eight or "snowman" appearance is created. The pulmonary vascularity is greatly increased. The ECG shows right axis deviation and severe right atrial and RV hypertrophy. At cardiac catheterization, the oxygen

Plate 5.4

Congenital Heart Disease

ANOMALOUS PULMONARY VENOUS CONNECTION (Continued)

content of the right SVC blood is found to be very high, indicating a massive left-to-right (L → R) supracardiac shunt, and the blood oxygen content is almost uniform in all cardiac chambers.

The diagnosis of TAPVC to the left SVC can be confirmed easily by selective injection of a contrast medium into the pulmonary trunk. After passage of the contrast through the lungs, the anomalous veins opacify quite satisfactorily. Computed tomographic angiography (CTA) and cardiac MRI can also define the anatomic pathology of persistent left SVC.

TAPVC to Coronary Sinus

The pulmonary veins join to form a very short, wide, common vessel that empties into the hugely dilated coronary sinus in TAPVC to the coronary sinus (see Plate 5.3). The clinical picture and ECG findings are similar to those just described for left SVC. The radiographic appearance is different, in that the upper mediastinum is not widened. The right atrium may be huge. Cardiomegaly and plethora of the lung fields are seen. Cardiac catheterization fails to show the high oxygen content of the SVC; otherwise, radiograph findings are similar to those in TAPVC to the left SVC. Angiocardiography is much less helpful, and the anomalous connection to the coronary sinus may be difficult to demonstrate with certainty. CT and MRI help define the anatomic pathology.

Other types of TAPVC (e.g., to right atrium or to several different sites) are infrequently seen as isolated malformations but also may be seen in association with other severe cardiac defects.

Infradiaphragmatic Type

In an unusual form of TAPVC, generally occurring as an isolated anomaly, the pulmonary veins drain into the portal venous system. This is generally referred to as *infradiaphragmatic* TAPVC; the other TAPVCs are classified as *supradiaphragmatic*. With infradiaphragmatic TAPVC the pulmonary veins join to form a single long vessel that descends in front of the esophagus and courses with it through the esophageal hiatus, to enter the proximal portal venous system, generally the left gastric vein. Usually, there is a stenotic area in the preesophageal vein just before it enters the portal venous bed. Along with the need for pulmonary venous blood to traverse the hepatic capillary bed before entering the right atrium by the hepatic veins, this stenosis causes severe pulmonary venous hypertension and is responsible for the characteristic clinical picture and laboratory findings, which are quite different from those seen in the various supradiaphragmatic TAPVCs. Plate 5.3 shows the infradiaphragmatic anomaly as seen from the back.

Severe symptoms appear soon after birth, and almost all infants with infradiaphragmatic TAPVC die within a few days or weeks. The symptoms include clear persistent cyanosis, marked dyspnea, and serious feeding difficulties. Cardiac failure becomes evident very early and is almost impossible to treat successfully. These infants are obviously very sick but show no abnormal cardiac findings. The heart is not enlarged, and a murmur, if present, is faint. The ECG is normal or near-normal. The chest radiograph is characteristic but not pathognomonic because it is also seen in other anomalies in which pulmonary venous obstruction occurs. There is evidence of severe pulmonary venous hypertension; the

SURGERY FOR ANOMALOUS PULMONARY VENOUS RETURN

Procedure for total anomalous pulmonary venous return to left superior vena cava

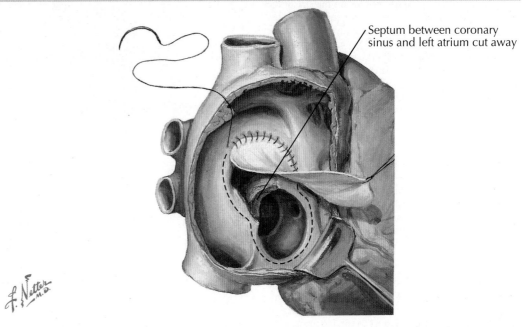

Preoperative angiocardiogram:
LBV = left brachiocephalic vein
SVC = superior vena cava
LSVC = left superior vena cava
PT = pulmonary trunk; RA = right atrium
RV = right ventricle

Right brachiocephalic vein (right innominate vein)

Left brachiocephalic vein (left innominate vein)

Right superior vena cava

Atrial septal defect closed and septum drawn to right, thus enlarging left atrium

Left superior vena cava ligated and divided

Left pulmonary veins

Right pulmonary veins

Pulmonary venous pool anastomosed to left atrium

Procedure for anomalous pulmonary venous return to coronary sinus

Septum between coronary sinus and left atrium cut away

hilar markings are pronounced and fuzzy, and the lungs show a reticulated appearance.

Surgical Treatment

The treatment of TAPVC is surgical to redirect pulmonary vein flow entirely to the left atrium (Plate 5.4). In most types of total anomalous pulmonary venous return, the pulmonary veins return to a common confluence behind the left atrium. The common pulmonary

vein confluence is connected to the back of the left atrium, resulting in a normal connection of pulmonary veins to the left atrium. All other pulmonary vessels to the supracardiac or infracardiac areas are tied off. Any coexisting ASD is closed. Older children and adults generally have good surgical results. The repair results in normal circulation; the pulmonary veins return as normal to the left atrium without abnormal connections or septal defects.

Plate 5.5

Cardiovascular System: VOLUME 8

ANOMALIES OF THE ATRIA

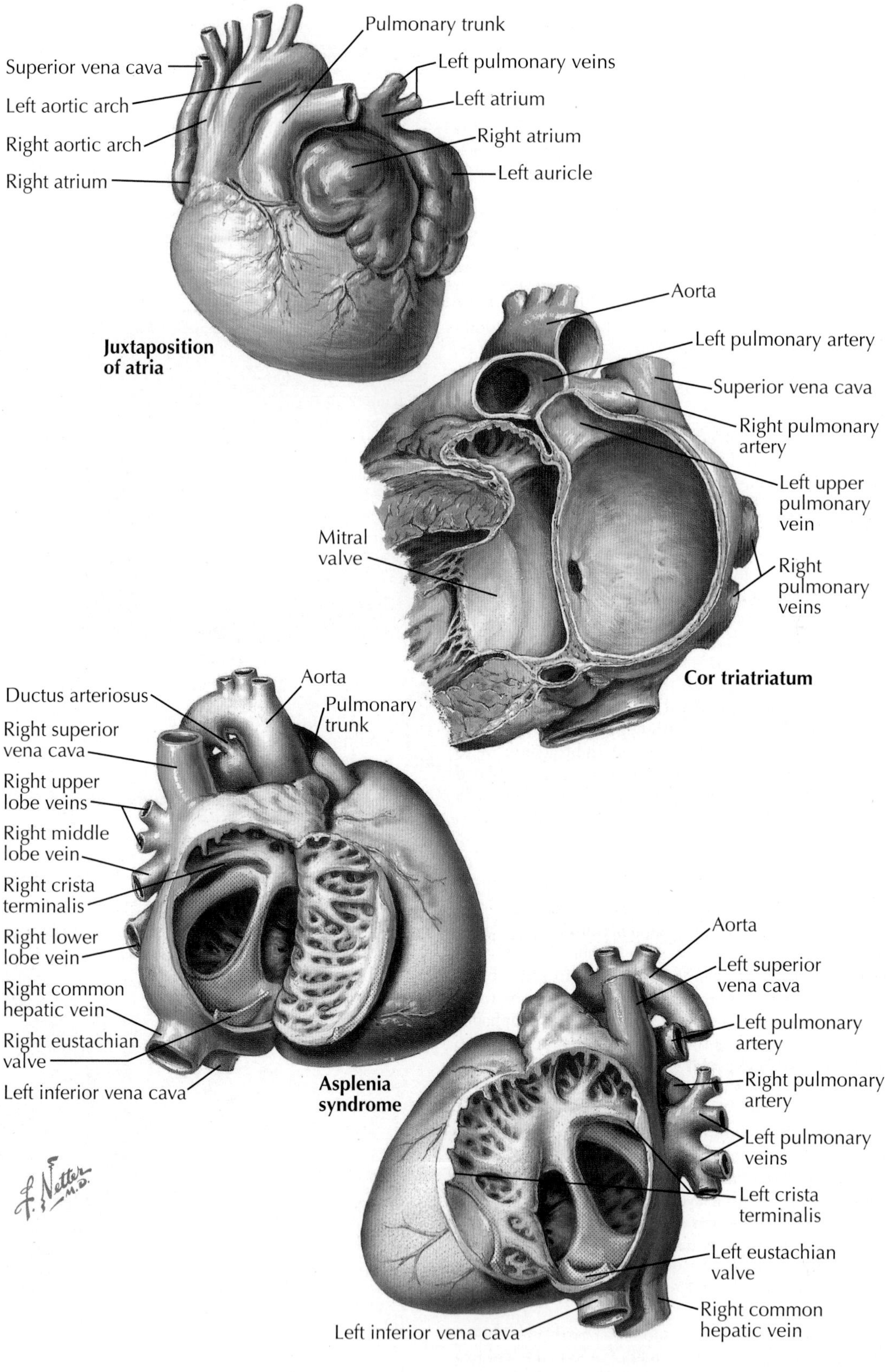

JUXTAPOSITION OF THE ATRIAL APPENDAGES

In juxtaposition of the atrial appendages (auricles), the main bodies of the atria are normally located, but there is levoposition of the right atrial appendage. Instead of being to the right of the arterial trunks, the right atrial appendage crosses behind them to appear on their left, interposing itself between the great arteries and the left atrial appendage. Juxtaposition of the atrial appendages has no functional significance because it causes no hemodynamic disturbance itself. Its presence, however, always indicates the coexistence of other major cardiac anomalies. Transposition of the great vessels and a ventricular septal defect (VSD) are invariably present, and atresia of the tricuspid valve is common. Plate 5.5 also depicts a double aortic arch.

COR TRIATRIATUM

In the rare cor triatriatum, a fibromuscular septum divides the left atrium into a posterosuperior part receiving the pulmonary veins and an anteroinferior part giving access to the mitral valve and left atrial appendage (Plate 5.5). Cor triatriatum is probably caused by incomplete incorporation of the embryonic common pulmonary vein into the left atrium. The original pulmonary venous ostium is represented by an opening of variable size. Rarely, the septum is imperforate, and the distal pulmonary venous compartment drains through a defect into the right atrium or an anomalous vessel into the systemic venous system. Usually the fossa or foramen ovale is located between the anteroinferior compartment and right atrium.

The severity of symptoms depends on the size of the opening between the two compartments of the left atrium. Respiratory difficulties and dyspnea may be marked, and cardiac failure develops early. If the os is very small, death occurs within the first year of life; if it is larger, symptoms appear later and closely resemble those seen in mitral stenosis; that is, chronic cough, dyspnea, fatigability, chest pain, and hemoptysis. Cyanosis may be present, and there is marked cardiomegaly. A mild or moderate systolic murmur is usually heard, but a diastolic murmur is seldom present. The ECG usually suggests RV hypertrophy because the pulmonary pressure is elevated. Cor triatriatum is easily diagnosed with transthoracic cardiac ultrasound and other imaging modalities. Surgical repair is relatively simple; the anomalous membrane is excised.

ASPLENIA SYNDROME

Congenital absence of the spleen rarely occurs alone. Other visceral anomalies are present in most patients, about 60% of whom have typical asplenia syndrome (Plate 5.5). The most important feature of asplenia syndrome is the tendency for normally asymmetric organs (e.g., liver, lungs) to develop more or less symmetrically. The stomach may be located on either side or rarely in the midline. Both lungs are usually trilobed and resemble a normal right lung. The heart is generally severely malformed. A single or common ventricle is usually present, and an endocardial cushion defect of the complete type is often found. Transposition of the great vessels is the rule, usually associated with pulmonary stenosis. The atrial septum is reduced to a peculiar triangular band of muscle that crosses the common atrioventricular orifice. In typical cases, both the right atrium and the left atrium morphologically resemble a

Juxtaposition of atria

Cor triatriatum

Asplenia syndrome

normal right atrium (*isomerism* of atria), meaning that both sinus horns have been incorporated into their corresponding atria. A coronary sinus is therefore absent. TAPVC is typically present. The great systemic veins also tend to develop symmetrically, at times with a bilateral SVC and a large vein entering on each side of the atrial floor, representing a bilateral persistence of the proximal vitelline veins. One of these drains a lobe of the liver (common hepatic vein), and the other drains

the opposite lobe and the remainder of the IVC bed. The site of the viscera is impossible to determine (*situs ambiguus*, or heterotaxy syndrome).

The diagnosis of asplenia syndrome should be suspected in any infant with CHD associated with some form of partial visceral heterotaxy, particularly if cyanosis is present. Howell-Jolly and Heinz bodies are typically present in the peripheral blood smear. The prognosis is poor.

Plate 5.6

Congenital Heart Disease

ATRIAL SEPTAL DEFECTS

Ostium secundum defect

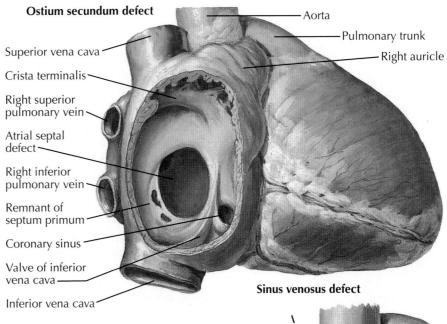

- Aorta
- Pulmonary trunk
- Right auricle
- Superior vena cava
- Crista terminalis
- Right superior pulmonary vein
- Atrial septal defect
- Right inferior pulmonary vein
- Remnant of septum primum
- Coronary sinus
- Valve of inferior vena cava
- Inferior vena cava

Sinus venosus defect

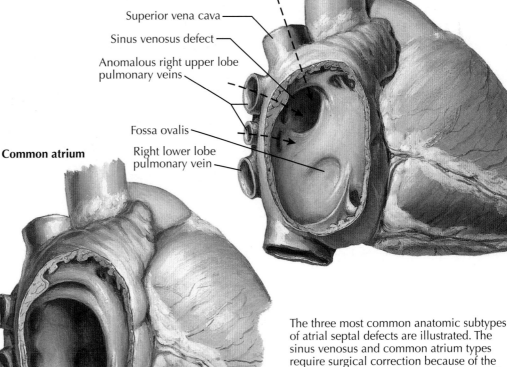

- Superior vena cava
- Sinus venosus defect
- Anomalous right upper lobe pulmonary veins
- Fossa ovalis
- Right lower lobe pulmonary vein

Common atrium

The three most common anatomic subtypes of atrial septal defects are illustrated. The sinus venosus and common atrium types require surgical correction because of the lack of septal rims to anchor a device and/or the proximity to vital structures.

DEFECTS OF THE ATRIAL SEPTUM

The atrial septum normally consists of two overlapping, closely adjacent components. Each forms an incomplete partition. The right-side component, corresponding to the embryonic *septum secundum,* is muscular and firm and has a posteroinferior oval-shaped opening, the *foramen ovale*. The left-side component, derived from the embryonic *septum primum,* is fibrous and thin and has a somewhat round opening anterosuperiorly, the *ostium secundum*. Together, the two components act as a one-way flap valve, allowing the flow of blood from *right to left* (normal before birth) but not from left to right. After birth, with the establishment of pulmonary circulation, the increased amount of blood entering the *left atrium* elevates the pressure in that chamber, thereby closing the flap valve. In most cases, this functional closure is eventually followed by anatomic closure; that is, the two components of the septum fuse. In the minority of cases where fusion fails, an increase in the *right atrial* pressure due to congenital cardiac anomalies, or any other condition that elevates RV and right atrial pressure, causes the right atrial blood to flow again into the left atrium. Such a *probe-patent foramen ovale,* however, should not be considered a form of atrial septal defect; it causes no hemodynamic abnormalities by itself. In ASD there is an abnormal opening in the atrial septum allowing blood to flow either way; a predominantly left-to-right shunt usually exists. With associated anomalies or other conditions tending to increase right atrial pressure, the shunt is always from right to left, as in tricuspid valve atresia, or an initially left-to-right shunt reverses, as occurs after pulmonary vascular changes with pulmonary hypertension.

OSTIUM SECUNDUM DEFECT

Of the two main types of ASD, the *secundum* type is more common and is one of the most frequently seen congenital cardiac anomalies (Plate 5.6). The normal resorptive process that leads to the formation of the ostium secundum in the embryo is exaggerated, and

most of the septum primum disappears. Most secundum ASDs are large, and the resulting left-to-right shunt is generally substantial, causing a several-fold increase in pulmonary blood flow. Both the right atrium and the RV dilate and hypertrophy, and the pulmonary arteries enlarge considerably. Even though pulmonary venous return and therefore blood flow in the left atrium are increased, the left atrium does not enlarge because resistance to emptying into the LV is higher than to the RV, and thus it can

readily "bleed off" through the defect into the more compliant right atrium. Systemic blood flow is generally at a low-normal rate or occasionally diminished.

The clinical features of ostium secundum ASD are not remarkable, considering the size of the defect and the magnitude of the shunt (see Plate 5.7). Only rarely are infants with ASD symptomatic; in fact, this anomaly is so well tolerated that disabling symptoms usually do not occur until adulthood, when it is the most common congenital cardiac defect. In children and young adults,

Plate 5.7   Cardiovascular System: VOLUME 8

SURGERY FOR ATRIAL SEPTAL DEFECTS

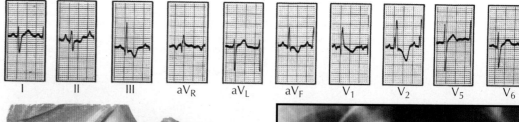

I   II   III   aV$_R$ aV$_L$ aV$_F$ V$_1$ V$_2$ V$_5$ V$_6$

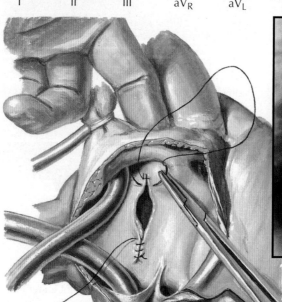

Direct suture of ostium secundum defect

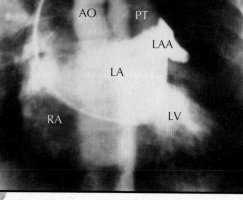

Preoperative angiocardiogram: AO = aorta; PT = pulmonary trunk; LAA = left atrial appendage; LA = left atrium; RA = right atrium; LV = left ventricle

Application of patch for closure of sinus venosus defect (broken line indicates intended line of suture continuation)

DEFECTS OF THE ATRIAL SEPTUM (Continued)

the only symptoms are mild fatigability and dyspnea on exertion. Many patients are not even aware of the significance of ASD, recognizing the defect only in retrospect after it has been corrected surgically and they have more energy and breathe more easily. Growth and development are generally normal. The heart is only slightly or moderately enlarged, and a thrill is extremely uncommon in isolated ASD. A left lower parasternal "heave" is often present, but a precordial bulge is seen only in patients with marked cardiomegaly. The murmur heard in ASD is not loud but rather systolic, medium pitched, and of the ejection type, which is best heard at the base to the left of the sternum. The ASD murmur is caused not by the left-to-right shunt itself, but by the increased amount of blood passing through the otherwise normal pulmonary valve. A similar mechanism is thought to cause the faint, short diastolic murmur heard in the tricuspid valve area (tricuspid flow murmur). Characteristically, the second sound at the upper left sternal border is split, and the splitting is fixed. Unlike the variable splitting heard in normal children, the interval between the aortic (A$_2$) and pulmonic (P$_2$) components of S$_2$ remains constant through all phases of respiration; P$_2$ is often louder than A$_2$. An ejection click is rare in children but may be present in adults, indicating the presence of pulmonary hypertension.

The classic chest radiograph features of secundum ASD are mild to moderate cardiomegaly, prominent right-sided heart border caused by right atrial enlargement, evidence of RV enlargement, prominent pulmonary artery segment at left upper heart border caused by dilation of the pulmonary trunk, and marked hypervascularity of the lung fields. On fluoroscopy, distinct hilar pulsations can easily be seen, called the "hilar dance." The left atrium is never enlarged, and therefore the esophagus is not displaced posteriorly.

The ECG features are usually unmistakable. Right axis deviation is the rule, although the axis may be normal or rarely even oriented to the left. Prominent, peaked P waves may be seen in leads II and aV$_F$ and in

the right precordial leads. Most cases show an rSr' or an rSR' pattern over the right precordium, indicating mild to moderate RV enlargement. An rR', an Rs, and particularly a qR pattern, not typically seen in children, indicate more severe RV hypertrophy, as seen with the development of pulmonary vascular changes and hypertension.

At cardiac catheterization, it is usually easy to enter the left atrium through the secundum defect, particularly when this is carried out from the femoral venous

circulation. A distinct increase in oxygen content of the right atrium and an early opacification of the right atrium, on selective left atrial angiocardiography, demonstrate the presence of an ASD. RV and pulmonary artery pressures are normal or only slightly elevated in most children and young adults. Pulmonary hypertension may be present occasionally in early infancy or late in the disease course. A slight (10–15 mm Hg) pressure gradient across the pulmonary artery valve is common and does not, as a rule, indicate organic

Plate 5.8   Congenital Heart Disease

SEPTAL OCCLUDER DEVICE

The Amplatzer Septal Occluder is deployed from its delivery sheath, forming two disks, one for either side of the septum, and a central waist available in varying diameters to seat on the rims of the atrial septal defect.

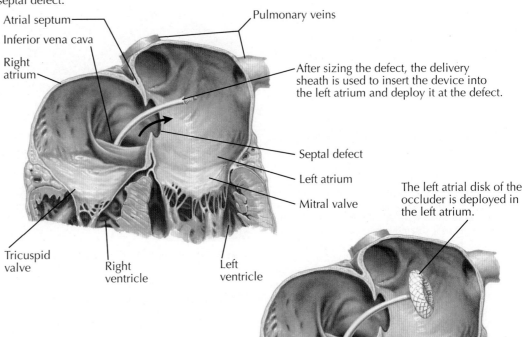

Atrial septum —
Inferior vena cava —
Right atrium —

Pulmonary veins

After sizing the defect, the delivery sheath is used to insert the device into the left atrium and deploy it at the defect.

Septal defect
Left atrium
Mitral valve

Tricuspid valve   Right ventricle   Left ventricle

The left atrial disk of the occluder is deployed in the left atrium.

DEFECTS OF THE ATRIAL SEPTUM (Continued)

pulmonary valve stenosis because it disappears after surgical closure of the defect.

In general the clinical, chest radiograph, ECG, and cardiac ultrasound findings are so characteristic that many cardiologists do not hesitate to refer patients with ASD to a surgeon without catheterization or angiocardiographic studies. Medical treatment is often not required, but symptoms (e.g., arrhythmias) should be treated as in any other cardiac condition. In children, cardiac failure rarely occurs, except in infants with very large defects. Bacterial endocarditis, the bane of many types of CHD, is extremely rare in uncomplicated ASD.

Surgical treatment ensures complete cure and should always be advised because surgery is easily done, employing cardiopulmonary bypass, and carries minimal risk. The ASD can usually be closed by direct suture. Because the defect is so well tolerated, surgery can safely be postponed until the child is 8 to 10 years or older. Percutaneous approaches using a septal occluder device (e.g., Amplatzer) have now become the transcatheter procedures of choice in patients, replacing the need for cardiopulmonary bypass (Plate 5.8).

COMMON ATRIUM

Extremely large secundum defects, involving practically all of the septum and referred to as *common atrium,* are seldom seen. The symptoms tend to be more pronounced, and slight arterial desaturation may be present because of easy mixing of blood at the atrial level. A prosthesis, consisting of a free pericardial graft, is usually necessary to close the defect (see Plate 5.6).

SINUS VENOSUS DEFECT

In the sinus venosus type of ASD, the region of the *fossa ovalis* is normal, the defect being located high in the septum at the ostium of the *superior vena cava,* which tends to straddle the defect (see Plate 5.6). Partial anomalous pulmonary venous return is almost always present. Such anomalous veins usually drain the right

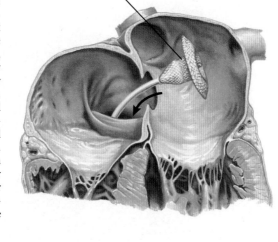

Once the left atrial disk and part of the connecting waist are deployed, the device is carefully pulled back until the left atrial disk touches the septum and the waist is in the septal defect.

C. Machado
— M.D.

The right atrial disk is deployed and the placement of the occluder is checked by echocardiography. Then the device is released.

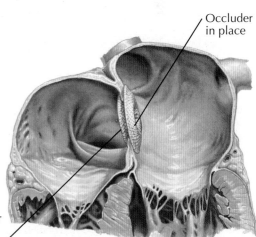

Occluder in place

upper lobe and the middle lobe. The embryology of this much rarer kind of atrial septal defect is not clear. The clinical picture and the radiographic and ECG findings are similar to those described above.

Surgical correction of this defect may require the use of a *pericardial patch* to reroute the anomalous venous return to the left atrium and simultaneously close the ASD without compromising the lumen of the superior vena cava or the pulmonary veins.

"OSTIUM PRIMUM" DEFECT

A third variety of anomalous interatrial communication is the "ostium primum" defect. Although some of its clinical features resemble other types of ASD, ostium primum ASD differs significantly in other ways, and it is not truly a defect of the atrial septum proper. The primum ASD is caused by a developmental anomaly of the embryonic atrioventricular endocardial cushions (see Plates 5.9 and 5.10).

Plate 5.9

Cardiovascular System: VOLUME 8

ENDOCARDIAL CUSHION DEFECTS

The group of anomalies known as *endocardial cushion defects* (ECDs) is of interest to not only the cardiologist but the embryologist, pathologist, and surgeon as well. All ECD types are primarily caused by a developmental defect of the atrioventricular endocardial cushions. Normally, the endocardial cushions fuse with each other and bend to form an arc, the convexity of which is toward the atrial side. The atrial septum fuses with the apex of the arc, thus dividing it into two approximately equal parts. The right half contributes to the ventricular septum, the atrioventricular septum, and the medial or septal cusp of the tricuspid valve. The left half of the fused cushions forms the aortic or anterior cusp of the mitral valve.

In ECD the cushions partly fuse or do not fuse, and the arc is usually not formed (Plate 5.9). This results in the following pathologic features characteristic of ECDs, shared by all types to varying degree:

- The aortic cusp of the mitral valve is cleft, and its origin is concave instead of convex, as in the normal heart.
- The interventricular septum has a peculiar, scooped-out appearance.
- The LV outflow area is narrower and longer than normal.
- The superior-inferior diameter of the ventricles is increased at the base.
- Imaging may show a large characteristic interatrial communication, a ventricular communication, or both.

If fusion of the cushions fails completely, the atrioventricular ostia form a large, single ostium (*complete type of endocardial cushion defect*, also called persistent common atrioventricular canal), and there is a large, central septal defect that allows free communication between all four chambers. The common atrioventricular valve consists of the normal left mural (posterior) mitral valve cusp, the anterior and posterior tricuspid valve cusps, and two large cusps that cross the defect and have developed from the unfused endocardial cushions. Either cusp or both of these cusps may be attached to the top of the ventricular septum by short chordae tendineae. The specimen illustrated in Plate 5.9 also has a persistent left superior vena cava.

If the cushions fuse only centrally, there is a division of the atrioventricular canal into right and left atrioventricular ostia, but the mitral valve (and often the septal cusp of the tricuspid valve) is cleft (*partial* ECD). Several types of ECD are distinguished, mainly depending on whether there is an *interventricular* or *interatrial* communication. The partial form, with only an interatrial communication, is known as the "ostium primum" type of ASD, as previously discussed. Again, the communication does not really correspond to the embryonic ostium primum, its position being similar to that of the atrioventricular septum of the normal heart. It must be emphasized that the atrial septum in ECDs typically is normally developed and complete, although

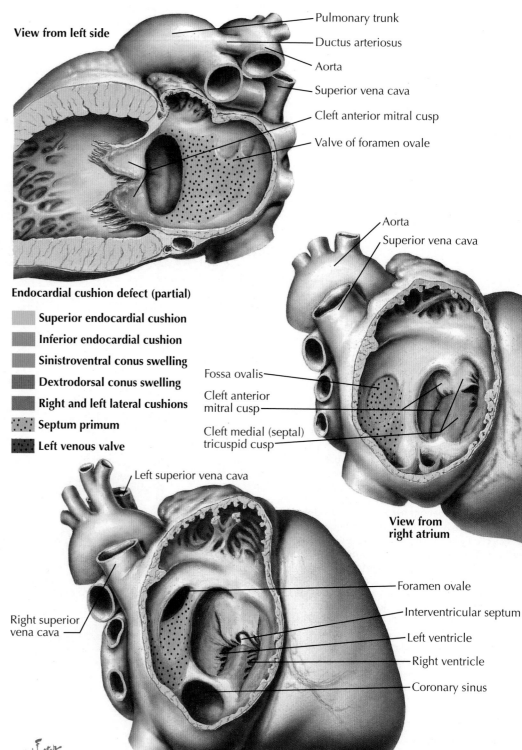

ENDOCARDIAL CUSHION DEFECTS: ANATOMY AND EMBRYOLOGY

View from left side

- Pulmonary trunk
- Ductus arteriosus
- Aorta
- Superior vena cava
- Cleft anterior mitral cusp
- Valve of foramen ovale

Endocardial cushion defect (partial)

- ▨ Superior endocardial cushion
- ▨ Inferior endocardial cushion
- ▨ Sinistroventral conus swelling
- ▨ Dextrodorsal conus swelling
- ▨ Right and left lateral cushions
- ▨ Septum primum
- ▨ Left venous valve

- Aorta
- Superior vena cava
- Fossa ovalis
- Cleft anterior mitral cusp
- Cleft medial (septal) tricuspid cusp

View from right atrium

- Left superior vena cava
- Right superior vena cava
- Foramen ovale
- Interventricular septum
- Left ventricle
- Right ventricle
- Coronary sinus

Endocardial cushion defect (complete)

associated ASDs do occur. The cleft mitral valve is usually incompetent. Even in cases of complete ECD, the valve may be competent.

The clinical manifestations of the ostium primum type of ECD largely resemble those seen in uncomplicated ASD. Symptoms tend to appear earlier in life, however, and growth retardation, fatigability, dyspnea, and respiratory infections are often more pronounced. Pulmonary vascular changes, resulting in RV and pulmonary artery hypertension, are more common and are

likely to occur earlier. A thrill is not uncommon, and auscultation again finds the systolic murmur at the left upper sternal border and the fixed splitting of S_2, as in ASD. In addition, however, in just over half the cases, a high-pitched, blowing, systolic murmur of mitral insufficiency is present at or within the apex and transmitted to the axilla.

On chest radiography the heart tends to be somewhat larger than in ASDs. The heart may assume a configuration of LV enlargement, with the apex turned

Plate 5.10

Congenital Heart Disease

SURGERY FOR OSTIUM PRIMUM AND CLEFT MITRAL VALVE

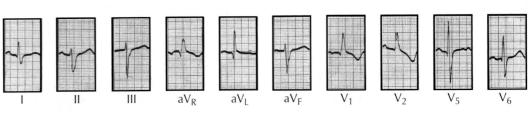

I   II   III   aV_R   aV_L   aV_F   V_1   V_2   V_5   V_6

ENDOCARDIAL CUSHION DEFECTS (Continued)

down and out in the presence of significant mitral insufficiency. Even with mitral insufficiency, however, there is no left atrial enlargement unless the interatrial communication is small or absent. Other chest radiograph features are similar to those seen in primum ASD.

The ECG shows a left deviation of the QRS axis in the frontal plane, usually between 0 and −60 degrees, but sometimes more to the left. In the complete type of ECD, the QRS axis may be located in the right upper quadrant. The precordial leads are similar to those seen in ASD, but the evidence for RV enlargement tends to be more pronounced, and the left precordial leads may show a pattern of LV hypertrophy resulting from mitral incompetence. The left axis deviation seen in ECD apparently is not related to possible LV hypertrophy and seems to be caused by an abnormal anatomic position of the conduction system. Conduction system abnormalities such as heart block can occur.

Cardiac ultrasound can confirm the diagnosis of an ostium primum ASD and easily demonstrates mitral and tricuspid regurgitation, if present. Cardiac MRI also can define the anatomic pathophysiology. Cardiac catheterization findings are similar to those in ASD and usually are not helpful in differentiating the two entities. Angiocardiography, on the other hand, is an extremely valuable tool because a selective LV angiogram shows a configuration not observed in any other cardiac anomaly. The scooped-out ventricular septum and the long, narrow LV outflow area are readily apparent during diastole, whereas during systole the two halves of the cleft mitral valve cusp are seen to bulge into the left atrium, with a notch indicating the position of the cleft. Mitral insufficiency, if present, is also readily demonstrated.

The *complete* type of ECD usually causes severe problems early in infancy, including repeated respiratory infections, feeding difficulties, growth retardation or serious failure to thrive, dyspnea, and congestive heart failure. Most of these children die within the first 2 years of life. Cyanosis is rare unless there is an associated obstruction of the RV outflow tract, respiratory infection, or heart failure. Cardiomegaly develops rapidly after birth. In general, the larger the ventricular component, the sicker the child is; if this component is small, the clinical manifestations resemble those of the partial ostium primum type. A well-documented association exists between ECDs, particularly the complete type, and Down syndrome, which is seen in 35% to 40% of patients with a complete ECD.

The treatment of ECDs consists of open surgical correction of the malformation, always employing a cardiopulmonary bypass. Although technically much more difficult than closure of a simple ASD, the procedure now carries an acceptably low mortality rate if the

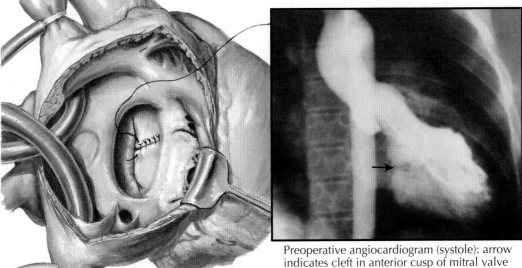

Suture of cleft in mitral valve

Preoperative angiocardiogram (systole): arrow indicates cleft in anterior cusp of mitral valve

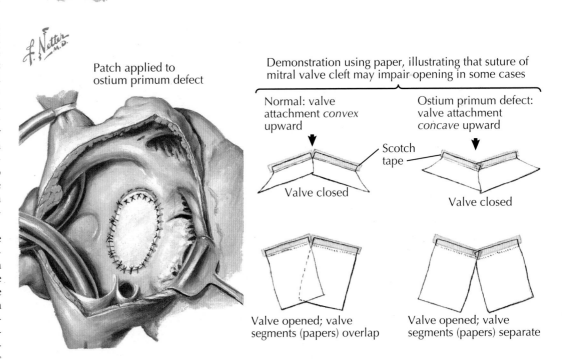

Patch applied to ostium primum defect

Demonstration using paper, illustrating that suture of mitral valve cleft may impair opening in some cases

Normal: valve attachment *convex* upward

Ostium primum defect: valve attachment *concave* upward

Scotch tape

Valve closed

Valve closed

Valve opened; valve segments (papers) overlap

Valve opened; valve segments (papers) separate

anomaly is the partial type. The interatrial communication is accurately closed by employing a prosthesis of appropriate size. Direct suture should not be done in most cases because it may cause distortion of the left atrioventricular ostium and thereby aggravate mitral insufficiency. Traditionally, the cleft in the anterior cusp of the mitral valve has been sutured to create a more or less normal cusp and reduce insufficiency when present or prevent its development. Although suture of the cleft in cases with marked mitral incompetence seems

justified, the wisdom of carrying out such a procedure in patients with a competent valve is highly debatable. In fact, suture of a competent cleft may well be contraindicated because it will interfere with the ability of the cusp to open freely and completely and thus produce mitral stenosis (Plate 5.10).

Correction of the complete forms of endocardial cushion defect is technically more difficult and, in some cases, impossible. In addition, children with ECD are generally smaller and more disabled.

Plate 5.11

Cardiovascular System: VOLUME 8

ANOMALIES OF THE TRICUSPID VALVE

Of the congenital tricuspid valve anomalies, only two—tricuspid valve atresia and Ebstein's anomaly—are clinically significant. Tricuspid regurgitation and stenosis occurring as isolated lesions are extremely rare. Some forms of septal defects, such as endocardial cushion defects or VSDs, may involve the tricuspid valve's medial cusp, rendering this cusp insufficient or allowing for a direct shunt from the LV to the right atrium. Tricuspid valve stenosis usually accompanies pulmonary atresia or severe stenosis when the ventricular septum is intact. Actually, the tricuspid valve in these patients, although small and often with thickened cusps, is normally formed, and the stenosis is a secondary hypoplasia.

TRICUSPID ATRESIA

Although uncommon, tricuspid atresia is seen often enough to have considerable clinical importance. Next to transposition of the great arteries, tricuspid atresia is the most common cause of pronounced cyanosis in the neonatal period, and the degree of cyanosis is usually more marked than in cases of transposition. Only rarely is there a recognizable, small tricuspid annulus, which then forms the rim of an imperforate membrane. Usually there is only a dimple, or no indication of a tricuspid valve, in the floor of the right atrium.

Several subtypes of tricuspid atresia are distinguished based largely on whether there is an associated transposition of the great vessels (with or without pulmonary stenosis) and whether the VSD, which is almost always present, is large or small. Of the various types, tricuspid atresia without transposition and with a relatively small VSD is by far the most common. Unfortunately, this type also carries one of the worst prognoses; the great majority of infants die in the first year and usually in weeks or months if not treated appropriately. The right atrium is dilated, and either the foramen ovale is patulous or an ASD exists. If the atrial septum is minimally patent, balloon atrial septostomy can be performed to widen a minimal patent foramen ovale or very small ASD. This allows blood to flow into the left side of the heart and thus to the systemic circulation. The mitral valve is large, as is the LV. Usually there is no trace of a RV inflow portion, and the infundibulum generally is present and thin walled. Although uncommon, pulmonary valve stenosis may be seen in association with tricuspid atresia.

Characteristic clinical features include the early appearance of moderate to marked cyanosis, progressing with time and increasing with crying. Cerebral hypoxic spells, similar to those seen in tetralogy of Fallot, are occasionally seen, consisting of a sudden deepening of cyanosis, crying, lethargy, and at times unconsciousness. The episodes usually last only a few minutes but may lead to death of the infant (Plate 5.11).

TRICUSPID ATRESIA

Features of tricuspid atresia

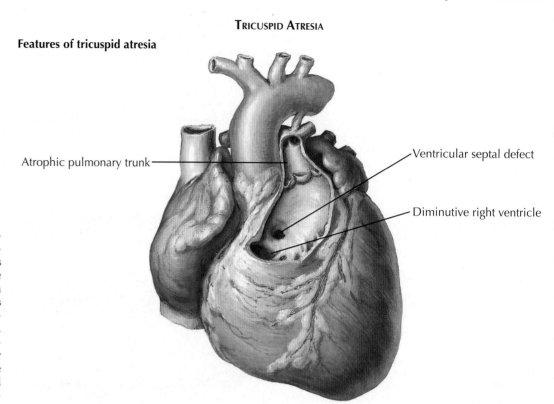

Atrophic pulmonary trunk

Ventricular septal defect

Diminutive right ventricle

Final anatomic aspect of the classic two-stage procedure created by Francis Fontan for ventricularization of the right atrium

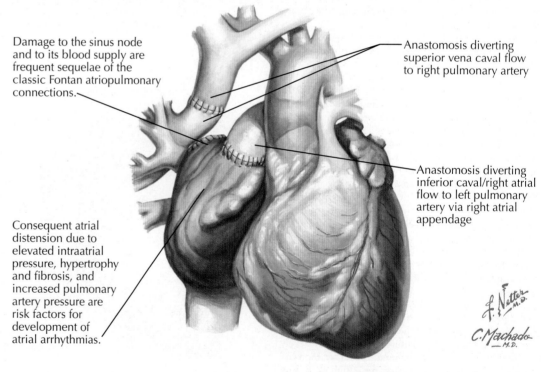

Damage to the sinus node and to its blood supply are frequent sequelae of the classic Fontan atriopulmonary connections.

Anastomosis diverting superior vena caval flow to right pulmonary artery

Anastomosis diverting inferior caval/right atrial flow to left pulmonary artery via right atrial appendage

Consequent atrial distension due to elevated intraatrial pressure, hypertrophy and fibrosis, and increased pulmonary artery pressure are risk factors for development of atrial arrhythmias.

Clubbing of the digits is never present at birth and takes time to develop; it is generally not well marked until about 3 months of age. The few children who live for any length of time usually have dyspnea on exertion (or even at rest) and fatigability. Occasionally a child may squat, but this is not a characteristic feature as in tetralogy of Fallot. Cardiomegaly is typically absent in patients of tricuspid atresia with no precordial bulge. A systolic thrill is rare. The apical heart sounds are unremarkable; S_2 at the base is normal or slightly increased and single, with P_2 greatly diminished or absent as a result of the reduced pulmonary blood flow. Typically, there is a harsh systolic murmur of moderate intensity, best heard at about the third left interspace parasternally.

On chest radiography the heart is either normal in size or only very slightly enlarged. The right border of the heart is prominent because of the enlarged right atrium; the left border may have a peculiar angulated or squared-off appearance, and the pulmonary artery

Plate 5.12   Congenital Heart Disease

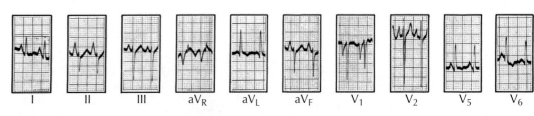

GLENN SURGERY FOR TRICUSPID ATRESIA

ANOMALIES OF THE TRICUSPID VALVE (Continued)

segment is reduced or absent. The vascularity of the lung fields is diminished. The ECG is much more helpful in arriving at a diagnosis. Left axis deviation, LV hypertrophy, and right atrial hypertrophy are invariably present. These are so typical for tricuspid atresia and so unusual in other types of cyanotic CHD that any cyanotic baby showing left axis deviation and LV hypertrophy on the ECG, and without cardiomegaly, should be considered to have tricuspid atresia. The P waves are generally tall and peaked (often very tall), indicating right atrial enlargement. Cardiac ultrasound and MRI can easily define the anatomic pathology, including shunts, valve regurgitation, and ventricular function.

Cardiac catheterization to obtain hemodynamic data generally should not be done; it contributes little to what is already known or suspected on clinical grounds, merely adding another stressful procedure for the very sick infant to undergo. If cardiac catheterization and angiography must be done, a simple venous angiocardiogram or a selective right atrial angiocardiogram confirms the diagnosis. Opacification of the right atrium is rapidly followed by visualization of the left atrium, LV, and great vessels. Generally, there is a typical, more or less triangular filling defect between the opacified right atrium and the LV. Cardiac magnetic resonance angiography (MRA) with contrast can confirm the anatomy as well. This area is normally occupied by the inflow portion of the RV. An LV injection in the lateral position shows the diminutive RV outflow portion to be filling by way of the VSD.

Treatment is surgical and can be only palliative. The surgery focuses on increasing pulmonary blood flow, which can also be accomplished in the newborn using prostaglandin E_1 (PGE$_1$). PGE$_1$ relaxes smooth muscle in the ductus arteriosus and keeps it patent to provide temporary blood flow from the aorta to the pulmonary artery. This palliation allows time for patients with tricuspid atresia to mature to the point where a surgical procedure can be performed safely. Blalock-Taussig (subclavian to pulmonary artery anastomosis), classic Glenn (right atrium to pulmonary artery), or a Fontan (variations of vena cava to pulmonary artery) procedure provides flow to the pulmonary circulation in these patients, who depend on pulmonary blood flow for survival. These surgical procedures require the pulmonary artery pressure to be low for flow to enter the pulmonary circulation from the vena cava or right atrium.

A side-to-side anastomosis of the ascending aorta to the pulmonary artery can substitute for the Blalock-Taussig shunt. In the Glenn procedure, the proximal pulmonary artery is ligated, as is the superior vena cava, between the anastomotic site and the right atrium (Plate 5.12). This operation has the considerable advantage

of bringing blood directly from a large systemic vein to the right lung, thus entirely bypassing the right side of the heart. Unfortunately, it is not suitable in very small infants, who are at the highest risk and comprise the majority of cases of tricuspid atresia, because the low-pressure shunt between the small vessels has a strong tendency to thrombose, with disastrous results. This is also characteristic, but to a lesser extent, of the Blalock-Taussig operation. The Fontan procedure is another

option to transfer venous blood directly into the pulmonary artery (see Plate 5.11).

Of the other (much rarer) forms of tricuspid atresia, those with a moderately large VSD and a normal to slightly increased pulmonary vascular resistance carry a much better prognosis and may not require surgery. A form that has a fairly good prognosis is that associated with transposition of the great vessels and a mild to moderate subpulmonic stenosis.

Superior vena cava
Right pulmonary artery
Temporary internal shunt
Right pulmonary veins
Right atrium
Schema of completed shunt procedure

Preoperative angiocardiogram: AO = aorta; LAA = left atrial appendage; LA = left atrium; RA = right atrium; LV = left ventricle

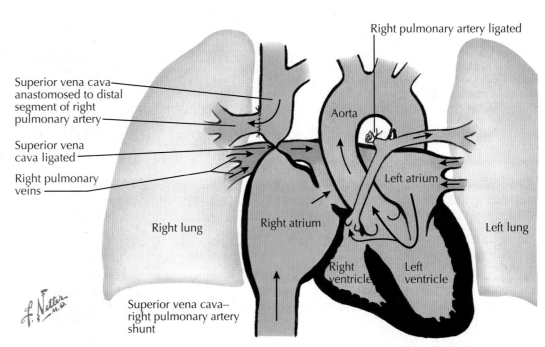

Plate 5.13

Cardiovascular System: VOLUME 8

EBSTEIN'S ANOMALY

ANOMALIES OF THE TRICUSPID VALVE (Continued)

EBSTEIN'S ANOMALY

As an isolated malformation, Ebstein's anomaly of the tricuspid valve is less common than tricuspid atresia. However, Ebstein's malformation is of considerable clinical importance because most patients reach childhood, adolescence, or even adulthood, and therefore it must be much better tolerated than tricuspid atresia. In principle, Ebstein's anomaly consists of a downward displacement of the tricuspid valve "origin." The valve cusps, except for the medial two-thirds of the anterior cusp, appear to originate from the RV wall, often as low as the junction of the inflow and outflow portions of the RV, instead of from the tricuspid annulus. The valve tissue is almost always redundant and wrinkled, and the chordae tendineae are poorly developed or absent (Plate 5.13).

Embryologically, Ebstein's malformation can be considered an abnormality in the undermining process of the RV wall, which normally leads to liberation of the inner layer of ventricular muscle. This process should continue until the atrioventricular junction is reached. Much of the apical portion of the valve "skirt" thus formed is normally resorbed, until only papillary muscles and narrow strands remain. The latter become fibrous (chordae tendineae), as do the valve cusps themselves. In Ebstein's anomaly, the process of undermining apparently is incomplete and does not reach the annulus. Individual cases vary greatly in this respect, and instead of cusps, chordae tendineae, and papillary muscles, there often are sheets of valve tissue with few or no chordae tendineae incorporating the papillary muscles. The anterior cusp is "liberated" very early in embryonic life, which may explain why this cusp always originates normally. The actual valve opening, located close to the crista supraventricularis, is usually much smaller than the normal tricuspid ostium, and the valve is almost always incompetent.

The downward displacement of the valve divides the RV into two parts: (1) an "atrialized" part between the normal annulus and the abnormal valve origin and (2) the normal outflow portion of the RV. The size of the "atrialized" portion of the RV varies greatly, and its wall may be fibrous and paper thin or muscular and normally formed. Rarely, the valve is imperforate, or its free portion is practically nonexistent. The pulmonary valve may be stenotic or rarely atretic.

The clinical features are highly diverse, an expression of the considerable variability of Ebstein's pathology. In general, the larger and thinner walled the atrialized RV part, the smaller the remaining normally developed RV part will be. Also, the greater the insufficiency of the tricuspid valve, the more serious the hemodynamic situation will be. In severe cases, symptoms (cyanosis, dyspnea, feeding difficulty) may begin in the neonatal period (see Plate 5.14). The early occurrence of heart

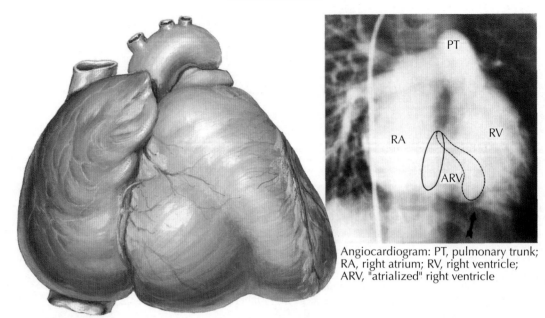

Angiocardiogram: PT, pulmonary trunk; RA, right atrium; RV, right ventricle; ARV, "atrialized" right ventricle

Ebstein's malformation: Heart viewed from right side

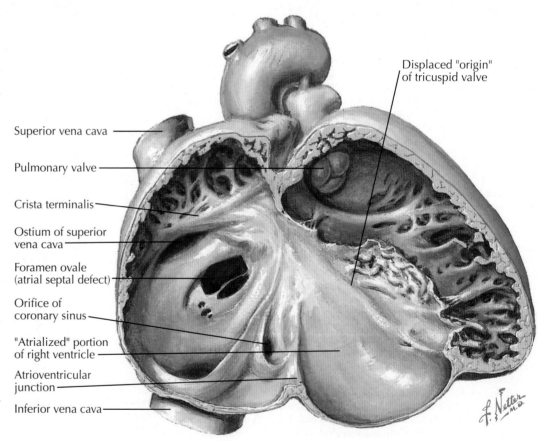

Superior vena cava

Pulmonary valve

Crista terminalis

Ostium of superior vena cava

Foramen ovale (atrial septal defect)

Orifice of coronary sinus

"Atrialized" portion of right ventricle

Atrioventricular junction

Inferior vena cava

Displaced "origin" of tricuspid valve

failure is an ominous sign and is usually followed by death within weeks. In milder cases, symptoms may not appear until later in childhood. Occasionally, the degree of malformation is slight and is compatible with a fairly active and normal life. Cyanosis and clubbing are usually present in older children, who tend to be underdeveloped and thin. Cyanosis in infancy often subsides temporarily, only to reappear later. Fatigue is a prominent symptom, along with exercise intolerance and dyspnea on effort. Cardiac arrhythmias are very common, usually consisting of some form of supraventricular tachycardia.

The patient with Ebstein's anomaly almost always has considerable cardiomegaly on both the left and right sides because of enlargement of the right atrium and the "atrialized" RV, and the peripheral pulses are weak. The apical impulse is diffuse and poorly felt. A precordial bulge and thrill are unusual. S_1 is of normal intensity and often is split, with the second component loud; S_2 is generally normal. A loud, early diastolic S_3 is heard

Plate 5.14

Congenital Heart Disease

ANOMALIES OF THE TRICUSPID VALVE (Continued)

along the left lower sternal border, and S_4 may be present. A mild to moderate systolic murmur is usually present along the left lower sternal border and may be accompanied by a diastolic murmur. The systolic murmur sometimes may have a curious scratchy quality, resembling that of a pericardial friction rub.

Chest radiography shows moderate to marked cardiomegaly, and the heart is often box or funnel shaped, mainly because of tremendous right atrial enlargement and displacement and dilation of the RV outflow tract. The pulmonary vascular markings are decreased, and the main pulmonary artery segment is small or absent. Left atrial enlargement is never seen in Ebstein's anomaly. Rarely, the heart may be almost normal in size and shape, indicating a mild degree of malformation.

The characteristic ECG displays right axis deviation, low voltage, and widened QRS complexes in the limb leads and the right precordial leads and, in the latter, a right bundle branch block pattern with "splintering" of the complexes. A pattern of RV hypertrophy is rarely seen, and LV hypertrophy is invariably absent. Tall, peaked P waves are usually seen in leads II, aV_F, and V_1 to V_3, and the PR interval is usually prolonged. Wolff-Parkinson-White syndrome (see Plate 2.23) is relatively common in Ebstein's anomaly.

Cardiac ultrasound or MRI can confirm the diagnosis of Ebstein's anomaly. With cardiac catheterization there is a distinct tendency for arrhythmias to occur, but the procedure can be used to establish the diagnosis and determine the degree of severity. The catheter tends to coil in the right atrium and thus outlines its tremendous size. The pressure in the atrialized portion of the RV is low and in general resembles that measured in the right atrium. RV pressures are normal, except in the rare case with associated pulmonary stenosis and resulting elevated RV pressure. If an electrode catheter is used, pressure tracings and intracavitary ECGs can be recorded simultaneously. Placement of the catheter in the distal portion of the RV will show typical RV pressure and ECG tracings. On pulling back into the atrialized part of the RV, the ECG tracings do not change significantly, whereas the pressure drops. In these circumstances, a ventricular intracardiac electrocardiogram may be recorded with an atrial pressure pulse. On further withdrawal into the right atrium, the ECG complexes assume a right atrial configuration with large P waves, and the pressure tracings show no further change (see Plate 5.13).

On selective right atrial angiocardiography, contrast successively opacifies the smooth-walled right atrium, the atrialized RV part, and often (after some delay) the trabeculated RV outflow portion. The diaphragmatic right border of the heart may have a trilobed, scalloped appearance. Injection into the RV outflow outlines the "incomplete" RV and regurgitation across the tricuspid valve.

Medical treatment is indicated mainly in patients with Ebstein's anomaly who have congestive heart failure

TYPES OF EBSTEIN'S ANOMALY

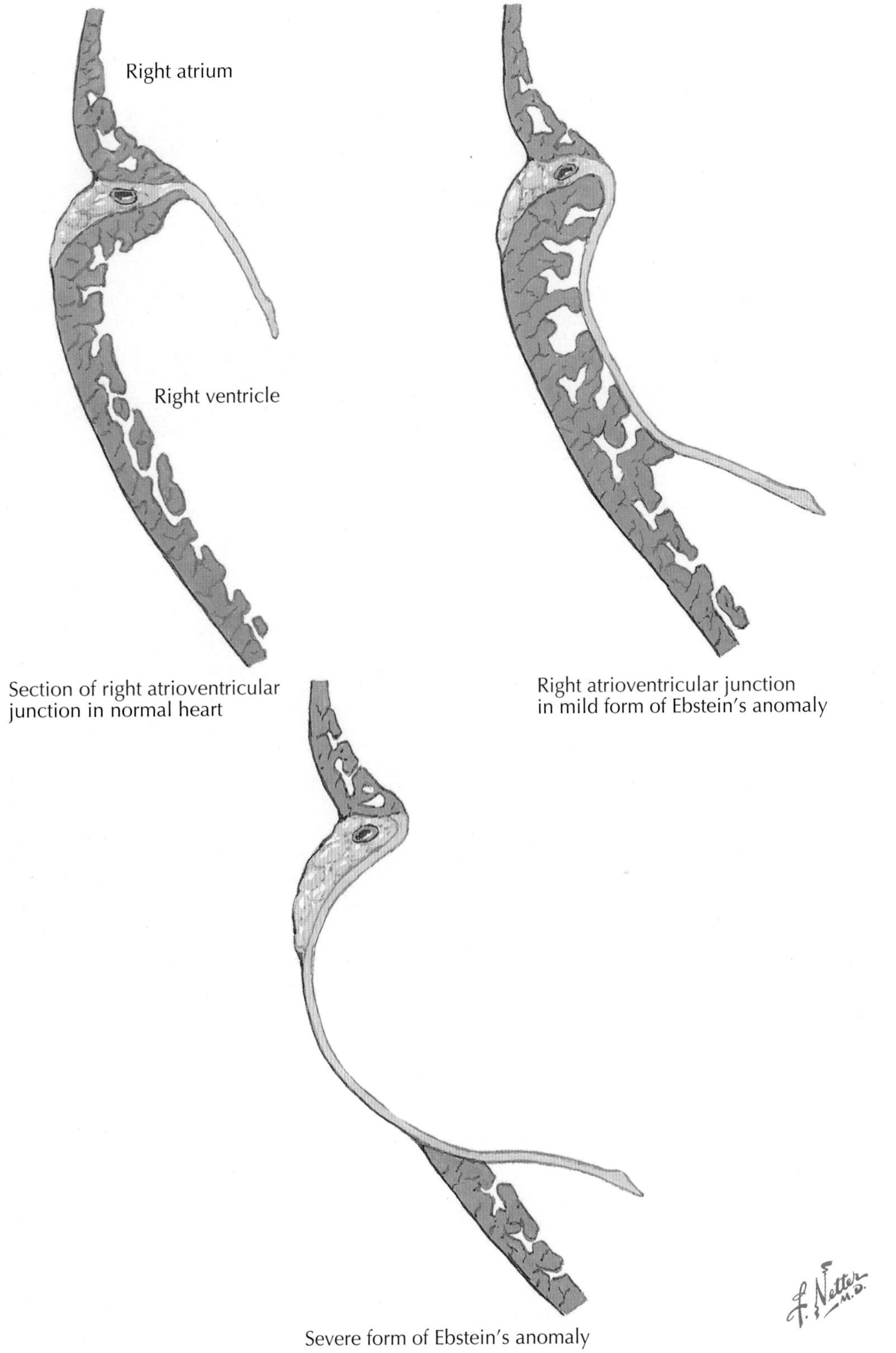

Right atrium

Right ventricle

Section of right atrioventricular junction in normal heart

Right atrioventricular junction in mild form of Ebstein's anomaly

Severe form of Ebstein's anomaly

or paroxysmal supraventricular tachycardia. Therapy consists of the usual anticongestive measures: digitalis, diuretics, oxygen, sedation, bed rest, and reduced salt intake. Angiotensin-converting enzyme inhibitors or angiotensin receptor blockers and beta-blocker therapy should be considered in patients with heart failure, as well as antiarrhythmics to control the tachycardia.

Surgical treatment is complicated and usually palliative. The choice of procedure depends on whatever pathology is present. In general, surgery should be advised only for patients with Ebstein's anomaly who are symptomatic and incapacitated. Rehabilitation of incapacitated patients has been achieved by prosthetic replacement of the anomalous valve and, in suitable cases, by resection or plication of the nonfunctioning atrialized part of the RV. An ASD, if present, should probably be closed at the same time to achieve the full benefit of the procedure. If the tricuspid valve is replaced, long-term anticoagulation must be achieved.

Plate 5.15

Cardiovascular System: VOLUME 8

ANOMALIES OF THE VENTRICULAR SEPTUM

VENTRICULAR SEPTAL DEFECTS ("MEMBRANOUS")

Of the anomalies involving VSDs, those located beneath the aortic valve, the membranous VSDs, are by far the most common. Not only are these defects frequently seen in association with other cardiac anomalies, but even when occurring as isolated lesions, the membranous VSDs constitute the most important and also the most common type of congenital heart disease. This is not surprising considering the complex embryologic history of the subaortic portion of the ventricular septum. This is the last part of the septum to close, a closure effected by the fusion of components from the embryonic muscular septum, endocardial cushions, and conal swellings. Anomalous development of any one or several of these contributors will lead to a defect of the ventricular septum. Therefore, although located in the same general area, membranous VSDs may vary considerably in position and size. Some are found immediately beneath the right and posterior aortic valve cusps; these probably are caused mainly by deficiency of the conus septum and, because of a lack of support for the aortic valve cusps, may lead to prolapse of one or both cusps, causing aortic regurgitation. Other membranous VSDs mainly caused by deficiency of the right limb of the endocardial cushions, or failure of otherwise normally developed endocardial cushions to fuse with the ventricular septum and conus septum, are located a few millimeters away from the aortic valve, leaving a rim of muscular or fibrous tissue. All of these defects are located in the general area where the *membranous septum* is found in the normal heart and thus are usually rather loosely referred to as "membranous septal defects."

Small Defects and Shunts

The clinical features vary, as might be expected in an anomaly with a diverse pathologic anatomy. Children who have small defects and shunts are well developed and asymptomatic, and the ECG is normal. Chest radiographs also are generally normal, although occasionally the vascular pattern may be slightly increased, with evidence of some left atrial enlargement. Such cases are referred to as having "maladie de Roger." A harsh systolic murmur, often well localized and, at times, quite loud, is heard best over the lower left parasternal area or (sometimes) somewhat higher up. A thrill may be palpable. Treatment is generally not indicated unless the anomaly is complicated by endocarditis, which fortunately occurs only rarely.

Large Defects

Large VSDs may cause symptoms in early infancy. Growth failure is usual in such cases; weight gain may be distressingly slow, and the children are pale, delicate looking, and scrawny. Feeding difficulties, respiratory infections, and congestive failure are common, and the infants may spend more time in the hospital than at home. There is cardiomegaly, and a loud, harsh, holosystolic murmur audible over the left lower sternum, accompanied by a thrill, is almost invariably present. An apical diastolic rumble, ascribed to torrential blood flow across the mitral valve, is often also heard.

The chest radiograph shows cardiomegaly, mainly caused by biventricular and left atrial enlargement; marked hypervascularity of the lungs, with a prominent

Defect of membranous ventricular septum (viewed from right ventricle)

Defect

Defect of membranous ventricular septum (viewed from left ventricle)

Defect

Aneurysm

Aneurysm of membranous septum

Ventricular septal defect ECG ➡

| I | II | III | aV$_R$ | aV$_L$ | aV$_F$ | V$_1$ | V$_2$ | V$_3$ | V$_4$ | V$_5$ | V$_6$ |

Radiograph: Ventricular septal defect in a 5-year-old boy

AO PT

←VSD

RV LV

LV angiocardiogram

pulmonary trunk and main pulmonary arteries; and a relatively small aorta. ECG generally reveals right axis deviation and evidence of biventricular enlargement. This often takes the form of large, biphasic QRS complexes in the mid precordial leads (Katz-Wachtel phenomenon). Cardiac ultrasound and MRI easily confirm the diagnosis of VSD and can define its anatomic pathology and location.

Cardiac catheterization readily demonstrates a marked increase in the oxygen content of the RV blood samples,

and the catheter may enter the LV or aorta through the VSD, especially when the catheter is advanced from the superior vena cava. Catheters advanced from the inferior vena cava generally do not cross the VSD. The RV and pulmonary artery pressures are elevated and may reach systemic levels. The pulmonary hypertension is caused in part by some increase in pulmonary vascular resistance but mostly by the greatly increased pulmonary blood flow, which may be several times that of the systemic blood flow. The injection of a

Plate 5.16

Congenital Heart Disease

ANOMALIES OF THE VENTRICULAR SEPTUM (Continued)

radiopaque medium selectively into the pulmonary trunk, after passage through the lungs, demonstrates the interventricular shunt. A selective LV angiogram will give even clearer pictures of the shunt.

Therapeutically, infants with large VSDs may present a serious problem. Every effort should be made to carry them through the first year, after which many improve greatly, probably because of the relative decrease in size of the VSD. If medical treatment is unsuccessful, a pulmonary banding procedure may be done, or in some cases a percutaneous approach may be used to close the VSD with a device. With banding, a plastic-like band is placed around the pulmonary trunk, just above the valve, and tightened until the diameter of the vessel is reduced by about two-thirds and the pressure distally has dropped closer to normal. Usually, there is a concomitant rise in aortic pressure, indicating a more favorable pulmonary/systemic blood flow ratio. The surgical results may be excellent, although many failures occur as well. In any case, banding is a temporary procedure followed by closure of the defect later, at which time the band is removed.

Moderate-Sized Defects

Fortunately, most children with moderately sized VSDs do not have the stormy infancy previously described, although respiratory infections are prevalent and many patients are small for their age. Dyspnea on exertion is also common. Congestive heart failure occurs rarely in older children, however, and the physician should always consider the possibility of a complicating lesion, such as prolapse of an aortic valve cusp causing aortic regurgitation, or bacterial endocarditis. A harsh, rather loud, holosystolic murmur accompanied by a thrill is generally best heard along the lower left sternal border. An apical diastolic murmur of moderate intensity (mitral flow murmur) is usually audible at the apex.

Clinical examination and chest radiography usually show moderate cardiomegaly; the pulmonary vasculature is distinctly increased, and the left atrium is enlarged. The ECG typically shows a normal or right axis deviation with a pattern of so-called LV diastolic overloading, consisting of deep Q waves, very tall R waves, and often tall, peaked T waves in the left precordial leads. Evidence for biventricular enlargement is also common. Cardiac ultrasound and MRI can define the size and position of the VSD. Cardiac catheterization findings are similar to those described above; however, the RV and pulmonary artery pressures are generally only slightly or moderately elevated and show little tendency to rise during childhood. An LV *angiogram* is easily done in this age group, and it will clearly demonstrate the size and position of the defect.

Treatment of patients with moderate-sized VSDs is surgical and consists of closure of the defect transatrially using direct suture or a prosthesis and cardiopulmonary bypass (see Plate 5.17). The surgical risk is low, but heart block caused by injury to the atrioventricular bundle can occur infrequently.

Pulmonary Hypertension

Some patients with VSDs either have always had, or develop as young adults, marked pulmonary hypertension because of vascular changes in the lungs. The pulmonary vascular resistance equals or exceeds systemic vascular resistance, and the shunt across the defect is (or becomes) bidirectional or mainly from right to left,

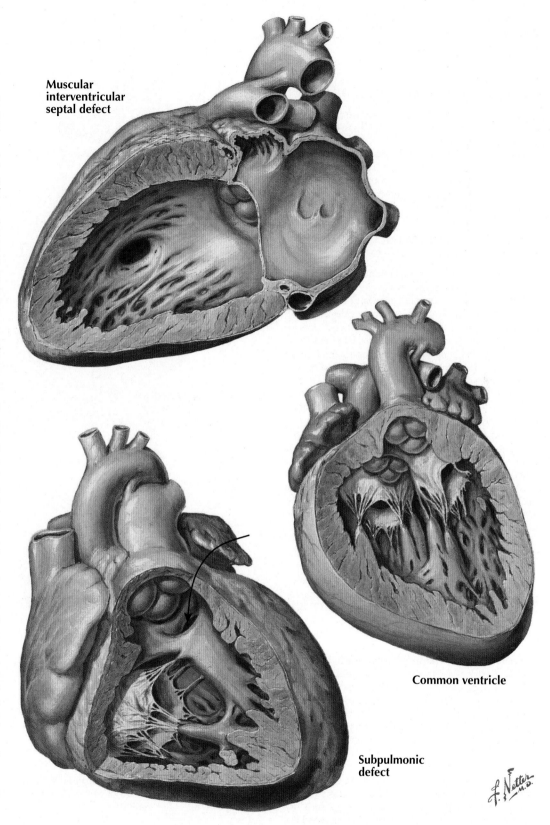

Muscular interventricular septal defect

Common ventricle

Subpulmonic defect

causing cyanosis and digital clubbing. In some patients a murmur is barely audible, an expression of the presence of equal pressures in the two ventricles and minimal net shunt. P_2 is loud and snapping, and the pulmonary valve may become incompetent, resulting in a diastolic murmur at the left upper sternal border.

Chest radiography reveals little or no cardiomegaly. The pulmonary artery and the branches are usually dilated and the lung fields are clear. ECG reveals right axis deviation and RV hypertrophy.

Prostaglandins, endothelin receptor antagonists, phosphodiesterase type 5 inhibitors, and activators of soluble guanylate cyclase are used to decrease pulmonary artery pressure in many patients with VSD with hypertension, especially those with some evidence of pulmonary artery constriction. Surgical closure of the defect carries a prohibitive mortality (~100%) and is contraindicated. Lung transplantation may be the only surgical procedure to reduce symptoms and prolong life.

Plate 5.17

Cardiovascular System: VOLUME 8

ANOMALIES OF THE VENTRICULAR SEPTUM (Continued)

ANEURYSM OF MEMBRANOUS SEPTUM

Aneurysms of the membranous septum are being diagnosed with increasing frequency as selective LV angiocardiography, echocardiography, CT, and MRI are increasingly done. The aneurysm may be intact or may contain one or more perforations (see Plate 5.15). The aneurysm itself produces no symptoms, unless large enough to cause RV outflow obstruction or unless an aortic cusp prolapses into it; both are rare complications.

MUSCULAR INTERVENTRICULAR SEPTAL DEFECTS

Defects of the muscular interventricular septum may occur anywhere in the septum (see Plate 5.16). These defects may be single or multiple and any size. If located in the trabeculated apical part of the septum, the defect may go undetected. Some defects have a "Swiss cheese" appearance. In the adult population without CHD, ventricular septal rupture secondary to acute myocardial infarction can produce comparable signs and symptoms as the congenital variety, and the prognosis is poor. The symptoms and signs depend on the combined size of the defects as well as the degree of ventricular dysfunction. Treatment is surgical or with a percutaneous closure device.

A special form of muscular interventricular septal defect is located beneath the two arterial valves and is caused by malalignment of the truncus and conus septa, which do not meet each other and therefore cannot fuse. The truncus septum is deviated to the left, and the pulmonary artery overrides the anteriorly located defect. The murmur tends to be located somewhat higher than usual and may sound superficial.

COMMON VENTRICLE

In a common ventricle the entire septum is absent except for a low muscular ridge, usually present along the posteroinferior ventricular wall (see Plate 5.16). Both atrioventricular valves enter the common chamber, and both structurally resemble the normal mitral valve. The two posterior papillary muscles, together with the low muscular ridge, may form a single muscle mass. The two great arteries are transposed, and both may originate from the common chamber, or one (usually the aorta) may spring from a small outflow chamber separated from the main ventricular body by a muscular septum-like ridge. Associated pulmonary stenosis often occurs and, if not too severe, generally improves the prognosis. Ventricular inversion is common and is present in the specimen illustrated here.

The clinical features depend largely on the presence of pulmonary stenosis; patients with stenosis present similar to those with tetralogy of Fallot (see Plate 5.18). If there is no stenosis, the symptoms and signs are those of a large VSD, except that the thrill and the loud systolic murmur are not present. A systolic murmur at the base is probably caused by a large pulmonary blood flow across the normal pulmonary valve. As in VSD, an apical diastolic rumble may be heard. Vascular changes in the lung develop early, resulting in a high resistance to blood flow and pulmonary hypertension.

On chest radiography, the heart is normal in size if pulmonary stenosis is present, and the pulmonary vasculature is diminished. In patients without pulmonary stenosis, cardiomegaly may be present, associated with an increase in the pulmonary vasculature. In patients with severe pulmonary hypertension as a result of the intrapulmonary vascular changes, cardiomegaly is mild or absent; the hilar vessels are large, but peripherally the markings are diminished. There are no characteristic ECG findings associated with the common ventricle, and the QRS axis and precordial lead patterns vary greatly. Selective angiocardiography establishes the diagnosis, as does the cardiac echocardiography, MRI, or CTA.

At present, treatment of common ventricle can be only palliative; correction is not possible for anatomic and hemodynamic reasons. Patients with mild to moderate pulmonary stenosis require no surgical treatment and may do well for many years. Patients with severe pulmonary stenosis may have a Blalock-Taussig shunt or an anastomosis from vena cava to pulmonary artery. In young children without stenosis, a pulmonary artery banding procedure may be considered.

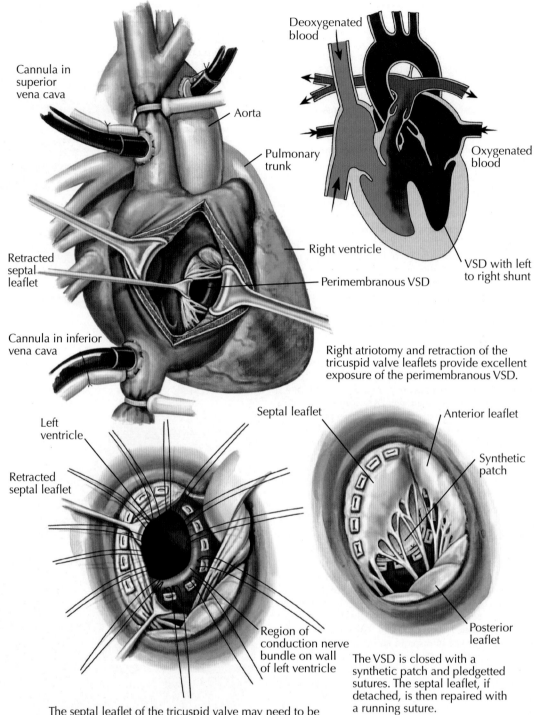

TRANSATRIAL REPAIR OF VENTRICULAR SEPTAL DEFECT

Cannula in superior vena cava

Deoxygenated blood

Aorta

Pulmonary trunk

Oxygenated blood

Right ventricle

Retracted septal leaflet

Perimembranous VSD

VSD with left to right shunt

Cannula in inferior vena cava

Right atriotomy and retraction of the tricuspid valve leaflets provide excellent exposure of the perimembranous VSD.

Septal leaflet

Anterior leaflet

Left ventricle

Synthetic patch

Retracted septal leaflet

Region of conduction nerve bundle on wall of left ventricle

Posterior leaflet

The VSD is closed with a synthetic patch and pledgetted sutures. The septal leaflet, if detached, is then repaired with a running suture.

The septal leaflet of the tricuspid valve may need to be bisected to permit placement of pledgetted sutures at its junction with the VSD. Superficial sutures are placed along the inferior border of the VSD to prevent injury to the conduction system.

K. Carter

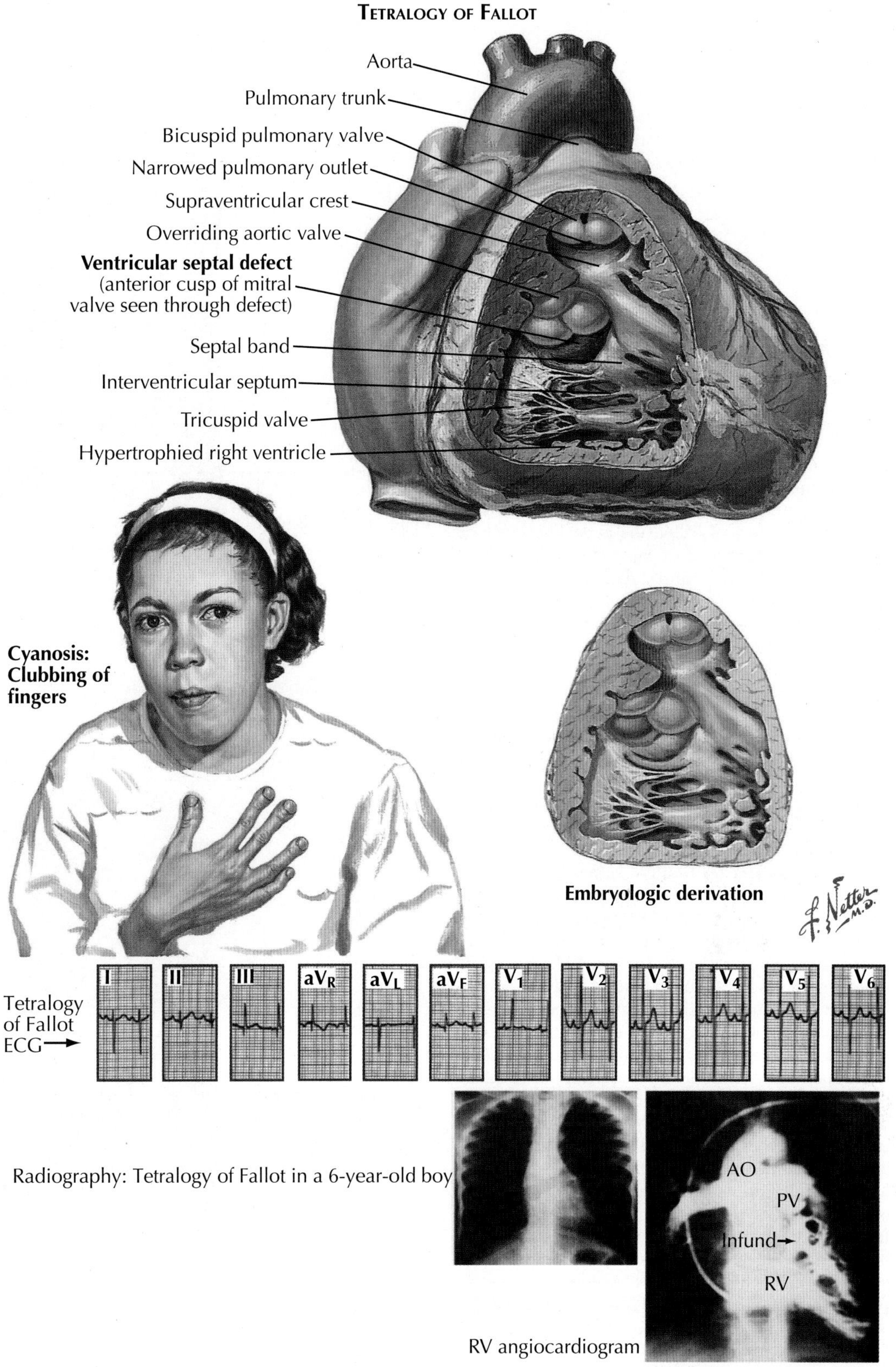

Plate 5.18

Congenital Heart Disease

TETRALOGY OF FALLOT

- Aorta
- Pulmonary trunk
- Bicuspid pulmonary valve
- Narrowed pulmonary outlet
- Supraventricular crest
- Overriding aortic valve
- **Ventricular septal defect** (anterior cusp of mitral valve seen through defect)
- Septal band
- Interventricular septum
- Tricuspid valve
- Hypertrophied right ventricle

ANOMALIES OF RIGHT VENTRICULAR OUTFLOW TRACT

TETRALOGY OF FALLOT

Tetralogy of Fallot is by far the most common form of cyanotic congenital heart disease that is compatible with life. Patients reaching adulthood are uncommon but not rare.

Classically, as described by Fallot, the four abnormalities that constitute the complex are RV outflow tract stenosis (or atresia), VSD, aortic straddling of the VSD (seems to originate from both ventricles), and RV hypertrophy (Plate 5.18). Anatomically, there is classically RV infundibular stenosis, but the pulmonary valve, although frequently *bicuspid,* is stenotic in only about 40% of patients. Nonstenotic valves may be hypoplastic, as part of a general hypoplasia of the pulmonary trunk. Stenotic valves may be bicuspid, tricuspid, or dome shaped, without well-defined cusps. The degree of infundibular stenosis ranges from complete atresia to barely detectable. The VSD is usually large, offering little or no resistance to blood flow and involving not only the area of the membranous septum but also the adjacent, more anterior portions of the ventricular septum. The aortic straddling of the VSD, although variable, is always unmistakable, and the aorta often appears to originate primarily from the RV. The RV is always hypertrophied, reflecting the high RV pressure, which is identical to LV pressure.

From a developmental point of view, tetralogy of Fallot is a simple anomaly caused by a single embryologic error (see Plate 5.18). The *conus septum* is located too far anteriorly, particularly in its lower part, dividing the conus into a smaller, anterior RV part (thus the infundibular stenosis) and a larger posterior part. The conus cannot form the crista supraventricularis and participate in closure of the interventricular septum. This in turn makes it impossible for the aortic valve to seat itself in its normal position, with its free edge so far removed from the tricuspid valve that the aortic valve cannot contribute to the formation of the tricuspid valve. This is why the medial papillary muscle is absent and the tricuspid valve is abnormally formed in tetralogy of Fallot. The *truncus septum* is also usually displaced anteriorly, accounting at least in part for the small pulmonary trunk and disproportionately large ascending aorta.

The clinical picture depends mainly on the degree of RV outflow obstruction, which usually is moderate, at least initially. The shunt across the ventricular septum is mainly from left to right (*acyanotic* tetralogy of Fallot). Therefore many children with tetralogy are not clinically cyanotic during the first few months of life but become so as they grow and as the stenosis worsens. More venous blood enters the aorta directly from the RV, and the pulmonary blood flow decreases in a

Cyanosis: Clubbing of fingers

Embryologic derivation

Tetralogy of Fallot ECG →

Radiography: Tetralogy of Fallot in a 6-year-old boy

AO
PV
Infund →
RV

RV angiocardiogram

relative sense. At first, cyanosis is obvious only with exertion or crying, but generally within the first few years of life the children become cyanotic even at rest, and clubbing of the fingers and toes develops (see Plate 5.18). Occasionally, the infundibular stenosis is so mild that cyanosis never develops ("pink" tetralogy). These children, particularly in infancy, may behave more like patients who have a VSD with large left-to-right shunts.

At the other extreme are cases where the infundibulum and/or pulmonary valve are atretic or severely stenotic. Such infants are generally cyanotic from birth, although the severity of the condition may be masked by a short-lived patency of the ductus arteriosus, which temporarily maintains good pulmonary circulation. Unfortunately, however, the ductus usually closes within the first 2 weeks of life, often causing

Plate 5.19

Cardiovascular System: VOLUME 8

ANOMALIES OF RIGHT VENTRICULAR OUTFLOW TRACT (Continued)

rapid deterioration of the infant's condition, so that surgical intervention to increase pulmonary blood flow becomes imperative.

A worrisome phenomenon can occur in young children with tetralogy of Fallot, the hypoxic episode or "blue spell." A period of crying suddenly leads to a marked increase in cyanosis, dyspnea, and unconsciousness, sometimes with convulsions. Such episodes may occur only occasionally or as often as several times a day and may last for minutes or hours. The spells tend to be associated with bowel movements or feeding and occur early in the day, although the episodes can happen at any time for no apparent reason. Hypoxic events are serious and may be fatal. The hypoxia results from a sudden spasm of the RV infundibulum and a corresponding decrease in pulmonary blood flow. Although more common in frankly cyanotic infants, hypoxic episodes may also occur in the less severe forms of tetralogy.

Squatting is characteristically assumed by children of walking age with cyanotic tetralogy of Fallot. Squatting usually follows some degree of physical exertion, which may simply be walking. The posture rapidly restores arterial oxygen saturation by an incompletely understood mechanism, although the increased arterial vascular resistance during squatting may decrease right-to-left shunting. Dyspnea and hyperpnea on exertion are common, as in all forms of cyanotic CHD. These children typically are underdeveloped with clubbing of the fingers and toes, except in the first few months of life. There is usually no prominence of the left side of the chest, and a thrill is palpable at the lower left sternal border in most patients.

On auscultation, S_1 is normal and A_2 is loud, but P_2 is diminished or absent. In acyanotic or mildly cyanotic forms of tetralogy of Fallot, P_2 may be present, and S_2 may then be widely split. The systolic murmur is usually loud and of the stenotic crescendo-decrescendo type, ending before or at aortic closure. In general, the more severe the tetralogy, the shorter the murmur is; occasionally, no murmur is heard at all. Likewise, during a hypoxic episode, the murmur may be less obvious or may disappear altogether, only to return on recovery.

The chest radiograph characteristically shows the heart to be normal in size (see Plate 5.18). The apex is elevated, and the pulmonary segment is small or concave—the boot-shaped heart ("coeur en sabot"). The aortic arch is prominent, and the pulmonary vasculature may be diminished. The aortic arch is located on the right side in about 2.5% of cases. The ECG characteristically shows right axis deviation and RV hypertrophy of the systolic overload type, with tall R waves in the right precordial leads. Transition is usually early and rather sudden in V_2 or V_3 and is an expression of the heart's small size. Additional evidence of LV hypertrophy may be present in the left precordial leads in pink tetralogy, when the ventricular shunt is mainly or exclusively from left to right (see Plate 5.18).

On cardiac catheterization the pressures in the ventricles are usually equal and at systemic levels; RV and LV pressure tracings are identical and of normal configuration. Evidence of bidirectional shunting across the VSD shows that the right-to-left component is usually dominant. Arterial oxygen saturation varies considerably among patients. The aorta is often entered easily from the RV, when the catheter is advanced from either the SVC or IVC and pulmonary artery pressure is low.

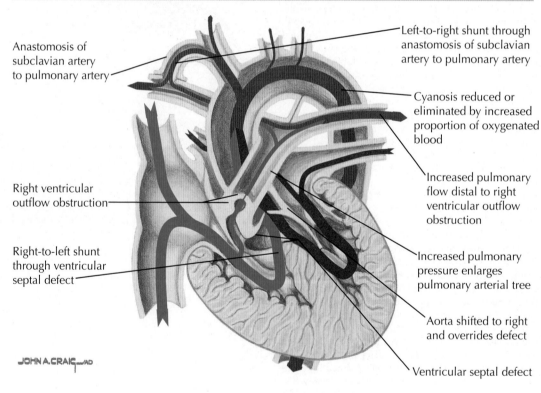

Pathophysiology

Intense cyanosis caused by high proportion of deoxygenated blood

Right ventricular outflow obstruction

Decreased pulmonary flow

Small pulmonary trunk

Right-to-left shunt through ventricular septal defect

Aorta shifted to right and overrides defect

Right ventricular hypertrophy

Ventricular septal defect

Blalock-Taussig Operation (palliative)

Anastomosis of subclavian artery to pulmonary artery

Left-to-right shunt through anastomosis of subclavian artery to pulmonary artery

Cyanosis reduced or eliminated by increased proportion of oxygenated blood

Right ventricular outflow obstruction

Increased pulmonary flow distal to right ventricular outflow obstruction

Right-to-left shunt through ventricular septal defect

Increased pulmonary pressure enlarges pulmonary arterial tree

Aorta shifted to right and overrides defect

Ventricular septal defect

JOHN A.CRAIG—AD

Plate 5.20

Congenital Heart Disease

CORRECTIVE OPERATION FOR TETRALOGY OF FALLOT

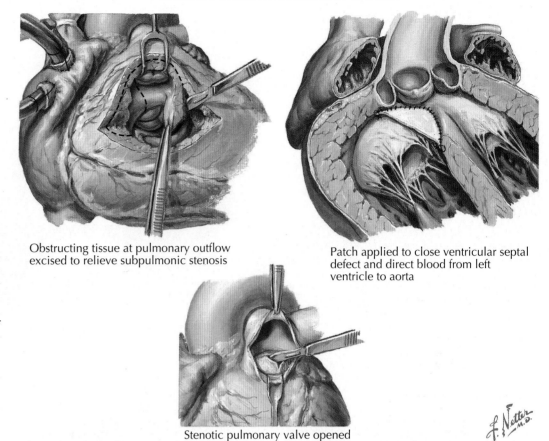

Obstructing tissue at pulmonary outflow excised to relieve subpulmonic stenosis

Patch applied to close ventricular septal defect and direct blood from left ventricle to aorta

Stenotic pulmonary valve opened

ANOMALIES OF RIGHT VENTRICULAR OUTFLOW TRACT (Continued)

Angiocardiography is especially valuable to the surgeon in delineating the anatomy of RV outflow and determining the size and position of the pulmonary artery. Cardiac ultrasound and MRA are also helpful. The prognosis depends on the severity of RV outflow obstruction. Infants who are cyanotic at or shortly after birth seldom survive the first year unless surgery is performed. Those with lesser forms of tetralogy of Fallot may live for many years and, although physically disabled in many ways, are usually alert and do well intellectually. The more common and serious complications are bacterial endocarditis, cerebral vascular accident (CVA, stroke) caused by thrombosis or severe hypoxia, and brain abscess. Central nervous system symptoms appearing in patients older than 2 years with cyanotic CHD almost always indicate the presence of a brain abscess. It is extremely rare in infants. On the other hand, CVA seldom occurs in patients older than 2 years. The etiology of brain abscesses and cerebral thrombosis may be related to shunting of blood from the venous system to the arterial system (see Plate 5.18).

Treatment of patients with tetralogy of Fallot is both medical and surgical. Heart failure is extremely uncommon beyond infancy but may occur in babies and should be treated in the usual manner. Hypoxic spells are often dramatically relieved by the administration of morphine and oxygen and squatting. Cyanotic children with normal or near-normal hemoglobin levels are usually anemic and should be given iron therapy until hemoglobin has increased to 15 to 17 g/dL (gm%). Once popular in patients with high hematocrit levels, venesection is now known to increase the symptoms and signs of hypoxia. Venesection should be done in small increments with caution, and then only in symptomatic patients with extremely high hematocrit (≥80 mL/dL).

Blalock-Taussig and Brock Operations

Surgical treatment is much more important in tetralogy of Fallot. Any cyanotic infant or child too young for correction but with significant symptoms should have the benefit of some type of palliative procedure. An end-to-side subclavian artery–pulmonary artery shunt, the *Blalock-Taussig operation*, is the procedure of choice in patients after infancy (see Plate 5.19). Technically straightforward, the surgery carries minimal risk of creating too large a shunt, which might lead to heart failure. In infants, who have small vessels, the Blalock-Taussig procedure is much less satisfactory; the shunt often thromboses immediately, or the infant rapidly outgrows it, necessitating a second operation on the opposite side. Creation of a direct side-to-side ascending aorta–pulmonary artery shunt may be preferable, known as the *Waterston* (Waterston-Cooley) *operation*.

Right Blalock shunt

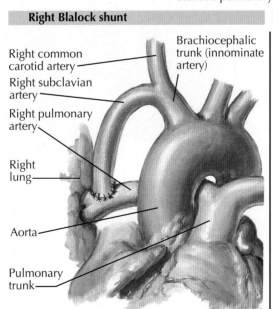

Right common carotid artery

Right subclavian artery

Right pulmonary artery

Right lung

Aorta

Pulmonary trunk

Brachiocephalic trunk (innominate artery)

Brock operation

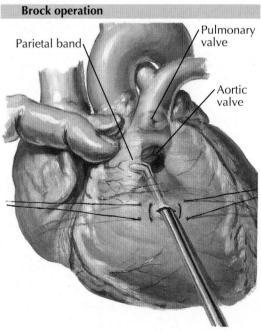

Parietal band

Pulmonary valve

Aortic valve

The older Potts procedure, with anastomosis from descending aorta to pulmonary artery, was found to be so difficult and dangerous to undo when done at a later age that it has been abandoned.

An alternate procedure that may be done in young infants and that may be preferable to some surgeons for older children as well is the *Brock operation* (Plate 5.20). This consists of removing at least some of the stenosing infundibular muscle tissue through an

RV stab wound, cutting the pulmonary valve as well if it is stenotic. The Brock procedure is performed blindly, is difficult to do adequately, and carries risks, particularly to the aortic valve.

The results of correction of tetralogy of Fallot are dramatic. The RV (pulmonary) outflow obstruction must be adequately relieved, which involves excision of as much obstructing muscle tissue as possible and possibly the use of an outflow patch to widen the infundibulum and at

Plate 5.21

Cardiovascular System: VOLUME 8

REPAIR OF TETRALOGY OF FALLOT

ANOMALIES OF RIGHT VENTRICULAR OUTFLOW TRACT (Continued)

times the pulmonary root and trunk as well. The VSD is closed, employing a second patch of appropriate size (Plate 5.21).

In the most severe forms of tetralogy of Fallot, in which the patient has atresia or near-atresia of the RV outflow tract, correction may not be possible. A permanent superior vena cava–right pulmonary artery shunt often provides excellent palliative therapy. A conduit from the RV to the pulmonary artery *(Rastelli procedure)* may also improve oxygenation.

EISENMENGER COMPLEX

Patients with Eisenmenger complex have a large VSD similar to that seen in tetralogy of Fallot, and the aorta straddles the VSD (see Plate 5.22). However, the crista supraventricularis is not significantly displaced, although it is hypoplastic and occasionally nearly absent. As in tetralogy, the tricuspid valve is abnormally formed in this anomaly. There is no RV outflow obstruction, so the pulmonary artery is large. The anomaly is rare, and the term *Eisenmenger syndrome* arose to designate situations where a left-to-right shunt, regardless of its level, changed gradually to a predominantly right-to-left shunt, with severe pulmonary hypertension caused by pulmonary vascular changes and a concomitant rise in pulmonary vascular resistance (PVR). Pathologically, the Eisenmenger complex may be differentiated from a simple VSD by noting the anomalous tricuspid valve. In a simple VSD, the tricuspid is normally formed, and a medial papillary muscle is present. At times, differentiation of the Eisenmenger complex from acyanotic tetralogy of Fallot is difficult, because in tetralogy of Fallot, as in all forms of tetralogy, the crista may not only be displaced but also be hypoplastic. Embryologically, the anomaly is caused by hypoplasia of the conus septum.

In young children the clinical picture of Eisenmenger complex is that of a VSD with a large left-to-right shunt and RV and pulmonary artery hypertension. As might be expected, P_2 is very loud, and an ejection click is usually present. Pulmonary vascular changes develop early, and older children become increasingly cyanotic.

On chest radiography, cardiomegaly and increased pulmonary vascularity are seen in young children. In older patients, the heart is only slightly enlarged or normal and the vascular pattern of the peripheral lung fields is attenuated, while the main pulmonary arteries remain large. Initially the ECG typically shows biventricular enlargement in older patients increasingly resembling the pattern seen in tetralogy of Fallot. At *cardiac catheterization*, the RV and pulmonary artery pressures are high and equal to the systemic pressure, and, even in acyanotic patients with a predominant

left-to-right shunt, some systemic arterial desaturation may be detectable by oximetry. *Angiocardiography* occasionally demonstrates the hypoplastic crista.

Pulmonary banding should be carried out early in an effort to prevent the development of pulmonary hypertension and increased PVR. Once a right-to-left shunt is established, surgery is contraindicated, and in the severely symptomatic patient lung transplantation should be considered.

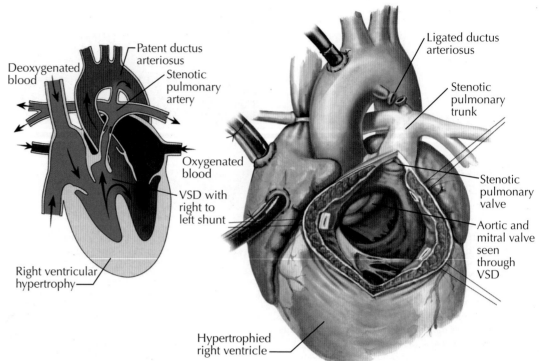

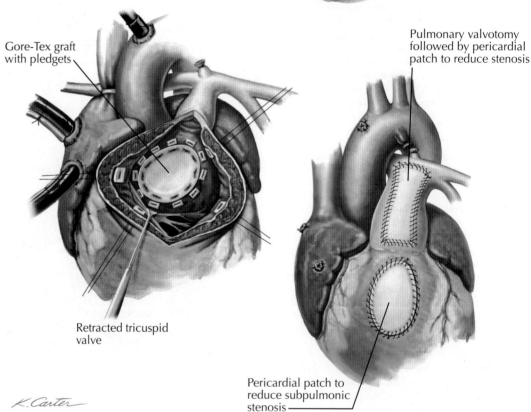

K. Carter

DOUBLE-OUTLET RIGHT VENTRICLE

In the double-outlet RV, both the aorta and the pulmonary artery originate from the RV (see Plate 5.22). The pulmonary artery is normally located; the aorta arises from the ventricle to the right of and posterior to the pulmonary artery. Pulmonary valvular with infundibular stenosis is common and usually severe. A muscular band of varying width derived from the bulboventricular flange separates the aortic valve from the mitral

Plate 5.22

Congenital Heart Disease

ANOMALIES OF RIGHT VENTRICULAR OUTFLOW TRACT (Continued)

valve. A VSD is always present, forming the sole outlet for the LV. Embryologically, double-outlet RV probably results from a persistent bulboventricular flange, which keeps the aortic and mitral valves separated and prevents the normal transfer of the aorta to the LV. The conus septum cannot develop in its normal relation to the right atrioventricular valve, so it cannot contribute to the formation of the AV valve.

Clinical and chest radiograph findings for double-outlet RV are similar to Eisenmenger complex. The ECG shows biventricular or predominantly RV enlargement, and the QRS axis usually is oriented to the right and superiorly. When pulmonary stenosis is present, the double outlet may be mistaken for tetralogy of Fallot. Cardiac catheterization demonstrates systemic RV pressures and may show mild systemic arterial desaturation, even in acyanotic children. The aortic blood always has higher oxygen saturation than the pulmonary artery blood. Angiocardiographically, the aorta is far to the right, the aortic valve is too "high," and the aorta and pulmonary artery are almost in the same frontal plane. These features can be seen with cardiac ultrasound, CTA, and MRI.

Treatment for double-outlet RV is surgical. As in Eisenmenger complex, pulmonary banding should be done early in patients without pulmonary stenosis. Correction is feasible (in those who do not have prohibitive PVR changes) by connecting the VSD and the adjacent right-side aorta by a half-shell–shaped patch. Occasionally, enlargement of the VSD will be required. Where pulmonary with infundibular stenosis is present, outflow tract enlargement with a prosthesis is usually also necessary because of the severity of the pulmonary stenosis as well as the obstructive effect of the anterior bulge of the subjacent tunnel patch. A major right coronary conal artery is often present and should be taken into account in placing the ventriculotomy; not knowing its position may be dangerous in some patients with pulmonary stenosis.

A special form of double-outlet RV, in which the VSD is located anteriorly beneath the pulmonary valve, is known as the *Taussig-Bing complex*. The pulmonary valve overrides the defect, and at cardiac catheterization the saturation of the pulmonary artery blood is higher than that of the aorta. Corrective surgery consists of completing the transposition of the pulmonary artery to the LV by patch closure of the VSD and intraatrial venous transposition, as described by Mustard. Although the result is a hemodynamic improvement, whether the RV can sustain the systemic circulation for a normal life span remains conjectural. Again, the degree of PVR must be considered in selecting patients for surgery.

EISENMENGER COMPLEX AND DOUBLE-OUTLET RIGHT VENTRICLE

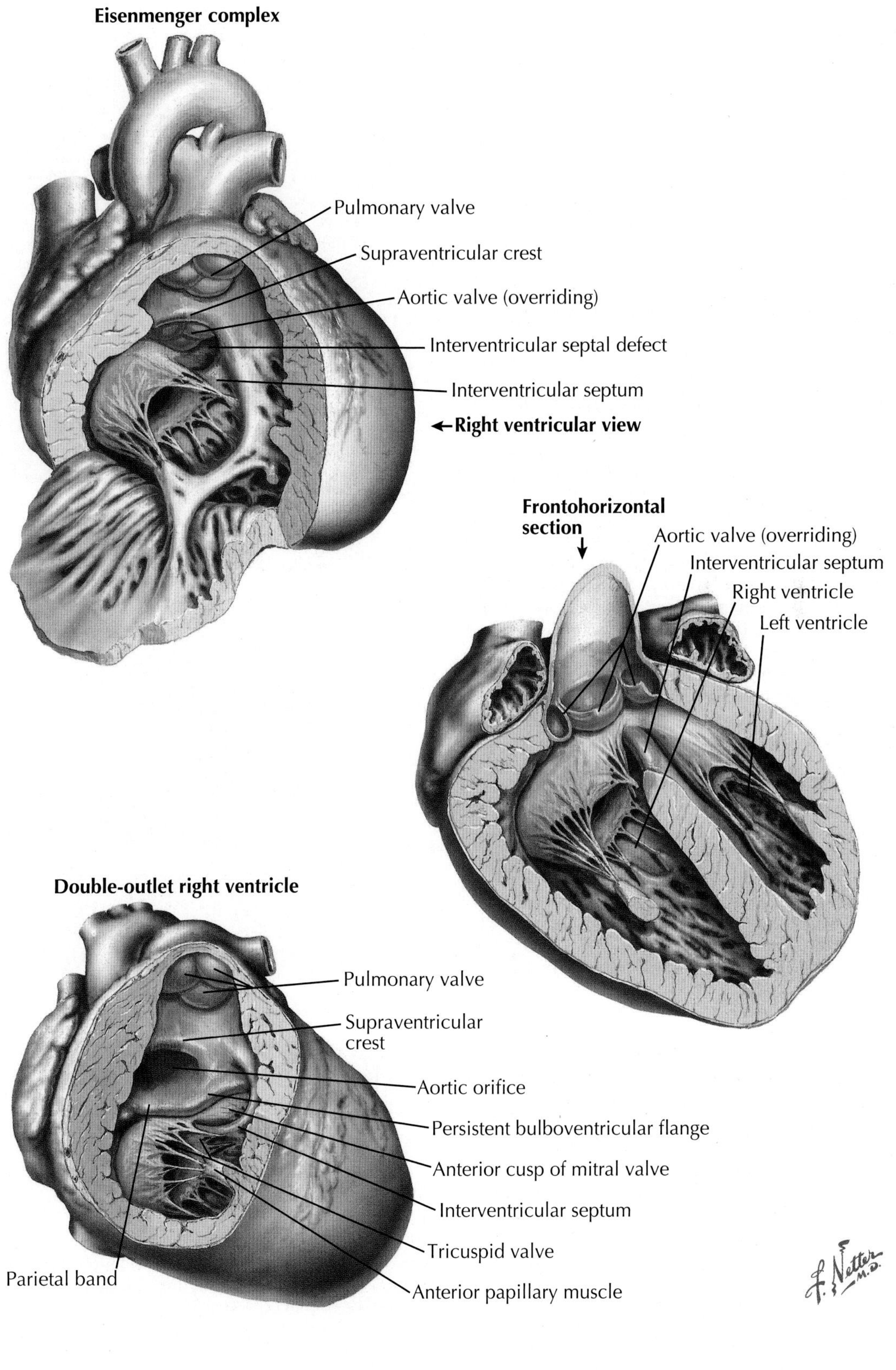

Eisenmenger complex

- Pulmonary valve
- Supraventricular crest
- Aortic valve (overriding)
- Interventricular septal defect
- Interventricular septum

← **Right ventricular view**

Frontohorizontal section
- Aortic valve (overriding)
- Interventricular septum
- Right ventricle
- Left ventricle

Double-outlet right ventricle

- Pulmonary valve
- Supraventricular crest
- Aortic orifice
- Persistent bulboventricular flange
- Anterior cusp of mitral valve
- Interventricular septum
- Tricuspid valve
- Anterior papillary muscle

Parietal band

RIGHT VENTRICULAR OUTFLOW OBSTRUCTION WITH INTACT VENTRICULAR SEPTUM: PULMONARY STENOSIS

RV outflow obstruction with intact ventricular septum is usually caused by stenosis of the pulmonary valve. "Pure" subvalvular (infundibular) stenosis is rare and may be the result of an abnormality in the architecture of the RV outflow musculature or part of the myocardial-dysplasia syndrome and associated with hypertrophic cardiomyopathy.

The pathologic anatomy of the pulmonary artery root and valve varies in isolated or pure pulmonary valvular stenosis (see Plate 5.23). Typically, the valve is more or less dome or cone shaped, with the valve ostium located at the apex of the dome. Rudimentary fused commissures are present near the base of the

Plate 5.23

Cardiovascular System: VOLUME 8

PULMONARY VALVULAR STENOSIS AND ATRESIA

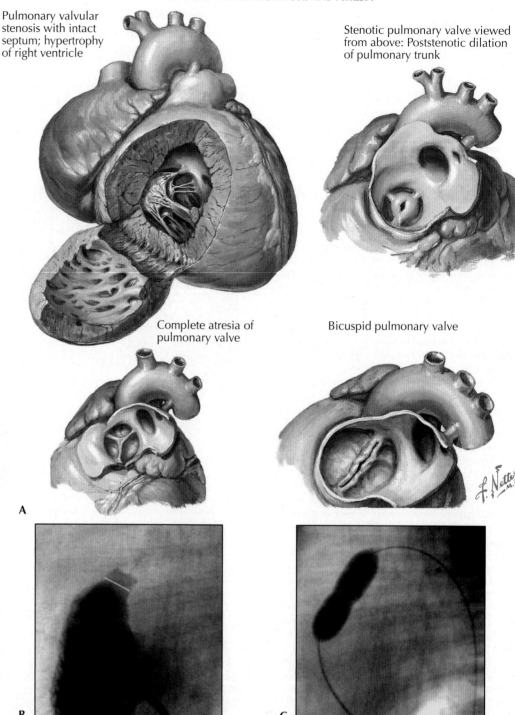

Pulmonary valvular stenosis with intact septum; hypertrophy of right ventricle

Stenotic pulmonary valve viewed from above: Poststenotic dilation of pulmonary trunk

Complete atresia of pulmonary valve

Bicuspid pulmonary valve

(A) The anatomic features of congenital pulmonary stenosis and atresia are illustrated. **(B)** A lateral-view right ventricular angiogram in a neonate with critical pulmonary valve stenosis shows the doming valve with an annulus diameter of 5.9 mm and a tiny poststenotic jet. **(C)** A lateral view of an 8-mm-diameter balloon dilation catheter fully inflated across the annulus. The balloon has been passed over a guidewire that had been placed across the ductus to the descending aorta.

ANOMALIES OF RIGHT VENTRICULAR OUTFLOW TRACT (Continued)

dome, and the sinuses of Valsalva are hypoplastic. In other cases, the valve cusps are fairly normal but thickened, and the commissures are fused for a variable distance or, occasionally, completely obliterated (pulmonary valve atresia). The valve may be bicuspid or tricuspid. A *bicuspid* (but not stenotic) pulmonary valve causes little or no functional disturbance and has minimal clinical significance, but it may be prone to endocarditis. Unlike the aortic valve, calcification does not occur in the pulmonary valve later in life. Even in relatively mild cases of pulmonary stenosis, RV hypertrophy is present. If the stenosis is severe, the hypertrophy becomes immense, and the tricuspid valve is often hypoplastic and thickened and may be incompetent.

The clinical features vary considerably depending on the degree of stenosis. Children with mild or moderate pulmonary stenosis are well developed, are not cyanotic, and are asymptomatic, except perhaps for fatigue and dyspnea on exertion. In those with severe stenosis, cyanosis is common and usually caused by a right-to-left shunt at the atrial level through a patent foramen ovale. A tricuspid regurgitant murmur may be present in these children, which accounts for increased right atrial pressure and thus allows a right-to-left shunt through a patent foramen ovale. Heart failure is rare but may occur, generally in infancy. A forceful precordial heartbeat may be palpable, and a thrill is usually felt at the base, to the left of the sternum, in the suprasternal notch. In the same areas a typically loud, diamond-shaped systolic murmur is audible, often preceded by an ejection click if the stenosis is mild or moderate. If present, both A_2 and P_2 of S_2 are clearly split in proportion to the severity of the stenosis. Good correlation exists between ECG findings and degree of stenosis. The ECG may be normal in mild cases, but clear evidence of RV hypertrophy usually is present. In general, the more severe the stenosis, the more the QRS axis shifts to the right and the taller the R waves become in the right precordial leads. The T waves are usually inverted in the right precordial leads but may be upright, even if the corresponding QRS complex looks unimpressive. In severe cases the sequence of R and S waves may be reversed in the precordial leads.

On chest radiography the heart is normal or only slightly enlarged, except in severe cases of considerable enlargement, particularly in the presence of right-sided heart failure. The vasculature is normal or somewhat diminished, and there is poststenotic dilation of the pulmonary trunk and left pulmonary artery, except when the stenosis is subvalvular or extreme. At cardiac catheterization the RV pressure is elevated, up to 200 mm Hg or more in severe cases; pulmonary artery pressure is normal or decreased. The arterial blood is desaturated in severe cases in which a right-to-left shunt is present at

the atrial level. Selective RV angiocardiography is helpful in outlining the particular anatomy present, as is cardiac ultrasound and MRI.

No treatment is indicated in patients with mild pulmonary stenosis. In the more severe cases, the treatment is surgical and consists of relieving the obstruction using open cardiopulmonary bypass procedures. Closed transventricular pulmonary valvotomy is indicated as an emergency procedure in infants with severe stenosis

who are cyanotic, have syncopal episodes, or are in heart failure. In infants it is advisable to relieve the stenosis, at least partially, by the transventricular approach, if RV pressure is 100 mm Hg or higher. Catheter-based balloon valvuloplasty is a preferred option, and the results are excellent. Even if no clear symptoms are present, this is done in an effort to prevent the development of massive RV hypertrophy, which may make the surgery difficult and hazardous in older children.

Plate 5.24

Congenital Heart Disease

AORTIC ATRESIA, BICUSPID AORTIC VALVE, AND AORTIC VALVULAR STENOSIS

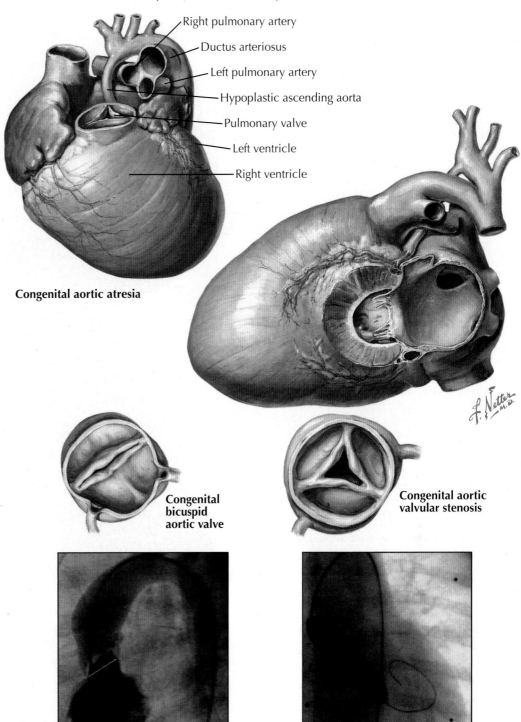

Right pulmonary artery

Ductus arteriosus

Left pulmonary artery

Hypoplastic ascending aorta

Pulmonary valve

Left ventricle

Right ventricle

Congenital aortic atresia

Congenital bicuspid aortic valve

Congenital aortic valvular stenosis

Left: A lateral-view left ventricular angiogram shows the doming aortic valve with a valve annulus diameter of 9.6 mm and poststenotic dilation of the ascending aorta. **Right:** Anteroposterior view of a 9-mm-diameter balloon dilation catheter fully inflated across the annulus. The balloon has been passed over a guidewire that had been placed retrograde across the valve and looped in the left ventricular apex.

ANOMALIES OF THE LEFT VENTRICULAR OUTFLOW TRACT

BICUSPID AORTIC VALVE

Aortic valve anomalies are common. A bicuspid (but not stenotic) aortic valve causes no symptoms in children or young adults, and the only finding is a systolic murmur in the aortic area (Plate 5.24). Later in life, however, such valves almost invariably become thickened and calcified, with resultant significant stenosis. In a bicuspid aortic valve, the two cusps are unequal in size, with the larger cusp approximately equally divided by an abortive raphe. A truly bicuspid valve, equally divided, is uncommon.

AORTIC VALVULAR STENOSIS

Stenotic aortic valves are usually also bicuspid (Plate 5.24). A developed tricuspid valve with partially fused commissures is occasionally seen. Poststenotic dilation of the ascending aorta is common. Stenotic aortic valves calcify later in life. The clinical picture varies with the degree of stenosis. Severe aortic stenosis may cause cardiac failure and death early in infancy. More often, however, aortic stenosis is well tolerated, and both children and young adults are usually asymptomatic and well developed. Symptoms consist of fatigue, chest pains, and syncope. Cardiac failure is rare in children. Obvious cardiomegaly is uncommon, but a precordial or apical "slow-rising heave" is usually present. A loud, typically harsh systolic ejection murmur, preceded by an ejection click and often accompanied by a thrill, is best heard at the second interspace, to the right of the sternum, and is transmitted well to the apex and along the carotid arteries. A suprasternal thrill is always palpable.

Chest radiography shows that the heart is normal or mildly enlarged, with a rounded left border in most cases. A poststenotic dilation of the ascending aorta may be present. The ECG is normal in mild and moderately severe cases. *Normal radiographs and ECGs do not necessarily indicate mild aortic stenosis.* On the other hand, clear ECG evidence of LV hypertrophy generally indicates significant obstruction. The vectorcardiogram is more sensitive in aortic stenosis because the QRS forces in the horizontal plane are found to be directed far posteriorly. The only accurate means of evaluating the severity of aortic stenosis is cardiac catheterization to determine the pressure gradient across the aortic valve. Cardiac Doppler ultrasound can assess severity of aortic stenosis by measuring velocity across the aortic valve and along with angiocardiography is useful in distinguishing valvular aortic stenosis from subvalvular LV outflow obstruction. Cardiac ultrasound, CTA, and MRI are also helpful.

Imaging will also indicate whether the aortic root is hypoplastic, making surgery more difficult unless aortic replacement or reconstruction is done.

The prognosis during childhood and adolescence is good. Sudden death, the only major complication other than bacterial endocarditis, does occur, but its incidence is minimal in patients with aortic stenosis and a normal ECG. Nevertheless, aortic stenosis of other than a mild degree is the only congenital cardiac anomaly in which the patient's activities, particularly participation

Plate 5.25

Cardiovascular System: VOLUME 8

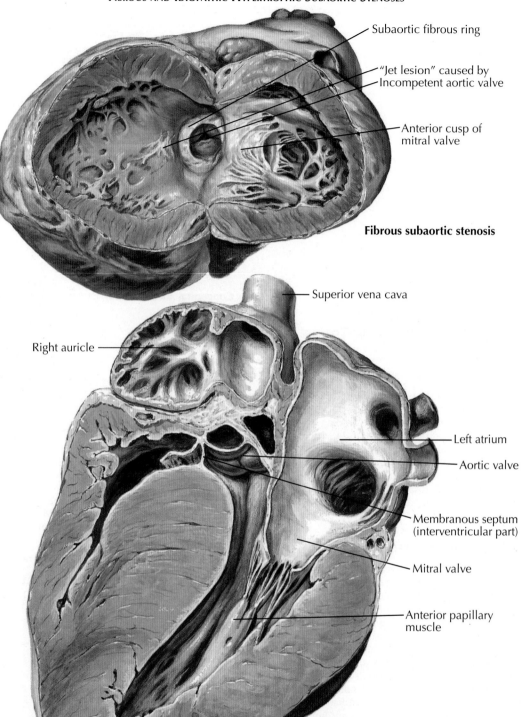

FIBROUS AND IDIOPATHIC HYPERTROPHIC SUBAORTIC STENOSES

Subaortic fibrous ring

"Jet lesion" caused by Incompetent aortic valve

Anterior cusp of mitral valve

Fibrous subaortic stenosis

Superior vena cava

Right auricle

Left atrium

Aortic valve

Membranous septum (interventricular part)

Mitral valve

Anterior papillary muscle

Idiopathic hypertrophic subaortic stenosis (posterior view)

ANOMALIES OF THE LEFT VENTRICULAR OUTFLOW TRACT (Continued)

in competitive sports, should be restricted. Surgery is reserved for patients who are symptomatic, show deterioration on the ECG, or have high pressure gradients across the aortic valve.

AORTIC ATRESIA

In patients with aortic atresia, the aortic valve is completely atretic or severely stenotic, and the ascending aorta is extremely hypoplastic (see Plate 5.24). The aorta serves merely to bring blood to the coronary arteries. The aorta is always fed by a widely patent ductus arteriosus. The ventricular septum is generally intact, and the LV is diminutive or occasionally absent. Its endocardium is fibroelastic, thickened, and pearly white, resembling enamel. The mitral valve usually is tiny but normally formed; rarely it is atretic or absent. Left atrial blood shunts across an ASD or more often across a foramen ovale whose valve has prolapsed to the right into the right atrium.

Prognosis is poor, and unless a Norwood procedure is performed, the infant will die within weeks of birth. The surgery can be divided into three main stages (see Plate 5.26).

HYPERTROPHIC CARDIOMYOPATHY

In hypertrophic cardiomyopathy (HCM), no discrete stenosis of the subvalvular region is demonstrable anatomically. The anomaly represents one manifestation of a condition characterized by enormous hypertrophy of the ventricular musculature. Most frequently, this involves the LV wall, particularly the septum (asymmetric septal hypertrophy) but the RV may also be hypertrophied, as in the specimen shown in Plate 5.25, which depicts the anterosuperior half of the heart as seen from below and behind. Several members in a family may be affected.

Clinically, patients with HCM can present with a variety of symptoms depending on the severity of their obstruction, including syncope, dyspnea, chest pain, and sudden cardiac death (SCD). Sudden death is common,

particularly in the adolescent during strenuous athletic competition. The clinical picture resembles aortic stenosis, with important differences. Usually there is a systolic murmur, heard best at the lower left sternal border rather than in the aortic area and possibly related to mitral insufficiency. No ejection click occurs. Mitral insufficiency may be an associated finding and tends to be maximal rather late in systole. The peripheral pulses are usually easily palpable and may seem brisk because the initial phase of ventricular ejection is normal, giving the typical

rapid rise in arterial pressure. With further contraction, the aortic subvalvular area is suddenly narrowed severely (systolic anterior motion of anterior leaflet of mitral valve), and the arterial pressure drops while the proximal ventricular pressure rises. Finally, as the outflow part of the LV relaxes again, the remainder of the blood can be discharged into the aorta. This causes a second hump in the arterial pressure tracing.

Chest radiography shows that the heart is mildly to moderately enlarged, with a rounded left border. The

Plate 5.26

Congenital Heart Disease

Norwood Correction of Hypoplastic Left Heart Syndrome

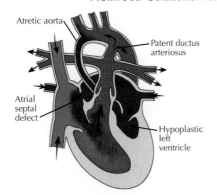

Atretic aorta

Patent ductus arteriosus

Atrial septal defect

Hypoplastic left ventricle

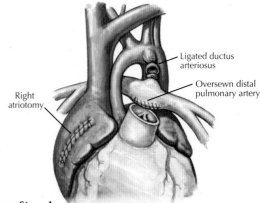

Right atriotomy

Ligated ductus arteriosus

Oversewn distal pulmonary artery

Stage I
Hypothermic cardiopulmonary bypass and right atriotomy are utilized to excise the interatrial septum. The main pulmonary artery is transected and a "neoaorta" is created.

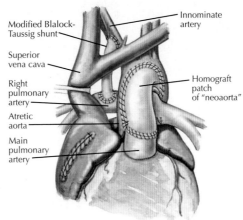

Modified Blalock-Taussig shunt

Innominate artery

Superior vena cava

Right pulmonary artery

Homograft patch of "neoaorta"

Atretic aorta

Main pulmonary artery

The main pulmonary artery and a cryopreserved aortic homograft create a neoaorta. Pulmonary blood flow is established through a systemic-to–pulmonary artery shunt.

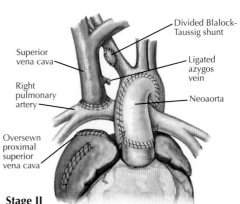

Divided Blalock-Taussig shunt

Superior vena cava

Ligated azygos vein

Right pulmonary artery

Neoaorta

Oversewn proximal superior vena cava

Stage II
At about 6 months of age, after pulmonary vascular resistance falls, a bidirectional Glenn shunt is necessary to reduce volume load on the right ventricle. The previous Blalock-Taussig shunt is divided.

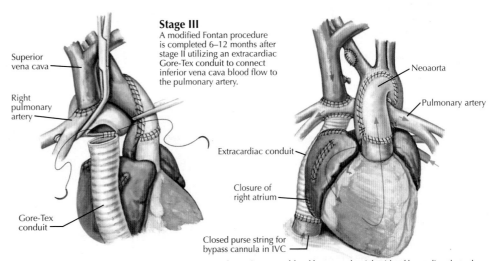

Stage III
A modified Fontan procedure is completed 6–12 months after stage II utilizing an extracardiac Gore-Tex conduit to connect inferior vena cava blood flow to the pulmonary artery.

Superior vena cava

Right pulmonary artery

Gore-Tex conduit

Neoaorta

Pulmonary artery

Extracardiac conduit

Closure of right atrium

Closed purse string for bypass cannula in IVC

Systemic venous blood bypasses the right side of heart directly to the pulmonary arteries and lungs. Oxygenated blood is pumped from the left to right atrium through a septotomy. The "neoaorta" directs oxygenated systemic blood flow from the right ventricle.

K. Carter

Anomalies of the Left Ventricular Outflow Tract (Continued)

pulmonary vasculature is normal. The ECG shows LV hypertrophy, even when minimal or no pressure gradient is demonstrable in the aortic subvalvular area. If present at cardiac catheterization or during cardiac Doppler ultrasound, a pressure gradient may be localized in the body of the ventricle, at the level of the apices of the hypertrophied papillary muscles, or in the subaortic area. The pressure gradient may vary considerably in severity from day to day and is increased, or induced when not present initially, by exercise or by the infusion of isoproterenol, inhalation of amyl nitrite, or other arterial vasodilators. Angiocardiographically, or with cardiac ultrasound, cardiovascular magnetic resonance imaging (CMR), or CTA, the LV is thick walled with a peculiar appearance in systole. Mitral incompetence is typically present. Currently, echocardiography and CMR are most commonly used for screening of patients and their families.

Treatment options depend on the individual patient but include medications, device therapy with implantable cardioverter-defibrillators to prevent SCD, surgical myectomy, alcohol septal ablation, and heart transplantation.

Traditional medical therapy includes medications such as beta blockers, verapamil, disopyramide as a negative inotrope, antiarrhythmic drugs to prevent atrial fibrillation, anticoagulation if indicated for atrial fibrillation, and angiotensin-converting enzyme inhibitors, angiotensin receptor blockers, and diuretics for those with advanced heart failure. A new drug, mavacamten, was recently approved by the U.S. Food and Drug Administration for use in HCM.

Implantable cardioverter-defibrillator implantation is very effective in preventing SCD and should be carefully considered in patients who are high risk for SCD or who have already presented with SCD or sustained ventricular tachycardia.

Surgical myectomy and alcohol septal ablation for the relief of mechanical LV outflow area obstruction are both currently available treatment options for selected patients. Surgical myectomy has been available for over 50 years, and when performed in high-volume, experienced centers has an excellent outcome with a low surgical mortality. Alcohol septal ablation is a newer percutaneous alternative that should also only be performed in experienced centers. Because the procedure is dependent on coronary arterial anatomy, the outcomes are less uniform, although the mortality rate and complication profile are the same as that for surgical myectomy. Transplantation is considered for these patients when there are no other options available. Genetic counseling should be recommended for all patients. In summary, HCM has excellent treatment options resulting in normal longevity in many when appropriately diagnosed.

Plate 5.27

Cardiovascular System: VOLUME 8

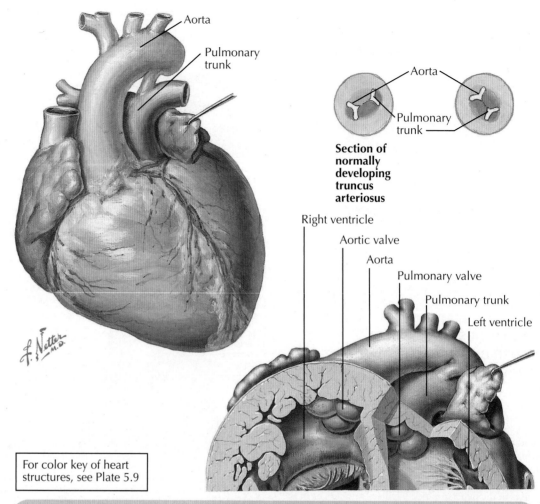

Aorta

Pulmonary trunk

Aorta

Pulmonary trunk

Section of normally developing truncus arteriosus

Right ventricle

Aortic valve

Aorta

Pulmonary valve

Pulmonary trunk

Left ventricle

For color key of heart structures, see Plate 5.9

TRANSPOSITION OF THE GREAT VESSELS

An abnormal anteroposterior relationship of the two arterial trunks, with one or both vessels arising from the wrong ventricle, is extremely common and often forms a component of complex cardiac anomalies. In simple, complete *transposition of the great vessels,* the aorta arises anteriorly from the RV and the pulmonary trunk arises posteriorly from the LV, with the two arterial trunks running parallel to each other. This discussion considers only the complete type of transposition, without associated anomalies other than a septal defect, patent ductus arteriosus, or pulmonary stenosis (Plate 5.27).

The anteroposterior relationship between the aorta and the pulmonary artery varies, but most often in transposition of the great vessels, the pulmonary artery lies posterior and to the left of the aorta. In uncomplicated cases, the ventricles are normally formed. The aortic valve, however, lies slightly more to the right of the pulmonary valve than in a normal heart. In less than half of cases, the ventricular septum is intact, and no other anomalies are present.

The great morphologic similarity of hearts that have isolated transposition of the great vessels suggests that the anomaly is simple; that is, it is caused by a single embryologic error. Furthermore, with normally formed ventricles, the error probably occurs in the truncus arteriosus. Two pairs of truncus swellings usually develop. Of these, the major pair executes the partitioning of the truncus arteriosus, and the intercalated valve swellings merely form a pair of arterial cusps. Transposition may result if the wrong truncus swellings become the major pair; the pulmonary and aortic intercalated valve swellings form the truncus septum and align themselves, respectively, with the sinistroventral and dextrodorsal conus swellings. The result is that the aorta arises from the RV anteriorly, and the pulmonary artery arises from the LV posteriorly. The conus septum develops normally and therefore its derivatives—the crista supraventricularis, medial part of tricuspid valve, and medial papillary muscle—are normal.

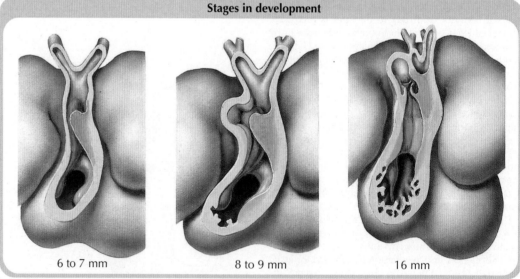

Stages in development

6 to 7 mm

8 to 9 mm

16 mm

Transposition of the great vessels, the most frequent cause of cardiac failure in early infancy, particularly with an intact septum, shows the following clinical features. If a VSD is present, failure occurs usually after a few weeks or months. If pulmonary stenosis is also present, it may be delayed much longer or may occur only late, as a terminal event. Cardiomegaly is absent at birth but is usually already marked within the first 2 weeks of life. The anteroposterior diameter of the chest is increased, and a left precordial bulge is common. Cyanosis may be

present from birth or may appear within the first few days or weeks of life. It appears earlier, is more intense, and progresses more rapidly if associated anomalies, which provide for mixing between the circulations, are absent. Conversely, children with a large ASD or VSD may not become cyanotic for many months or even a few years in exceptional cases. Cyanosis increases with crying, but this intensification usually is not as pronounced as in cardiac anomalies where venoarterial shunting is associated with diminished pulmonary

Plate 5.28

Congenital Heart Disease

MUSTARD AND BLALOCK-HANLON OPERATIONS

Mustard operation

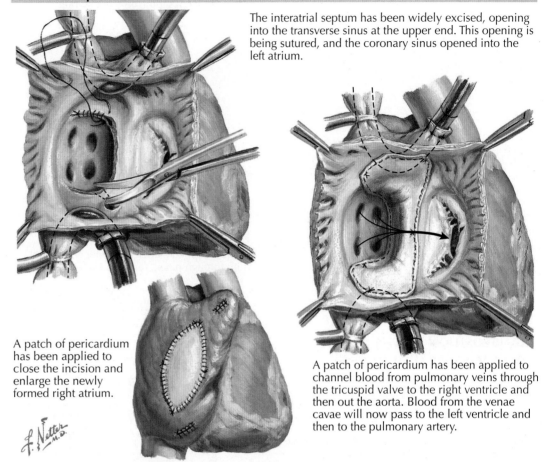

The interatrial septum has been widely excised, opening into the transverse sinus at the upper end. This opening is being sutured, and the coronary sinus opened into the left atrium.

A patch of pericardium has been applied to close the incision and enlarge the newly formed right atrium.

A patch of pericardium has been applied to channel blood from pulmonary veins through the tricuspid valve to the right ventricle and then out the aorta. Blood from the venae cavae will now pass to the left ventricle and then to the pulmonary artery.

TRANSPOSITION OF THE GREAT VESSELS (Continued)

blood flow (e.g., tetralogy of Fallot). Although the birth weight is usually normal, weight gain is poor, and infants who survive for some time become progressively more underweight. Dyspnea and rapid, shallow respirations are usually present.

The second heart sound at the base is loud because of the proximity of the aortic valve to the chest wall. S_2 may appear single because of poor transmission of P_2 resulting from the far-posterior location of the pulmonary valve. In cases with an intact ventricular septum, a murmur is usually absent or, if present, is not loud. If a VSD is present, a murmur is almost always audible and may be quite loud but is often not harsh or pansystolic. A diastolic mitral flow murmur may be present. In patients with associated pulmonary stenosis, a moderately loud systolic murmur, often accompanied by a thrill, is audible at the base.

The chest radiographic findings are usually typical. The heart is enlarged and characteristically egg shaped, and the upper mediastinum is narrow because the aorta and pulmonary artery lie almost in the same sagittal plane. The pulmonary vasculature is increased, with corresponding left atrial enlargement. In cases with pulmonary stenosis, there is little or no cardiomegaly, and the vasculature is normal or diminished. The ECG typically shows right axis deviation, right atrial hypertrophy, and RV hypertrophy. In the newborn period, it may be difficult to detect ECG abnormalities unless qR patterns are present in the right precordial leads. Additional evidence for LV hypertrophy is usually seen in patients with a large VSD or patent ductus arteriosus.

Although the diagnosis usually can be made clinically, confirmation by angiocardiography, cardiac ultrasound, MRI, or CTA may be required, especially when the picture is obscured by associated anomalies. A peripheral venous angiocardiogram is easily done and indicated in extremely sick infants, but selective angiocardiography is more precise and preferred.

The prognosis in simple transposition of the great vessels is extremely poor, and the great majority of infants

Blalock-Hanlon operation

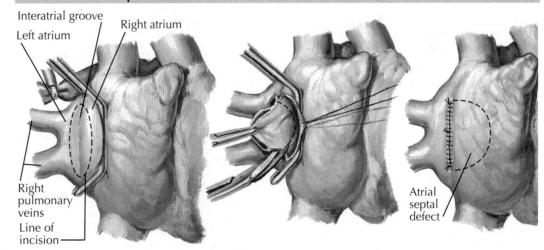

Interatrial groove

Right atrium

Left atrium

Right pulmonary veins

Line of incision

Clamp has been applied to exclude the interatrial groove and right pulmonary veins.

Clamp has been momentarily loosened to permit the interatrial septum to be drawn out and excised.

Atrial septal defect

A large atrial septal defect has thus been created.

die within the first 3 months of life. It is considerably better if an ASD or VSD with pulmonary stenosis is also present.

SURGICAL TREATMENT OF TRANSPOSITION OF GREAT VESSELS

Medical treatment is useful only in combating cardiac failure, and surgery is usually performed early. In

infants this consists of the creation of an ASD, the *Blalock-Hanlon procedure,* which provides satisfactory palliation in patients who survive (Plate 5.28). Also, an ASD can be created "medically" using the *Rashkind procedure.* A balloon-tipped catheter is introduced by the femoral vein and passed through the foramen ovale into the left atrium. After inflation of the balloon with dilute radiopaque fluid, the catheter is withdrawn forcefully, thus tearing the thin valve of

Plate 5.29

Cardiovascular System: VOLUME 8

BALLOON ATRIAL SEPTOSTOMY AND ARTERIAL REPAIR OF TRANSPOSITION OF THE GREAT ARTERIES

Balloon atrial septostomy (technique)

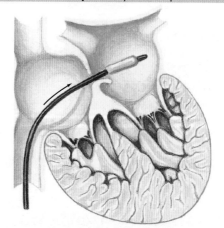

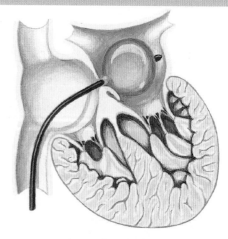

1. Balloon-tipped catheter introduced into left atrium through patent foramen ovale

2. Balloon inflated

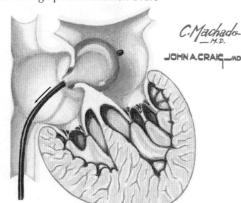

C. Machado
_M.D._

JOHN A. CRAIG_MD

3. Balloon withdrawn producing large septal defect

4. Large septal defect allows mixing of oxygenated and deoxygenated blood

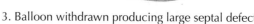

Arterial repair of transposition of the great arteries

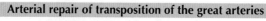

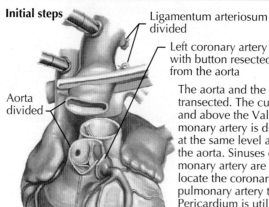

Initial steps

Ligamentum arteriosum divided

Left coronary artery with button resected from the aorta

Aorta divided

Final steps

Coronary arteries anastomosed to neoaorta

Distal pulmonary artery

Aorta repaired with pericardial patches

The aorta and the pulmonary artery are transected. The cut of the aorta is slanted and above the Valsalva sinuses. The pulmonary artery is divided above its valve at the same level as the transection of the aorta. Sinuses of the aorta and pulmonary artery are excised to translocate the coronary ostia from the pulmonary artery to the neoaorta. Pericardium is utilized to reconstruct the neopulmonary artery sinuses.

TRANSPOSITION OF THE GREAT VESSELS (Continued)

the foramen ovale (Plate 5.29). This procedure can be carried out even in small, sick infants, and it may be lifesaving.

Various methods of anatomic, or at least functional, correction have been devised. The *Mustard operation* (atrial switch) uses cardiopulmonary bypass to remove the atrial septum and suture a pericardial graft into the atrium so that the pulmonary venous blood is directed toward the right (systemic) ventricle and the systemic venous blood toward the left (pulmonary) ventricle. Atrial switch is most successful in children older than 2 years in whom the ventricular septum is intact and the only associated lesion is a naturally occurring or artificially created ASD. The Mustard procedure provided good palliative results but now is infrequently used because of problems developing during adolescence or early adulthood.

The *Jatene procedure* (arterial switch) is now often used to treat transposition of the great vessels (Plate 5.29). If pulmonary stenosis or VSD is present, correction is much less satisfactory, and the surgical mortality is high. Children with transposition and VSD rapidly become inoperable; the early development of pulmonary vascular changes results in a high PVR. Relief of the stenosis of the posteriorly positioned pulmonary artery valve is technically difficult and often is impossible to perform satisfactorily. In patients with a VSD and marked pulmonary stenosis, the creation of a palliative Blalock-Taussig shunt is preferred (see Plate 5.20, *bottom left*).

TRANSPOSITION OF GREAT VESSELS WITH INVERSION OF VENTRICLES (CORRECTED TRANSPOSITION OF GREAT VESSELS)

As in simple, complete transposition of the great vessels, the ascending aorta is situated anterior and parallel to the pulmonary trunk but arises anteriorly from the left-side ventricle, and the pulmonary trunk originates posteriorly from the right-side ventricle (see Plate 5.30).

Thus the transposition is at least functionally corrected; that is, the aorta receives arterial blood and the pulmonary artery receives venous blood. In addition to the reversed anteroposterior relationship of the great vessels, the left-right relationship of the ventricles is reversed. The right-side ventricle morphologically resembles a normal LV, and its atrioventricular valve is a mitral valve. (The valves always follow the ventricle.) The left-side ventricle structurally resembles an RV and contains a tricuspid valve. The morphology and position of the atria are normal.

The left AV valve is usually abnormal and incompetent. Ebstein's anomaly of the left-side tricuspid valve is common. Other associated defects are preexcitation of the ventricle (Wolff-Parkinson-White syndrome), VSD, pulmonary stenosis, and double-inlet (right-side) LV with a rudimentary left-side (RV) outflow chamber from which the aorta arises.

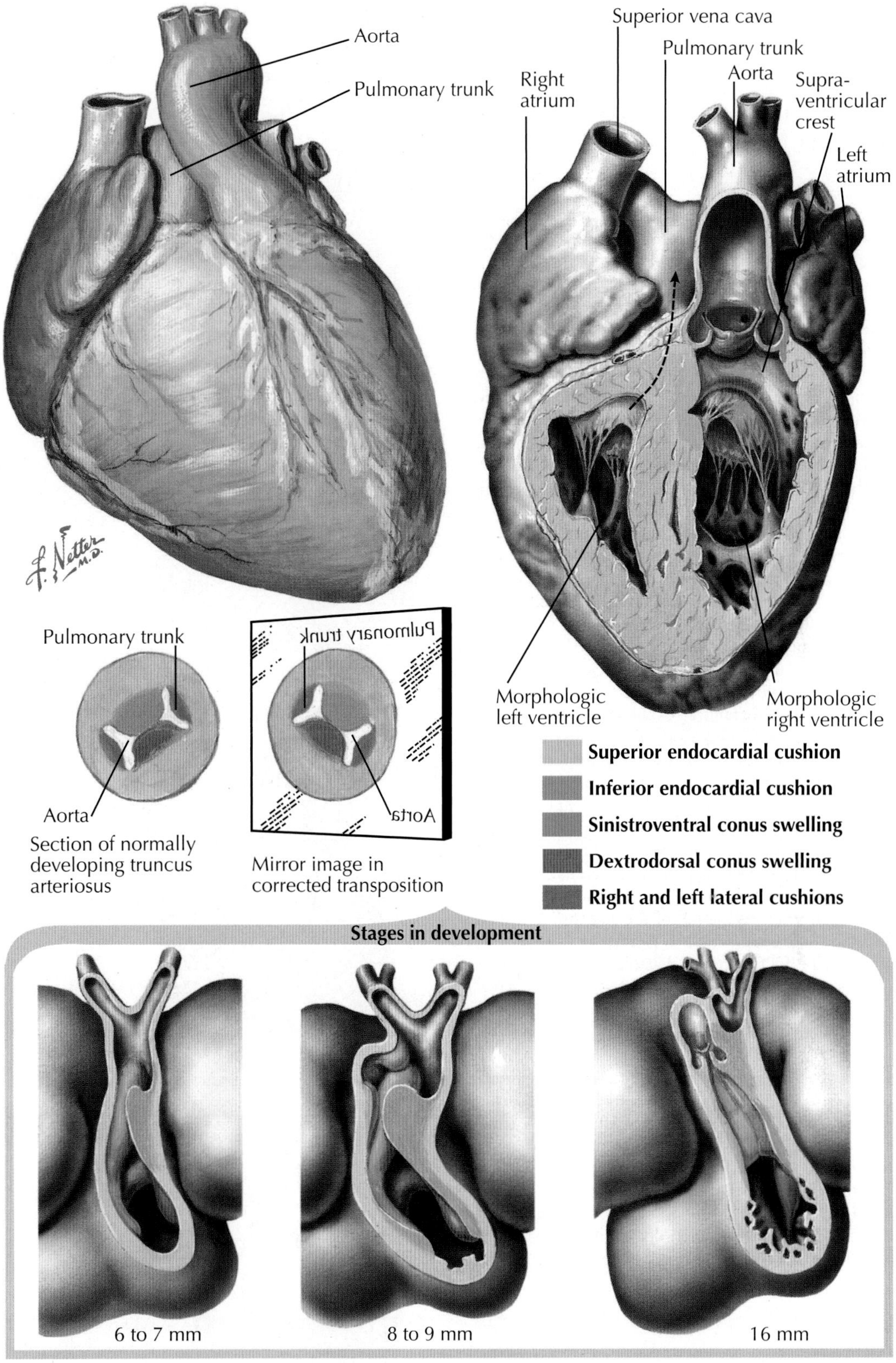

Plate 5.30

Aorta

Pulmonary trunk

Superior vena cava

Pulmonary trunk

Right atrium

Aorta

Supra-ventricular crest

Left atrium

TRANSPOSITION OF THE GREAT VESSELS (Continued)

Corrected transposition can be understood as caused by a single embryologic error. If very early, the cardiac tube bends to the left rather than the right, and the bulboventricular loop internally develops normally, but in mirror image, then all structures derived from the bulboventricular part of the heart (e.g., AV valves, ventricles, proximal great arteries) will become inverted. Only the intrapericardial, freely movable part of the embryonic heart can participate in the inversion; the fixed, extrapericardial parts (atria, sinus venosus, truncoaortic sac) cannot. Therefore the atria develop and are located normally. Development of the truncoaortic sac itself proceeds normally; because the inverted truncus arteriosus is partitioned in mirror image, the end result is transposition of the great vessels, with the aorta arising anteriorly from a left-side RV and the pulmonary trunk posteriorly from a right-side LV.

The clinical features of transposition with ventricular inversion are determined largely by the character and severity of associated anomalies. Conduction disturbances, with varying degrees of heart block, are common and may occur in the absence of VSD or other gross defects. In the rare uncomplicated cases, S_2 at the base to the left of the sternum is loud because of the anterior location of the aortic valve. A low-grade systolic murmur of uncertain origin may be audible at the base. Other auscultatory findings may also vary.

Chest radiographs may show features suggesting corrected transposition. The vascular pedicle may be narrow, as in simple complete transposition. Of more significance is an indentation of the left side of a barium-filled esophagus, caused by the enlarged, posteriorly located pulmonary trunk. The left upper heart border may be unusually straight or even convex because of the anterior and leftward position of the ascending aorta. Other radiographic features vary greatly and are determined by the associated lesions. The ECG often shows differing amounts of heart block, and the presence of congenital complete heart block in an otherwise asymptomatic child should suggest corrected transposition. Reversal of

Pulmonary trunk

Aorta

Section of normally developing truncus arteriosus

Pulmonary trunk

Aorta

Mirror image in corrected transposition

Morphologic left ventricle

Morphologic right ventricle

Superior endocardial cushion

Inferior endocardial cushion

Sinistroventral conus swelling

Dextrodorsal conus swelling

Right and left lateral cushions

Stages in development

6 to 7 mm

8 to 9 mm

16 mm

the initial ventricular activation is evident in the ECG by the absence of a Q wave in leads I, aV$_L$, and the left precordial and a qR or QS pattern in the right precordial leads. Associated defects will modify the ECG.

At cardiac catheterization, the diagnosis may be suspected because of the unusually medial and posterior position of the tip of the venous catheter, if it can be made to enter the pulmonary trunk, and the anterior and far-leftward position of the arterial catheter if it is

passed into the ascending aorta. Angiocardiography is more valuable than cardiac catheterization and easily establishes the diagnosis, as does cardiac ultrasound, CMR, and CT angiography.

The prognosis of the very rare, uncomplicated transposition cases without conduction disturbances should be good. In complicated cases, prognosis depends on the severity of the associated anomalies, which also determine the type of procedure if surgery is indicated.

Plate 5.31

Cardiovascular System: VOLUME 8

ANOMALIES OF THE TRUNCUS SEPTUM

In truncus septum anomalies, a large single vessel arising from the heart gives off the coronary and pulmonary arteries and the aortic arch with its usual branches. The truncal valve is generally tricuspid but may be *quadricuspid* or bicuspid. A large VSD is always present and located anteriorly. Several types of truncus septum anomaly are known, as determined by how the pulmonary arteries arise from the common trunk. In the most common form, a short main stem left coronary artery bifurcates into a right and a left pulmonary artery. More rarely, these arteries arise independently from the trunk, or the pulmonary arteries, as such, are absent (Plate 5.31).

The clinical features of the most common truncus septum defect depend largely on the pulmonary vascular bed. If PVR in this bed is high, pulmonary blood flow will be the same as or less than systemic flow. The child is cyanotic and has polycythemia, finger clubbing, dyspnea on exertion, and easy fatigability. If PVR is still low (usually in infants and very young children), pulmonary blood flow is greatly increased. Cyanosis is only mild or absent, but the infants are dyspneic and have feeding difficulties, frequent respiratory infections, and growth failure. Congestive heart failure is common. With the development of a high PVR in the few surviving children, the left-to-right shunt gradually diminishes, and the heart decreases in size. The patient's general condition improves, but cyanosis appears and generally is progressive. Some patients remain almost acyanotic for many years, whereas others are among the most deeply cyanotic individuals ever seen.

A systolic murmur is best heard at the third or fourth intercostal space to the left of the sternum and is preceded by an ejection click. S_1 is normal; S_2 is very loud and may be followed by a diastolic murmur, which is usually caused by incompetence of the truncal valve. A continuous machinery murmur, so characteristic of patent ductus arteriosus, is unusual.

The chest radiograph findings vary. In children with large left-to-right shunts, the heart is large, at times with an upturned apex, and the vascularity is much increased. The left upper heart border is usually concave, and the aortic knob is large. As the magnitude of this shunt diminishes with increased PVR, the cardiomegaly and pulmonary plethora also decrease. The ECG shows a normal or, more commonly, a right axis deviation and either RV hypertrophy or, in a case with large left-to-right shunts, biventricular or rarely only LV hypertrophy; tall peaked P waves are common. Retrograde aortic angiography can establish the diagnosis.

TRUNCUS ARTERIOSUS REPAIR

If left untreated, truncus arteriosus can be fatal. Surgery to repair truncus arteriosus is generally successful, especially if the repair occurs before 2 months of age (Plate 5.31). Surgery is required to close the VSD with a patch and separate systemic from pulmonary blood flow. This prevents pulmonary hypertension and damage to the lung. The pulmonary arteries are then disconnected from the single great vessel, and a conduit with a valve is placed from the RV to these pulmonary arteries (Rastelli repair).

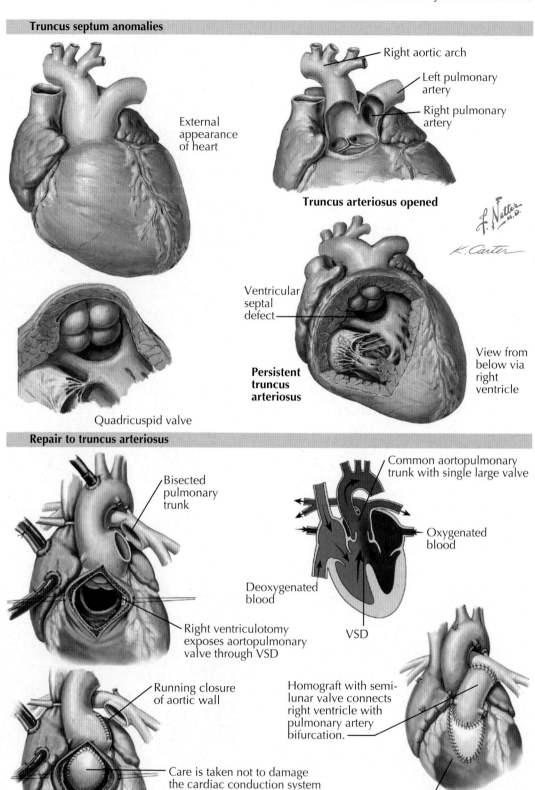

Truncus septum anomalies

External appearance of heart

Right aortic arch

Left pulmonary artery

Right pulmonary artery

Truncus arteriosus opened

Quadricuspid valve

Ventricular septal defect

Persistent truncus arteriosus

View from below via right ventricle

Repair to truncus arteriosus

Bisected pulmonary trunk

Right ventriculotomy exposes aortopulmonary valve through VSD

Running closure of aortic wall

Care is taken not to damage the cardiac conduction system when sewing Gore-Tex graft over inferior rim of the VSD.

Common aortopulmonary trunk with single large valve

Oxygenated blood

Deoxygenated blood

VSD

Homograft with semilunar valve connects right ventricle with pulmonary artery bifurcation.

Pericardial patch over closure of right ventriculotomy

AORTICOPULMONARY SEPTAL DEFECT

This is a rare congenital anomaly, usually characterized by the presence of a large defect between the ascending aorta and the pulmonary trunk (Plate 5.31). Initially, the clinical features are those of a large left-to-right shunt at the ventricular or arterial level and are roughly intermediate in severity between those of persistent truncus arteriosus and patent ductus arteriosus. The ECG usually shows a pattern of biventricular hypertrophy, at least in childhood, and the chest radiography resemble those seen in a large patent ductus arteriosus. Retrograde aortography is diagnostic. The prognosis without *surgical treatment*, though more favorable than that of truncus arteriosus, is still rather poor, and the mortality during the first year of life is significant. Fortunately, surgical repair of the defect, employing a cardiopulmonary bypass, can be carried out rather easily, but it should be done at an early age, before a marked increase in PVR renders the patient inoperable.

Plate 5.32

Congenital Heart Disease

ANOMALOUS LEFT CORONARY ARTERY AND ANEURYSM OF SINUS OF VALSALVA

The anomalous origin of both coronary arteries from the pulmonary artery is extremely rare and is not compatible with postnatal life. A similar, equally rare anomaly involving the right coronary artery (RCA) causes no symptoms.

ANOMALOUS LEFT CORONARY ARTERY

More common but still infrequently seen is the anomalous origin of the left coronary artery (LCA) from the pulmonary artery (see Plate 5.32). Because pressures in the aorta and pulmonary artery are equal before birth and oxygen saturation of the blood in these vessels is much the same, the anomaly is of no consequence prenatally.

After birth, with the normally occurring fall in pulmonary artery pressure, perfusion of the anomalous LCA is greatly reduced, resulting in myocardial ischemia. Given time, the normally present but small intercoronary anastomoses expand. The normal RCA and its branches become dilated and tortuous, but the LCA remains small and thin walled. The potential benefit for the LV myocardium from the developing large intercoronary anastomoses, however, is largely lost because of stealing of the blood into the low-pressure pulmonary artery, with minimal blood reaching the myocardium itself. The LV dilates greatly, and its myocardium becomes fibrotic, particularly in its anterolateral and apical parts. The endocardium is thickened and fibroelastotic, and calcifications may be present.

In infants, the main clinical features of anomalous LCA are congestive heart failure with episodes of distress, characterized by pallor, restlessness, slight cyanosis, dyspnea, and sweating. The attacks may be precipitated by feeding or straining and are thought to be ischemic. Between episodes, the child is happy and asymptomatic until the onset of congestive heart failure. The heart is considerably enlarged, but any murmur is insignificant. Symptoms usually do not appear until the babies are 4 to 6 weeks old, and most die within the next few weeks. Occasionally the child's condition improves, and the cardiomegaly recedes. A minority of cases are asymptomatic in early childhood and may present themselves later with signs of mitral insufficiency. Sudden death is common.

There are no characteristic radiographic findings with anomalous LCA. There is general cardiomegaly in infants, and the pulmonary vasculature is normal, or evidence may indicate pulmonary venous congestion. In older patients the heart is normal in size or only moderately enlarged. The ECG in symptomatic infants typically shows the pattern of anterolateral myocardial infarction and usually LV hypertrophy. In older children and adults, the ECG generally indicates only LV hypertrophy. Cardiac catheterization is not helpful, but aortography and selective coronary angiography confirms the diagnosis.

Treatment is surgical: ligation of the defective artery at its origin to prevent further runoff ("coronary steal"). Current surgical procedures establish revascularization by creating a coronary artery system using either a left subclavian artery–coronary artery anastomosis, a saphenous vein bypass graft, aortopulmonary window and intrapulmonary tunnel extending from anomalous ostium to the window, or direct reimplantation. With a patent coronary artery system established, most patients experience normalization of LV systolic function, thereby improving long-term survival.

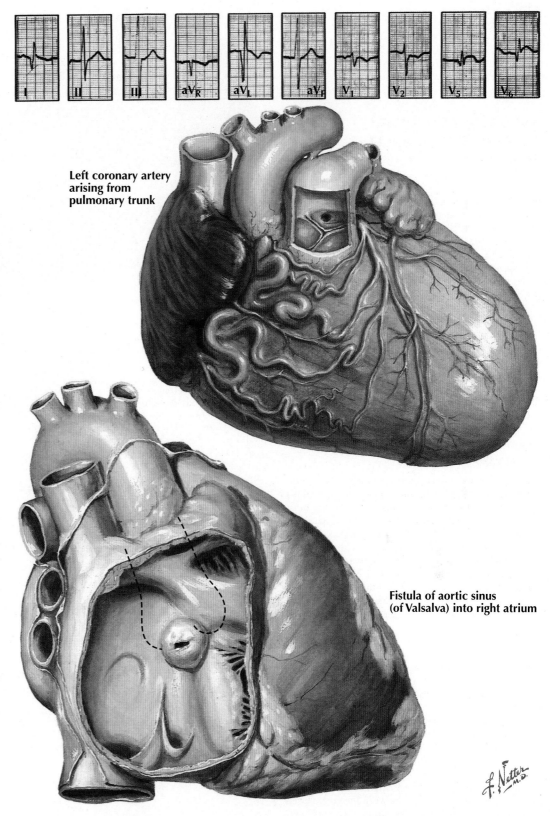

Left coronary artery arising from pulmonary trunk

Fistula of aortic sinus (of Valsalva) into right atrium

ANEURYSM OF AORTIC SINUS OF VALSALVA

An aortic sinus of Valsalva aneurysm is caused by a congenital weakness of the bottom of the right coronary sinus or less often the noncoronary sinus (Plate 5.32). The aneurysm itself does not usually cause symptoms. Rarely, conduction disturbances are present, including complete heart block. Rupture of a congenital aortic sinus aneurysm, occurring usually in young adults, is into a cardiac chamber, generally the RV or right atrium. The sudden onset of an often large aortocardiac shunt may precipitate congestive heart failure or may be rapidly fatal. Therefore the clinical features are often dramatic: dyspnea, chest pain, bounding pulses, and a machinery murmur accompanied by a thrill over the lower precordial area.

Chest roentgenograms are normal in intact aneurysms; after rupture, cardiomegaly usually develops rapidly, and the vasculature is increased. The ECG is not specific. Retrograde aortography establishes the diagnosis of aortic sinus aneurysm.

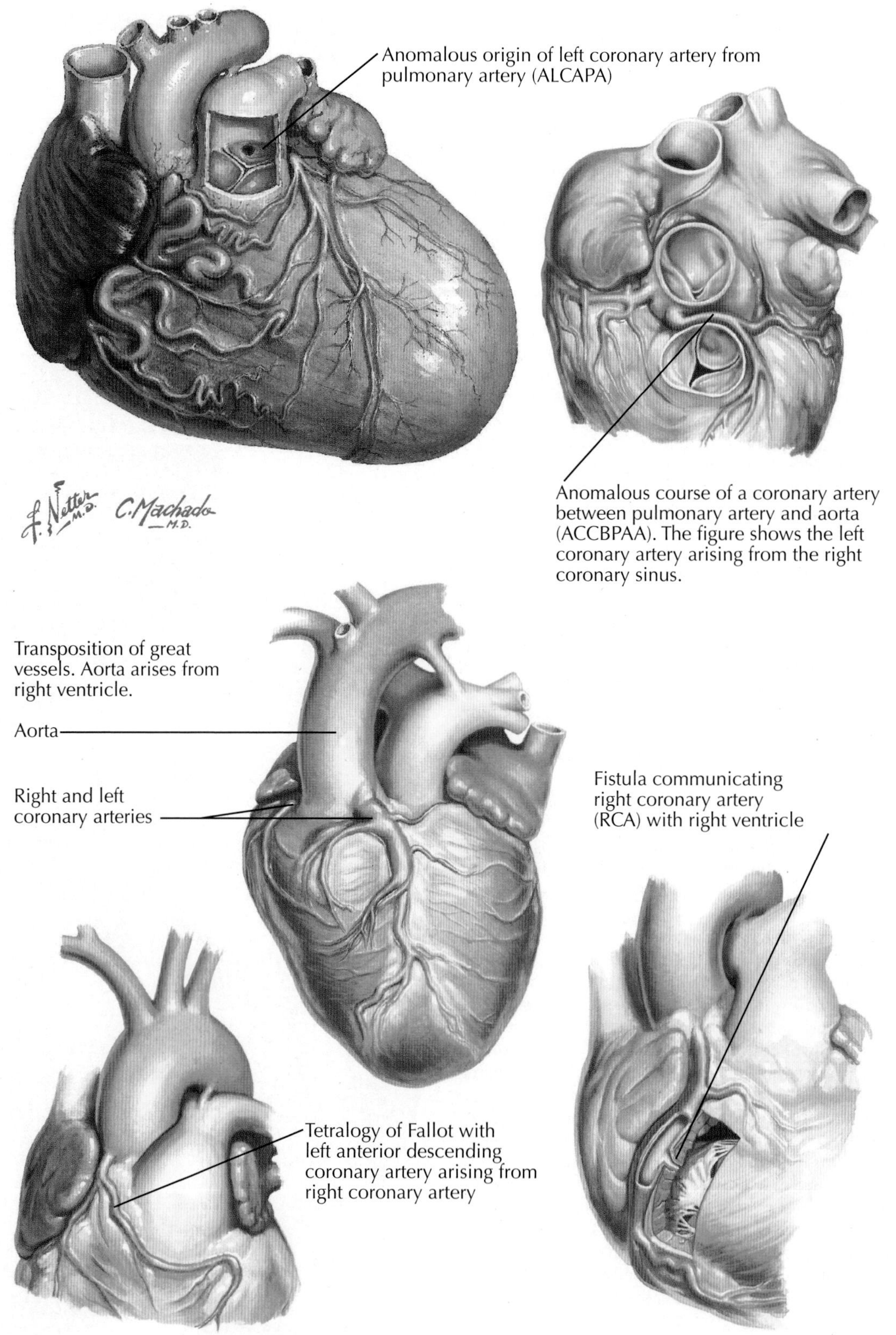

Plate 5.33

Cardiovascular System: VOLUME 8

ANOMALOUS CORONARY ARTERIES SEEN IN ADULT PATIENTS

In general, the coronary artery anomalies considered benign in terms of development of major adverse coronary cardiac events include (1) separate origin of the left anterior descending and circumflex arteries from the left sinus of Valsalva, (2) ectopic origin of the circumflex artery from the right sinus of Valsalva, (3) ectopic coronary origin from the posterior sinus of Valsalva, (4) anomalous coronary origin from the ascending aorta, (5) absent circumflex artery, (6) intracoronary communications, and (7) small coronary artery fistula. Coronary anomalies associated with serious sequelae (e.g., myocardial ischemia, myocardial infarction, syncope, cardiac arrhythmias, congestive heart failure, sudden death) include ectopic coronary origin from the pulmonary artery, ectopic coronary origin from the opposite aortic sinus, single coronary artery, and large coronary fistula.

ADULTS WITH CORONARY ARTERY ANOMALIES

Predicting adverse events in patients with coronary anomalies is at best an educated guess. Because adults with anomalies are survivors, the anomalies are most often incidental findings in symptomatic patients, usually caused by coronary artery disease (CAD) found in other vessels (e.g., origin of circumflex coronary from right sinus of Valsalva). Other patients may have CAD with anomalous RCA of origin from the pulmonary artery or huge congenital coronary artery aneurysms. A few patients have had coronary stenosis in an anomalous coronary artery, which then could undergo angioplasty.

The most common congenital anomaly seen in adult patients is an *anomalous circumflex coronary artery*, which comes from the right sinus of Valsalva as a separate orifice or arises off a branch of the RCA. This anomalous circumflex vessel typically is retrocardiac and therefore probably benign. At coronary angiography in the catheterization laboratory, it may be difficult to determine whether the artery is anterior to the great vessels, posterior to the great vessels, between the great vessels, or intramural within the aorta; CT coronary angiography can easily determine this.

As a general rule, any artery originating from either sinus of Valsalva and passing between the great vessels or taking an intramural course through the aorta may be at risk and may cause SCD. The potential for poor outcomes from an anomalous coronary artery thus depends on the course of the anomalous vessel. Compression can occur (Laplace's law), or if the artery takes off at an acute angle, the ostia of the anomalous coronary artery can be severely narrowed.

Again, it is often challenging to diagnose the position of the anomaly during catheter-based coronary angiography, because it is difficult to see the relationship to the great vessels. CT angiography allows evaluation of not just artery caliber and lumen but also

Anomalous origin of left coronary artery from pulmonary artery (ALCAPA)

Anomalous course of a coronary artery between pulmonary artery and aorta (ACCBPAA). The figure shows the left coronary artery arising from the right coronary sinus.

Transposition of great vessels. Aorta arises from right ventricle.

Aorta

Right and left coronary arteries

Fistula communicating right coronary artery (RCA) with right ventricle

Tetralogy of Fallot with left anterior descending coronary artery arising from right coronary artery

course and relationship to adjacent structures, as well as the takeoff angle of the anomalous vessel from the sinus of Valsalva.

Potentially Serious Coronary Anomalies

An anomalous RCA that comes off either the left sinus of Valsalva or branches of the single LCA can be retroaortic, but in the vast majority of patients it tracks between the aortic and pulmonary artery or even may track intramurally in the aorta. The latter two courses may result in major adverse cardiac events, although data are sparse. In contrast, an anomalous LCA originating from the right sinus of Valsalva or branches of a single RCA can be retroaortic, anterior, or intramural. In most patients, however, the anomalous LCA courses between the aorta and pulmonary artery and thus may be more dangerous than other coronary arteries of ectopic origin.

Plate 5.34

Congenital Heart Disease

PATENT DUCTUS ARTERIOSUS

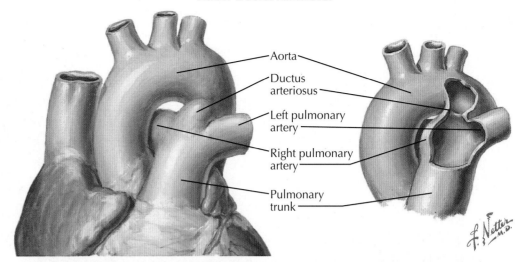

Aorta

Ductus arteriosus

Left pulmonary artery

Right pulmonary artery

Pulmonary trunk

The internal anatomy of a typical "type A" ductus arteriosus, demonstrating the conical aortic ampulla and narrowing near the pulmonary end, making coil placement feasible

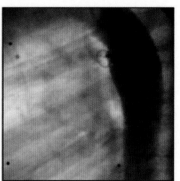

A lateral-view aortogram showing residual leakage through a patent ductus arteriosus that had been partially closed with a Rashkind umbrella occluder years previously. Three platinum markers can be seen on the aortic umbrella of the Rashkind device.

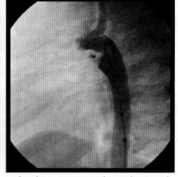

Follow-up lateral-view aortogram after snare-assisted coil delivery showing complete closure

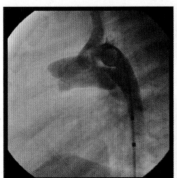

Lateral aortogram showing a typical conical ductus opacifying the pulmonary artery.

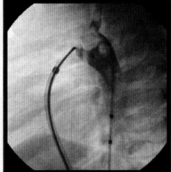

An Amplatzer Duct Occluder has been delivered through a long transvenous sheath, and a test angiogram confirms proper position.

A final aortogram after release of the occluder shows complete closure.

ANOMALIES OF AORTIC ARCH SYSTEM

PATENT DUCTUS ARTERIOSUS

As an isolated anomaly, patent ductus arteriosus (PDA) is one of the most common and most benign types of congenital heart disease. The anomaly represents a continued patency of a channel—the ductus arteriosus—that connects the origin of the left pulmonary artery to the aorta and, in fetal life, allows most of the RV blood to bypass the nonfunctioning lungs. After birth and with onset of respiration, its usefulness ends, and the ductus normally closes, at least functionally, within hours after birth. It is not known why, in some babies, the ductus arteriosus remains patent. PDA is a common cardiovascular anomaly in the rubella syndrome, which occurs in children whose mothers had German measles during the first 2 months of pregnancy. PDA is often associated with other cardiac anomalies, and in some patients (e.g., those with aortic atresia) it is always present (see Plates 5.24 and 5.26).

The clinical features of uncomplicated PDA are characteristic in the majority of cases. The ductus arteriosus is rather small, and there are few or no symptoms in early childhood. Growth and development are normal. The heart is normal in size or may be enlarged slightly to moderately, depending on the magnitude of the shunt across the ductus arteriosus. A thrill is often palpable over the left upper sternal border, usually systolic in time, but may continue into diastole. There is a characteristic machinery or fistulous-type murmur that starts shortly after S_1, increases in intensity, and decreases again after the end of systole. The characteristic features of the murmur result from aortic pressure being higher than pulmonary artery pressure during all phases of the cardiac cycle, because PVR is considerably lower than resistance in the systemic vascular bed. The easy and rapid runoff of blood during diastole into the low-resistance pulmonary vascular bed results in a wide pulse pressure and explains the bounding peripheral pulses typically present in children with PDA.

In premature infants, intravenous indomethacin may help close a PDA by stimulating the muscles inside the ductus to constrict.

Some infants with a large ductus arteriosus may become symptomatic early in life or may even progress to congestive heart failure (Plate 5.34). The symptoms and physical findings resemble those seen in babies with a large VSD and massive left-to-right shunt.

The chest radiographic findings are similar to those in VSD, but the aortic arch, instead of being small, is usually large. The ECG is normal in almost half the cases; the remainder show LV hypertrophy of the volume-overload type or, in a minority of cases, biventricular hypertrophy. The clinical findings are generally so characteristic that cardiac catheterization and angiocardiographic studies are not necessary. When in doubt, aortograms reveal the ductus arteriosus. Treatment is simple and consists of surgical division of the PDA or percutaneous occlusion. Surgical repair is usually recommended for infants younger than 6 months who have large defects that are

Plate 5.35

Cardiovascular System: VOLUME 8

ABERRANT RIGHT SUBCLAVIAN ARTERY

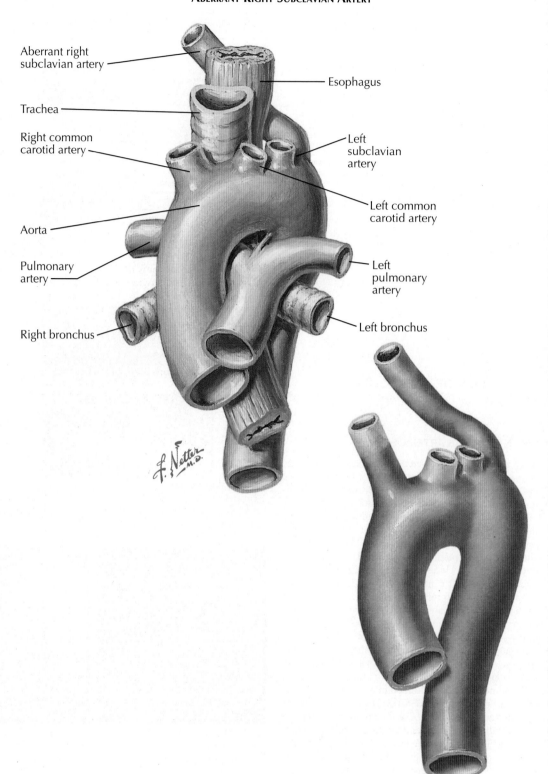

Aberrant right subclavian artery

Esophagus

Trachea

Right common carotid artery

Left subclavian artery

Left common carotid artery

Aorta

Pulmonary artery

Left pulmonary artery

Right bronchus

Left bronchus

ANOMALIES OF AORTIC ARCH SYSTEM (Continued)

causing symptoms. PDA may also be repaired by a cardiac catheterization procedure using occluder devices. Closure is contraindicated once the patient has become cyanotic because of shunt reversal.

ABERRANT RIGHT SUBCLAVIAN ARTERY

An anomalous right subclavian artery, originating from the descending aortic arch as a last branch and crossing behind the esophagus to the right arm, is common both as an isolated anomaly and in association with other defects. The anomaly can be explained by postulating a disappearance of the right fourth aortic arch, which normally forms the most proximal part of the right subclavian artery, and persistence of the normally disappearing right dorsal aorta (Plate 5.35).

An anomalous right subclavian artery can be detected radiographically because it causes a posterior and oblique indentation of the barium-filled esophagus at the level of the fourth thoracic vertebra. This anomaly has been blamed for causing *dysphagia lusoria* but rarely does so. Usually it is an incidental finding.

In an embryo with crown-to-rump length of 7 to 8 mm, the first two pairs of aortic arches have disappeared, as such. The fifth pair, never well developed in humans, has had only a fleeting existence. The remaining third, fourth, and sixth pairs of arches are well developed, originate from the truncoaortic sac, and encircle the developing esophagus and tracheobronchial tree to join the right and left dorsal aortas. All of these aortic arches are normally retained, except for the distal portion of the right sixth arch, which has already disappeared in a 14-mm embryo. The establishment of a normal aortic arch system involves the involution of three additional vessel segments.

The encirclement of the trachea and esophagus by the aortic arch system in an early embryo does not constrict these structures because of the wide opening in the arterial ring. With further development, however, the arteries shorten and widen and the ring becomes tighter, leading to compression of the esophagus and the trachea unless the ring system is opened. To do this, only the distal portion of one of the dorsal aortas needs to disappear. If the distal right dorsal aorta persists as a major channel, a vascular ring can be prevented only if both the distal right sixth arch and the right dorsal aortic segment between the right fourth and sixth arches disappear. This simply results in an anomalous right subclavian artery. However, if only the right distal sixth arch vanishes, a *double aortic arch* is formed. If only the segment of dorsal aorta between the fourth and sixth arches is removed, the result will be a *right-side ductus of the posterior type*.

DOUBLE AORTIC ARCH

In patients with double aortic arch, the two arches may be equal in size but usually are not (see Plate 5.36).

Plate 5.36   Congenital Heart Disease

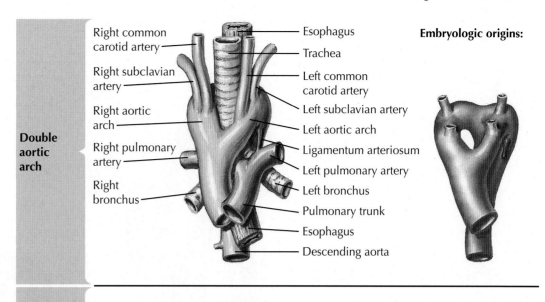

Double aortic arch

Right common carotid artery
Right subclavian artery
Right aortic arch
Right pulmonary artery
Right bronchus

Esophagus
Trachea
Left common carotid artery
Left subclavian artery
Left aortic arch
Ligamentum arteriosum
Left pulmonary artery
Left bronchus
Pulmonary trunk
Esophagus
Descending aorta

Embryologic origins:

Right aortic arch and left ductus arteriosus: anterior type

Right common carotid artery
Right subclavian artery
Right aortic arch
Right pulmonary artery
Right bronchus

Esophagus
Trachea
Left subclavian artery
Left common carotid artery
Ligamentum arteriosum
Left brachiocephalic trunk
Left pulmonary artery
Left bronchus
Pulmonary trunk
Esophagus
Descending aorta

Right aortic arch and left ductus arteriosus: posterior type

Right common carotid artery
Right subclavian artery
Right aortic arch
Right pulmonary artery
Right bronchus

Esophagus
Trachea
Left common carotid artery
Left subclavian artery
Ligamentum arteriosum
Left pulmonary artery
Left bronchus
Pulmonary trunk
Esophagus
Descending aorta

ANOMALIES OF AORTIC ARCH SYSTEM (Continued)

Most often the right-side arch is dominant, regardless of whether the descending aorta courses to the right or more frequently to the left of the spine. At times the left arch is atretic. In most cases the ductus (ligamentum) arteriosus is on the left side, but it may be on the right. Rarely there is a bilateral ductus arteriosus. Left and right common carotid and subclavian arteries arise from their corresponding arches.

The clinical symptoms of double aortic arch reflect obstruction of the trachea and esophagus, and the severity depends on the tightness of the vascular ring. Symptoms generally are present in childhood, often in early infancy, and occasionally patients are asymptomatic and the ring is discovered incidentally. Wheezing, cough, inspiratory stridor, repeated respiratory infections, and aspiration pneumonia are common problems. Extension of the head and back tends to relieve respiratory difficulties, and infants often spontaneously assume such a position of hyperextension. Dysphagia varies in severity, often increasing or appearing when the child begins to take solid foods. Chest radiographic examination, including esophagogram, is important to demonstrate the ring's constriction of both the esophagus and the trachea.

Surgery is indicated in symptomatic patients and at times must be done as an emergency procedure. It consists of division of the smaller or atretic arch. If present, a ductus arteriosus or ligament on the same side also should be divided. Otherwise, the patient will be left with a vascular ring of a different type, formed by the right arch, left ductus arteriosus, and pulmonary artery.

RIGHT AORTIC ARCH WITH LEFT-SIDE CONTRALATERAL DUCTUS ARTERIOSUS

This condition may or may not cause symptoms. If the ductus originates from the bifurcation of the (here left-side) innominate artery, no ring is formed. However, if the ductus arteriosus arises *posteriorly* from a diverticulum

(representing the left dorsal aorta) of the descending arch, a ring is formed by the right arch, left ductus arteriosus, and pulmonary artery (Plate 5.36). Symptoms of right aortic arch with left-side contralateral ductus arteriosus are similar to those already described for aortic arch anomalies but generally appear later and tend to be less severe. This type of anomaly can also occur in mirror-image fashion in patients with a left aortic arch. Treatment

is simple and consists of division of the ductus arteriosus or ligament.

OTHER AORTIC ARCH ANOMALIES

Other variants of aortic arch anomalies involving the third or fourth arches occur, but as long as no constricting ring is formed, these defects only occasionally

Plate 5.37

Cardiovascular System: VOLUME 8

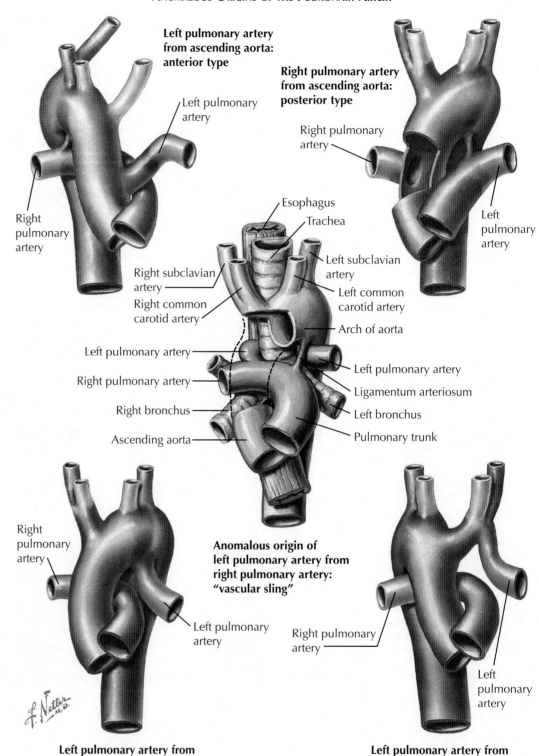

ANOMALOUS ORIGINS OF THE PULMONARY ARTERY

Left pulmonary artery from ascending aorta: anterior type

Left pulmonary artery

Right pulmonary artery from ascending aorta: posterior type

Right pulmonary artery

Esophagus

Trachea

Right subclavian artery

Right common carotid artery

Left subclavian artery

Left common carotid artery

Arch of aorta

Left pulmonary artery

Right pulmonary artery

Left pulmonary artery

Ligamentum arteriosum

Right bronchus

Left bronchus

Ascending aorta

Pulmonary trunk

Left pulmonary artery

Right pulmonary artery

Anomalous origin of left pulmonary artery from right pulmonary artery: "vascular sling"

Left pulmonary artery

Right pulmonary artery

Left pulmonary artery

Left pulmonary artery from left ductus arteriosus: left aortic arch

Left pulmonary artery from left ductus arteriosus: right aortic arch

ANOMALIES OF AORTIC ARCH SYSTEM (Continued)

cause symptoms and are of little clinical importance. Anomalies of the aortic arch system that mainly involve the sixth arches are uncommon and usually referred to as cases of "absent" left or right pulmonary artery, which is misleading. The embryonic pulmonary arteries proper arise as branches of the sixth arches and actually have appeared before the ventral and dorsal primordia of the sixth arches have joined each other to complete these arches. In most cases of "absent" pulmonary artery, the derivatives of the (intrapulmonary) embryonic pulmonary arteries are present, even though they may have lost contact with the pulmonary trunk and receive their blood supply from a systemic arterial source. It is true that complete absence of a pulmonary artery and its terminal branches, with the lung supplied solely by anomalous systemic arteries arising from the aorta beyond the arch, is rare. Cases of "absent" pulmonary artery fall into one of two categories: either the distal pulmonary artery of the involved lung is continuous with a large artery originating from the ascending aorta, or it is supplied by a ductus arteriosus.

PULMONARY ARTERY ARISING FROM ASCENDING AORTA

This anomaly may be of the *anterior* or *posterior* type. The pathogenesis of these two types is entirely different. As indicated in Plate 5.37, the *anterior type* of pulmonary artery consists of the left fourth arch, a segment of the dorsal aorta, distal part of the left sixth arch, and the left embryonic pulmonary artery. It is always contralateral to the aortic arch and can occur with either a right or a left aortic arch, and the subclavian artery contralateral to the aortic arch can be expected to arise anomalously from the descending aortic arch. The *posterior type* of artery consists of the proximal portion of the sixth arch and the embryonic pulmonary artery. Apparently, at the time of partitioning of the truncus

and truncoaortic sac, it was left "stranded." It may be expected to be located always on the right side (in situs solitus individuals) with either a right or a left aortic arch, and the branching pattern of the aortic arch vessels is normal, unless another independent anomaly of these vessels is present. A pulmonary artery arising from the ascending aorta is generally large. The clinical features are similar to those seen in other conditions with anomalous communications at the arterial level and depend on the magnitude of the shunt. The

diagnosis of pulmonary artery from ascending aorta can best be established by angiocardiography.

PULMONARY ARTERY ARISING FROM DUCTUS ARTERIOSUS

If the proximal segment of one of the sixth arches disappears early, the corresponding embryonic pulmonary artery will be supplied instead by the *distal* sixth arch segment; that is, it will be supplied by the ductus

Plate 5.38

Congenital Heart Disease

ANATOMIC FEATURES OF AORTIC COARCTATION IN OLDER CHILDREN AND NEONATES

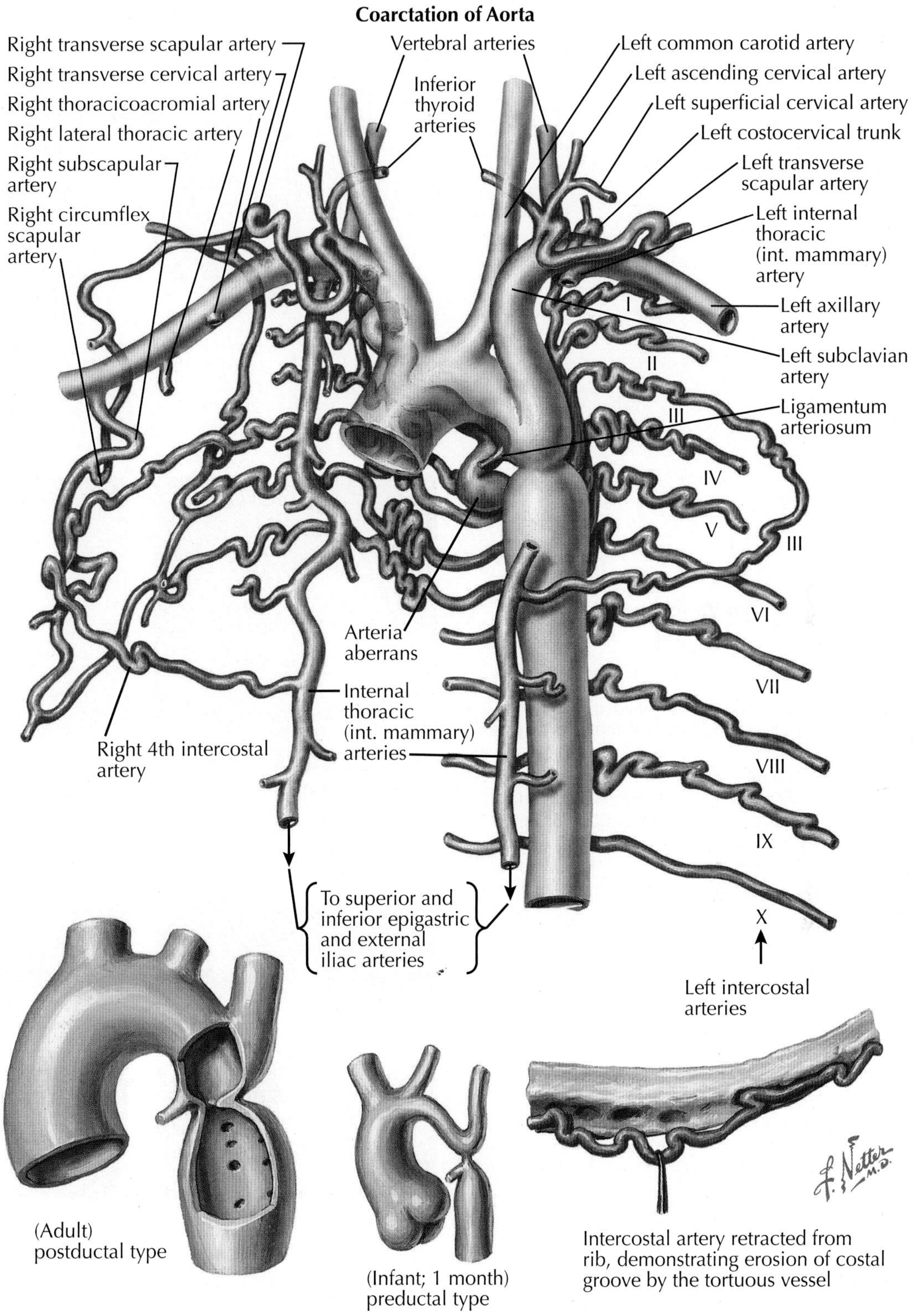

Coarctation of Aorta

Right transverse scapular artery
Right transverse cervical artery
Right thoracicoacromial artery
Right lateral thoracic artery
Right subscapular artery
Right circumflex scapular artery
Vertebral arteries
Inferior thyroid arteries
Left common carotid artery
Left ascending cervical artery
Left superficial cervical artery
Left costocervical trunk
Left transverse scapular artery
Left internal thoracic (int. mammary) artery
Left axillary artery
Left subclavian artery
Ligamentum arteriosum
Arteria aberrans
Internal thoracic (int. mammary) arteries
Right 4th intercostal artery
To superior and inferior epigastric and external iliac arteries
Left intercostal arteries

(Adult) postductal type

(Infant; 1 month) preductal type

Intercostal artery retracted from rib, demonstrating erosion of costal groove by the tortuous vessel

ANOMALIES OF AORTIC ARCH SYSTEM (Continued)

arteriosus (see Plate 5.37). Such a ductus arteriosus originates from the aortic arch if the arch is on the same side or from the innominate artery if the aortic arch is on the opposite side. The ductus arteriosus tends to close, and a large left-to-right shunt therefore is not usually present. In many cases this duct obliterates completely, and the involved lung then is supplied by bronchial artery collaterals.

LEFT PULMONARY ARISING FROM RIGHT PULMONARY ARTERY ("VASCULAR SLING")

An anomalous left pulmonary artery arising from the right pulmonary artery is an interesting malformation. The vessel always comes off the posterior aspect of the right pulmonary artery at the level of the right main bronchus and carina, running between the trachea and the esophagus to the left lung. The ductus arteriosus is located normally on the left side. Other cardiovascular anomalies may be associated. In some cases, tracheobronchial anomalies have been reported, including complete tracheal rings or a right upper lobe bronchus arising independently from the trachea some distance above the carina ("bronchus suis"). No dysphagia is present, but severe respiratory difficulties usually manifest at an early age. Inspiratory stridor and expiratory stridor generally are pronounced, and emphysema or atelectasis and pneumonitis of the right upper lobe, or even of the entire right lung, are usual. Lateral chest radiography may show an ovoid mass separating the barium-filled esophagus and air-filled lower trachea. Although not pathognomonic, this finding should strongly suggest the presence of a "vascular sling." A pulmonary artery angiogram establishes the diagnosis (see Plate 5.37). Treatment is surgical and consists of detaching the anomalous vessel from the right pulmonary artery, followed by reimplantation into the main pulmonary artery. The prognosis without treatment is poor; most infants die within the first year of life.

COARCTATION OF AORTA

Coarctation of the aorta is a congenital narrowing of the descending aorta that usually occurs in the area of the ductus arteriosus, which may be patent (Plate 5.38). If the coarctation is located proximal to the ductus arteriosus, it is called *preductal*; if located distal, the coarctation is termed *postductal*. Preductal coarctation is usually associated with other intracardiac anomalies, and the ductus arteriosus is often widely patent

(PDA). The preductal type is most often seen in infants. Postductal coarctation is usually not associated with other intracardiac defects, except for aortic valve anomalies, and is the type usually found in older children and adults.

The coarctation may be mild but usually is tight or even atretic, and the distal aorta receives most of its blood through collaterals. These collaterals are generally extremely abundant, particularly in older children

Plate 5.39

Cardiovascular System: VOLUME 8

COARCTATION OF AORTA

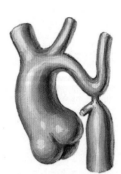

(Adult)
postductal type

(Infant; 1 month)
preductal type

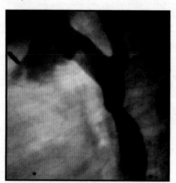

A lateral view aortogram showing a recurrent aortic coarctation distal to the left subclavian artery.

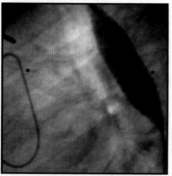

A balloon dilation catheter fully inflated in the site of narrowing, guided by a wire looped in the ascending aorta.

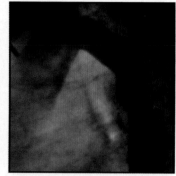

Follow-up aortogram showing marked improvement in the caliber of the aorta in the site of coarctation, without aneurysm formation or residual stenosis.

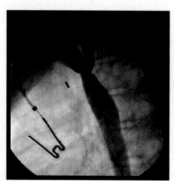

An aortogram showing a nondiscrete native coarctation.

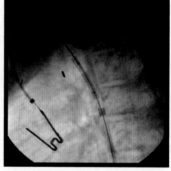

A stent is mounted on a balloon and positioned in the area of the coarctation.

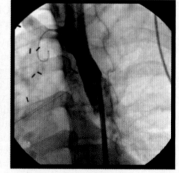

An aortogram after stent placement showing relief of the coarctation and "flaring" of the distal stent to oppose the aortic wall.

ANOMALIES OF AORTIC ARCH SYSTEM (Continued)

and adults. The main collateral routes are from branches of the subclavian arteries (internal thoracic, transverse scapular, transverse cervical) and the intercostal arteries. Other collateral routes are formed by cervical vessels at the thoracic inlet, the vertebral and anterior spinal arteries. Aortic valve anomalies are common in coarctation of aorta, occurring in about 80% or more of patients.

The clinical features of coarctation are characteristic in most patients. Symptoms are typically absent in childhood, and growth and development are normal (Plate 5.39). As a rule, coarctation of aorta is diagnosed indirectly and incidentally because the femoral pulses are diminished or absent, a chest radiograph shows rib notching, or the patient has hypertension. Some patients complain of coldness of the feet or headaches. In older adults, symptoms are mainly caused by long-standing hypertension. Bacterial endocarditis, generally of an anomalous aortic valve and rarely at the site of coarctation, may occur at any age beyond early childhood. Rupture of the aorta and intracranial hemorrhage are most often seen in young adults. Some patients develop difficulty in infancy leading to severe congestive heart failure. Associated cardiac defects may be responsible for the early decompensation, but this is not always the case. The most important findings are absent or greatly diminished femoral pulses; this is a pathognomonic sign in children and young adults because other conditions causing obstruction of the lower aorta are rare in these age groups. Hypertension in the proximal aortic bed usually is absent in young children but becomes increasingly common and severe with advancing age. Other findings are systolic murmur and visible or palpable pulsations around the scapulae and in the axillae and intercostal spaces.

Chest radiography shows a normal or enlarged heart (if no significant aortic valve disease is present); notching of the ribs in older children and adults, caused by erosion of the ribs by the tortuous dilated intercostal arteries; and often a notch in the left border of the upper descending aortic shadow, indicating the site of the coarctation. An esophagogram may outline the opposite (also notched) border of the coarcted aortic segment. MRI can also define the coarctation. In uncomplicated cases the ECG is either normal or more often shows LV hypertrophy. Cardiac catheterization is not essential. If information is desired concerning the status of the aortic valve or coronary arteries, or if other cardiac anomalies are suspected, cardiac catheterization is best postponed until after the coarctation has been corrected surgically or by percutaneous balloon dilation and stent deployment (Plate 5.39). Open-heart surgical techniques to repair aortic coarctation include resection with end-to-end anastomosis, patch aortoplasty, left subclavian flap angioplasty, and bypass graft repair. Balloon angioplasty/stent is also an option for initially treating aortic coarctation or for treating recoarctation after surgery (Plate 5.39).

Plate 5.40

Congenital Heart Disease

ENDOCARDIAL FIBROELASTOSIS AND GLYCOGEN STORAGE DISEASE

Endocardial fibroelastosis typically is a disease of early childhood, although it has occasionally been described in older children and even in young adults. The pathologic features are characteristic (Plate 5.40). The LV is hugely dilated and may be almost globular. The interior is coated by a shiny white layer representing the thickened endocardium, and the trabeculae are coarse and relatively few in number. The mitral and aortic valves may be thickened, rather stiff, and occasionally incompetent. Endocardial fibroelastosis also occurs in association with severe cardiac malformations, such as aortic stenosis or atresia, congenital mitral stenosis, and coarctation of aorta. Fibroelastosis is also seen in various forms of acquired valvar disease, presumably as a secondary lesion. Its distribution in these patients is variable and spotty.

The clinical picture is somewhat characteristic. The age of onset is generally between 2 and 7 months but can be earlier or later. Before onset, asymptomatic and perfectly healthy infants appear to develop symptoms of a cold, followed by irritability, refusal to feed, tachypnea, dyspnea, fever, and cough. Signs of cardiac failure, as evidenced by hepatomegaly, abdominal pain, generalized edema with puffy eyelids, and often the appearance of a systolic murmur, reveal the problem to be a more serious one. The heart can be greatly enlarged, with a gallop rhythm and tachycardia.

Chest radiography and cardiac ultrasound confirm the heart's size, with evidence of pulmonary venous congestion, with or without pneumonitis. The left upper lobe may be overinflated because of compression of the left main bronchus. The ECG shows left axis deviation or more frequently a normal axis and almost always evidence of LV hypertrophy with tall qR patterns and inverted T waves in the left precordial leads. Additional RV hypertrophy may be present in infants with marked failure, but this disappears after successful treatment. Arrhythmias and conduction disturbances are common. Cardiac catheterization and angiocardiography are usually not necessary, unless associated defects are suspected.

The treatment of endocardial fibroelastosis is the same as for chronic cardiac failure; its acute exacerbations are often precipitated by respiratory infections. Early and prolonged treatment with digoxin may be helpful; digoxin cessation may result in acute cardiac failure. Other therapeutic measures for acute failure and exacerbations of failure may be required, and precipitating factors such as infection and anemia demand immediate attention. Warfarin therapy should be considered if patients have thrombotic/embolic complications.

GLYCOGEN STORAGE DISEASE

Excessive deposition of glycogen in the tissues is caused by a hereditary error in carbohydrate metabolism. It is transmitted as an autosomal recessive gene and often occurs in siblings. Several types are distinguished, and the enzyme defect of most of these is known. In the cardiac variety, first described by Pompe, glycogen is deposited in abnormal amounts in all tissues but especially in the heart, which is enormously enlarged and globular, with tremendously thick and solid walls (Plate 5.40). Microscopically, large central vacuoles in the myocardial fibers, with a thin surrounding shell of cytoplasm, give the sections a peculiar lace appearance. Glycogen can be

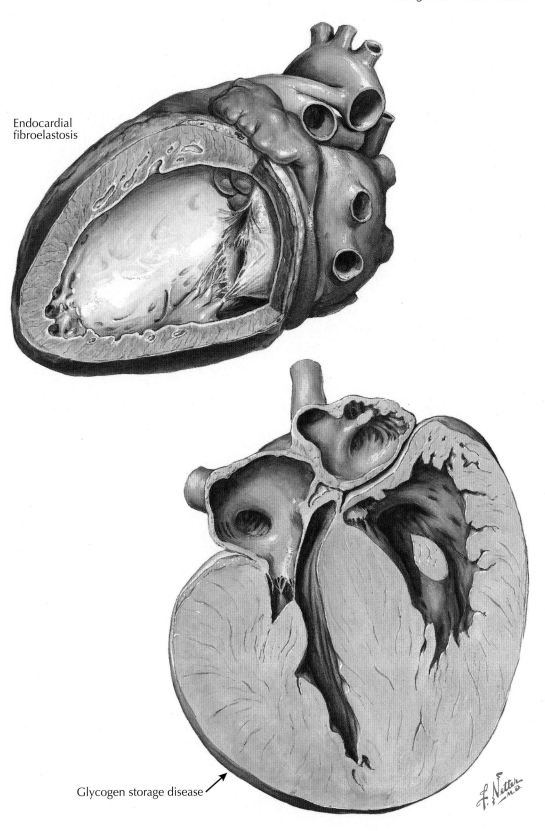

Endocardial fibroelastosis

Glycogen storage disease

demonstrated with various histochemical staining techniques. Clinically, the patient has marked cardiomegaly and muscular weakness. Congestive heart failure appears early in infancy. There may be macroglossia, also from abnormal glycogen deposition in the tongue muscle. Chest radiography reveals marked cardiomegaly, and the ECG characteristically shows a short PR interval, with or without Wolff-Parkinson-White syndrome, and LV hypertrophy. The prognosis is poor, and death usually occurs within the first year of life. However, enzyme replacement therapy in infantile-onset patients has been shown to decrease heart size, maintain normal heart function, and reduce glycogen accumulation. Alglucosidase alfa has received U.S. Food and Drug Administration approval for the treatment of infants and children with glycogen storage disease.

ACQUIRED HEART DISEASE

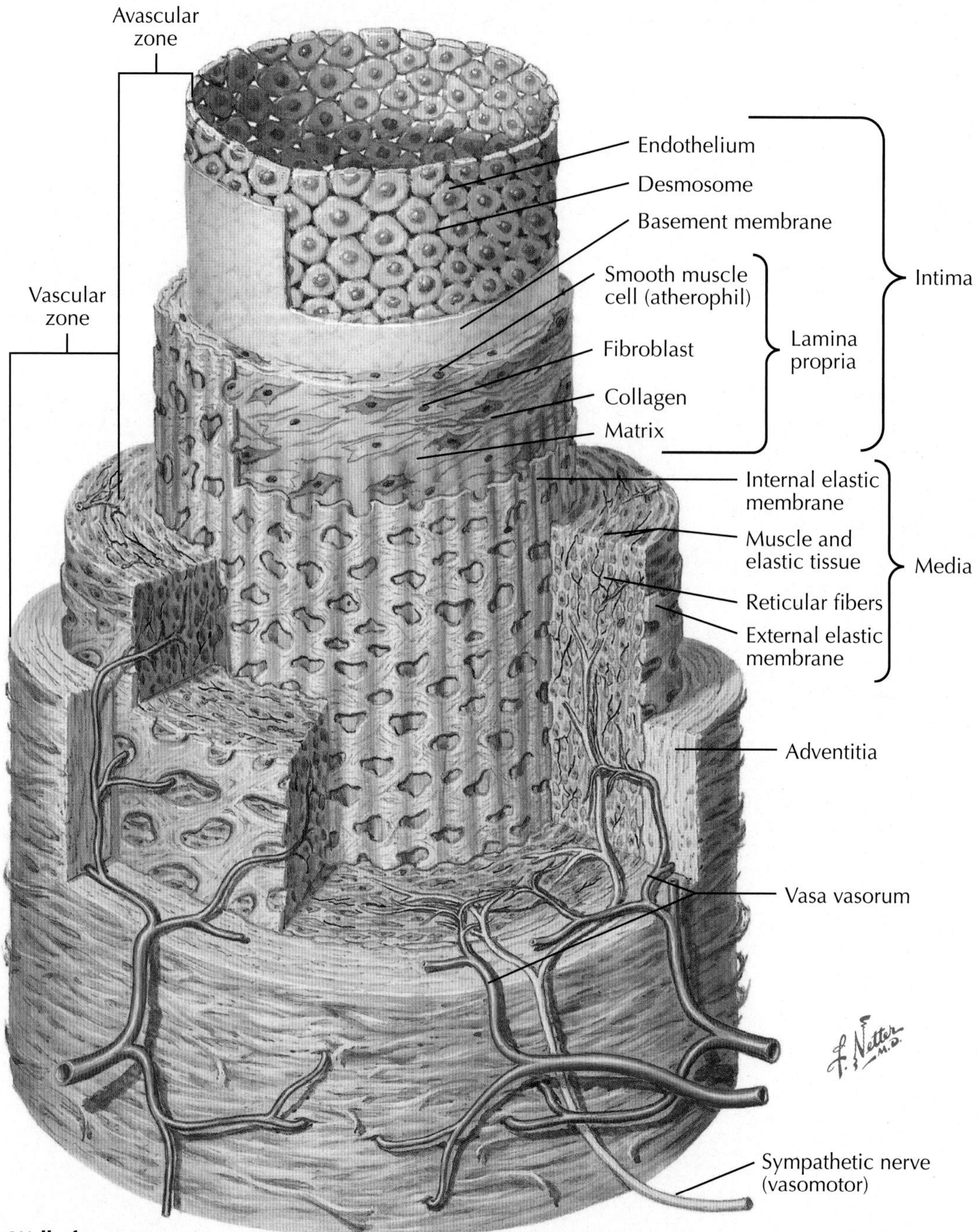

Plate 6.1

Cardiovascular System: VOLUME 8

STRUCTURE OF CORONARY ARTERIES

The coronary arteries are susceptible to atherosclerosis as well as its complications, particularly intravascular thrombosis, often resulting in myocardial infarction. *Atherosclerosis* is a form of arteriosclerosis characterized by initial involvement of the inner layer of the arterial wall, or *intima*. The intimal localization of early atheromas helps to differentiate the atherosclerosis type from other forms of arteriosclerosis, such as Mönckeberg medial sclerosis or periarteritis nodosa, that primarily involve the muscular or adventitial layers.

Recent histochemical, organ culture, and electron microscopy studies have found further evidence of the complexity of the arterial wall. As Plate 6.1 shows, a medium-sized muscular artery, such as a main coronary vessel, consists of a series of concentric tubes or coaxial coats of differentiated cellular and extracellular components in three layers: *tunica intima* or intima, *tunica media* or muscular, and *tunica adventitia*. In the intima, the innermost cell layer in direct contact with the bloodstream consists of a sheet of polygonal endothelial cells, usually less than 1 micron (µm) thick, except at the site of the cell nucleus, and elongated in a direction parallel to the vessel's axis. Many of these endothelial cells have pinocytotic vesicles of *caveolae* in their cytoplasm, abundant mitochondria, well-developed granular endoplasmic reticulum, and Golgi complexes. Microscopically, the areas of contact between endothelial cells vary from simple mutual contact of the cell membranes to well-defined intercellular bridges, or *desmosomes,* corresponding to the so-called intercellular cement lines described in earlier light microscopy studies. A distinct basement membrane separates these endothelial cells from the subendothelial space, which varies in thickness according to age of the patient as well as size of the artery. In fetal life and shortly after birth, the endothelium in the coronary arteries lies in direct contact with the internal elastic membrane, or *lamina,* without the subendothelial space, which appears by the end of the first decade of life.

In adulthood, the intima consists of a matrix of ground substance containing small amounts of acid mucopolysaccharides and elastic and collagen fibers separating scattered intimal cells, or *intimacytes*. Because of morphologic and cytochemical difficulties in classifying intimacytes, their response to in vitro incorporation of serum lipids is used to identify them. Some intimacytes, or *atherophils,* incorporate lipid rapidly and show ultrastructural characteristics of modified smooth muscle cells, with typical bundles of myofilaments in their cytoplasm, pinocytotic vesicles, and parts of limiting basement membrane on the cell

surface. On the other hand, cells called *fibrophils* are spindle shaped and have finger-like cytoplasmic projections, with no basement membrane and few pinocytotic vesicles. Occasionally, large mononuclear ovoid cells appear, containing cytoplasmic inclusions with "single-unit" acid phosphatase–positive granules or lysosomes resembling macrophages.

The *lamina propria* is separated from the underlying smooth muscle cells of the media usually by a well-developed internal elastic membrane of tenacious matrix containing fibrils about 500 angstroms (Å) in diameter with abundant fenestrations. This *internal elastic membrane* is usually wavy in cross sections, and the fenestrations are oval or round openings extending across its surface. The underlying tunica media is characterized by concentric layers of smooth muscle cells 10 to 25 µm in length and oriented transversely to the artery's main

axis. Individual smooth muscle cells are surrounded by a network of collagenous and elastic fibers, which continue without transition into both internal and external elastic membranes. The *external elastic membrane* separates the media from the adventitia and is characterized by the presence of loosely packed collagen and elastic fibers. Small blood vessels or *vasa vasorum* are also found, as well as both *sympathetic* and *parasympathetic* nerve fibers from the autonomic nervous system.

These morphologic and functional characteristics of the coronary arteries are modified early in the presence of the intimal changes characteristic of atherosclerosis. The most important clinical difference between coronary and aortic atherosclerosis is the high incidence of acute thrombosis in coronary vessels, with infarction resulting in irreversible damage to the underlying myocardium.

Avascular zone

Vascular zone

Endothelium
Desmosome
Basement membrane
Smooth muscle cell (atherophil)
Fibroblast
Collagen
Matrix
Intima
Lamina propria
Internal elastic membrane
Muscle and elastic tissue
Reticular fibers
External elastic membrane
Media
Adventitia
Vasa vasorum
Sympathetic nerve (vasomotor)

Wall of an artery: cutaway view

Plate 6.2

Acquired Heart Disease

PATHOGENESIS OF ATHEROSCLEROSIS

Histologic and functional characteristics of the intimal lining of the arteries help in understanding the histogenesis of spontaneous atheromas, often initiated shortly after birth, particularly the presence of different cell types in a ground substance matrix and the absence of a direct blood supply. The well-developed atherosclerotic plaque resulting from inflammatory and reparative processes is a complex lesion containing extracellular deposits of calcium salts, blood components, cholesterol crystals, and acid mucopolysaccharides. The initial changes, however, seem to occur at the cellular level, often accompanied by an abnormal intracellular storage of *lipids,* particularly cholesterol esters, fatty acids, and lipoprotein complexes. These findings on microscopy have strengthened the thesis that lipid infiltration from the bloodstream may be a significant factor in the growth of the atheromatous plaque. Furthermore, recognition by cytochemical techniques makes lipids helpful indicators of abnormal cell behavior, independent of their role in the etiology of atheroma.

Because of the frequency and severity of atherosclerosis, short-term organ culture techniques for the isolation of arterial intimal cells (intimacytes) identify susceptible cell populations, based on their response to incorporation of homologous serum lipids in vitro. Intimacytes from arteries, with and without histologic evidence of atherosclerosis, show two types of atherophils: genetically highly susceptible cells and genetically resistant cells to intracellular lipid accumulation.

In the presence of increased perfusion rates of plasma lipoproteins caused by local hemodynamic changes, hypertension, elevated serum lipids, or changes in endothelial surface permeability (trauma, fibrin deposition, platelet aggregation), *genetically susceptible atherophils* will be transformed into lipid-laden *atherocytes.* The secondary release of intracellular lipids from these cells will induce surrounding atherophils to incorporate them, creating a self-feeding process with cytologic changes that increase metabolic requirements, including oxygen consumption rates, which result in increased permeability of the cell membrane to lipids if not met. These events set up a cycle favoring further expansion of focal atherosclerotic changes. Collagen fibers are laid down by fibrophils, which are then transformed into *fibrocytes* surrounded by acid mucopolysaccharide deposits. This eventually results in a characteristic intimal hyperplasia after ground substance changes. These histologic lesions are self-perpetuating, resulting in the replacement of intimacytes by an acellular area of arterial intima that stimulates further surface involvement of the vascular wall in this interplay among deposition, inflammatory response, and scarring, with the eventual production of a typical atherosclerotic *plaque.*

In contrast, *genetically resistant atherophils,* even in the presence of elevated serum lipid levels, do not respond (or respond minimally) to an increased perfusion

of plasma lipids. If some atherocytes appear, they are few in number, and only superficial *fatty streaks* are developed, resulting in sparse intimal elevations with few fibrophils and no well-organized plaque. This type of cytologic response also seems less susceptible to the clinical complications of atherosclerosis, particularly thrombosis or rupture, because of the limited involvement of the vascular wall.

This approach to the pathogenesis of atherosclerosis emphasizes the clinical significance of the earliest possible identification of patients whose arteries are susceptible to atheroma, to modify or prevent environmental conditions that favor the acceleration of atherogenesis in the arterial intima cells. Local factors are also important in identification of the lesions, suggesting possible therapeutic approaches for their arrest or inhibition.

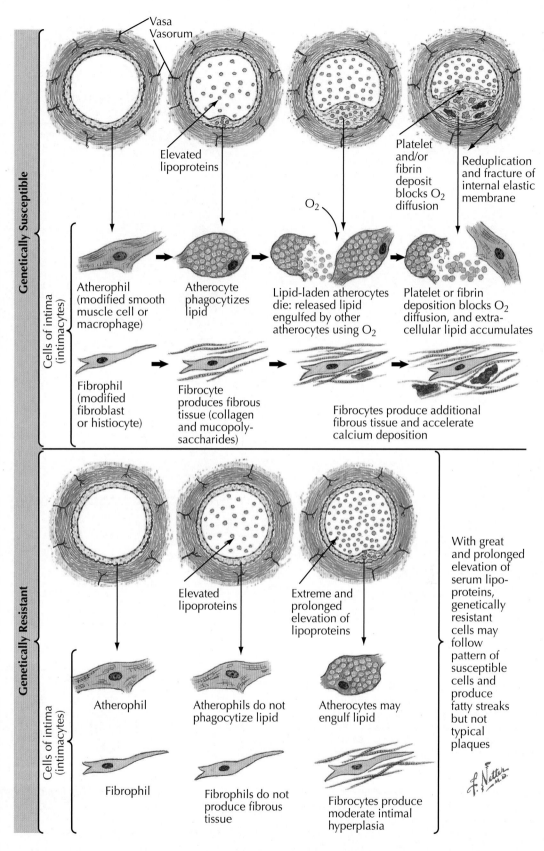

Genetically Susceptible

Cells of intima (intimacytes)

Vasa Vasorum

Elevated lipoproteins

O_2

Platelet and/or fibrin deposit blocks O_2 diffusion

Reduplication and fracture of internal elastic membrane

Atherophil (modified smooth muscle cell or macrophage)

Atherocyte phagocytizes lipid

Lipid-laden atherocytes die: released lipid engulfed by other atherocytes using O_2

Platelet or fibrin deposition blocks O_2 diffusion, and extracellular lipid accumulates

Fibrophil (modified fibroblast or histiocyte)

Fibrocyte produces fibrous tissue (collagen and mucopolysaccharides)

Fibrocytes produce additional fibrous tissue and accelerate calcium deposition

Genetically Resistant

Cells of intima (intimacytes)

Elevated lipoproteins

Extreme and prolonged elevation of lipoproteins

With great and prolonged elevation of serum lipoproteins, genetically resistant cells may follow pattern of susceptible cells and produce fatty streaks but not typical plaques

Atherophil

Atherophils do not phagocytize lipid

Atherocytes may engulf lipid

Fibrophil

Fibrophils do not produce fibrous tissue

Fibrocytes produce moderate intimal hyperplasia

Plate 6.3

Cardiovascular System: VOLUME 8

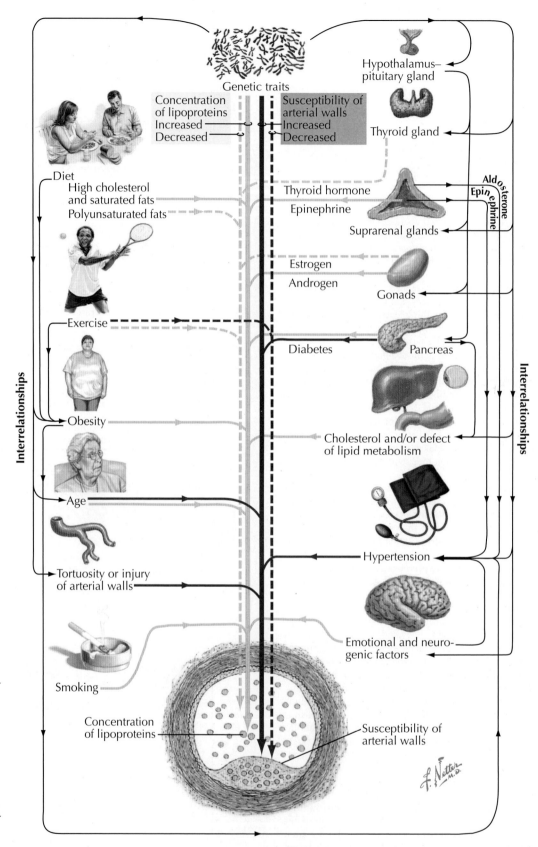

Genetic traits

Concentration of lipoproteins
Increased
Decreased

Susceptibility of arterial walls
Increased
Decreased

Hypothalamus–pituitary gland

Thyroid gland

Diet
High cholesterol and saturated fats
Polyunsaturated fats

Thyroid hormone
Epinephrine

Aldosterone
Epinephrine

Suprarenal glands

Estrogen
Androgen

Gonads

Exercise

Diabetes
Pancreas

Obesity

Cholesterol and/or defect of lipid metabolism

Age

Hypertension

Tortuosity or injury of arterial walls

Interrelationships

Interrelationships

Emotional and neurogenic factors

Smoking

Concentration of lipoproteins

Susceptibility of arterial walls

Risk Factors in Etiology of Atherosclerosis

In terms of mortality, the most serious problem facing more developed countries is atherosclerosis of the cardiac and cerebral blood vessels. There is no single cause of atherosclerosis, which is often labeled a multifaceted disease. Atherosclerosis reflects the culmination of many factors acting over a lifetime and usually clinically manifests only when angina pectoris, sudden cardiac death, myocardial infarction (MI), transient ischemic attack, or cerebrovascular accident (stroke) occurs. Heart failure is usually caused by MI.

Patients with a family history of premature manifestations of atherosclerosis may be at high risk for development of atherosclerotic disease. Older age, male sex, hypertension, diabetes, obesity, and tobacco smoking are associated with coronary atherosclerosis. Lack of exercise may interact with other clinical factors, and an exercise program (e.g., walking) is known to diminish symptoms in patients with known clinical manifestations of atherosclerosis. Excessive saturated fat in the diet is also involved in atherogenesis. High-fat diets increase blood lipid levels, particularly low-density lipoprotein (LDL) cholesterol. Elevated triglycerides and low levels of high-density lipoprotein (HDL) are also implicated in the etiology of atherosclerosis. Elevated serum uric acid may also contribute to atherogenesis, although further study is required. *Unsaturated*

fatty acids with two or more double bonds help reduce cholesterol blood levels when their relationship to *saturated* fatty acids is increased.

Current concepts of atherogenicity are complex and involve monocytes, platelets, macrophages, foam cells, endothelial cells, smooth muscle cells, oxidized LDL, and many other subcellular substances. Interested readers should refer to current literature and textbooks on the subject. In general, the physician or clinician can

profile a patient potentially prone to atherosclerosis, such as an adult male with hypertension who smokes cigarettes, exercises little, and has elevated blood cholesterol and triglyceride levels, low HDL levels, and abnormal glucose metabolism. Currently, in addition to diet and exercise, drugs used to treat lipid abnormalities include HMG CoA reductase inhibitors (statins), nicotinic acid preparations, ezetimibe, fibric acid derivatives, and bile acid sequestrants.

Plate 6.4

Acquired Heart Disease

TYPES AND DEGREES OF CORONARY ATHEROSCLEROTIC NARROWING OR OCCLUSION

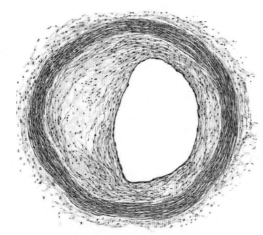

Moderate atherosclerotic narrowing of lumen

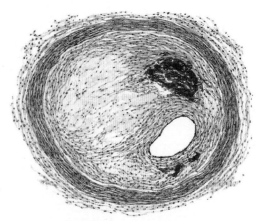

Almost complete occlusion by intimal atherosclerosis with calcium deposition

PATHOLOGIC CHANGES IN CORONARY ARTERY DISEASE

The earliest recognizable atheromatous changes in blood vessels are accumulation of aggregates of lipid-laden macrophages in the intima. The appearance of this lesion is similar to that seen in many experimental vascular lesions. Another apparently early phenomenon, difficult to correlate and possibly unrelated, is a subintimal deposit of collagen that often is primitive and thus rich in acid mucopolysaccharides. Lesions of this type shadow atherosclerosis wherever it occurs. The relationship of this vascular lesion to the type seen in Asian populations has not been elucidated, but this disorder does occur in Asian individuals. A further complication of this lesion is the deposition of fibrin on or within its superficial layers.

As more lipid accumulates, an atheromatous plaque with many constituents is formed. This plaque may involve only a segmental portion of the artery or its entire circumference. When the macrophages die, their lipid is released and becomes an inflammatory irritant. Fibrin accumulates, as do other blood constituents; calcium deposits form; and fibroblasts proliferate. Stenotic lesions may accumulate more surface material with deposited layers of thrombus. These lesions regress with lipid-lowering agents and antiplatelet therapy.

Even a segmental atheroma can cause atrophy of the underlying arterial wall, and the concentric type seems associated with major destruction of the lamina and parts of the media. Such changes appear secondary to interference with the nutrients permeating the intima. The stages of atheroma reveal another major feature in the lesion's development: an inability to clear blood constituents that have permeated the media. This dynamic event is demonstrated by perfusing isolated segments of living canine arteries and observing the quantity of lipid in the vasa vasorum of the adventitia.

Hemorrhage into the lesion can result from surface blood dissecting into the plaque or from vasa vasorum bleeding. Thrombosis may occlude the artery; if the person survives, organization of the fibrin clot can progress and occasionally recanalize the artery. However,

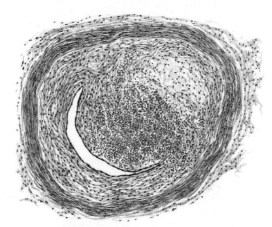

Hemorrhage into atheroma, leaving only a slit-like lumen

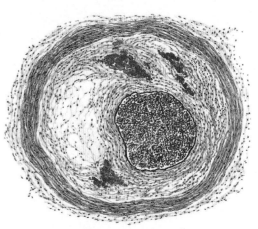

Complete occlusion by thrombus in lumen greatly narrowed by atheroma

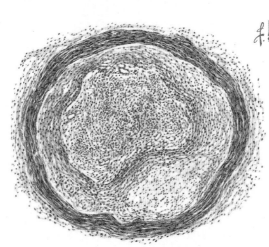

Organization of thrombus

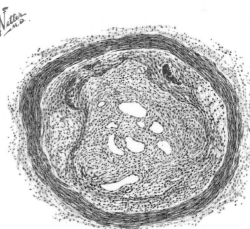

Organization with recanalization may occur

the ability of these small channels to supply any appreciable volume of blood beyond the area of obstruction is insufficient in most patients to revascularize the downstream myocardium. Rarely, an occluding thrombus completely disappears.

In addition to atheromatous and thrombus blockade of the coronary arteries, emboli can obstruct an otherwise normal coronary artery. Such emboli may

consist of thrombi, valvular calcification, pieces of tumor, and occasionally even small foreign bodies. Various types of aortitis can involve the proximal vessels; syphilis of the aortic wall can occlude the ostia. The atheroma is the main disorder, however, because of its *distribution*. The lesions closest to the aorta (proximal) are the plaques most likely to impede flow to the cardiac microcirculation.

Plate 6.5

Cardiovascular System: VOLUME 8

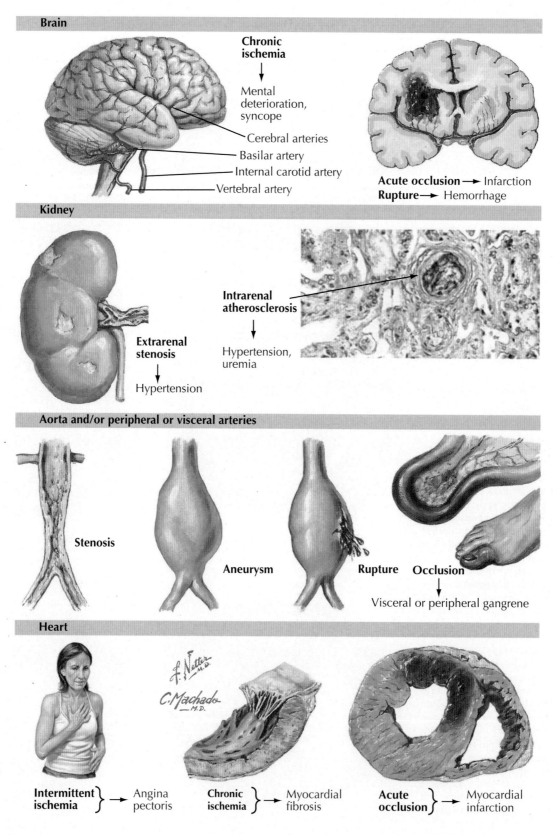

Brain

Chronic ischemia → Mental deterioration, syncope

Cerebral arteries
Basilar artery
Internal carotid artery
Vertebral artery

Acute occlusion → Infarction
Rupture → Hemorrhage

Kidney

Extrarenal stenosis → Hypertension

Intrarenal atherosclerosis → Hypertension, uremia

Aorta and/or peripheral or visceral arteries

Stenosis

Aneurysm

Rupture   Occlusion → Visceral or peripheral gangrene

Heart

Intermittent ischemia } → Angina pectoris

Chronic ischemia } → Myocardial fibrosis

Acute occlusion } → Myocardial infarction

END ORGAN DAMAGE BY VASCULAR DISEASE

The cerebral circulation is particularly vulnerable in patients who are hypertensive. Stroke is the major cause of death. Hypertensive vascular disease is usually a combination of hypertension and atherosclerosis, the latter accelerated by elevated blood pressure. Infarction of the brain is more common than subarachnoid bleeding. Bleeding results from rupture of microaneurysms of the small arteries or from trauma. The coronary vessels are next most vulnerable. Angina pectoris and MI are common results of accelerated atherosclerosis, necessitating concurrent treatment of the hypertension and atherosclerosis. Many patients reduce their high blood pressure and return to normal levels, only to have an MI or die of complications of atherosclerosis.

The results of the increased rate of atherogenesis are also seen in other large vessels besides the coronary arteries. Thus aneurysms of the aorta and renal arteries are common, leading to distal embolization, dissection, and possible rupture. Reducing blood pressure has a beneficial action on these lesions. Drugs, surgery, and interventions are now available to treat the clinical effects of both hypertension and atherosclerosis, although the goal should be prevention.

Plate 6.6

Acquired Heart Disease

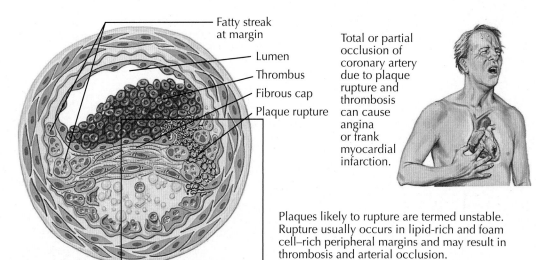

Fatty streak at margin
Lumen
Thrombus
Fibrous cap
Plaque rupture

Total or partial occlusion of coronary artery due to plaque rupture and thrombosis can cause angina or frank myocardial infarction.

Plaques likely to rupture are termed unstable. Rupture usually occurs in lipid-rich and foam cell–rich peripheral margins and may result in thrombosis and arterial occlusion.

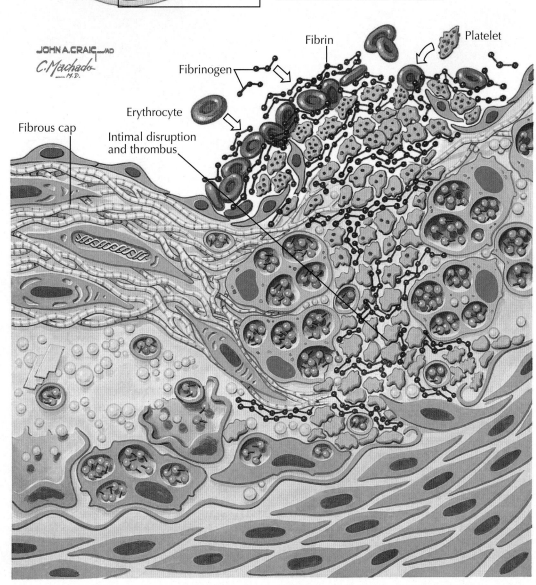

Fibrin
Platelet
Fibrinogen
Erythrocyte
Fibrous cap
Intimal disruption and thrombus

Unstable Plaque Formation

Plaques likely to rupture are called "unstable" and are the main cause of acute coronary syndromes. Plaques with a thin cap and a lipid core associated with inflammation and cap fatigue may be associated with rupture at the edges of the plaque. The plaques are rich in lipids and foam cells, found at the peripheral margins. On rupture, plaques extrude thrombogenic material, which then can trigger thrombosis on the plaque, in turn occluding the coronary artery and resulting in MI.

If the vessel only is almost occluded, a condition known as *unstable angina* may result. Risk factors such as cigarette smoking, hypertension, diabetes mellitus, and dyslipidemia contribute to endothelial injury, causing smooth muscle cell proliferation, inflammation, and deposition of lipid within the blood vessel wall. These events may lead to the development of unstable plaques. Other physical factors may alter plaque composition and make a plaque vulnerable to rupture; cold temperature (32°C–34°C) may promote the crystallization of liquid cholesterol, and these sharp crystals may perforate the cap. Cytokines, growth factors, and oxidative stress are other factors in progression of atherosclerosis and instability.

Thrombosis related to these plaques may be caused by endothelial erosion or plaque disruption. In general, plaque erosion occurs over high-grade stenoses, whereas thrombosis related to plaque disruption is often seen in patients with few stenoses. In addition, multiple triggers of plaque disruption are probably related to increased tension, bleeding originating from the vasa vasorum, bending and twisting of the arteries, and increased systolic and pulse pressures.

Plate 6.7

Cardiovascular System: VOLUME 8

Angiogenesis occurs by the budding of new blood vessels. Hypoxia and inflammation are the two major stimuli for new vessel growth.

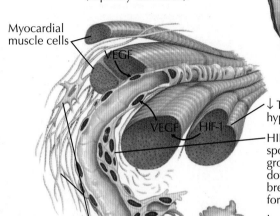

Obstructed coronary artery

Ischemic myocardium (shaded area)

Angiogenesis
(capillary formation)

Myocardial muscle cells

VEGF

VEGF   HIF-1

Fibroblasts and extracellular matrix

Sprouting capillary

↓ Tissue O$_2$ tension promotes release of hypoxia-inducible factor 1 (HIF-1).

HIF-1 binds to the DNA sequence of the gene responsible for the expression of vascular endothelial growth factor (VEGF), which induces mitosis of endothelial cells that, in turn, activates pathways to break down the extracellular matrix, opening space for the sprouting vessel to grow.

Lasting myocardial ischemia leads to an inflammatory reaction. Macrophages (transformed monocytes) produce cytokines such as basic fibroblast growth factor (bFGF), VEGF, and transforming growth factor β (TGF-β).

Recruited pericytes contribute to stabilize the three-dimensional structure of the new vessel.

Newly formed blood vessels connect to each other, forming loops and expanding the capillary network.

Pericytes

Restored extra-cellular matrix

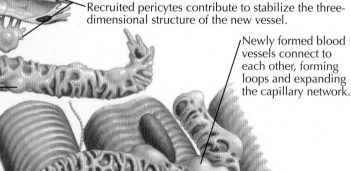

ANGIOGENESIS AND ARTERIOGENESIS

Unfortunately, the terms *angiogenesis* and *arteriogenesis* are often confused and interpreted to have the same meaning. These processes are really two separate entities representing blood vessel changes in the heart.

ANGIOGENESIS

Angiogenesis is essentially the budding of new blood vessels from sprouts of existing vessels to expand the capillary network (the *microcirculation*). Current investigations focus on creation of new blood vessels in areas of critical need, as in patients with large areas of infarcted myocardium surrounded by ischemic zones. The two major stimuli for new vessel growth are *hypoxia*, which activates hypoxia-inducible factor 1, and *inflammation*, which stimulates macrophages to secrete cytokines in patients with MI, including basic fibroblast growth factor (bFGF) and transforming growth factor β (TGF-β). As a result, newly formed blood vessels arise. This is particularly evident in animal models and is being tested in human trials (e.g., stem cell therapy in patients with MI).

ARTERIOGENESIS

In arteriogenesis, collateral vessels are recruited to increase blood flow to ischemic tissue. Coronary artery collateral vessels are thought to be stimulated and generated as a result of "demand ischemia" in areas of the myocardium. For example, the distal portion of a left anterior descending (LAD) coronary artery with high-grade stenosis or obstruction may receive blood from the right coronary artery (RCA) through septal collaterals or from the posterior descending coronary artery. Another potential source of collateralization is from the conus branch of the RCA, essentially one

coronary artery supplying another artery, by either capillary-sized (microcirculation) collaterals or large muscular collaterals that are epicardial vessels (e.g., conus artery of RCA). This blood vessel is known to provide collateral blood flow to a severely stenotic proximal LAD artery.

Collaterals are not seen in patients without evidence of myocardial ischemia, possibly because no dormant

collateral vessels are present. Also, in patients with balloon occlusion of an epicardial vessel and resultant myocardial ischemia, collateral flow through a previously dormant collateral vessel can be seen immediately. This indicates that these collateral vessels are dormant and visualized only when there is demand ischemia. Collateral vessels easily visualized with coronary angiography are categorized under arteriogenesis.

Plate 6.8

Acquired Heart Disease

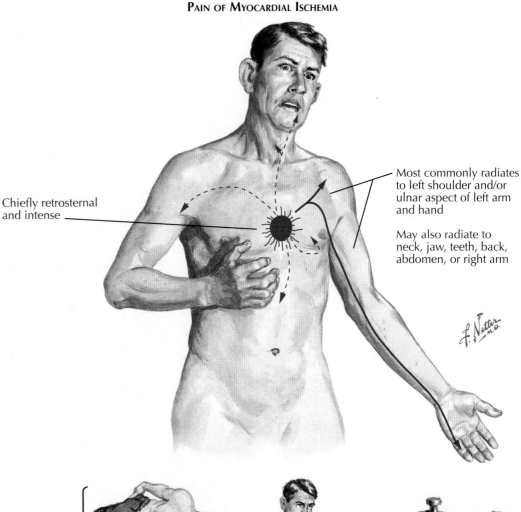

PAIN OF MYOCARDIAL ISCHEMIA

Chiefly retrosternal and intense

Most commonly radiates to left shoulder and/or ulnar aspect of left arm and hand

May also radiate to neck, jaw, teeth, back, abdomen, or right arm

OVERVIEW OF MYOCARDIAL ISCHEMIA

In patients without myocardial ischemia, myocardial oxygen demand is balanced by myocardial oxygen supply. Determinants of myocardial oxygen supply are related to aortic diastolic pressure, left ventricular end-diastolic pressure (LVEDP), and coronary artery resistance. Determinants of myocardial oxygen demand are related to heart rate, systolic blood pressure (BP), left ventricular (LV) tension, and LVEDP. Myocardial ischemia related to balloon occlusion of a coronary artery involves a sequence of decreased coronary blood flow, as detected by perfusion scintigraphy; altered regional flow/demand ratio resulting in decreased coronary sinus oxygen saturation; LV diastolic relaxation abnormalities, detected by cardiac ultrasound; systolic contraction abnormalities, detected by cardiac ultrasound or angiography; increased LVEDP; ST-segment depression on electrocardiography; and angina pectoris or its equivalent symptoms (e.g., breathlessness).

At the cellular level, the current hypothesis is that myocardial ischemia increases the late sodium current, which increases the sodium content of the myocardial cells. The sodium/calcium exchanger then increases the calcium content of the cell. As a result, the LV stiffens, increasing LVEDP, which decreases endomyocardial blood flow, propagating the myocardial ischemia.

Myocardial ischemia and its usual manifestation angina pectoris result from an imbalance between myocardial oxygen supply and myocardial oxygen demand. Myocardial ischemia manifested by angina pectoris can be acute or chronic. In general, patients with an *acute* clinical presentation have a crescendo pattern of angina and are considered to be in an unstable or "acute coronary syndrome" state.

Common descriptions of pain

Vise-like

Constricting

Crushing weight and/or pressure

Other manifestations of myocardial ischemia

Fear

Perspiration

Shortness of breath

Nausea, vomiting

Weakness, collapse, coma

Although most patients with myocardial ischemia are symptomatic, 25% may be asymptomatic. However, most symptomatic patients have many episodes of asymptomatic myocardial ischemia. Laboratory manifestations of myocardial ischemia other than electrocardiographic (ECG) changes are abnormalities of perfusion, as indicated by nuclear studies, and transient regional wall motion abnormalities, usually detected by echocardiographic studies or other noninvasive imaging techniques (e.g., magnetic resonance imaging [MRI]). Clinical manifestations of myocardial ischemia are generally chest discomfort (angina pectoris), arrhythmias, and LV dysfunction in both systole and diastole.

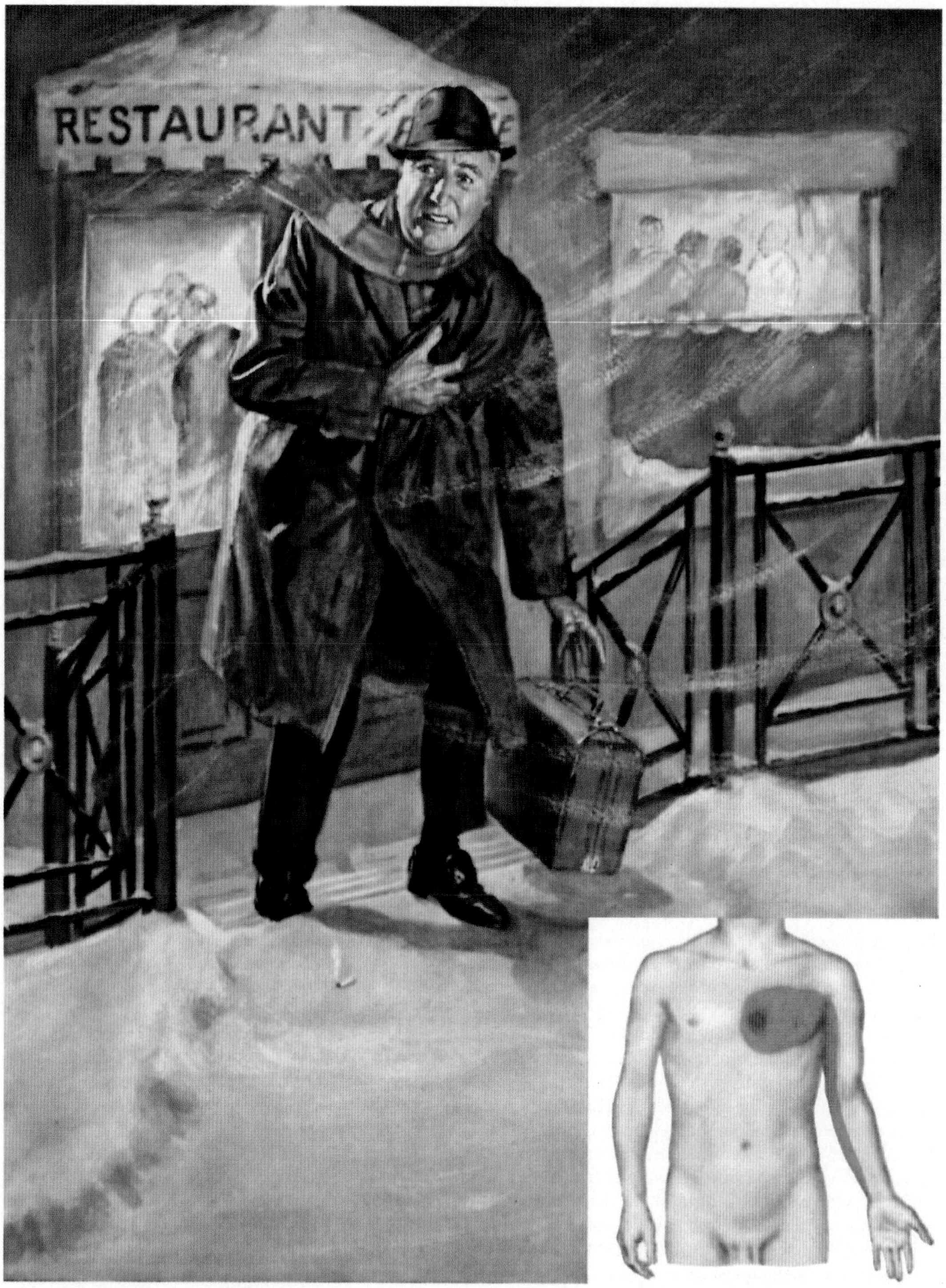

Plate 6.9

Cardiovascular System: VOLUME 8

ANGINA PECTORIS

Angina pectoris ("strangling of the chest") was first described as a serious symptom by Heberden in 1768, although he did not associate angina with coronary artery disease, as discovered later by Jenner. Angina is usually of short duration, associated with effort or emotion, and usually relieved in minutes by rest or sublingual nitroglycerin administration.

Angina pectoris varies somewhat from patient to patient, but the usual description of symptoms includes a feeling of a heavy weight, oppression, or a choking sensation under the middle of the chest and pain extending occasionally to the arms, especially the left, and almost never to the back and rarely to the neck and jaw. Many patients do not describe angina as a pain but rather as a discomfort in the chest. It is produced, as a rule, by effort or emotion, especially in cold weather and particularly after meals or smoking. Angina rarely lasts more than 2 or 3 minutes and is relieved in a few minutes by sublingual nitroglycerin, which is also often used preventively, particularly if the patient knows a given situation will provoke cardiac pain. Angina must be differentiated particularly from gastrointestinal, musculoskeletal, and costochondritic origins of the discomfort.

Angina pectoris and the pain of acute MI are caused by the same disease process, but the prolonged pain in angina is associated with coronary artery occlusion and not the coronary artery stenosis of MI. The prognosis in the patient with angina pectoris varies greatly, but with medical management, many patients can continue to lead a normal life. Over months or years, their angina pectoris may diminish or disappear through natural development of collateral circulation to the ischemic zone of myocardium. However, angina is always an important symptom and may be life-threatening because of the potential for ventricular arrhythmias. Treatment

Common precipitating factors in angina pectoris: Heavy meal, exertion, cold, smoking

Characteristic distribution of pain in angina pectoris

of angina pectoris always includes medical therapy and often includes percutaneous coronary intervention (PCI, angioplasty/stent) or surgical bypass of a stenotic artery. Diet, blood pressure control, lipid management, nitrates, β-blockers, angiotensin-converting enzyme (ACE) inhibitors, aspirin or other antiplatelet agents, smoking cessation, and exercise are considered optimal therapy before and after a revascularization procedure.

Prevention of the underlying disease that causes angina pectoris is paramount. For those at risk, as shown by family history and high serum cholesterol, the avoidance of obesity, a diet low in animal fat, routine exercise (if no heart disease), and smoking cessation should be the first priority in any health promotion and heart disease prevention program and should start in childhood.

Plate 6.10

Acquired Heart Disease

CORONARY ARTERY SPASM

In 1959, Prinzmetal and colleagues described a syndrome of "variant angina" and postulated that the mechanism of chest pain in patients with this finding was due to coronary artery spasm associated with fixed coronary obstruction.

The first observation of coronary artery spasm during coronary angiography was reported by Gensini and others in 1963. Many individuals have contributed to the vast amount of the accumulated literature on coronary artery spasm, but Maseri and colleagues have provided elegant pathophysiologic investigations in patients presenting with angina at rest.

FEATURES OF CORONARY ARTERY SPASM

Changes with coronary spasm provoked by ergonovine are similar to those occurring during spontaneous coronary spasm. Various terms are used to classify coronary spasm, such as *spontaneous, induced, ischemic, nonischemic,* and *catheter induced.*

Arteriograms demonstrate the following features of coronary artery spasm: shape, length, location of the spastic segment, multivessel spasm migration of the site of spasm, and the relationship of spasm to underlying coronary artery disease.

ETIOLOGY OF CORONARY ARTERY SPASM

No single cause has yet been found for coronary artery spasm, although both human and animal investigations have suggested that coronary spasm is a heterogeneous and complex disorder with multiple possible pathophysiologic mechanisms that may act singly or in concert at a given time in a given patient.

Various stressors have been used to provoke coronary spasm, including exercise, cold pressure testing, hyperventilation, histamine, and ergonovine.

DEATHS DUE TO CORONARY ARTERY SPASM

There have been a few cases in which patients died. More patients and a longer follow-up are necessary to appreciate the prognostic value of provoked and spontaneous coronary artery spasm in these patients.

PAIN DUE TO CORONARY ARTERY DISEASE

In patients with coronary artery spasm, pain is not generally preceded by an increase in heart rate and blood pressure but is preceded by a regional fall in oxygen saturation in the coronary venous system as well as a decrease in regional coronary blood flow as measured by coronary venous flow techniques.

In patients with reproducible effort angina, it is likely that ischemia is a result of increased oxygen demand above the supply fixed by coronary arthrosclerosis. It cannot be stated whether vasospasm when present in conjunction with advanced coronary stenoses is the cause or the effect of coronary spasm.

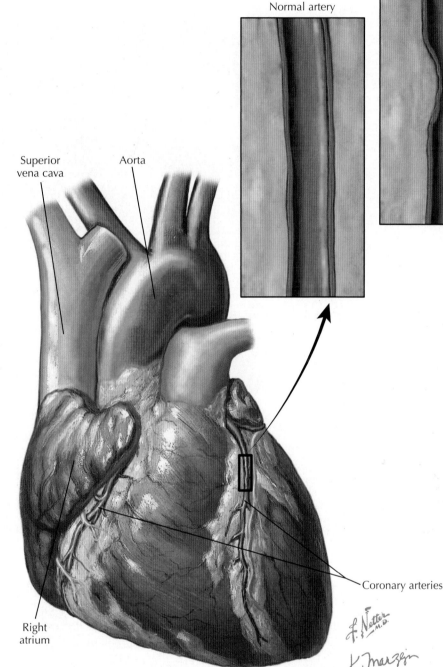

Normal artery

Constricted artery

Superior vena cava

Aorta

Coronary arteries

Right atrium

TREATMENT

Acute

Acute treatment of coronary artery spasm is generally easy either with intravenous (IV) or sublingual nitrates and calcium antagonists, especially the calcium antagonists that lower heart rate; that is, diltiazem or verapamil.

Long-Term

It is possible that inflammatory or immunologic processes involving blood vessels may contribute alone or in combination to the production of myocardial ischemia due to coronary vasoconstriction.

Vessels denuded of endothelium are missing endothelium-derived relaxing factor (EDRF) and as a result tend to constrict.

ROLE OF ATHEROSCLEROSIS

Atherosclerotic plaques may disrupt endothelium and decease EDRF, thus providing a link between atherosclerosis and coronary spasm.

In recent years, there seems to be a decrease in the number of patients with coronary artery spasm. This may be related to the fact that many of these patients are treated with long-term calcium antagonists and aggressive lipid-lowering drugs.

Plate 6.11

Cardiovascular System: VOLUME 8

Myocardial ischemia, demonstrated by stress test

At rest

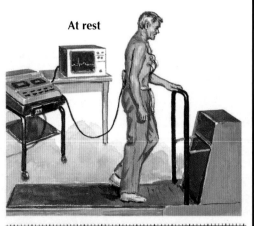

Exercise

Incline and speed of treadmill progressively increased

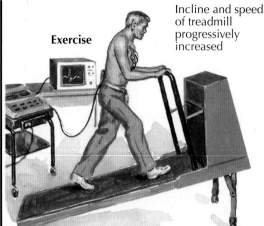

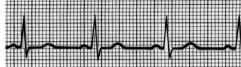

Heart rate normal for resting state

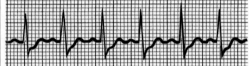

Heart rate accelerated

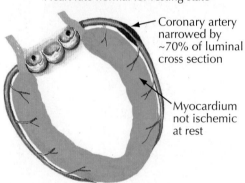

Coronary artery narrowed by ~70% of luminal cross section

Myocardium not ischemic at rest

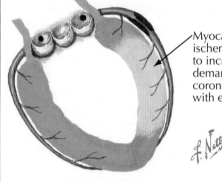

Myocardium ischemic due to increased demand for coronary flow with exercise

DETECTION OF MYOCARDIAL ISCHEMIA

The simplest and least expensive way to diagnose the presence or absence of myocardial ischemia and to quantitate functional impairment in patients with chronic stable angina is exercise stress testing with ECG monitoring. Exercise testing is typically performed using a treadmill or bicycle to provoke chest discomfort and obtain diagnostic evidence of myocardial ischemia. It is important to record 12 leads before, during, and after exercise testing to detect transient changes suggesting ischemia. Under resting conditions, the heart rate is usually normal and the ST segment on the electrocardiogram usually isoelectric. Thus the 12-lead ECG may be normal even if a coronary artery has 70% stenosis, the usual percentage that results in myocardial ischemia when myocardial oxygen demand is increased. The ECG is normal because the myocardium is not ischemic under these resting conditions; myocardial oxygen supply is balanced by demand, and the patient does not report angina pectoris or equivalents such as breathlessness. The treadmill increases speed and incline progressively, thus stressing the patient, who needs to increase heart rate and blood pressure to maintain appropriate cardiac output to meet the demand. During bicycle exercise, resistance to pedaling is increased to accomplish the same increase in heart rate and blood pressure. Patients who develop myocardial ischemia show the classic ECG changes of ST-segment depression. In the patient with 70% stenosis, under conditions of increased myocardial oxygen demand, the balance of oxygen supply and increased demand will be upset, and myocardial ischemia will result. In

Normal ECG. No ST-segment depressions

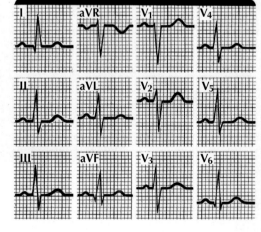

ST-segment depression in leads overlying ischemic zone

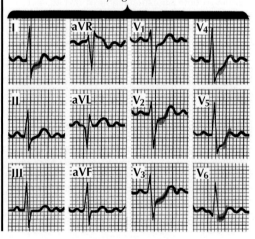

some patients, myocardial ischemic changes on the ECG may not be accompanied by angina pectoris, termed *silent* myocardial ischemia. Despite the lack of symptoms, the prognostic importance of silent or asymptomatic myocardial ischemia is the same as symptomatic disease.

Chronic stable angina is often called *stable ischemic heart disease*. Myocardial ischemia results when the oxygen needs of the myocardium exceed the supply of oxygen derived from coronary blood flow. The oxygen needs of the myocardium are increased by aggravating or precipitating factors such as hypertension, tachycardia, heart failure, hypermetabolic state, and sympathomimetic drugs. Myocardial oxygen demand depends on heart rate, blood pressure, and LV size, thickness, and contraction. Other factors, such as severe anemia, may result in tachycardia and increased oxygen demand.

Plate 6.12

Acquired Heart Disease

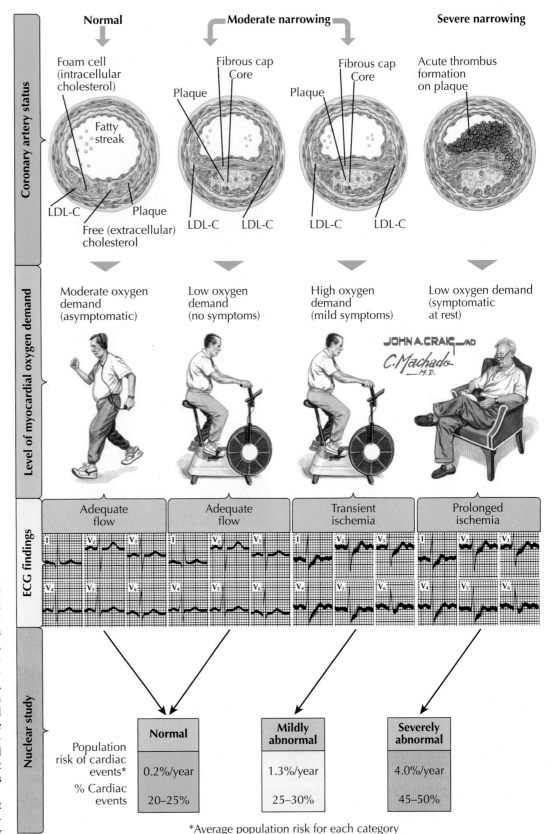

DEGREE OF FLOW-LIMITING STENOSES

Patients with normal coronary arteries have no flow-limiting epicardial stenoses and remain asymptomatic under conditions of moderate oxygen demand, or even high oxygen demand in most cases. Patients with moderate narrowing caused by coronary atherosclerosis may also be asymptomatic or symptomatic (angina, myocardial ischemia) depending on the degree of flow-limiting stenosis to the myocardium. When flow is adequate under moderate myocardial oxygen demand, the ECG may be normal with isoelectric ST segments in all 12 leads. However, when there is high myocardial oxygen demand in this same patient with moderate coronary atherosclerosis, ECG changes in the appropriate leads (e.g., aV_L, V_2–V_6) in patients with left-sided coronary disease demonstrate abnormal ST-segment shifts during transient ischemia and abnormal changes during prolonged ischemia at rest.

Thus a normal ECG correlates with widely patent coronary arteries providing adequate flow and no evidence of ischemia. Similarly, moderate coronary artery disease (CAD) under mild stress conditions shows no ECG changes. Under high oxygen demand in patients with moderate CAD, however, transient ST-segment shifts can be found. In addition, patients with severe narrowing often have symptoms and ECG changes under resting or near-resting conditions or during trivial exercise, particularly with severe high-grade proximal stenoses (e.g., left main or proximal LAD stenosis). These patients usually have severe proximal multivessel epicardial CAD.

If done to detect myocardial perfusion abnormalities, nuclear imaging studies are usually normal if the coronary arteries have mild or no stenosis. If there is moderate stenosis with high oxygen demand, myocardial perfusion may be mildly abnormal. The treatment and prognostic implications are related to the severity and extent of the perfusion defects. For severely abnormal myocardial perfusion in patients with high-grade stenoses, aggressive medical therapy is often combined with PCI (angioplasty with stenting) or bypass surgery.

To make appropriate decisions about prognosis and therapy in the patient with symptomatic CAD, knowledge of coronary pathology must be coupled with physiologic assessment of the lesions.

Plate 6.13

Cardiovascular System: VOLUME 8

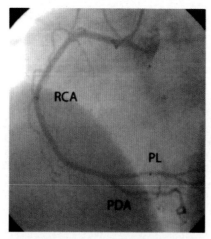

Angiogram of normal right coronary artery (RCA) and normal posterolateral (PL) and posterior descending (PDA) branches

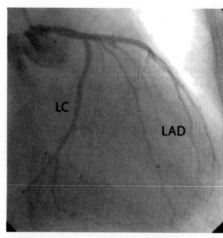

Angiogram of normal left anterior descending coronary artery (LAD) and left circumflex (LC) artery

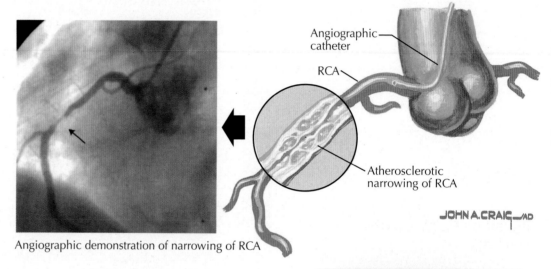

Angiographic demonstration of narrowing of RCA

JOHN A. CRAIG—AD

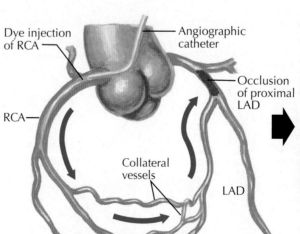

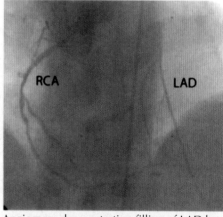

Angiogram demonstrating filling of LAD by dye injected into RCA via collateral vessels

Left-Sided Heart Angiography

Left-sided heart catheterization and angiography includes injection of iodinated radiopaque contrast into the aorta, left ventricle, and coronary arteries to visualize the status of the aorta and its branches, presence or absence of aortic insufficiency, patency of conduit coronary bypasses, LV function and anatomy, and condition of the coronary circulation. Coronary angiography is a precise method of determining the extent, location, and severity (percentage stenosis) of CAD. Multiple views of the coronary arteries are necessary to assess the significance of a specific lesion and the distribution of the right coronary, circumflex, and anterior descending arteries and the septal and diagonal distal circulation. The classic views of the right and left coronary arteries are the right anterior oblique and left anterior oblique projections. Multiple angulated views (caudal and cranial) are particularly important if PCI (angioplasty) is planned. One must remember that catheter-based coronary angiography is *lumenography;* only the vessel's lumen is seen. The vascular wall must be visualized by intravascular ultrasound or optical coherence tomography; despite its limitations, this is a prerequisite for coronary artery surgery and in many patients allows determination of management: medical therapy (alone or plus angioplasty/stent) or bypass surgery.

Ventriculography is part of the evaluation of patients undergoing coronary angiography, to obtain the best possible assessment of ventricular function. I prefer to have ventriculography performed in the right anterior oblique and left anterior oblique views to assess the global function of the ventricle, particularly in patients with LV dysfunction.

Plate 6.14

Acquired Heart Disease

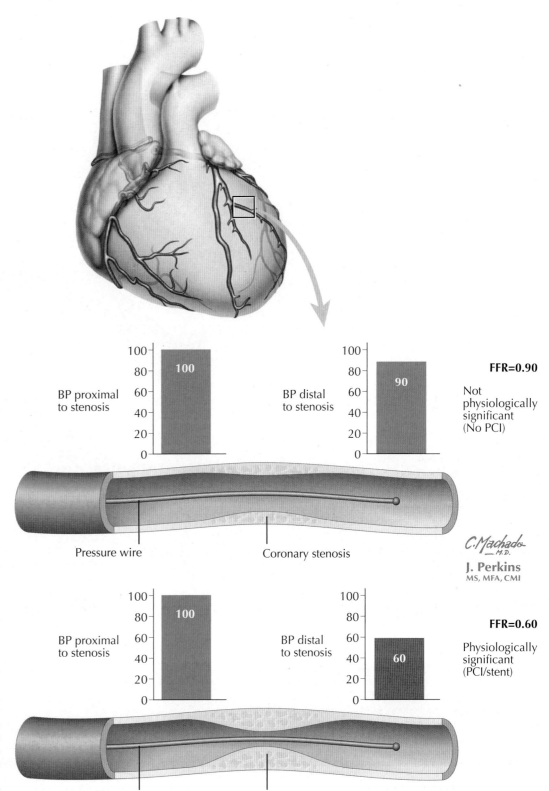

FRACTIONAL FLOW RESERVE

In the catheterization laboratory, interventional cardiologists can determine the physiologic significance of a specific coronary artery stenosis by passing a small wire (0.014-inch pressure guidewire) with a pressure transducer at the tip, through the stenosis in question, which allows them to measure systolic BP proximal and distal to the stenosis. The systolic BP distal to the stenosis is divided by the pressure proximal to the stenosis; the resulting fraction is the percentage of BP decrease across the stenosis. Measurements are made at baseline and after infusion of adenosine, which increases coronary blood flow. For example, if BP across the stenosis drops by 50%, the fractional flow reserve (FFR) will be 0.50. The formula is FFR $= Pd/Pa$, where Pd is pressure distal to the stenosis and Pa is pressure proximal to the stenosis. This technique is particularly useful when the visual estimate of the clinical significance of a specific stenosis by angiography is uncertain.

If FFR is combined with intravascular coronary ultrasound, the interventional cardiologist will be able to determine the physiologic significance of the stenosis as well as the nature of the plaque being investigated; that is, stable or unstable vulnerable plaque. FFR could also be called "functional flow reserve" because it supports that measurements reflect the pathophysiologic significance of a stenosis. The technique obviously requires cardiac catheterization and a specially designed pressure guidewire in which the pressure is measured proximal to and distal to a given epicardial coronary artery stenosis. Based on clinical trials, a cutoff point of 0.75 to 0.80 has been used to indicate a significant pathophysiologically important coronary artery stenosis.

In my view, this measurement is equivalent to our measurements of noninvasively measured ankle–brachial index, in which a difference in pressure between the arm and leg suggests pathologic decrease in leg perfusion. An advantage is that this technique can provide immediate information for angioplasty/stent being considered for an epicardial stenotic vessel. If FFR is less than 0.75, the stenosis appears to be causing downstream myocardial ischemia, and angioplasty/stent seems appropriate. The DEFER clinical trial used FFR to determine whether PCI with stenting was necessary in patients with FFR greater than 0.75. In these patients, stenting of the coronary stenosis did not influence clinical outcome. In another study guided by FFR, fewer stents were used in patients who had FFR in the normal range. After 1 year, death, MI, or repeat revascularization occurred less in the FFR group, and hospital stay was shorter with less procedural cost.

Plate 6.15

Cardiovascular System: VOLUME 8

STENT DEPLOYMENT

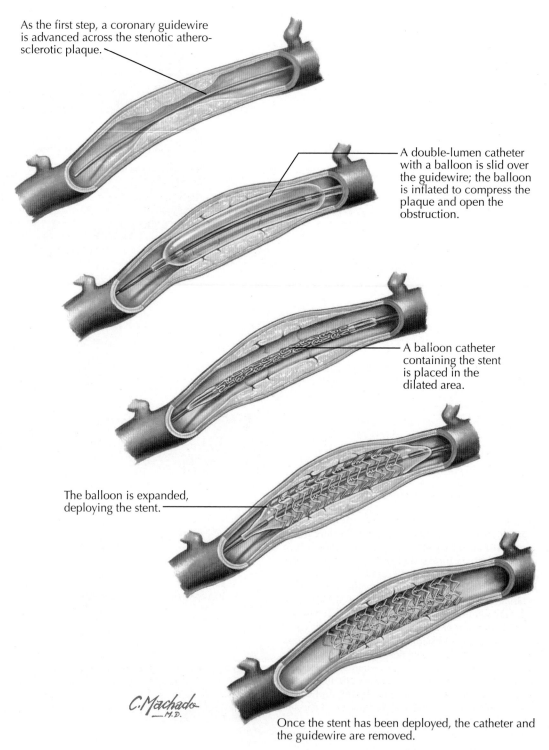

As the first step, a coronary guidewire is advanced across the stenotic atherosclerotic plaque.

A double-lumen catheter with a balloon is slid over the guidewire; the balloon is inflated to compress the plaque and open the obstruction.

A balloon catheter containing the stent is placed in the dilated area.

The balloon is expanded, deploying the stent.

Once the stent has been deployed, the catheter and the guidewire are removed.

CHRONIC ANGINA REVASCULARIZATION PROCEDURES

Revascularization involves either PCI, as first performed by Gruenzig in 1978, or coronary artery bypass graft (CABG) surgery.

PERCUTANEOUS CORONARY INTERVENTION FOR CHRONIC ANGINA

Stent Deployment

PCI is performed through a guiding catheter introduced into the ostium of a coronary artery. A guidewire is advanced into the catheter and passed across the stenosis, and a balloon catheter is then placed at the stenosis. The balloon is inflated and the stenosis dilated. If a stent surrounds the balloon, as the balloon is inflated, the stent is deployed and forms a scaffold to maintain patency of the artery (Plate 6.15). Stents can be bare metal or drug eluting. The balloon is deflated and removed, and the stent remains in place.

Rotational Atherectomy and Distal Protection Device

Other devices such as rotational atherectomy can be used before stenting, particularly in calcified stenoses (see Plate 6.16). A diamond-coated burr is used to fragment the plaque, widening the stenosis. Occasionally, distal protection devices are used to filter some of the detritus and atherosclerotic debris that migrate distally.

SURGERY FOR CHRONIC ANGINA DISEASE

In 1968, Favaloro performed the first successful CABG at the Cleveland Clinic, where Sones had done the first selective coronary angiogram in 1958. Selective coronary angiography permitted for the first time a realistic appraisal of the patient suspected of having coronary disease because it established the presence or absence of disease, localized an existing myocardial perfusion deficit, and assessed LV functional status. Postoperatively, Sones' technique allowed assessment of the disease course as well as surgical success or failure. This procedure also led to percutaneous catheter–based myocardial revascularization procedures.

Before CABG was developed, several procedures were used that are no longer performed, including implantation of the internal thoracic artery directly into the myocardium (Vineberg procedure) and a Vineberg variant (Sewell procedure) in which the internal thoracic artery with a pedicle (including artery, vein, muscle, and fibrous tissue) was implanted into the myocardium.

Plate 6.16

Acquired Heart Disease

ROTATIONAL ATHERECTOMY AND DISTAL PROTECTION DEVICE

Rotational atherectomy

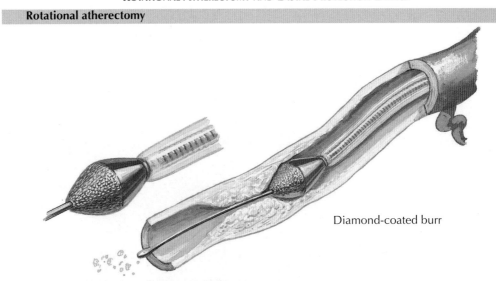

Diamond-coated burr

Distal protection device: coronary filter

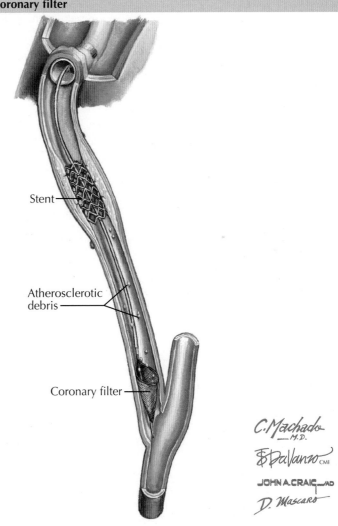

Stent

Atherosclerotic debris

Coronary filter

CHRONIC ANGINA REVASCULARIZATION PROCEDURES (Continued)

VENTRICULAR ANEURYSMECTOMY

Ventricular aneurysm may occur in patients who sustain a large MI. Postinfarction aneurysm usually affects the anterior wall and the LV apex perfused by the left anterior descending branch of the left coronary artery. Aneurysm of the inferior left ventricle rarely occurs, although an infarction of sufficient magnitude to produce a ventricular aneurysm usually results in mitral incompetency secondary to papillary muscle dysfunction.

Ventricular aneurysmectomy is usually an elective procedure that is not undertaken until several months after MI, unless the patient has intractable heart failure, intractable ventricular arrhythmias, or severe mitral regurgitation not responsive to acute vasodilator therapy. Early intervention in these patients greatly increases the surgical risk.

CORONARY ARTERY BYPASS GRAFTS

The concept of direct coronary artery surgery uses the saphenous vein graft or an internal thoracic artery to bypass a proximally stenotic coronary artery. CABG requires target vessels either free of disease or minimally diseased. Vein graft conduits are "free grafts" and connect the ascending aorta to the coronary vessel. In contrast, internal thoracic artery conduits remain connected to the subclavian artery and connect to the coronary artery distal to the stenosis. CABG not only promotes perfusion of the distal microcirculation of the epicardial vessel but also provides perfusion of other stenotic vessels by enhancing flow through collateral circulation.

Follow-up Studies

Angiograms months or years after CABG show patency in a high percentage of grafted vessels. However, not all saphenous vein grafts are as patent at 10 years as they were initially. The use of the internal thoracic artery as a conduit to bypass a proximal stenosis has proved to be the best CABG procedure to date. Often, bilateral internal thoracic arteries are used. Although rare, this type of conduit can stenose or thrombose, probably related to technical intraoperative problems.

Plate 6.17

Cardiovascular System: VOLUME 8

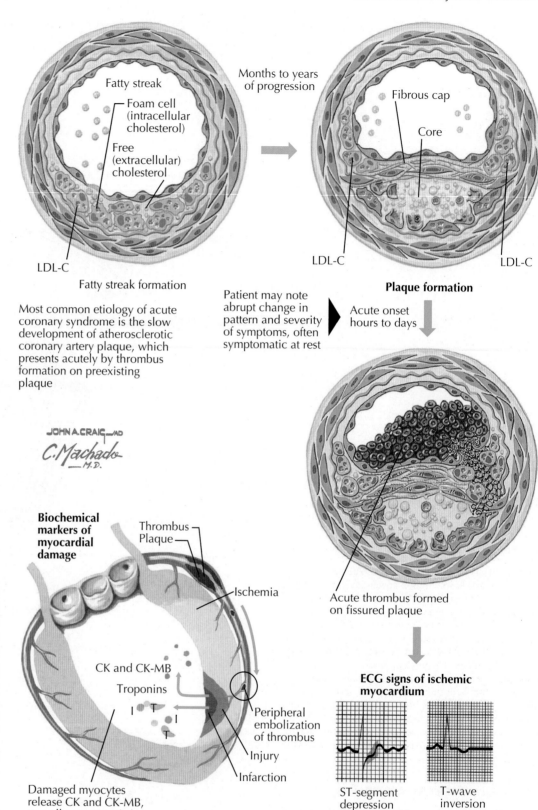

Fatty streak

Foam cell
(intracellular
cholesterol)

Free
(extracellular)
cholesterol

LDL-C

Fatty streak formation

Most common etiology of acute
coronary syndrome is the slow
development of atherosclerotic
coronary artery plaque, which
presents acutely by thrombus
formation on preexisting
plaque

Months to years
of progression

Fibrous cap

Core

LDL-C

LDL-C

Plaque formation

Patient may note
abrupt change in
pattern and severity
of symptoms, often
symptomatic at rest

Acute onset
hours to days

JOHN A. CRAIG—MD

C. Machado
—M.D.

Acute thrombus formed
on fissured plaque

**Biochemical
markers of
myocardial
damage**

Thrombus
Plaque

Ischemia

CK and CK-MB

Troponins

I   T
        I
   T

Peripheral
embolization
of thrombus

Injury

Infarction

Damaged myocytes
release CK and CK-MB,
as well as contractive
proteins troponins T and I

**ECG signs of ischemic
myocardium**

ST-segment
depression

T-wave
inversion

PATHOPHYSIOLOGY OF ACUTE
CORONARY SYNDROMES

Patients with acute coronary syndrome (ACS) present
in three different ways: unstable angina, non–ST-segment
elevation myocardial infarction, and ST-segment elevation MI. Potential causes for the development of an
ACS include extracardiac factors in the patients with
severe coronary atherosclerosis, such as hypertension,
tachycardia, and anemia. In 1858 Virchow proposed
that injury to the inner wall of a blood vessel, possibly
caused by fat, might lead to inflammation and secondary plaque formation, similar to current theory. ACS is
also caused by plaque disruption resulting in transient
platelet aggregation and release of vasoactive substances in diseased vessels, dynamic or intermittent
coronary artery thrombosis, hemorrhagic dissection
into an atheromatous plaque, and progression of coronary stenoses from plaque healing.

Acute coronary syndromes result from myocardial
ischemia initiated by two primary factors: platelet and
thrombus formation and resulting intense vasoconstriction from accumulation of local thromboxane A_2
and serotonin, reduction of local concentrations of
EDRF, and inhibitors of platelet aggregation. These
events are usually preceded by rupture or erosion of the
lipid-laden plaque and involve the balance between
thrombosis and thrombolysis. Patients with ACS may
stabilize clinically, but this may not be associated with
stabilization of the plaque. Identifying these patients
requires observation for recurrent ischemia and assessment of troponin levels and possibly C-reactive protein

levels. Abnormal test results indicate increased risk for
future cardiac events.

The acute coronary syndromes are not a homogeneous condition. Clinical variables evident in many
patients include ECG changes, release of creatine kinase and troponins, C-reactive protein level, and differences in LV function, as well as pathology on coronary
angiography. In patients with ACS, the TIMI risk score

helps to predict the risk for death, MI, or recurrent
ischemia at 14 days. The risks are age older than
65 years, three risk factors for CAD, prior 50% coronary stenosis, ST-segment change on admission, angina
twice in 24 hours, aspirin use within 7 days, and increased serum cardiac markers. The more risk factors
present, the higher the rate of composite endpoints in
14 days.

Plate 6.18

Acquired Heart Disease

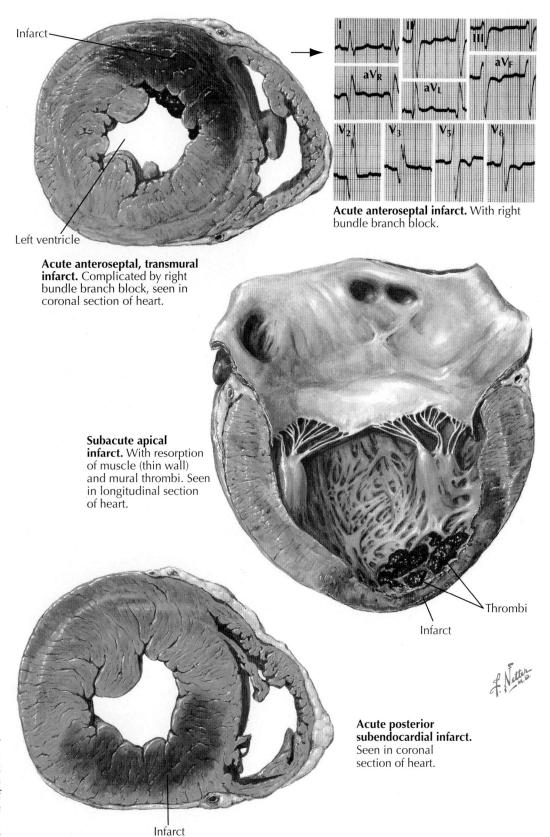

Infarct

Left ventricle

Acute anteroseptal, transmural infarct. Complicated by right bundle branch block, seen in coronal section of heart.

Acute anteroseptal infarct. With right bundle branch block.

Subacute apical infarct. With resorption of muscle (thin wall) and mural thrombi. Seen in longitudinal section of heart.

Thrombi

Infarct

Acute posterior subendocardial infarct. Seen in coronal section of heart.

Infarct

MYOCARDIAL INFARCTION: CHANGES IN THE HEART

Myocardial infarction can result in an extensive panorama of changes. Death of the cardiac muscle may occur in a single zone or as multiple foci scattered diffusely throughout the heart. The latter can be found after suboptimal perfusion of the heart using a pump oxygenator, in which all the minute necrotic foci are of the same age. More often, however, the multiple minute foci can be found as destroyed zones of varying ages. In the acute phases, these microinfarcts may be extremely difficult to see and may be recognizable only microscopically as areas showing variable myofibril destruction and replacement by collagen. Chronically, these small foci may be minute white patches salted throughout the myocardium.

A larger myocardial infarct shows a variety of changes that depend in part on the duration of the patient's survival after the episode. The earliest changes are associated with the resulting paralysis of vessel walls, engorgement of the capillaries, and migration of polymorphonuclear leukocytes (PMNs). Some autolytic changes then occur, and the dead muscle fibers can be recognized as showing a loss of striations and an increase in eosinophilia, fragmentation, and the gradual disappearance of nuclei. The dead muscle becomes an irritant, and more PMNs appear. Finally, the subsequent activities of repair include macrophage infiltration and replacement fibrosis. If the infarct is minute, such a sequence is of relatively short duration, but if large, remnants of necrotic muscle may be found several years later. It appears that such dead tissue has been effectively sealed away from physiologic activities.

The infarct may be named according to the *area of the heart* involved. Most posterior infarcts affect areas of the septum as well, and many anterior infarcts involve anterior portions of the septal wall, termed *anteroseptal*

Plate 6.19

Cardiovascular System: VOLUME 8

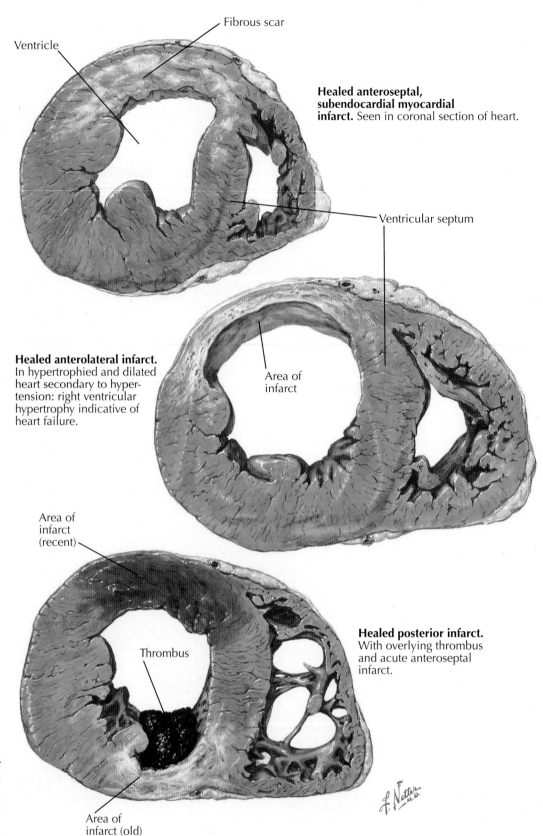

Ventricle

Fibrous scar

Healed anteroseptal, subendocardial myocardial infarct. Seen in coronal section of heart.

Ventricular septum

Healed anterolateral infarct. In hypertrophied and dilated heart secondary to hypertension: right ventricular hypertrophy indicative of heart failure.

Area of infarct

Healed posterior infarct. With overlying thrombus and acute anteroseptal infarct.

Area of infarct (recent)

Thrombus

Area of infarct (old)

MYOCARDIAL INFARCTION: CHANGES IN THE HEART
(Continued)

and *posteroseptal* (see Plate 6.18). A *lateral* infarct is found in a small percentage of the cases. The sequence of events—muscle death, removal, and repair—may or may not result in thinning of the myocardium. Infarcts may also be classified according to the *thickness of the ventricular wall* involved. If all layers are affected (transmural), the term ST-segment elevation myocardial infarction (STEMI) is used, most often associated with occlusion of the coronary artery. In about 90% of these lesions, occlusion is demonstrated, as contrasted with a lesser incidence in non–ST-segment MI. In NSTEMI, the zone of infarction is usually limited to the endocardial surface of the ventricle. *Mural thrombosis* may be a more common accompaniment of either STEMI or NSTEMI because both infarcts involve the endocardium.

A major problem with coronary artery disease is the lack of many correlations between CAD and MI in a patient who has died. Although the appearance of a lesion in the anterior descending or the main left coronary artery is a common finding in sudden cardiac death and occasionally may be the only lesion discovered, the status of the underlying cardiac muscle is not known because morphologic MI cannot be demonstrated. In about 25% of MIs encountered at autopsy—either acute or chronic but especially chronic—no history can be elicited as to when such a disorder occurred. In hearts with acute MI, only about half show occlusion of the coronary artery, although the other half exhibit a significant to marked *stenosis* of the infarcted vessel. In addition, when the immediate cause of death is believed to be CAD, no recent acute MI is found (Plate 6.19).

Exercise may be extremely valuable in all of these patients with MI. Studies indicate that although the

Plate 6.20

Acquired Heart Disease

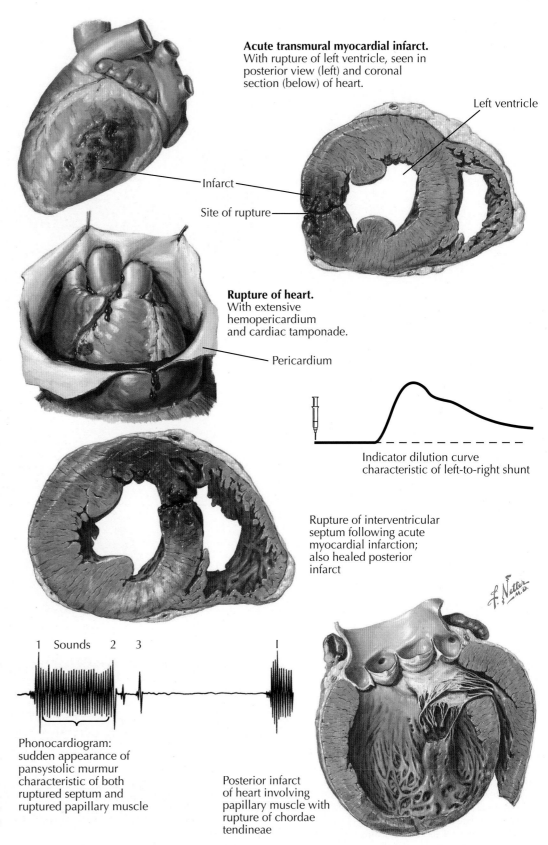

Acute transmural myocardial infarct.
With rupture of left ventricle, seen in posterior view (left) and coronal section (below) of heart.

Left ventricle

Infarct

Site of rupture

Rupture of heart.
With extensive hemopericardium and cardiac tamponade.

Pericardium

Indicator dilution curve characteristic of left-to-right shunt

Rupture of interventricular septum following acute myocardial infarction; also healed posterior infarct

1   Sounds   2   3

Phonocardiogram: sudden appearance of pansystolic murmur characteristic of both ruptured septum and ruptured papillary muscle

Posterior infarct of heart involving papillary muscle with rupture of chordae tendineae

MYOCARDIAL INFARCTION: CHANGES IN THE HEART (Continued)

incidence of MI is not decreased, its severity is less in those who have maintained cardiac fitness.

Acute damage to areas of the conduction system, such as hemorrhage or infarction, can be demonstrated in only some cases. However, other complications are common. The immediate results of the changes in the circulatory status and constituents of the blood apparently can lead to a deposition of thrombus at numerous sites, including the coronary arteries, with a further extension of the MI. Mural thrombi form on the endocardium (probably related to healing of infarcted tissue), in the atrium (much more common on the left than the right), and possibly at all sites where previous atheromas had existed. Therefore cerebral anoxia can result not only from the decreased cardiac output but also from superimposed thrombosis during the early stages. Thrombosis also occurs in the systemic veins.

Embolism is a natural sequela of thrombosis, and systemic embolization occurs in an unknown number of patients with thrombi in the left side of the heart. *Cerebral* embolism is the most severe and damaging, although *saddle* embolism of the distal aorta is also serious, as is embolization in an extremity. Smaller emboli may produce any focal embolus, including splenic and renal arteries. Less often, *mesenteric* embolism may occur, which can be a medical disaster if not recognized early. Unfortunately, mural thrombi persist for a long period, and systemic embolization may occur at various periods after apparent recovery from the acute infarction. Pulmonary embolism is also often related to venous stasis.

Plate 6.21

Cardiovascular System: VOLUME 8

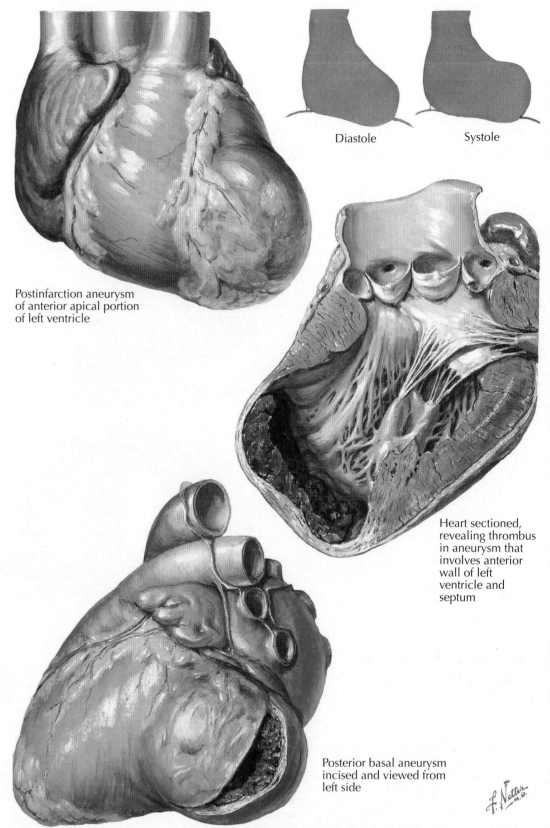

Diastole

Systole

Postinfarction aneurysm
of anterior apical portion
of left ventricle

Heart sectioned,
revealing thrombus
in aneurysm that
involves anterior
wall of left
ventricle and
septum

Posterior basal aneurysm
incised and viewed from
left side

MYOCARDIAL INFARCTION: CHANGES IN THE HEART (Continued)

As with the hypertensive heart in failure, the hypoxic heart can dilate, with resultant valvular insufficiency and subsequent regurgitation.

Rupture of the heart (ventricular septal defect, papillary muscle, free wall) is another variable autopsy finding (see Plate 6.20). The incidence of cardiac rupture ranges from 1% to 10% in deaths from acute MI. The area of rupture often shows a large increase in PMNs and at a much later time than such cellular elements are usually encountered; ruptures of the heart usually occur in the first week. The classic patient prone to rupture is hypertensive, is having a first infarction, and has no visible collaterals to the infarcted artery. In addition to free rupture of the heart into the pericardial cavity and the resulting cardiac tamponade, rupture of the interventricular septum occasionally occurs. Rarely, papillary muscles rupture.

The posterior papillary muscle is more likely to rupture than the anterior muscle because it does not have dual blood supply.

As a chronic complication, anterior and apical *aneurysm* may be more prone to mural thrombi, and thus the patient is continually exposed to the risk of embolism (Plate 6.21).

In addition to all the complications of embolism, cardiac aneurysm, sudden death, and rupture of the heart, there is the problem of *reinfarction*. Some hearts demonstrate not only the zone of a previous infarct but also areas of new infarct. The new infarct may be adjacent to the previous one or can occur in a different area of other coronary arteries.

Plate 6.22

Acquired Heart Disease

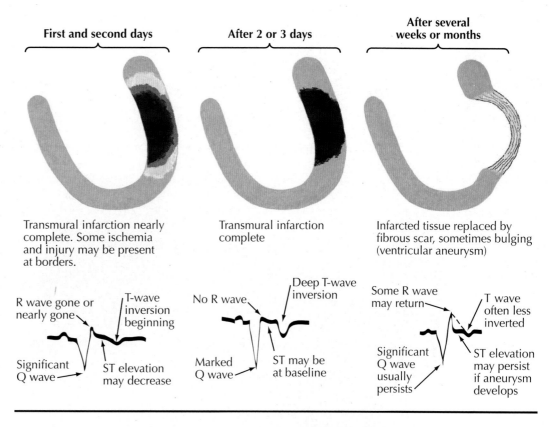

MANIFESTATIONS OF MYOCARDIAL INFARCTION

First and second days

Transmural infarction nearly complete. Some ischemia and injury may be present at borders.

R wave gone or nearly gone

T-wave inversion beginning

Significant Q wave

ST elevation may decrease

After 2 or 3 days

Transmural infarction complete

No R wave

Deep T-wave inversion

Marked Q wave

ST may be at baseline

After several weeks or months

Infarcted tissue replaced by fibrous scar, sometimes bulging (ventricular aneurysm)

Some R wave may return

T wave often less inverted

Significant Q wave usually persists

ST elevation may persist if aneurysm develops

First several days

Some subendocardial muscle dies, but lesion does not extend through entire heart wall.

R wave persists but may diminish somewhat

T-wave inversion may occur

Q wave not significant

ST often returns to baseline

After several weeks or months

Lesion heals. Some subendocardial fibrosis may occur but does not involve entire thickness of heart wall.

ST segment and T wave } may or may not return to normal

Q wave not significant

Key

Myocardial ischemia

Myocardial injury

Myocardial death (infarction)

Fibrosis

MANIFESTATIONS OF MYOCARDIAL INFARCTION

PATHOLOGIC AND ECG MANIFESTATIONS OF MYOCARDIAL INFARCTION

In patients with acute MI, particularly with STEMI, pathologic changes in the heart may reveal necrosis from endocardium to the subepicardial myocardium. In the first 24 hours, the ECG manifestations are variable, but usually the R wave is gone or almost gone, a Q wave is present, the ST segment is elevated, and the T wave may be inverted (Plate 6.22). Several days later, pathology may reveal a complete infarction of the ventricular wall (transmural). The ECG continues to show Q waves, no R wave, and T-wave inversion. The ST segments may return to baseline in some cases. Several weeks or months later, the infarcted tissue may be replaced with fibrous scar, which occasionally results in a bulging ventricular aneurysm. If the aneurysm is obvious on ventriculography or cardiac ultrasound, the ST segment may be elevated. Other ECG changes usually persist (e.g., Q wave; inverted T waves, less than earlier seen), and the R wave may somewhat return.

In contrast, a patient with NSTEMI in the first 24 hours shows subendocardial necrosis, and the ECG often reveals persistent R wave, small Q wave, isoelectric ST segment, and T-wave inversion. The infarcted myocardium is surrounded by a periinfarction ischemic zone. Days, weeks, or months later, the subendocardial necrosis heals, and subendocardial fibrosis replaces infarcted myocardium. This fibrosis is limited to the subendocardial area and does not extend transmurally to the epicardium. The ECG changes may or may not return to normal.

Plate 6.23

Cardiovascular System: VOLUME 8

EFFECTS OF MYOCARDIAL ISCHEMIA, INJURY, AND INFARCTION ON ECG

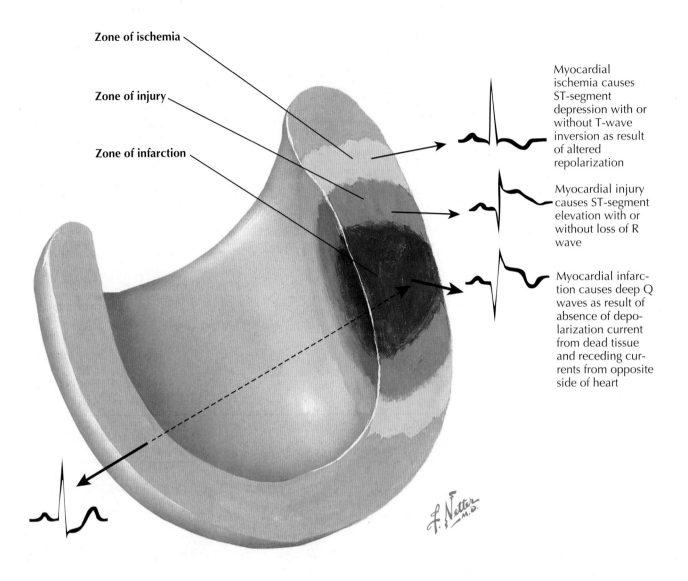

Zone of ischemia

Zone of injury

Zone of infarction

Myocardial ischemia causes ST-segment depression with or without T-wave inversion as result of altered repolarization

Myocardial injury causes ST-segment elevation with or without loss of R wave

Myocardial infarction causes deep Q waves as result of absence of depolarization current from dead tissue and receding currents from opposite side of heart

MANIFESTATIONS OF MYOCARDIAL INFARCTION (Continued)

ISCHEMIC INJURY AND INFARCTION: ECG LOCALIZATION

In the myocardial region of an occluded coronary artery, ECG changes caused by ischemia, injury, and infarction can be identified (Plate 6.23). ECG abnormalities are highly suggestive but not diagnostic of acute MI. In the patient who has large Q waves, ST-segment elevation, and T-wave inversion in several ECG leads, the diagnosis of an evolving MI is highly suspect; however, not all patients with MI have these classic changes. Some patients present with severe chest pain and only T-wave inversion or a significant ST-segment depression, as well as elevation of cardiac markers (NSTEMI). In contrast, other patients have had obvious Q waves develop on the ECG and prominent ST-segment elevation (STEMI). All MIs begin in the subendocardial area and extend transmurally. The development of Q waves and ST-segment elevation probably relates to the transmural degree of wall involvement; the more involvement toward the epicardium, the more likely the appearance of Q waves and ST-segment elevation.

The site of the infarction can be localized in general by the ECG abnormalities. Thus anterior and anterolateral MIs generally display ECG abnormalities of the precordial leads as well as leads I and aV_L. However, all variations of these ECGs can occur, and there may be changes from V_1 to V_6 (including lead I) and aV_L, or changes may occur only in leads I and aV_L and the early precordial leads. In contrast, the diaphragmatic or inferior MI generally shows ST elevation in leads II, III, and aV_F.

CARDIAC MARKERS AND DIAGNOSIS OF ACUTE MYOCARDIAL INFARCTION

Cardiac markers are essential for the diagnosis of acute myocardial infarction but do not appear immediately in the bloodstream if an occlusion occurs. Creatine kinase (CK), CK isoenzymes (e.g., CK-MB), and troponin T are measurably abnormal about 4 hours after occlusion. Troponin T is the most sensitive and specific marker for acute myocardial infarction at the present time and probably is the only cardiac marker necessary to make the diagnosis of acute myocardial infarction; however, renal failure can result in the elevation of all cardiac markers in the absence of an acute myocardial infarction.

Clinically, if the cardiac markers are normal at admission to the emergency department (ED), when the patient is having acute cardiac pain and ST-segment elevation, the MI likely has occurred recently, within 3 or 4 hours. However, if the cardiac marker is elevated, the occlusion and STEMI likely occurred more than 4 hours before ED evaluation. The onset and duration of increase in CK enzymes and troponin T after a coronary occlusion vary, but in the patient with STEMI the occlusion usually occurred recently if initial serum values are normal. If a revascularization procedure is performed early in the course of acute MI, the cardiac markers may increase much more than if a revascularization procedure had not been performed, most likely from washout of the markers from the perfused myocardium.

Plate 6.24

Acquired Heart Disease

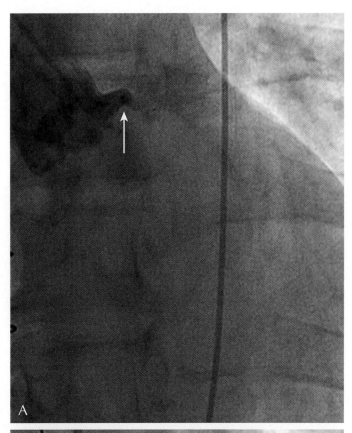

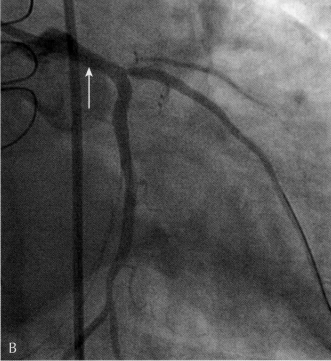

A. Left main trunk occlusion (*arrow*) in a patient with a prior bypass graft to the left anterior descending artery before PCI. **B.** Left main trunk after PCI and reperfusion of left main trunk, LAD, and circumflex arteries.

Recanalization of Occluded Coronary Artery in Acute Myocardial Infarction

Rapid opening of the infarcted artery is generally accepted as critical to increase patient survival, preferably using PCI. However, thrombolytic therapy remains a viable option in hospitals when PCI capability is not immediately available. Percutaneous recanalization of an occluded coronary artery by balloon angioplasty and stent placement in patients with STEMI is the standard of practice. The appropriate management of acute STEMI currently is door-to-balloon ("D2B") time—from ED arrival to passage of a guidewire into the infarcted artery. D2B time is easily and accurately measured and documented. D2B time less than 90 minutes is an acceptable goal. The rationale is that short D2B time results in less myocardial necrosis. A favorable outcome correlates well with minimal necrosis and ejection fraction (EF) greater than 40%. An unfavorable outcome correlates with a large amount of necrosis and EF less than 40%.

TIMING OF VESSEL OCCLUSION

In canine studies, MI size versus duration of coronary occlusion was measured with the circumflex coronary artery ligated. Thus the actual time of onset of coronary occlusion was identified and the time course of myocardial necrosis measured. Myocardial cells started to die about 20 minutes after onset of ischemia, with cell death complete by 6 hours.

Theoretically in the human, if mortality reduction is plotted against extent of salvage of myocardium from 0 to 3 hours, a steep reduction in percentage mortality occurs, and by 3 hours the myocardial salvage is greatly reduced. After 3 hours, the percentage mortality reduction is similar to that found at 3 hours. Unfortunately, the exact time of vessel occlusion is not known in human MI.

Plate 6.25

Cardiovascular System: VOLUME 8

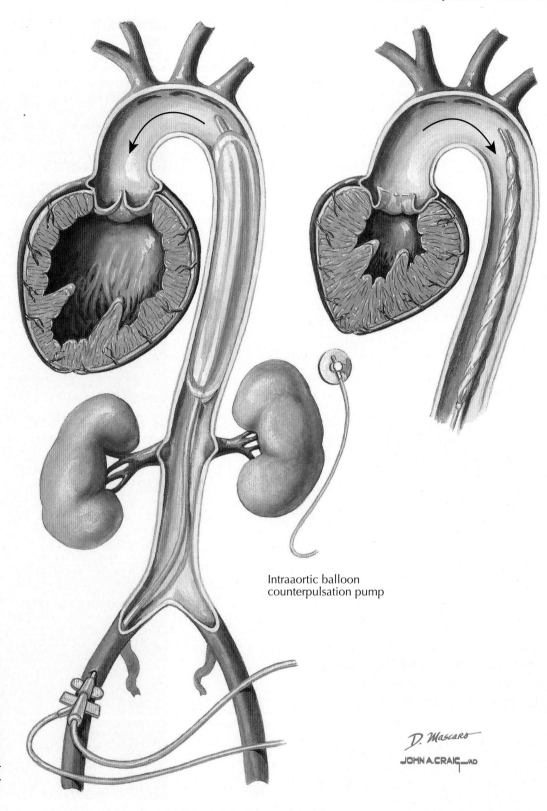

Intraaortic balloon
counterpulsation pump

D. Mascaro

JOHN A. CRAIG—AD

INTRAAORTIC BALLOON COUNTERPULSATION

Counterpulsation is the only technique that will lower aortic systolic pressure and increase aortic diastolic pressure. To accomplish intraaortic balloon counterpulsation (IABCP), a catheter with a cylindrical polyethylene balloon (~40 mL in adult device) is introduced into the aorta, deflated, and extended to just below the left subclavian artery and above the renal arteries, to avoid obstructing either vessel. When visualized on chest radiography or fluoroscopy, the tip of the catheter is placed at the level of the bifurcation of the right and left main bronchi, again to avoid occluding subclavian and renal arteries. Balloon expansion with helium occurs actively during diastole, and collapse of the balloon occurs actively during systole. Intraaortic pressure is measured at the catheter tip.

Timing of balloon expansion and collapse is controlled by either ECG or pressure waveform during the cardiac cycle. When the balloon is expanded in diastole, aortic diastolic pressure increases, as does coronary perfusion pressure, which theoretically increases myocardial blood flow. When the balloon is collapsed during systole, LV afterload reduction occurs, probably a suction effect that unloads the left ventricle and increases cardiac output. When counterpulsation is working correctly, the elevated diastolic aortic pressure likely is interpreted as high blood pressure, and the baroreceptor reflexes tend to lower systolic pressure, thus decreasing myocardial oxygen demand.

The clinical indications for IABCP are cardiogenic shock of any etiology, acute mitral regurgitation that does not respond to nitroprusside, acute ventricular septal defect, and refractory acute coronary syndromes (ischemia or arrhythmias). Less clear indications relate to preprocedural use in patients considered high risk for a revascularization procedure such as PCI or CABG (e.g., high-grade left main coronary artery stenosis). IABCP should not be used in patients with aortic insufficiency; the increase in diastolic pressure will increase the degree of aortic insufficiency. IABCP cannot be used in patients whose aorta cannot be accessed because of severe peripheral vascular disease. Complications with IABCP are fortunately rare and include leg ischemia, aortic disruption, renal artery obstruction when the balloon is not properly placed, and bleeding.

Plate 6.26

Acquired Heart Disease

RHEUMATIC FEVER IN SYDENHAM CHOREA

RHEUMATIC FEVER

Although uncommon in the United States and other developed countries, rheumatic fever is common in developing countries and can affect people of all ages, except in the first years of life. The febrile onset is accompanied by severe but temporary arthritis and often by carditis affecting all three cardiac layers. The etiologic relationship of rheumatic fever to β-hemolytic streptococci is based on the following evidence:

- Most patients have a history of acute streptococcal sore throat 2 to 3 weeks before onset of arthritis.
- Incidence of rheumatic fever in any community parallels the incidence of streptococcal throat infections, epidemics of which are invariably followed by epidemics of rheumatic fever, with a lag period again of 2 to 3 weeks.
- High or rising titers of antibodies to streptococcal antigens may indicate a recent streptococcal infection. If the response to a single antigen is studied, such as antistreptolysin O titer, evidence of recent infection is found in about 70% of patients, increasing progressively with the more antibodies studied and reaching virtually 100% with a panel of four tests.

The frequency with which rheumatic fever follows a streptococcal infection varies from 3% in epidemics to about 0.3% in sporadic infections. This discrepancy is largely caused by the greater severity of epidemic types of infection, as revealed by clinical features and the antibody titers induced. When streptococcal infections of comparable severity are studied, the incidence of subsequent rheumatic fever, even in sporadic cases, is also about 3%.

The lesions of rheumatic fever do not result from direct invasion by streptococci. When adequate precautions are taken against contamination, organisms cannot be isolated from the joints or the heart. The events relating the primary infection to these lesions are still unclear, but circulating toxins released from the organisms are unlikely to be responsible, because then the clinical manifestations of rheumatic fever would coincide with the sore throat (as do the toxic symptoms of diphtheria). Furthermore, none of the many known streptococcal products produces comparable lesions in animals. The relationship between streptococcal infection and rheumatic fever is therefore most widely regarded as *immunologic*, with the lesions resulting from an *antigen–antibody reaction* in the affected tissues. This concept was supported by observations that lesions superficially resembling those of rheumatic carditis could be produced in rabbits by the injection of massive doses of foreign serum.

A comparable massive exposure to antigen is unlikely to occur in humans. Any *immunologic reaction* underlying the pathogenesis of rheumatic fever is more likely to be more specific, directly involving one or more of the antigens native to the affected tissues. Many strains of β-hemolytic streptococci contain an antigen in their cell walls that cross-reacts with an antigenic component of mammalian hearts, including the human. Furthermore, animals injected with such strains of streptococci produce antibodies that react with cardiac antigens. Similar antibodies have been found in a high proportion of patients with active rheumatic fever.

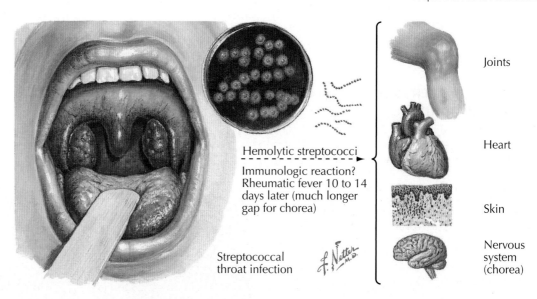

Hemolytic streptococci

Immunologic reaction? Rheumatic fever 10 to 14 days later (much longer gap for chorea)

Streptococcal throat infection

Joints

Heart

Skin

Nervous system (chorea)

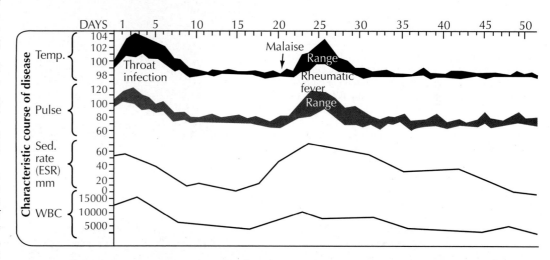

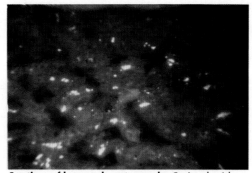

Section of human heart muscle. Stained with preimmune serum of rabbit (×200)

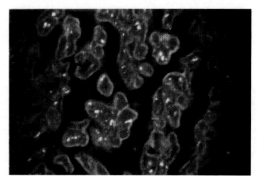

Human heart muscle. Stained with antiserum against type 6 matt group A streptococci (×200). Note fluorescence of subsarcolemmal region of muscle fibers.

However, despite the presence of firmly bound gamma globulin (presumably antibody) in the heart of many patients with rheumatic fever, circulating antibody correlates poorly with clinical severity. Cardiac damage in experimentally immunized animals is unconvincing; repeated infection in rabbits by different β-hemolytic streptococci most closely resembles human rheumatic carditis. Although the mechanism is still unclear, immunologic cross-reactivity with myocardial and other antigens is presently the most likely cause.

The clinical features of an acute attack may range from the trivial to the fulminating—from easily overlooked pallor and fatigue to an exquisitely painful arthritis with high fever, rash, and carditis sufficiently severe to lead to congestive heart failure. The temperature chart is characterized by a nonremittent type of fever with a pulse rate raised disproportionately. The arthritis is *migratory*, rarely lasting in any one joint for more than 1 or 2 days. Swelling is slight and accompanied by some flushing of the overlying skin. Large joints are more frequently affected than small joints, although

Plate 6.27

Cardiovascular System: VOLUME 8

RHEUMATIC FEVER IN SYDENHAM CHOREA (Continued)

these can become involved as well, and the clinical picture may then resemble rheumatoid arthritis.

Despite the many features common to rheumatic fever and rheumatoid arthritis, notably polyarthritis and subcutaneous nodules, these are distinct nosologic entities. If differentiation is difficult in the early stages, the difference in clinical evolution rapidly distinguishes rheumatic fever from arthritis, and even in the early stages, histology of the synovium or biopsied nodule can be helpful. The lesion in rheumatic fever is *capsular* rather than synovial, with areas of fibrinoid necrosis accompanied by focal infiltrations of histiocytes and lymphocytes.

The joint lesions, even when severe, are entirely reversible, and permanent damage does not result. This contrasts with the cardiac lesions, which can occasionally progress to mitral stenosis and its sequelae, even when initial damage is mild. Skin rashes are uncommon but can be characteristic, especially *erythema annulare,* a fleeting, ring-shaped, usually flat eruption typically found on the trunk. Each lesion spreads centrifugally, leaving a slight staining in the center. Another typical feature of rheumatic fever, seen especially in severe cases, is *subcutaneous nodules,* mainly confined to the tissues over bony prominences, where friction combined with pressure is apparently responsible for nodule development. The nodules are most conspicuous after 2 to 3 weeks, although their impending development is often preceded by a more diffuse, boggy thickening. Histologically, a typical nodule shows an area of fibrinoid composed of parallel or interlacing bands sparsely infiltrated with histiocytes and fibroblasts. The adjacent tissue is edematous and contains groups of small vessels surrounded by similar cells. Fibrous tissue is inconspicuous.

Permanent cardiac damage correlates closely with persistent or recurrent activity of rheumatic disease, so the detection of such activity is important. The most helpful test is the erythrocyte sedimentation rate, which is almost never normal in the presence of active disease, except in patients with congestive heart failure. The converse, however—a persistently raised erythrocyte sedimentation rate—does not necessarily imply continued activity, especially in young females. Therefore estimations of C-reactive protein may more accurately reflect the state of the disease activity. The greatest danger to the patient with a history of rheumatic fever is developing a new infection with β-hemolytic streptococci, because the risk of relapse is much greater than after an initial attack. The success of chemoprophylaxis has confirmed both the importance of such reinfection in the development of a relapse and the role of streptococci in rheumatic fever pathogenesis.

Environmental and genetic factors have been studied widely in an attempt to account for the considerable geographic variation in the incidence of rheumatic disease. The most impressive data are provided by Mills' map, showing the progressive decrease in mortality from rheumatic fever as one passes from the northern to the southern latitudes of the United States. Evidence of genetic factors besides female predominance is less precise, but the increased incidence of nonsecretors of

the blood group substances in patients with rheumatic fever indicates modest genetic influence. The dominant factor is environmental and related to the incidence and virulence of the local streptococci.

SYDENHAM CHOREA

The rheumatic nature of Sydenham chorea (St. Vitus dance), first recognized just over 100 years ago, is now

established by evidence similar to that for rheumatic fever as a poststreptococcal state. This is confirmed by the frequent subsequent development of rheumatic heart disease, in the absence of any clinical evidence of rheumatic fever. The outstanding clinical features are ataxia, incoordination, and weakness, accompanied by spontaneous movements that can be most clearly depicted by the photographic record of a penlight held in the patient's hand.

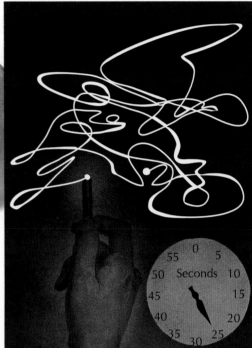

Erythema marginatum

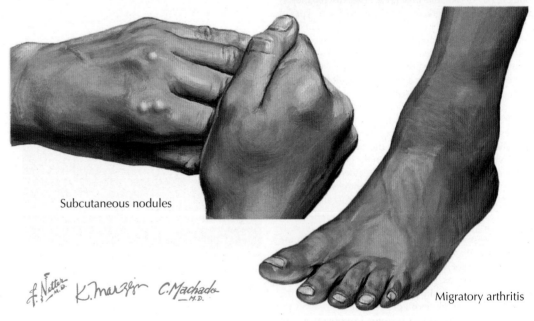

Sydenham chorea: spontaneous uncoordinated movements demonstrated by electric penlight held in patient hand

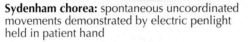

Subcutaneous nodules

Migratory arthritis

Plate 6.28

Acquired Heart Disease

RHEUMATIC HEART DISEASE: ACUTE PERICARDITIS AND MYOCARDITIS

Rheumatic heart disease is a complication of recurrent upper respiratory infection with group A β-hemolytic streptococci. Streptococcal products circulating from this source through the body cause a reaction in connective tissues called *rheumatic inflammation*. Predisposed sites include the heart, skin, and synovial membranes. In the latter two areas, inflammation usually heals by resolution, leaving no residual effects, but in the heart these recurrent respiratory infections may lead to severe deformities, usually of the valves.

Chronic rheumatic heart disease requires recurrent infections. Each attack of rheumatic inflammation goes through an active stage followed by healing. In the joints, active rheumatic involvement is characterized by migratory arthritis. In the skin, transitory subcutaneous nodules may appear. In the heart, each of the major anatomic components—the pericardium, myocardium, endocardium, and particularly the valves—may be involved.

ACUTE RHEUMATIC PERICARDITIS

Acute rheumatic pericarditis is characterized by variable exudation of serum and fibrin into the pericardial cavity. Large effusions of fluid may result in radiographic features of uniform cardiac enlargement and physical signs of pericardial effusion. Impairment of the inflow of blood to the heart, with resultant increased systemic venous pressure, may be evident through distention of the cervical veins. The fibrinous element of acute rheumatic pericarditis is manifested by particles of fibrin floating in the associated effusion and by the concentration of a fibrinous deposit on the visceral (epicardial) and parietal layers. The shaggy fibrin, evident when the two layers of the pericardium are separated, has given rise to the name "bread-and-butter heart" of rheumatic pericarditis. This gross feature is not specific, however, because it applies to any condition in which *fibrinous pericarditis* occurs. Histologically, during the active stage of rheumatic pericarditis, fibrin is deposited on the pericardial surfaces. Beneath this, capillaries and fibroblasts are mobilized and gradually enter the fibrin as granulation tissue. The pericardium shows edema and mild leukocytic infiltration. Specific Aschoff bodies, which characterize acute rheumatic myocarditis, are not usually seen in the pericardium.

ACUTE RHEUMATIC MYOCARDITIS

The specific histologic lesion of acute rheumatic carditis is usually restricted to the myocardium and takes the form of the Aschoff body. *Aschoff bodies* are reactive nodules within the connective tissue and therefore are predominantly found around blood vessels of the myocardium and in other bundles of connective tissue that separate myocardial fascicles. The primary lesion appears to be an alteration of collagen, which shows a coagulation-like change with eosinophilia, a process called *fibrinoid necrosis*. Secondary cellular reaction to the primary process in the collagen leads to the formation of the nodule. The involved cells include nonspecific phagocytes, myocardial histiocytes, and multinucleated cells (Aschoff giant cells). In the early Aschoff body, fibroblastic proliferation is not strongly evident, but as the lesion becomes older, the phagocytic cells become less numerous and are replaced by fibroblastic cells. Toward the end of the activity of an Aschoff body, the nodule may be entirely fibrous and acellular in nature.

The characteristic scant loss of muscle in acute rheumatic carditis is paradoxical in view of the frequent occurrence of myocardial failure during this stage of the disease.

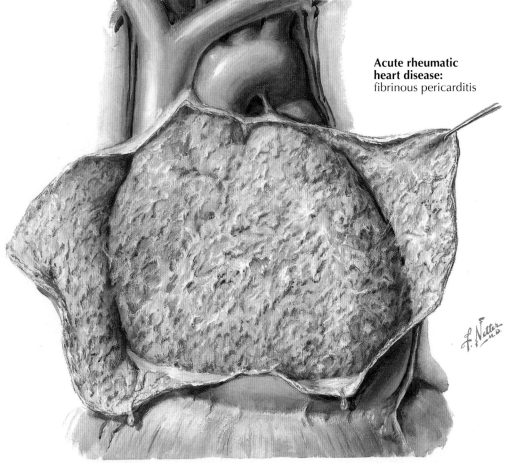

Acute rheumatic heart disease: fibrinous pericarditis

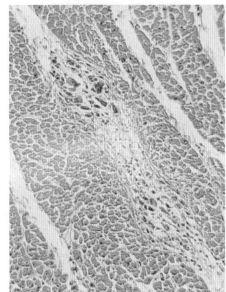

Characteristic distribution of myocardial Aschoff bodies. In interstitial tissue between fascicles of muscle.

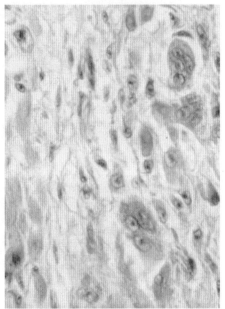

Well-developed Aschoff body. Composed of the variety of cells, including multinucleated Aschoff cells.

Plate 6.29

Cardiovascular System: VOLUME 8

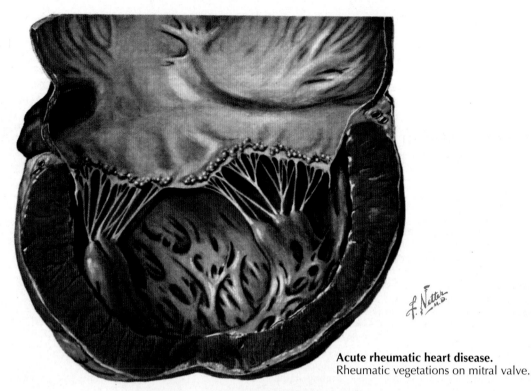

Acute rheumatic heart disease.
Rheumatic vegetations on mitral valve.

RHEUMATIC HEART DISEASE: ACUTE VALVULAR INVOLVEMENT

The gross changes exhibited in the cardiac valves as a manifestation of acute rheumatic involvement are highly characteristic. The mitral and aortic valves tend to be involved, whereas the tricuspid valve is affected only occasionally and the pulmonary valve classically not at all. The primary change in the valve is edema with minimal leukocytic infiltration. A secondary erosion of the valve cusp along the line of closure occurs as a complication of closing the edematous cusp. Fibrin and platelets are then deposited along the denuded area, accounting for the row of delicate, tan, translucent bead-like lesions that usually are confined to the line of closure. From the atrioventricular valves, the lesions may extend onto the chordae tendineae. Another characteristic feature of the gross changes in rheumatic valvulitis is the absence of destructive effects on the valve tissue or chordae tendineae, with minimal deformity of the valves at this stage.

Because *acute rheumatic valvulitis* is almost universally associated with acute rheumatic myocarditis, the gross effects of rheumatic myocarditis in the form of ventricular dilation are frequently evident. *Mitral insufficiency* may be present as a transient phenomenon during the acute stage of rheumatic carditis. The valvular disturbance is attributed primarily to the myocarditis and associated ventricular dilation rather than intrinsic disease of the mitral valve. The involvement of the aortic valve by acute rheumatic endocarditis causes little functional change. *Mitral regurgitation* during acute rheumatic carditis may be associated with an area of regurgitant "jet lesions" on the posterior wall of the left atrium, called MacCallum patches, considered a focus of response to regurgitation rather than primary rheumatic mural endocarditis.

Acute rheumatic valvulitis occurring at a given time may represent either the first attack or one of several recurrent insults. The structural changes observed in a patient with acute rheumatic endocarditis will depend on whether the attack is the first event or one of several recurrent episodes. Even with a first attack, evidence may show a healing response to the inflammatory process. In such cases there is little gross alteration, except for vegetations. The response to an initial attack has certain characteristics; in the cusp beneath the vegetation, various cells (e.g., fibroblasts, macrophages) are mobilized in a palisade manner. Fibroblasts and capillaries grow into the inflamed material, replacing the

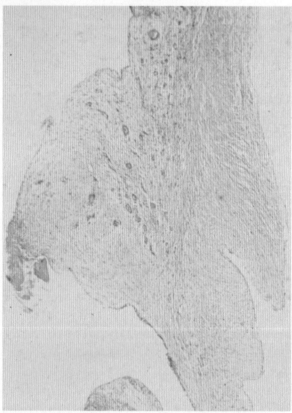

Photomicrograph of mitral valve in acute rheumatic endocarditis. Swelling along line of closure of the valve cusp represents healing of vegetative material, some of which still caps the summit of the swelling.

fibrin. This sets the stage for the *healed phase*, when the sites of the valve lesions are represented by fibrous nodules. In cases where the chordae tendineae also are involved by vegetative material, healing leads to chordal thickening and sometimes adhesions between the chordae tendineae. If an attack is one of several recurrent episodes, the characteristic changes of acute rheumatic valvulitis are superimposed on residua of

healed previous attacks, including cusp shortening, fibrous thickening along the line of closure, varying degrees of interadhesion between the chordae tendineae, shortening of the chordae, and vascularization of the cusps. If valvular insufficiency has resulted from earlier attacks of acute rheumatic endocarditis, an enlargement of the chambers specific for the type of such insufficiency may be observed.

Plate 6.30

Acquired Heart Disease

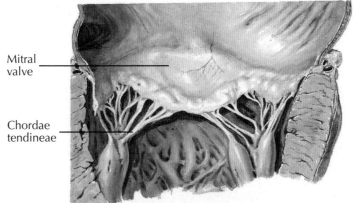

Mitral
valve

Chordae
tendineae

Mitral valve. Some fusion of chordae tendineae and thickening of cusps at contact areas; blood vessel growing into the cusps.

RHEUMATIC HEART DISEASE: RESIDUAL CHANGES OF ACUTE RHEUMATIC CARDITIS

Recurrent acute rheumatic carditis may lead to severe residual changes represented by stenosis or insufficiency of one or more valves. In some patients, however, the rheumatic process leaves only minor damage, or each involved valve exhibits only minor changes. Other patients have one or two valves that may show significant deformities. Minor residual changes of acute rheumatic carditis also may be observed in the myocardium and pericardium, regardless of the specific damage to the valves.

In the mitral valve, minor residual changes are represented by fibrous thickening along the line of closure of the cusps at the site of healed lesions of acute rheumatic valvulitis. Minimal shortening of the free aspect of the cusp may occur, making the insertion of chordae tendineae appear to be directly into the free edge of the cusp. Vascularization of the mitral valve is often seen as a sign of healed rheumatic involvement. Characteristically, the vascularization involves the anterior cusp. At its base, a vessel is seen to proceed toward the free aspect of the cusp, where it arborizes. Minor degrees of chordal shortening, thickening, and interadhesion may occur in competent valves. Also, minor degrees of fusion between the cusps at their commissures may be observed. In the tricuspid valve the minor residual effects are similar to those in the mitral valve.

In the aortic valve the minor residual changes include limited degrees of fibrous thickening along the line of closure, cusp shortening, and commissural fusion. Shortening of the cusps is demonstrated in the conventional view of the opened aortic valve by a greater depth of the aortic sinuses than in the normal valve. The most common clinical observation in a patient with mitral valvulitis and stenosis is aortic regurgitation. Aortic valve commissural fusion of a degree that allows near-normal function of the valve is usually confined to one commissure. This results in one conjoined cusp about twice the width of the second cusp, which is not adherent to its neighbors. An aortic valve so altered may be termed an *acquired bicuspid valve.* Although such a valve may be competent and also not stenotic, it fails to open with the freedom of a normal tricuspid aortic valve and is subject to the complication of slowly becoming calcified and stenotic. Another potential complication of the minor residual effects of rheumatic disease in the valves is infective endocarditis, particularly of the mitral and the aortic valves.

In hearts with only minor residual valvular disease of rheumatic endocarditis, the myocardium is grossly normal and not hypertrophied, but small myocardial scars may exist. The latter are the residua of Aschoff bodies and are represented by avascular and acellular scars in perivascular locations. In many cases the healing of Aschoff bodies may be so complete that it is difficult to determine whether a strand of connective

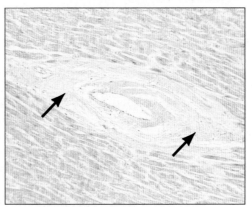

Photomicrograph of interstitial nodule of myocardium. Representing a healed Aschoff body (*arrows*).

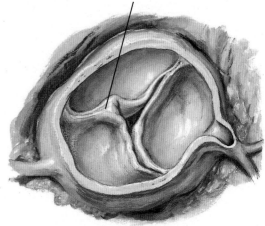

Fusion

Aortic valve. Fusion of right cusp and posterior cusp, resulting in a bicuspid valve that is still competent.

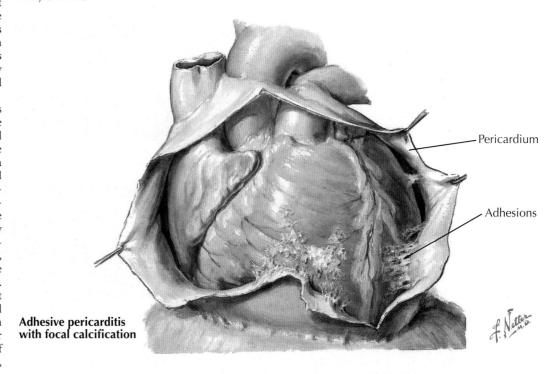

Adhesive pericarditis with focal calcification

Pericardium

Adhesions

tissue in the myocardium is normal supporting tissue or a residual scar.

The healed effects of acute rheumatic pericarditis are rarely if ever responsible for significant disturbances of the circulation, regardless of the form that healing may take. Usually, acute rheumatic pericarditis heals by resolution, leaving a smooth-lined, nonadhesive pericardium. In other cases, the fibrinous exudate is replaced focally or diffusely by fibrous adhesions. Even in uncommon instances where the entire pericardium is obliterated by fibrous adhesions, the adhesions are relatively thin and do not constitute a basis for cardiac constriction. In some cases of fibrous obliteration of the pericardial sac, focal plaques of calcium may be deposited in the adhesions, but even then there appears to be no constrictive effect.

Plate 6.31

Cardiovascular System: VOLUME 8

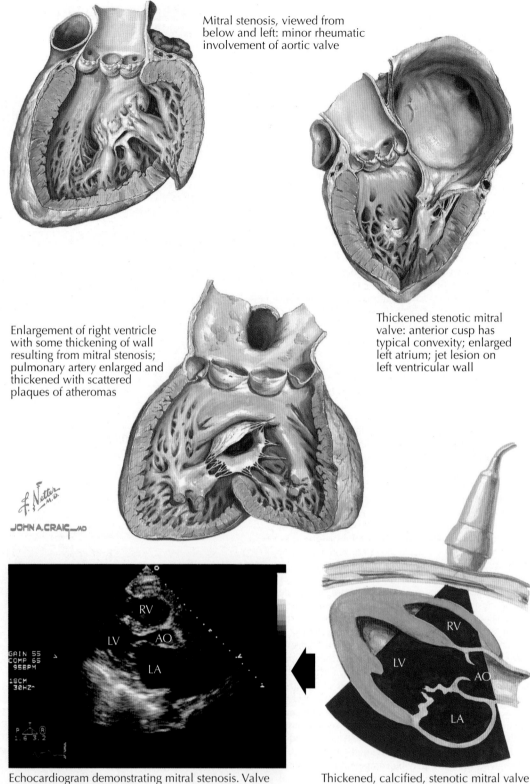

Mitral stenosis, viewed from below and left: minor rheumatic involvement of aortic valve

Thickened stenotic mitral valve: anterior cusp has typical convexity; enlarged left atrium; jet lesion on left ventricular wall

Enlargement of right ventricle with some thickening of wall resulting from mitral stenosis; pulmonary artery enlarged and thickened with scattered plaques of atheromas

Echocardiogram demonstrating mitral stenosis. Valve located between left atrium (LA) and left ventricle (LV) is thickened, with reduced orifice and intense signal due to excessive calcium.

Thickened, calcified, stenotic mitral valve demonstrated in echocardiographic study at left

MITRAL STENOSIS: PATHOLOGIC ANATOMY

Mitral stenosis is the most common serious effect of recurrent rheumatic fever and represents the culmination of recurrent attacks: a highly deformed and obstructed mitral valve. The healing valvular lesions of acute rheumatic fever cause not only fibrous thickening of the cusps but also, and more importantly, cusp interadhesions at the commissures and chordae tendineae changes. The healing of lesions on the chordae surfaces is responsible for their fusion, obliterating the spaces between the chordae. In the normal mitral valve, blood flows through the part of the orifice between the papillary muscles and also through the spaces between the chordae, lateral to the papillary muscles. After interchordal adhesion, the secondary pathways for flow are obliterated. The chordae tendineae also undergo recurrent inflammation, causing these strands to shorten, which is responsible for the cusps being held tautly in a downward position. The chordae related to each commissure exhibit a fan-like shape. The base of the fan is attached to the cusps, with the apex to the papillary muscle. As the chordae become shortened and pull the cusps downward, they draw the base of the fan toward the apex. This tends to hold the cusps together and

favors adhesion between the cusps at their commissures during healing of the valve lesions. The process of chordal shortening, with the resultant fixation of the cusps, is probably the major factor in restenosis after mitral valve commissurotomy.

The stenotic mitral valve shows a typical deformity of its anterior cusp, characterized by a convexity directed

toward the atrium. In the absence of valve calcification, during left ventricular diastole when the left atrial pressure exceeds the LV pressure, the cusp at the site of this deformity buckles toward the ventricle. This buckling could be responsible for the "opening snap" at the beginning of diastole (imagine a sailboat spinnaker catching the wind), considered classic for mitral stenosis.

Plate 6.32

Acquired Heart Disease

PATHOPHYSIOLOGY AND CLINICAL ASPECTS OF MITRAL STENOSIS

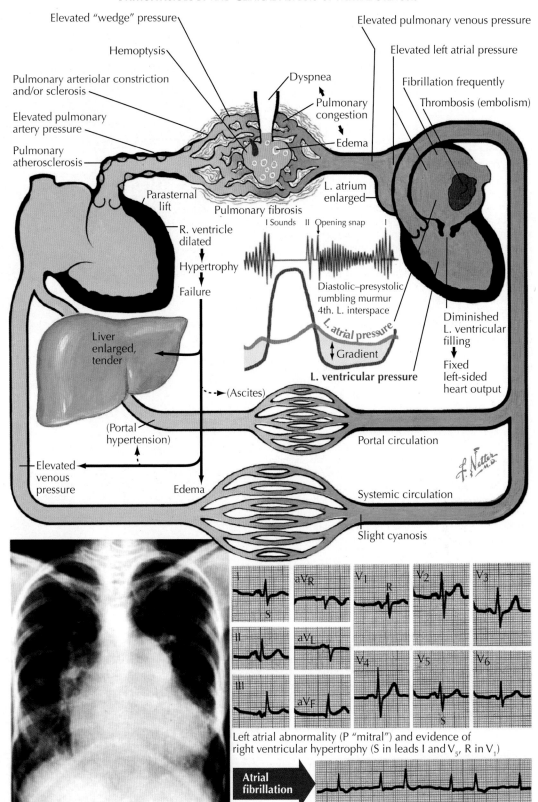

MITRAL STENOSIS: PATHOLOGIC ANATOMY (Continued)

During ventricular systole, the deformity buckles toward the atrium and impinges on the base of the posterior mitral cusp, to act as a flutter valve to prevent regurgitation through the valve.

The primary functional effect of mitral stenosis is obstruction at the mitral valve.

The pressure rises in the left atrium, in the entire pulmonary vascular bed, and in the right ventricle. These functional changes result in secondary structural effects that aid in the clinical diagnosis, including enlargement of the left atrium and the main pulmonary arteries and hypertrophy of the right ventricle. The left atrial pressure exceeds the left ventricular diastolic pressure. This effect, coupled with the presence of a narrow mitral orifice, is responsible for the narrow, high-velocity stream of blood passing through the mitral orifice that creates the diastolic rumble on auscultation. At the sites where such streams strike the LV wall, jet lesions may develop.

In patients with established mitral stenosis, functional studies indicate diminished cardiac output, which may be fixed. Therefore the heart may not respond with an increase in output with a demand for

increased tissue oxygenation. With exercise and even at rest in severe cases, there is a greater-than-normal extraction of oxygen at the systemic capillary level. This results in the characteristic increased arteriovenous oxygen difference in patients with mitral stenosis. The low cardiac output of mitral stenosis is reflected in the size of the left ventricle and the aorta. The LV cavity

usually is smaller than normal, and the wall usually is normal or thinner. The diameter of the aorta may be narrower.

Mitral stenosis has classic physical findings; an opening snap is followed by a diastolic rumble, with presystolic accentuation into a loud first heart sound. These findings can be confirmed by cardiac ultrasound.

Plate 6.33

Cardiovascular System: VOLUME 8

Aorta

Left pulmonary artery

Left main bronchus

Left upper pulmonary vein

Left atrium

Widening of angle of tracheal bifurcation by enlarged left atrium: compression of left upper lobe bronchus between left pulmonary artery and left upper pulmonary vein with resultant bronchial obstruction

Cross section of compressed bronchus

MITRAL STENOSIS: SECONDARY ANATOMIC EFFECTS

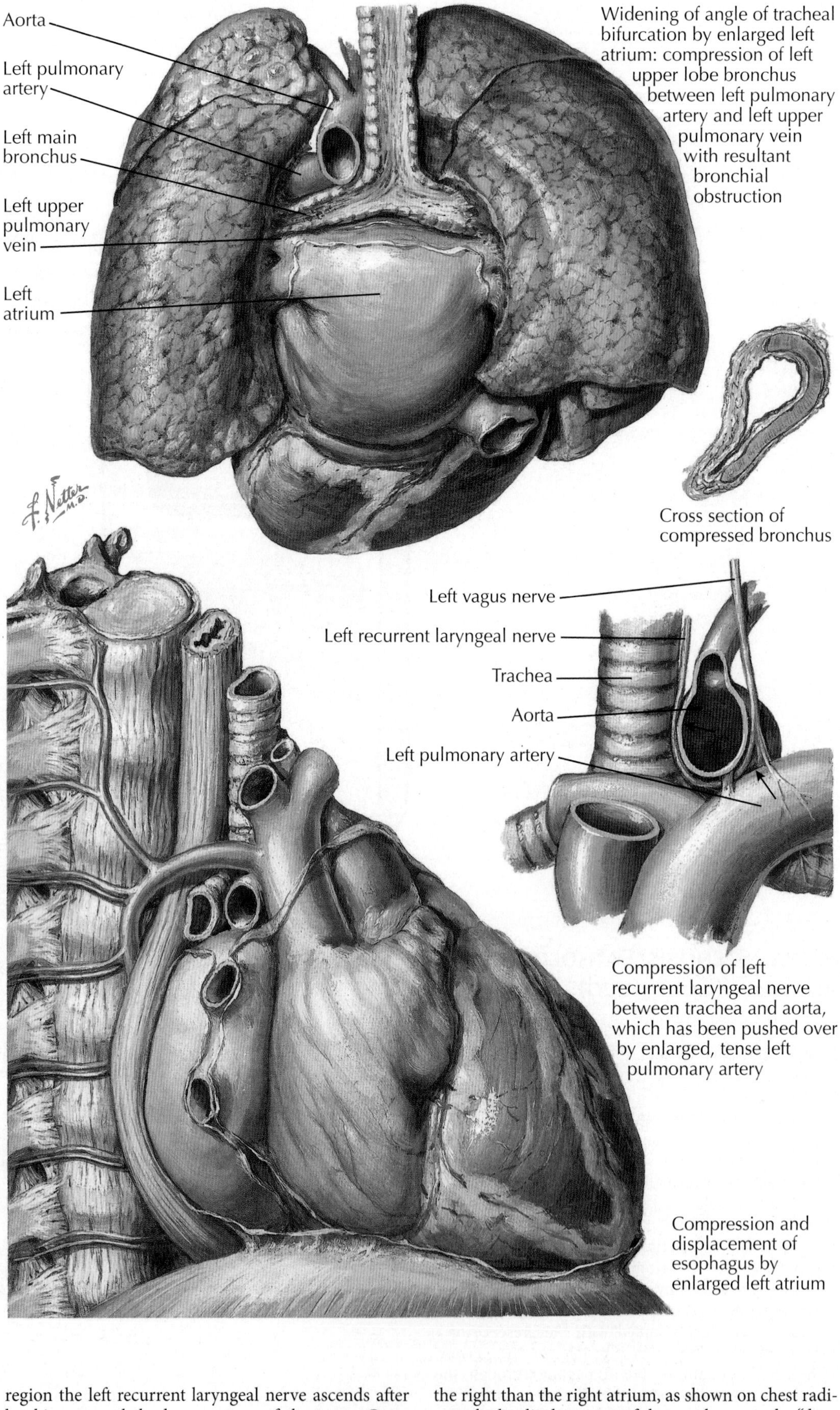

The primary functional effect of mitral stenosis is impaired flow across the mitral valve. This increases pressure in the left atrium, the entire pulmonary vascular system, and the right ventricle, causing secondary anatomic effects that include hypertrophy of the muscle in the left atrial wall and enlargement of the left atrial chamber. The wall of the right ventricle becomes hypertrophied, and the chamber may be of normal size or may be enlarged, probably a result of complicating congestive cardiac failure. Enlargement of the right ventricular chamber may in turn be responsible for dilation of the tricuspid orifice and secondary tricuspid regurgitation. Dilation of the major pulmonary arteries results from pulmonary hypertension, which also accentuates the second cardiac sound in the pulmonary area and contributes to atherosclerosis of the major pulmonary arteries.

The left atrium is located inferior to the *tracheal bifurcation*, in such a position that its superior aspect is separated from the inferior aspects of the two major bronchi by only two structures: the tracheobronchial lymph nodes and the pericardium. The tracheal bifurcation arches over the left atrium. When the left atrium becomes dilated, as in mitral stenosis, the angle of the tracheal bifurcation increases. This results mainly from an upward displacement of the left main bronchus, with the right main bronchus less affected. The close relationship between the left upper pulmonary vein and the left main bronchus may favor the latter's upward displacement. The increased angulation (widening of angle) of the tracheal bifurcation may be identified in thoracic radiographs and serves as a parameter in identifying left atrial enlargement.

Bronchial compression may also occur, more evident in the left main bronchus than in the right. In extreme degrees of compression, the normally rounded lower aspect of the left main bronchus is represented by a sharp edge. The impaired airway resulting from bronchial compression may cause recurrent pulmonary infections. This aspect of mitral stenosis may contribute to dyspnea, which is a common symptom in patients with this valvular disease.

Hoarseness results from paralysis of the left vocal cord and may be observed in the occasional patient with mitral stenosis. This sign must be taken as a complication of the associated pulmonary hypertension because it is also observed in patients with other forms of cardiac disease involving pulmonary hypertension. Left vocal cord paralysis is an ultimate effect of enlargement of the major pulmonary arterial system. The aortic arch and the left pulmonary artery lie within a C-shaped angle formed by the left side of the trachea medially, the left main bronchus inferiorly, and the left upper lobe bronchus laterally. Within this confined zone, an enlarged left pulmonary artery forces the aortic arch against the left side of the trachea. In this

Left vagus nerve

Left recurrent laryngeal nerve

Trachea

Aorta

Left pulmonary artery

Compression of left recurrent laryngeal nerve between trachea and aorta, which has been pushed over by enlarged, tense left pulmonary artery

Compression and displacement of esophagus by enlarged left atrium

region the left recurrent laryngeal nerve ascends after hooking around the lower aspect of the aorta. Compression of the recurrent laryngeal nerve as it courses between the trachea and aortic arch appears to explain the paralysis.

Enlargement of the left atrium is an important sign of mitral stenosis. This chamber may extend farther to the right than the right atrium, as shown on chest radiography by displacement of the esophagus and a "double" atrial shadow. The left atrium lies close to the esophagus, so the enlarged left atrium frequently causes posterior displacement of the esophagus. In extreme cases, the esophagus may also be displaced laterally, usually toward the right.

Plate 6.34

Acquired Heart Disease

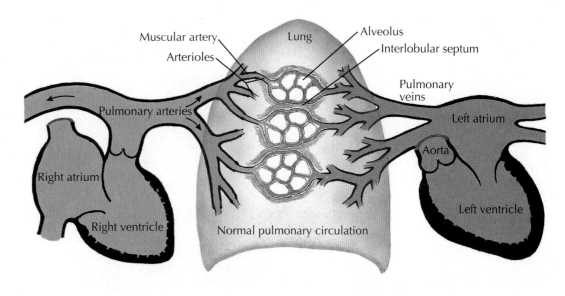

Normal pulmonary circulation

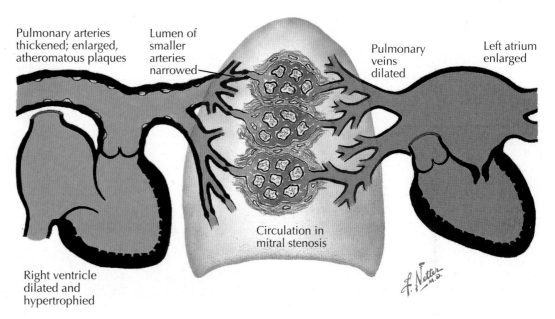

Circulation in mitral stenosis

MITRAL STENOSIS: SECONDARY PULMONARY EFFECTS

In mitral stenosis, obstruction at the diseased valve is reflected as an increase in pressure within the entire pulmonary vascular bed and right ventricle. In the normal pulmonary vascular bed, there is a low-grade differential of pressure across the arteriolar level. The small, thin-walled pulmonary arteries and arterioles are incapable of exerting high levels of vasospasm. In mitral stenosis, however, these small arterial vessels exhibit medial *hypertrophy* and appear to be capable of displaying considerable vasoconstriction, which is associated with greater pressure differences between pulmonary arterial and venous sides than normal. Pulmonary capillary bed pressure is determined by resistance to blood flow from the lungs (downstream stenotic mitral valve) and amount of blood flowing into the bed. If the hydrostatic pressure within the capillary bed rises to certain levels, pulmonary edema may result. The volume of flow into the capillary bed of the lung probably is determined by the degree of pulmonary arteriolar vasoconstriction, which may be seen as a protective phenomenon in mitral stenosis, guarding against flow to the degree that pulmonary edema might develop.

Although the mechanism of pulmonary arteriolar vasospasm stimulation is unknown, hypoxia may be the bottom-line cause, because oxygen does decrease pulmonary artery pressure, and when vasoconstriction is the cause, drugs such as calcium antagonists in high doses and sildenafil-like drugs also decrease pulmonary pressure in patients with evidence for pulmonary vasoconstriction. The pulmonary arteriolar bed may exert a constantly changing degree of vasoconstriction, depending on pulmonary capillary pressure.

Pulmonary arteriolar vasospasm is clinically significant in patients with tachycardia. Diastole is shortened, and in the presence of mitral stenosis, tachycardia is reflected in the retention of blood in the left atrium and in the pulmonary venous and capillary beds. Reduced blood flow into the capillary bed tends to maintain the capillary pressure at a lower level than would occur if no regulation were present. Under conditions of tachycardia, development of pulmonary edema may be ascribed to failure of the pulmonary arteriolar protective effect.

Among the structural changes in the pulmonary vascular bed is medial thickening of all classes of vessels, including the major arteries and veins. Intimal fibrous thickening may be apparent in venules, arterioles, and small arteries. These changes are nonspecific and should not be compared with the characteristic atherosclerosis, which may occur in the major pulmonary arteries. Intimal fibrous thickening of small arterial vessels is responsible for varying degrees of lumen narrowing. When present, severe changes are usually focal, with many vessels spared. This may relate to the phenomenon that pulmonary vascular disease of the degree seen in mitral stenosis does not preclude a fall

in pulmonary arterial pressure if the mitral stenosis is relieved.

In addition to distention of the pulmonary capillaries, the parenchyma of the lung in mitral stenosis may show several significant alterations, including cuboidal cells lining the alveoli, fibrosis of the alveolar walls, organization of a fibrinous exudate in the alveolar spaces, and occasional spicules of bone in the alveolar spaces. Dilation of the pulmonary lymphatics is apparent in the visceral pleura and in the interlobular septa, which probably contributes to the "straight lines" seen in the lower pulmonary lobes on chest radiographs of patients with mitral stenosis, known as Kerley B lines. This may be evidence of the assumed phenomenon in mitral stenosis that some of the fluid of the blood in the lungs is diverted to the right side of the heart by way of the lymphatics. *Hemosiderosis* is caused by recurrent hemorrhages from distended pulmonary alveolar capillaries, characteristically represented by the intraalveolar accumulation of macrophages laden with iron-containing pigment. Such accumulations are responsible for the stippled appearance of the lungs in the chest radiograph and are another clinical sign of mitral stenosis.

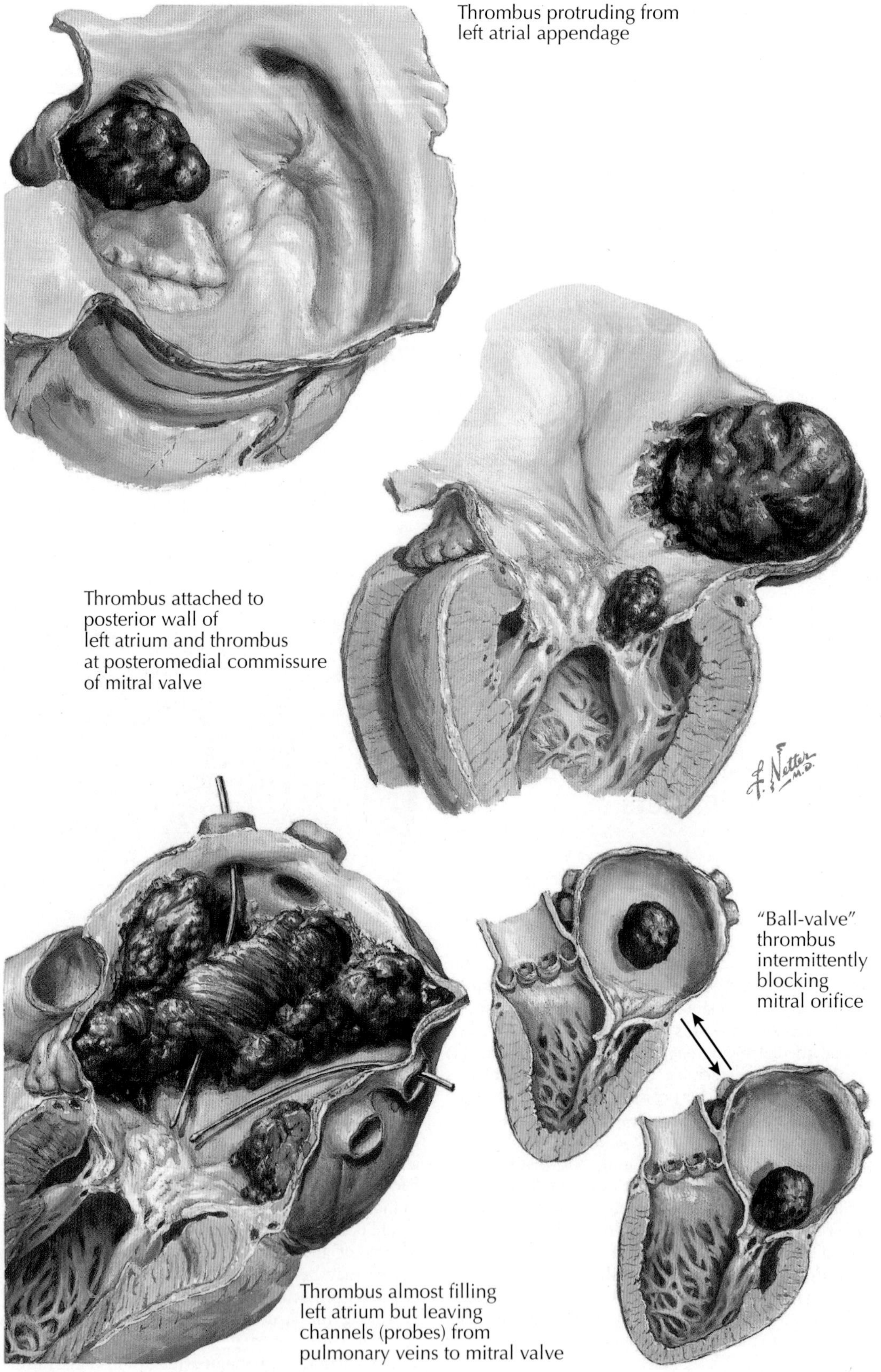

Plate 6.35

Cardiovascular System: VOLUME 8

Thrombus protruding from
left atrial appendage

Thrombus attached to
posterior wall of
left atrium and thrombus
at posteromedial commissure
of mitral valve

MITRAL STENOSIS: THROMBOEMBOLIC COMPLICATIONS

Thromboembolic complications are serious conse-quences of mitral stenosis and result from the common complication of left atrial thrombosis, a frequent second-ary effect of which is systemic embolism. The susceptibil-ity of the left atrium to develop thrombi in mitral stenosis relates to the incomplete emptying of the left atrium that may occur with each cardiac cycle and, in particular, whether this applies when atrial fibrillation is present. In this state, left atrial thrombosis and systemic embolism are significantly more common than in patients with mi-tral stenosis and sinus rhythm.

Two left atrial sites are predisposed to thrombosis when mitral stenosis is present and are well visualized on transesophageal cardiac ultrasound (Plate 6.35). These are the appendage of the mitral chamber and the posterior wall of the chamber, beginning just above the posterior cusp of the mitral valve. Thrombosis of the atrial appendage may be restricted to the append-age, or the thrombus may extend from the appendage into the main portion of the chamber. The thrombus may maintain its attachment to the wall of the main part of the left atrium and thus may be positioned for organization and firm attachment to the wall. More often, the part of the thrombus protruding from the atrial appendage in polypoid fashion into the cavity has little opportunity for attachment to the atrial wall. This type of thrombus is particularly vulnerable to fragmen-tation, thus serving as a basis for embolism.

Thrombi originating against the posterior wall of the left atrium are less common than thrombi of the atrial appendage. The predilection for thrombosis against the posterior wall may be associated with injury to this part of the left atrium by a jet-like stream of blood striking the wall, an expression of a minor degree of mitral insuf-ficiency. The distribution of thrombi in some patients with mitral stenosis is so extensive that the left atrium is

"Ball-valve"
thrombus
intermittently
blocking
mitral orifice

Thrombus almost filling
left atrium but leaving
channels (probes) from
pulmonary veins to mitral valve

described as "filled" with thrombi, although there is a characteristic distribution of the thrombotic material. As the flow from the pulmonary veins through the left atrium is maintained, the process of thrombosis spares the parts of the left atrial wall involved with blood flow-ing from the pulmonary veins toward the mitral valve. Factors related to extensive thrombosis of the left atrium

include severe mitral stenosis, older patients than usual, likelihood of left atrial wall calcification, and intractable pulmonary congestion. The severity of mitral stenosis and older patient age may in turn underlie changes in the left atrial wall, which predispose to extensive throm-bosis. These include fibrous endocardial thickening and left atrial wall calcification; radiographic evidence

Plate 6.36

Acquired Heart Disease

PRINCIPAL SITES OF EMBOLISM FROM LEFT ATRIAL THROMBOSIS

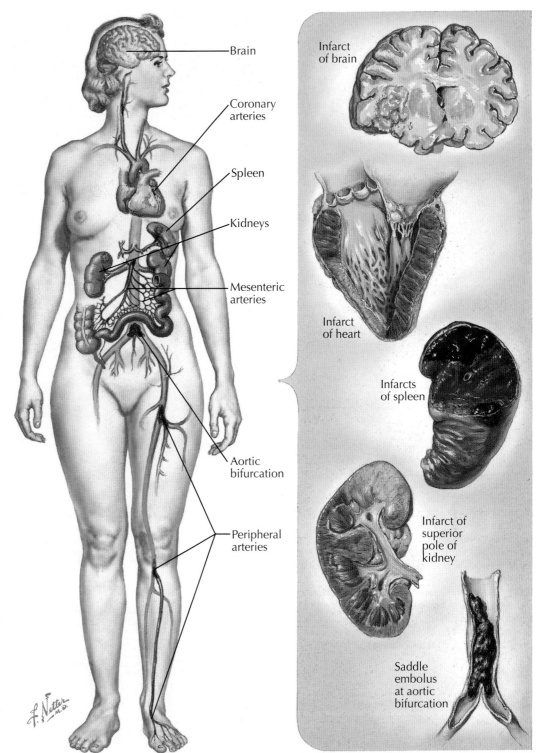

Brain

Coronary arteries

Spleen

Kidneys

Mesenteric arteries

Aortic bifurcation

Peripheral arteries

Infarct of brain

Infarct of heart

Infarcts of spleen

Infarct of superior pole of kidney

Saddle embolus at aortic bifurcation

MITRAL STENOSIS: THROMBOEMBOLIC COMPLICATIONS (Continued)

of calcification indicates that extensively distributed thrombi are likely harbored in the left atrium. The frequent presence of intractable congestive cardiac failure in patients with extensive left atrial thrombosis also may be related to stenosis severity and older patients, possibly reflected as myocardial failure because of a longer course for the primary disease process. Extensive thrombi occupy significant space in the left atrium and thus represent an obstructive factor in addition to the primary process at the mitral valve.

Another site for thrombosis leading to embolism is the mitral valve. Thrombosis of the mitral valve tends to involve one or both commissural areas in cases of valvular calcification. This relationship suggests that the basis for thrombosis of the mitral valve is fracture of calcific valvular tissue, leaving the nonendothelialized altered valvular substance exposed to the circulation as a nucleus for thrombosis to occur. Thrombosis of the valve tends to increase the degree of the mitral stenosis.

In a special form of left atrial thrombosis, a thrombus becomes detached from its site of origin, most often the atrial appendage, and remains as a loose body in the left atrium. As this mass moves about in the left atrium, it acquires a rounded or ovoid shape. It may engage the mitral orifice but is too large to pass through the stenotic valve. Thus, the mass acts as a ball valve and occludes the circulation during diastole; the patient may lose consciousness and die. Usually, however, the mass becomes dislodged from the mitral valve during systole; the circulation is reinstated, and the patient regains consciousness. In a patient with mitral stenosis, the clinical phenomenon of recurrent fainting attacks should lead to a strong suspicion of the "ball-valve" phenomenon (see Plate 6.35). A clinically similar state may be obtained in a patient with a primary myxoma of the left atrium.

In patients with mitral stenosis, embolism may occur in the pulmonary or the systemic vascular system. Pulmonary embolism is generally a complication of cardiac failure, and the usual source of emboli is the venous system of the legs, even though thrombosis of the right atrial appendage may occur, especially in patients in atrial fibrillation. Embolism of the systemic arterial system in mitral stenosis is most often a complication of thrombosis within the left atrium and less often on the stenotic mitral valve. Any of the tissues or organs supplied by the systemic arterial system may be affected (Plate 6.36). Depending on the size of the vessel occluded, involvement of the coronary arterial system by embolism may result in sudden death, clinical evidence of STEMI, or infarction associated with nonspecific electrocardiographic manifestations (NSTEMI). Infarction of the spleen is common. In some patients with splenic infarction, the process seems silent; others may develop acute left upper abdominal pain associated with leukocytosis.

Plate 6.37

Cardiovascular System: VOLUME 8

MITRAL BALLOON VALVULOPLASTY

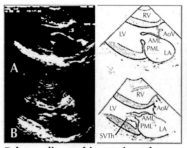

Echocardiographic scoring of mitral valve stenosis severity
Representative 2D echocardiograms from a patient with mitral stenosis with a mobile mitral valve and a low echo score (**A**) and from a patient with a high echo score (**B**)

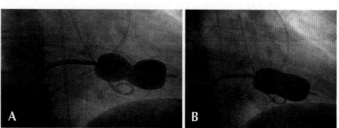

Inoue balloon mitral valvuloplasty. The Inoue balloon is seen partially inflated in the stenotic mitral stenosis orifice on the left (**A**) and fully inflated on the right (**B**). See text for description of the procedure.

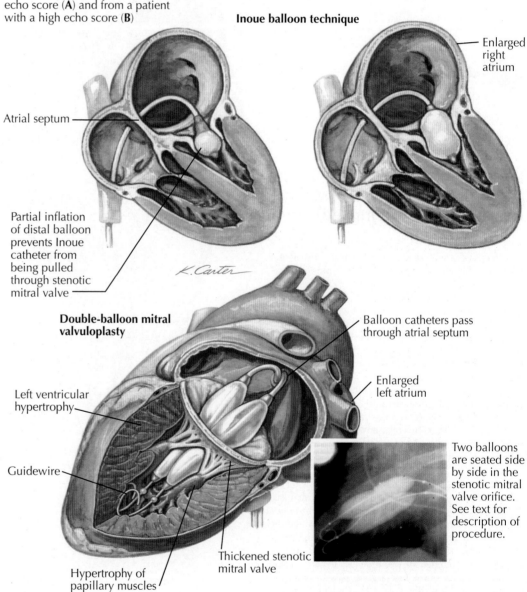

Inoue balloon technique

Enlarged right atrium

Atrial septum

Partial inflation of distal balloon prevents Inoue catheter from being pulled through stenotic mitral valve

K. Carter

Double-balloon mitral valvuloplasty

Balloon catheters pass through atrial septum

Enlarged left atrium

Left ventricular hypertrophy

Guidewire

Two balloons are seated side by side in the stenotic mitral valve orifice. See text for description of procedure.

Thickened stenotic mitral valve

Hypertrophy of papillary muscles

MITRAL STENOSIS: THROMBOEMBOLIC COMPLICATIONS (Continued)

Embolism in the kidneys with renal infarction is also common. As with the spleen, some episodes may be associated with acute abdominal pain and may be confused with conditions causing an "acute surgical abdomen." Under such circumstances, the frequent association of hematuria with renal infarction may help in the differential diagnosis. Embolism in the arteries of the gastrointestinal tract is most likely to involve the superior mesenteric artery, whereas the celiac and inferior mesenteric arteries are uncommon sites. Occlusion of the superior mesenteric artery leads to infarction of the entire small intestine (except duodenum) and right half of the colon. Embolism may occur in the branches of the extremities, but this is uncommon, at least in causing symptoms. An embolism of the aorta is more common, characteristically becoming impacted at the aortic bifurcation, a phenomenon called *saddle embolism.*

MITRAL BALLOON VALVULOPLASTY

Mitral balloon valvuloplasty entails passing a catheter with a special balloon from the right femoral vein to cross the interatrial septum through the foramen ovale into the left atrium and across the mitral valve (Plate 6.37). Using the Inoue balloon, the distal portion of the balloon is inflated and pulled against the valve cusps, and then the proximal portion is dilated to fix the center segment of the valve orifice. Finally, the central section is inflated transiently. Another technique uses a double balloon placed side by side in the stenotic valve orifice. Mitral balloon valvuloplasty is performed in select patients with mobile mitral valves, as determined by cardiac ultrasound. The procedure usually is performed with visualization by transesophageal ultrasound and fluoroscopy

and is successful, but complications can occur. The most serious complication is development of acute mitral regurgitation, usually caused by a tear in a valve leaflet or subvalvular apparatus. The transseptal puncture itself can result in complications, usually related to needle puncture of the atrium or the aorta.

Immediate results of the balloon procedure are reduction of the mitral valve gradient and relief of symptoms. Long-term follow-up data in these patients suggest that most patients are free from restenosis at 10 years; later results are less positive. Thus individual patients need long-term clinical follow-up, including cardiac ultrasound.

Plate 6.38

Acquired Heart Disease

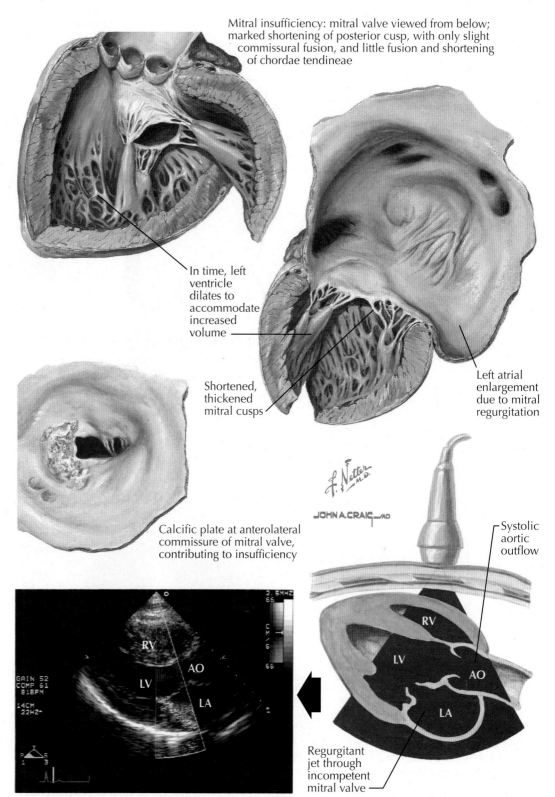

Mitral insufficiency: mitral valve viewed from below; marked shortening of posterior cusp, with only slight commissural fusion, and little fusion and shortening of chordae tendineae

In time, left ventricle dilates to accommodate increased volume

Shortened, thickened mitral cusps

Left atrial enlargement due to mitral regurgitation

Calcific plate at anterolateral commissure of mitral valve, contributing to insufficiency

Systolic aortic outflow

Regurgitant jet through incompetent mitral valve

Mitral Regurgitation

In some hearts, recurrent rheumatic mitral endocarditis results in chordal shortening and commissural fusion, changes that make the mitral valve stenotic but still competent. In other hearts, recurrent inflammation causes mitral valve incompetence. Cardiac ultrasound with color Doppler can demonstrate regurgitant flow through the incompetent mitral valve into the left atrium (Plate 6.38). The specific anatomic changes that result in mitral insufficiency include intrinsic shortening of the cusps, commissural calcification, and left atrial enlargement. Characteristically, in patients with rheumatic mitral insufficiency, the chordae tendineae may be somewhat thickened, but no significant shortening is usually present. Intrinsic shortening is more obvious in the posterior than in the anterior mitral cusp. Evidence of anterior cusp shortening is the conversion of its free edge from a convex to concave shape. As a cusp becomes contracted, the tissue near its free end retracts, resulting in a pattern with some chordae tendineae attaching directly to the free edge of the cusp. Cusp shortening is responsible for mitral insufficiency because tissue is inadequate to guard the mitral orifice.

Color Doppler study demonstrating systolic aortic outflow (blue/red) and multicolored jet of regurgitant flow through incompetent mitral valve into left atrium (LA)

Diagram of mitral regurgitation shown in Doppler color study at left

Some patients with mitral stenosis but no mitral regurgitation have commissural calcification. The involved commissures are held in a nearly closed position by the other changes responsible for mitral stenosis. In contrast, the mitral valve commissures are held in a nearly open position with calcification in patients who have mitral regurgitation. In fact, the calcification is responsible for fixation of the cusps in such a position

to make them incapable of making contact with the other in the area of the calcified commissure. If both commissures are calcified, the mitral valve is converted into a fixed structure that is open throughout the cardiac cycle.

Dilation of the left atrium is a primary effect of mitral insufficiency. Once established, however, left atrial enlargement may increase the degree of mitral valve

Plate 6.39

Cardiovascular System: VOLUME 8

PATHOPHYSIOLOGY AND CLINICAL ASPECTS OF MITRAL REGURGITATION

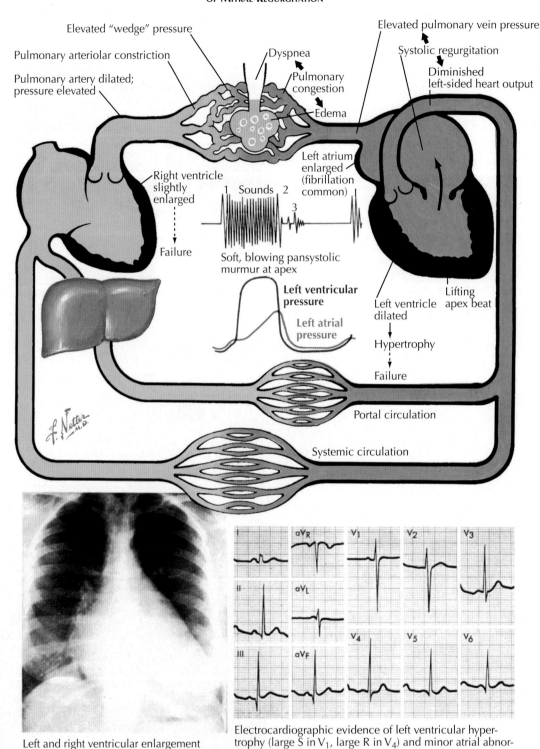

Elevated "wedge" pressure

Pulmonary arteriolar constriction

Pulmonary artery dilated; pressure elevated

Dyspnea

Pulmonary congestion

Edema

Elevated pulmonary vein pressure

Systolic regurgitation

Diminished left-sided heart output

Right ventricle slightly enlarged

Left atrium enlarged (fibrillation common)

Failure

1 Sounds 2

3

Soft, blowing pansystolic murmur at apex

Left ventricular pressure

Left atrial pressure

Left ventricle dilated

Lifting apex beat

Hypertrophy

Failure

Portal circulation

Systemic circulation

Left and right ventricular enlargement

Electrocardiographic evidence of left ventricular hypertrophy (large S in V_1, large R in V_4) and minor atrial abnormality (broad P)

aV_R V_1 V_2 V_3

II aV_L

V_4 V_5 V_6

III aV_F

MITRAL REGURGITATION (Continued)

incompetence when only one or neither commissure is fused. The aggravation of mitral insufficiency by left atrial enlargement depends primarily on the anatomic phenomenon of the left atrial wall and mitral cusps being one continuous structure. When the left atrium dilates, its posterior wall extends backward and downward, which in turn causes the posterior mitral cusp to be pulled posteriorly and away from the anterior cusp, increasing valve incompetence. In extreme cases the posterior cusp may be so displaced that it lies *over* the base of the left ventricle. The cusp is pulled posteriorly and downward by the left atrium while being restricted from its other end by the attached chordae tendineae. This results in fixation of the posterior cusp as it lies "hamstrung" over the LV base.

Mitral regurgitation is associated with enlargement of the LV cavity and moderate hypertrophy of the LV wall (Plate 6.39). Enlargement of the left atrium is constant, and the degree of enlargement is usually greater than in mitral stenosis. Examples of "giant left atrium" in association with mitral valvular disease are more apt to accompany mitral insufficiency than

mitral stenosis. Left atrial thrombosis occurs much less often in mitral insufficiency than in mitral stenosis, probably because of the constant washing of blood in this chamber and less likelihood that blood will be retained in the left atrium in mitral insufficiency than in mitral stenosis. The secondary effects on the esophagus, tracheal bifurcation, right ventricle, and pulmonary vascular bed are similar to those described for mitral stenosis.

On auscultation, the classic finding in mitral regurgitation is a holosystolic murmur associated with cardiomegaly, nonspecific ECG changes, left atrial enlargement, pulmonary congestion, pulmonary hypertension, right ventricular enlargement, and cardiomegaly on chest radiograph. Cardiac ultrasound using Doppler imaging will document the mitral regurgitation and provide semiquantitative assessment of the amount.

Plate 6.40

Acquired Heart Disease

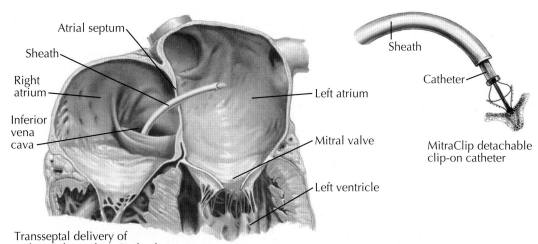

Atrial septum

Sheath

Right
atrium

Inferior
vena
cava

Left atrium

Mitral valve

Left ventricle

Transseptal delivery of
catheter above the mitral valve

Sheath

Catheter

MitraClip detachable
clip-on catheter

MITRAL VALVE CLIP

Percutaneous transseptal reduction of the mitral valve
orifice of a regurgitant mitral valve is a minimally invasive procedure to help reduce symptomatic severe mitral regurgitation in appropriate patients, especially
those who are deemed high risk for traditional surgical
repair. A clip device is used to mimic the surgical procedure (Alfieri) that creates a double orifice of the mitral valve resembling a bowtie. This creates a smaller
regurgitant orifice than the large orifice responsible for
severe mitral regurgitation. The procedure consists of
introducing a large sheath into the femoral vein and
advancing it to the inferior vena cava, right atrium, and
across the atrial septum into the left atrium. Under
transesophageal echocardiography guidance, the clip
position is then advanced across the mitral valve and
optimally positioned based on the mitral valve pathology. Next, the leaflets are grasped and the clip is closed
simulating the "bowtie" surgical stitch of Alfieri. Transesophageal echocardiography is then used to reassess
the mitral regurgitation, and, if adequate reduction is
obtained, the clip is released and left in place on the
mitral valve (Plate 6.40).

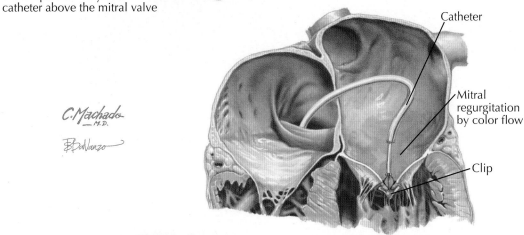

Catheter

Mitral
regurgitation
by color flow

Clip

Positioning of clip between anterior and
posterior mitral valve leaflets

Clip

Mitral valve clip in position at completion of
procedure

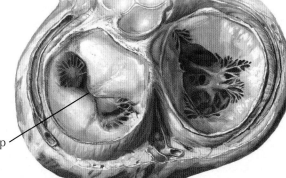

Leaflets held together by mitral valve clip

Plate 6.41

Cardiovascular System: VOLUME 8

Chordal Transfer, Sliding Annuloplasty, and Ring Annuloplasty

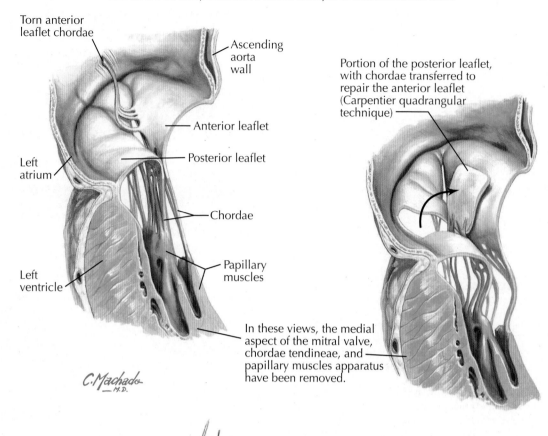

Torn anterior leaflet chordae

Ascending aorta wall

Anterior leaflet

Posterior leaflet

Left atrium

Chordae

Left ventricle

Papillary muscles

C. Machado
M.D.

Portion of the posterior leaflet, with chordae transferred to repair the anterior leaflet (Carpentier quadrangular technique)

In these views, the medial aspect of the mitral valve, chordae tendineae, and papillary muscles apparatus have been removed.

Anterior leaflet reconstructed

Insertion of a flexible annuloplasty ring may be indicated to reestablish the coaptation and strengthen the annular support.

Cut for sliding annuloplasty technique

In these views, the valvular apparatus is shown complete with chordae tendineae and papillary muscles.

Mitral Valve Repair

Most valve surgeons will attempt surgical repair of a regurgitant mitral valve by valve replacement or valve preservation using several evolving techniques, including the following:

- Ring annuloplasty to create a smaller orifice of the mitral valve ring, thus bringing the valve leaflets into closer apposition at closure.
- Resection of prolapsing portions of valve leaflets not supported by chordae tendineae to downsize a redundant valve leaflet, first done by Carpentier in France and essentially a quadrangular resection of the valve leaflet.
- Use of artificial chords or shortening of elongated chords to the appropriate physiologic size to approximate the normal architecture and closure of the valve leaflets during systole.
- Increasing or decreasing the mitral valve leaflet area by sliding annuloplasty.

Valve repair is the treatment of choice because of decreased risk of bleeding (anticoagulation is not necessary unless there is another indication such as increased risk of stroke from atrial fibrillation), decreased risk of stroke (a prosthetic valve is not used), and durability of the nonprosthetic valve (a prosthetic valve usually does not last as long as a repaired natural valve).

The cardiac surgeon must determine which procedure can be performed using criteria determined by transesophageal ultrasound and direct visualization of the valve apparatus at surgery. Approximately 90% of diseased valves from etiologies other than rheumatic

can be repaired, including degenerative disease resulting in elongation or rupture of the chordal apparatus and myxomatous degeneration such as mitral valve prolapse or floppy mitral valve, as described by Barlow of South Africa.

Evidence suggests that mitral valve repair, if feasible, should be done earlier rather than later, to prevent irreversible heart damage. Severe mitral regurgitation

determined by cardiac ultrasound, whether symptomatic or asymptomatic, warrants consideration of mitral valve repair, especially if the patient is in atrial fibrillation. Patients who undergo mitral valve repair must remember that they do not have an anatomically normal valve and that endocarditis prophylaxis must be considered when certain noncardiac procedures are performed.

Plate 6.42

Acquired Heart Disease

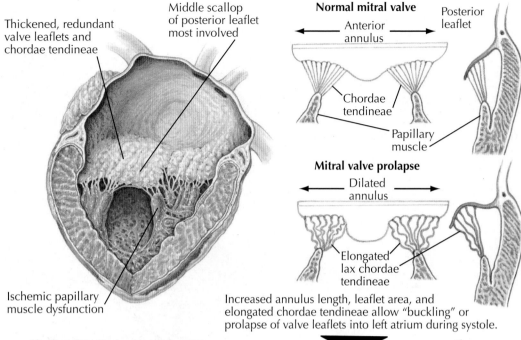

Thickened, redundant valve leaflets and chordae tendineae

Middle scallop of posterior leaflet most involved

Ischemic papillary muscle dysfunction

Normal mitral valve

Anterior annulus

Posterior leaflet

Chordae tendineae

Papillary muscle

Mitral valve prolapse

Dilated annulus

Elongated lax chordae tendineae

Increased annulus length, leaflet area, and elongated chordae tendineae allow "buckling" or prolapse of valve leaflets into left atrium during systole.

Findings in mitral valve prolapse

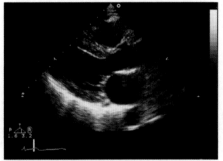

2D echocardiogram showing normal configuration of mitral valve leaflets in systole

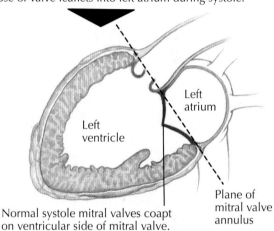

Left atrium

Left ventricle

Plane of mitral valve annulus

Normal systole mitral valves coapt on ventricular side of mitral valve.

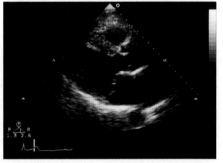

2D echocardiogram showing abnormal configuration of mitral valve leaflets in systole

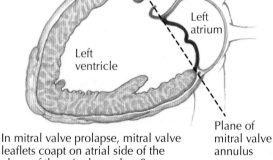

Left atrium

Left ventricle

Plane of mitral valve annulus

In mitral valve prolapse, mitral valve leaflets coapt on atrial side of the plane of the mitral annulus. Some mitral regurgitation may be present.

S. Moon, m.s.

MITRAL VALVE PROLAPSE

Mitral valve prolapse (MVP, ballooning mitral valve, Barlow syndrome) usually results from myxomatous degeneration of the valve, with thickened redundant leaflets and chordae tendineae, caused by the redundant valve tissue in ballooning or prolapse of the valve into the left atrium. If mitral insufficiency results from prolapse, physical examination reveals that the regurgitation is in late systole and is often preceded by a midsystolic click (late systolic murmur). The estimated prevalence of MVP is 2% to 3% of the population. MVP without mitral regurgitation can be determined on physical examination (isolated late systolic click) and is generally considered a benign condition. If mitral regurgitation is present, however, mortality depends on severity of the regurgitation and degree of LV dysfunction. Although infective endocarditis can occur on any valve, it is a rare event in patients with MVP without mitral regurgitation.

The diagnosis of MVP with mitral regurgitation is usually made on physical examination (late systolic click followed by a late systolic murmur) and is usually confirmed by cardiac ultrasound and Doppler imaging. Ultrasound features include an increase in the mitral annulus length, increased leaflet area, and elongated chordae tendineae. These features allow prolapse of the valve leaflets during ventricular systole. In the normal heart during systole, when the mitral valve closes, the coaptation of the valves occurs on the ventricular side of the mitral valve below the plane of the mitral valve annulus. During ventricular systole in the patient with MVP, the mitral valve leaflets coapt on the atrial side of the mitral valve annulus. Occasionally, minor mitral regurgitation can be seen on Doppler ultrasound.

Plate 6.43

Cardiovascular System: VOLUME 8

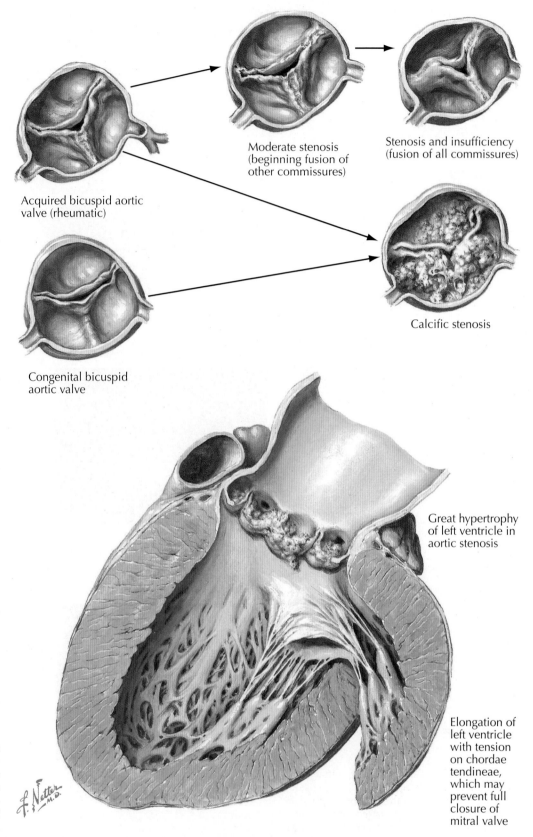

Acquired bicuspid aortic valve (rheumatic)

Moderate stenosis (beginning fusion of other commissures)

Stenosis and insufficiency (fusion of all commissures)

Congenital bicuspid aortic valve

Calcific stenosis

Great hypertrophy of left ventricle in aortic stenosis

Elongation of left ventricle with tension on chordae tendineae, which may prevent full closure of mitral valve

AORTIC STENOSIS: RHEUMATIC AND NONRHEUMATIC CAUSES

In the adult patient, obstruction at the aortic valve may be a direct result of recurrent rheumatic inflammation. In the younger adult patient, it may be a manifestation of the calcification of a bicuspid valve. In the older adult, the most common cause of aortic stenosis is progressive calcification of a trileaflet aortic valve. Diabetes, hypertension, hyperlipidemia, and chronic kidney disease may accelerate the development of calcific aortic stenosis.

In an aortic valve, various residua of rheumatic inflammation reduce the valve orifice (Plate 6.43). The simplest type of stenosis is characterized by fusion of two of the cusps at one commissure. The resultant pattern is that of an *acquired bicuspid aortic valve*. The orifice of the valve, although reduced, is usually sufficiently wide so as not to cause recognizable obstruction to the egress of blood from the left ventricle. In the next stage in severity, the cusps are fused at two of the commissures. The restricted motion of the cusps by the adhesions may reduce the orifice enough to cause significant aortic stenosis. The greatest restriction of motion is achieved with fusion of adjacent cusps at each commissure. Alteration of the aortic valve in this manner is always associated with some degree of cusp shortening. Fixation of the cusps makes the valve severely stenotic, and shortening is responsible for coexistent aortic insufficiency of a degree dependent on the extent of shortening.

The second way that rheumatic inflammation leads to aortic stenosis is through the inflammatory process, which operates indirectly by first establishing an acquired bicuspid valve, which in turn may become calcified. The resultant rigidity of the cusps makes the aortic valve stenotic.

The most common type of aortic valvular stenosis is the *calcific* form. This process may become established on the acquired bicuspid valve or may represent a complication of a congenital bicuspid valve (Plate 6.43). The most common etiology of calcific aortic valve stenosis is seen in elderly patients with

Plate 6.44   Acquired Heart Disease

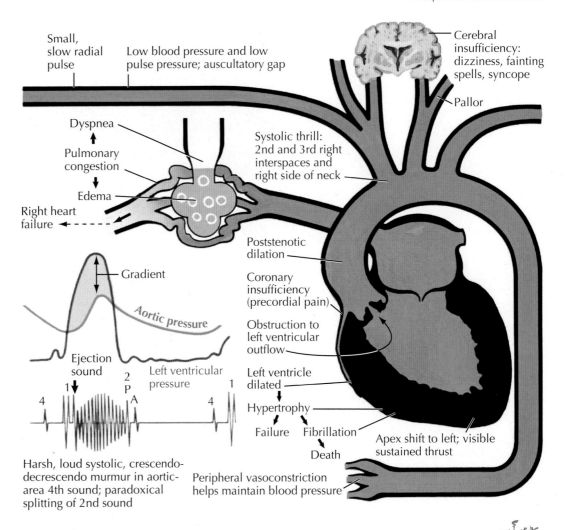

Small, slow radial pulse

Low blood pressure and low pulse pressure; auscultatory gap

Cerebral insufficiency: dizziness, fainting spells, syncope

Pallor

Dyspnea

Pulmonary congestion

Edema

Right heart failure

Systolic thrill: 2nd and 3rd right interspaces and right side of neck

Poststenotic dilation

Coronary insufficiency (precordial pain)

Obstruction to left ventricular outflow

Left ventricle dilated

Hypertrophy

Failure   Fibrillation

Death

Apex shift to left; visible sustained thrust

Gradient

Aortic pressure

Ejection sound

Left ventricular pressure

Harsh, loud systolic, crescendo-decrescendo murmur in aortic-area 4th sound; paradoxical splitting of 2nd sound

Peripheral vasoconstriction helps maintain blood pressure

AORTIC STENOSIS: RHEUMATIC AND NONRHEUMATIC CAUSES (Continued)

a tricuspid valve. Examination of involved valves shows that such valves are often bicuspid. A congenital bicuspid valve becomes a likely candidate for calcific aortic stenosis. This concept is supported by the intrinsic features of the valve. Also, some patients with calcific aortic stenosis have a malformation associated with a high incidence of congenital bicuspid valve, such as coarctation of the aorta.

Elderly individuals typically have some calcification of the aortic cusps, and some changes may be sufficient to cause a murmur such as that heard in aortic stenosis, but the signs of LV hypertrophy are usually absent. Such patients should be considered to have aortic sclerosis. Aortic stenosis is associated with elevated LV systolic pressure greater than aortic systolic pressure. LV hypertrophy follows, giving a conical shape to the left ventricle, which extends beyond the border of the right ventricle on chest radiographs (Plate 6.44).

In patients with aortic stenosis, coronary artery disease may be present to the same extent as seen in the general population. Areas of MI may be observed in those with normal coronary arteries but is usually associated with significant degrees of coronary artery disease. In an occasional case, coronary arterial narrowing results from embolism, the source of which

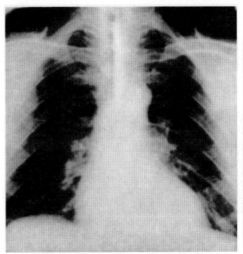

Left ventricular enlargement and moderate dilation of ascending aorta (poststenotic)

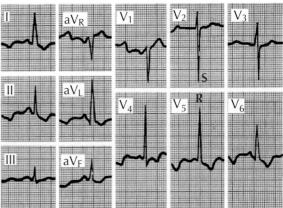

Evidence of left ventricular hypertrophy (large S in V_2, large R in V_5) and "strain" (inverted T and depressed ST in I, II, aVL, V_5, V_6)

may be calcific material in the diseased aortic valve or emboli from infective endocarditis of the aortic valve.

The pathophysiology and clinical features of aortic stenosis include a pressure gradient across the aortic valve resulting in LV outflow obstruction, LV hypertrophy, increased LVEDP, LV enlargement on ECG, and a harsh, loud, systolic crescendo-decrescendo murmur

in the aortic area. Pulmonary congestion can occur if left atrial pressure is elevated, which in turn increases pulmonary capillary wedge pressure. The carotid pulse is narrow and rises slowly (pulsus parvus and tardus). A systolic thrill can be palpated in the carotid arteries. Chest radiography can reveal dilation of the ascending aorta.

Plate 6.45

Cardiovascular System: VOLUME 8

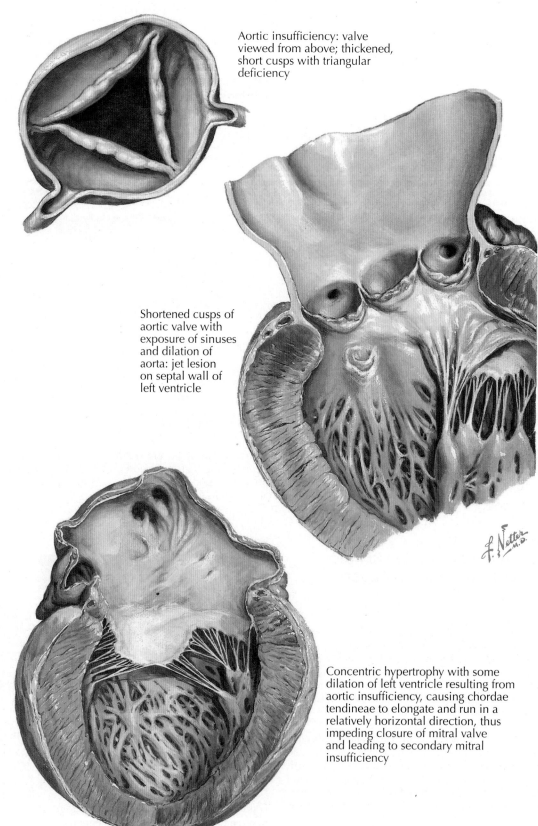

Aortic insufficiency: valve viewed from above; thickened, short cusps with triangular deficiency

Shortened cusps of aortic valve with exposure of sinuses and dilation of aorta: jet lesion on septal wall of left ventricle

Concentric hypertrophy with some dilation of left ventricle resulting from aortic insufficiency, causing chordae tendineae to elongate and run in a relatively horizontal direction, thus impeding closure of mitral valve and leading to secondary mitral insufficiency

Aortic Regurgitation: Pathology

If recurrent rheumatic inflammation affects the aortic cusps but spares the commissures, isolated aortic regurgitation may result. This functional change is derived from shortening of the scarred cusps. As each cusp is shortened, some of its "extra length," which makes the valve competent, is lost. With enough deformation the cusps become too short to make the valve competent. The incompetent orifice of the valve is then represented by a *triangular* opening bounded by the affected cusps (Plate 6.45).

Shortening of the cusps involves not only their width but also their length. Thus, when the left ventricle and the incompetent aortic valve are opened in the conventional pathologic dissection, more aortic sinuses are evident than with a normal aortic valve.

Secondary signs of aortic regurgitation include widening or dilation of the ascending aorta and alterations in the left ventricle. LV changes include hypertrophy and regurgitant jet lesions on the wall of the subaortic region. The jet lesions are responses to the trauma of the regurgitant stream striking the wall. These may be present on the septal wall of the outflow area or on the ventricular aspect of the anterior mitral valve leaflet. Characteristically, the fibrous tissue of the jet lesion is oriented in a cuspid pattern, the open parts of the cusps facing the source of the regurgitant stream. Jet lesions in the subaortic area provide important anatomic evidence for aortic regurgitation, and their location may correspond to the site of origin of the diastolic murmur of aortic regurgitation. The LV dilation and hypertrophy of aortic regurgitation may be extreme; in the heaviest hearts observed pathologically, aortic regurgitation is a common underlying problem. Along with thickening of the wall, the cavity becomes enlarged in both lateral and downward directions. The LV changes may be responsible for the development of *secondary mitral regurgitation* for the following reasons:

- In aortic regurgitation, as in aortic stenosis, while the left ventricle enlarges in a downward direction, the papillary muscles may be moved downward as well. The resultant tension on the chordae tendineae

Plate 6.46

Acquired Heart Disease

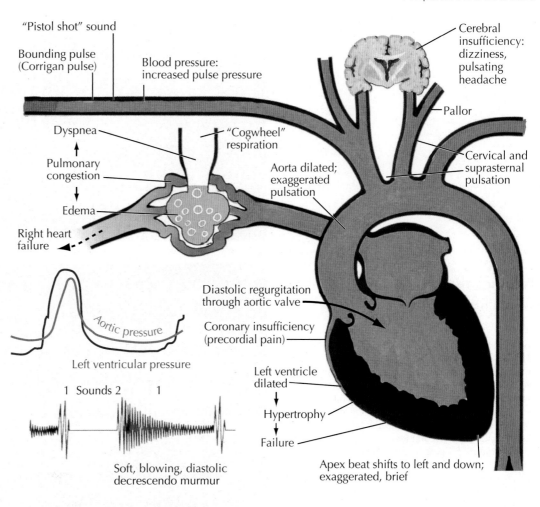

"Pistol shot" sound

Bounding pulse (Corrigan pulse)

Blood pressure: increased pulse pressure

Cerebral insufficiency: dizziness, pulsating headache

Pallor

Dyspnea

"Cogwheel" respiration

Cervical and suprasternal pulsation

Pulmonary congestion

Aorta dilated; exaggerated pulsation

Edema

Right heart failure

Diastolic regurgitation through aortic valve

Aortic pressure

Coronary insufficiency (precordial pain)

Left ventricular pressure

Left ventricle dilated

↓

Hypertrophy

↓

Failure

1 Sounds 2   1

Soft, blowing, diastolic decrescendo murmur

Apex beat shifts to left and down; exaggerated, brief

AORTIC REGURGITATION: PATHOLOGY (Continued)

of the mitral valve may be responsible for undue restraint on the mitral cusps, to such a degree that they cannot approximate each other adequately for closure of the mitral valve. Mitral regurgitation results.

- In aortic regurgitation, enlargement of the LV cavity is responsible for the lateral displacement of the papillary muscles. This tends to change the axis of the papillary muscles and the chordae tendineae from a near-vertical position, with respect to the long axis of the left ventricle, to an axis prone to an orientation toward the *horizontal* position. The change in direction of the pull of the papillary muscles may cause some dysfunction of the papillary muscle–chordal mechanism, with resultant mitral regurgitation.

The LV hypertrophy accompanying aortic regurgitation or aortic stenosis may be seen as a basis for increased resistance to LV filling. This manifestation is expressed functionally as elevated LVEDP, which in turn may be considered an obstruction to pulmonary venous flow and thus comparable to mitral stenosis. Left atrial, pulmonary capillary, and pulmonary arterial pressures are increased., and the parenchyma may simulate qualitatively that in mitral stenosis, although the degree of change is usually less in aortic valvular disease. The right ventricular hypertrophy accompanying aortic stenosis or aortic insufficiency may be derived similar to the right ventricular hypertrophy of mitral stenosis.

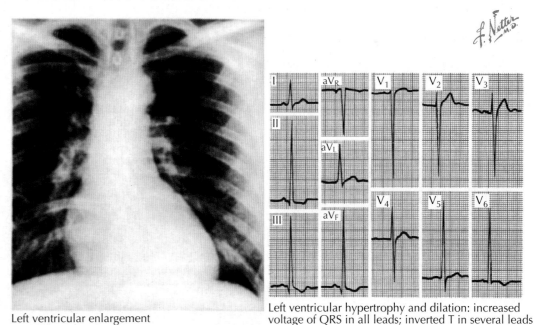

Left ventricular enlargement

Left ventricular hypertrophy and dilation: increased voltage of QRS in all leads; inverted T in several leads

Clinical manifestations also include diastolic regurgitation of blood through the aortic valve, which may result in inadequate filling of the coronary arteries, premature closure of the mitral valve (Austin-Flint murmur), mitral regurgitation, and pulmonary edema. A blowing, decrescendo diastolic murmur is heard best in the third left intercostal space (Erb's area). Because of

the aortic regurgitation, there can be a wide pulse pressure, bounding carotid and other artery pulsation, LV enlargement on physical examination and chest radiography, and LV hypertrophy on the ECG. A systolic murmur is usually audible, related to the large volume of blood flowing across a diseased valve in systole (Plate 6.46).

Plate 6.47

Cardiovascular System: VOLUME 8

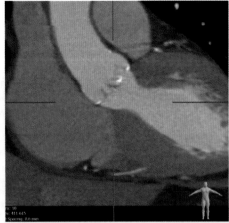

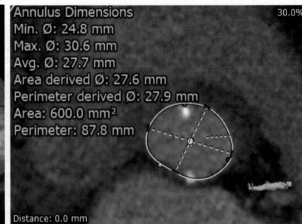

Left ventricular long axis

Aortic annulus

Transcutaneous Aortic Valve Replacement

The first transcutaneous aortic valve replacement (TAVR) was performed in 2002 in France by Cribier and has significantly grown since, with more than 275,000 implanted in the United States alone. In 2019 the total yearly volume of TAVR exceeded that of sub-cutaneous AVR, making TAVR the dominant form of aortic valve replacement in the United States. Catheter-based TAVR is most commonly delivered by a trans-femoral route of vascular access, though transapical, transsubclavian, transaortic, or even transcarotid approaches are also used based on the patient's anatomy. There are multiple valve platforms, but two major devices dominate the market: a self-expanding trileaflet porcine pericardial valve mounted on a metal frame (CoreValve, Medtronic) and a trileaflet valve of bovine pericardium mounted on a metal stent with expandable balloon (Sapien, Edwards Laboratories). The valves are carefully positioned and deployed to minimize interference with coronary ostia and to reduce the risk of post-deployment paravalvular aortic insufficiency and heart block. Computed tomography (CT) scans prior to placement are standard and used for choice of valve. Outcomes are excellent, and long-term data continue to accumulate in favor of TAVR. Initially, this technology was offered only to high-risk patients who were not candidates for open surgical replacement. It was then expanded to include intermediate-risk patients, and in 2019 the US Food and Drug Administration fully expanded approval of TAVR for use in low-risk patients.

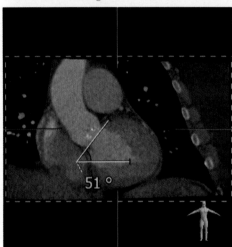

Aortic root angle CT

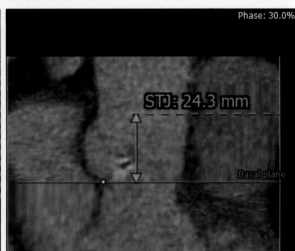

Sinus height triple image

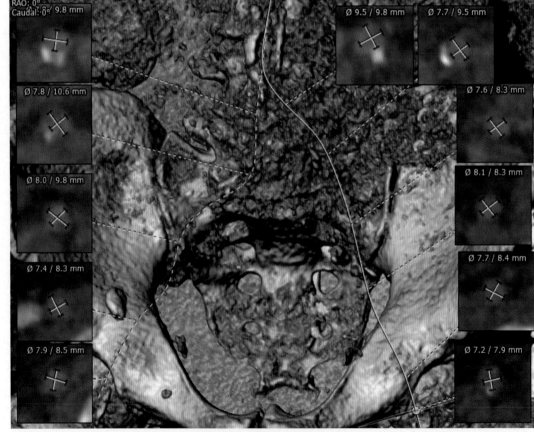

Iliac volume rendering

Images courtesy Michael R. Massoomi, MD

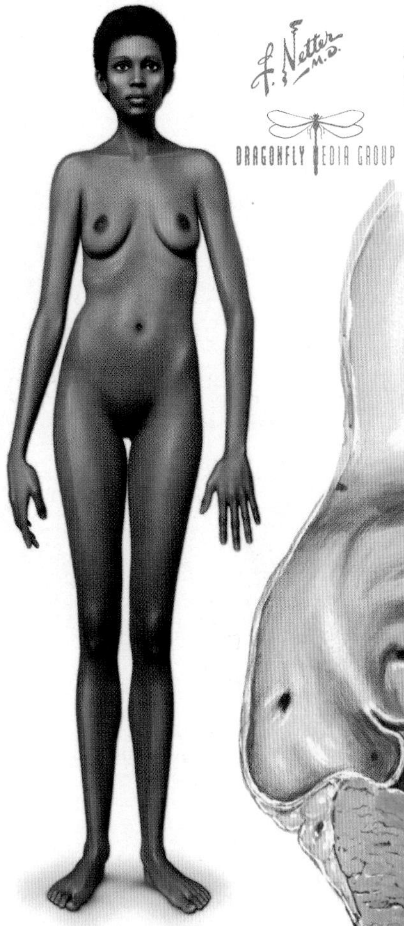

Plate 6.48

Acquired Heart Disease

Aortic valve. With a dilated annulus and incompetent orifice.

Dilated ascending aorta

Prolapsed leaflets of mitral valve

Dilation of ascending aorta and aortic ring; regurgitant lesion; "hooding" of mitral cusps; hypertrophy of left ventricle

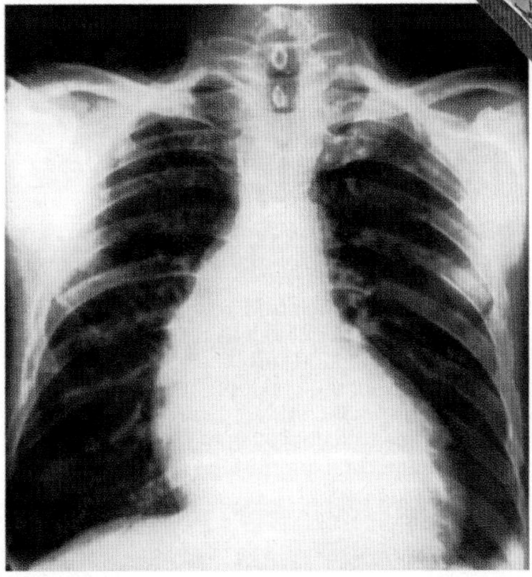

Cystic areas of medial necrosis

CYSTIC MEDIAL NECROSIS OF AORTA

Cystic medial necrosis (also called Erdheim disease) of the aorta is another cause of aortic regurgitation. In some patients the aortic valve may be competent, though other manifestations, such as mitral regurgitation or dissection of the aorta, may occur. Cystic medial necrosis is seen in elastic arteries and is characterized histologically by deposits within the media of amorphous basophilic accumulations, or *microcysts,* accounting for the "cystic" necrosis. Initially tiny and isolated lesions, the microcysts tend to coalesce and in extreme cases replace broad areas of the media. Though the microcysts are small, the elastic laminae of the aorta may be intact. In the presence of coalesced microcysts, however, the elastic laminae in a given area are interrupted, and such fibers then recoil. The histologic effect is that multiple areas of the media are devoid of elastic fibers. The overall gross effect of this process is an increase in the diameter of the aorta in the involved segments. In the aorta the greatest effect of cystic medial necrosis is evident from the root of the vessel distally to include the entire ascending aorta and varying extents of the arch.

Among patients with significant cystic medial necrosis of the aorta, variation occurs as to body habitus. In some this is normal, and the enlargement of the aorta is called *idiopathic dilation of the aorta.* Others exhibit distinct characteristics of body habitus and other effects that, collectively, are called Marfan syndrome. These patients characteristically are unusually tall and have correspondingly long bones of the arms, legs, feet, and hands. The arm span exceeds the total body height. These patients also have a high-arched palate, dislocation of the optic lenses, and a tendency toward emphysema. Biochemical abnormality may be detected by high urinary hydroxyproline levels.

Patients with extensive cystic medial necrosis of the aorta, including those with arachnodactyly, often have cardiovascular disease. Although certain congenital malformations of the heart have been identified, these

Marfan syndrome. Frequently associated with cystic medial necrosis.

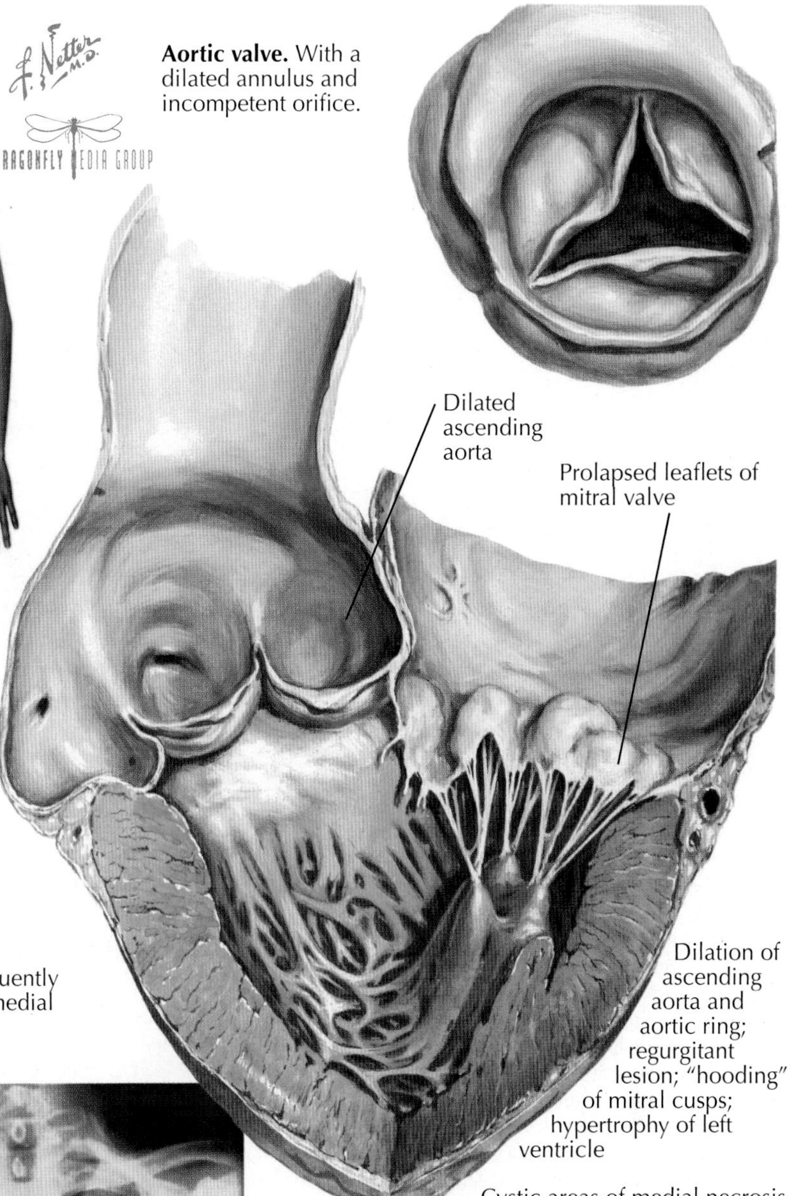

Dilated aortic root shown on chest radiograph

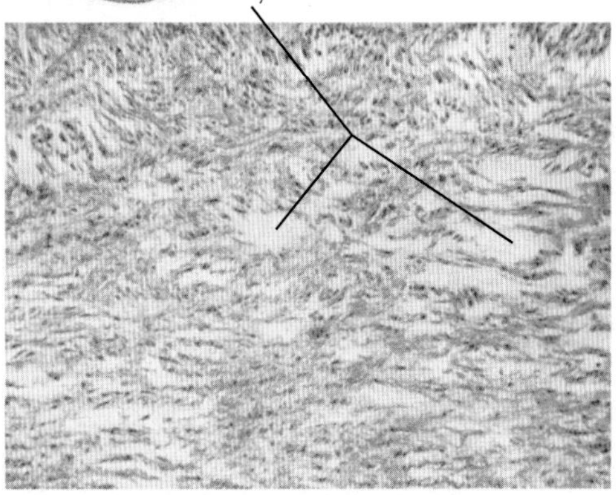

Aortic segment showing cystic medial necrosis

are not common, and the cardiovascular association may assist in making a diagnosis. Lesions involving the aorta, the aortic valve, the atrioventricular valves, and the pulmonary trunk appear to have a direct association with cystic medial necrosis.

The aortic valve effect is a common manifestation and results in aortic regurgitation. This functional abnormality may develop in several ways, most simply through extensive dilation of the aortic root, including each sinus of Valsalva. This process may be the sole cause of aortic valve incompetence. Some patients show extreme enlargement with prolapse of the aortic cusps, which compounds the effect of aortic dilation in causing aortic regurgitation.

Plate 6.49

Cardiovascular System: VOLUME 8

Abdominal aortic aneurysm (infrarenal)

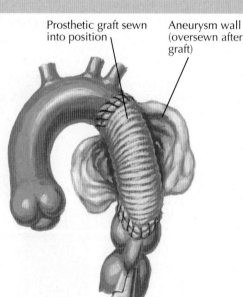

Aneurysm opened

Prosthetic graft sewn into position

Renal arteries

Aneurysm

Incision lines for opening aneurysm

JOHN A. CRAIG—AD

Indications for surgery include aneurysm diameter twice normal aorta, rapid enlargement, or symptomatic aneurysm

Graft

Aneurysm wall

Walls of aneurysm sewn over graft, forming sleeve

CYSTIC MEDIAL NECROSIS OF AORTA: SURGICAL MANAGEMENT

An aorta that harbors a significant degree of cystic medial necrosis tends to rupture. This complication takes three major forms. First, aortic rupture causes a simple *hemorrhage,* resulting in exsanguination or cardiac tamponade from hemopericardium. Second, the rupture results in a classic *aortic dissection,* with complications that may include coronary artery occlusion or occlusion of peripheral vessels. Third, the tear does not extend through the entire wall of the aorta and results in a localized intravascular *hematoma.* If present in the ascending aorta, this hematoma may distort the aortic valve sufficiently to initiate or exacerbate aortic regurgitation. Regardless of whether a localized dissection or an intramural hematoma is present, the ascending aorta dilated by cystic medial necrosis may cause some alteration in the shape of the heart on chest radiographs. Because the aortic origin is within the cardiac outline, however, major degrees of aortic dilation may go undetected unless ultrasound or CT images of the aorta are obtained.

The atrioventricular (AV) valves of patients with cystic medial necrosis of the aorta may show changes indicating the weakness of connective tissues. Characteristically, the valve substance between the insertion of the chordae tendineae tends to balloon up toward the atrium (myxomatous degeneration, mitral valve prolapse), and there may also be elongation of the chordae. These changes may account for incompetence of either the mitral or the tricuspid AV valve, although the mitral valve is affected more often. In the pulmonary artery, cystic medial necrosis manifests as dilation of the involved vessels. So-called idiopathic dilation of the pulmonary trunk may be a manifestation of cystic medial necrosis in this vessel.

Medical management of Marfan aortic disease consists of β-adrenergic blockade to decrease the force and velocity of contraction of the left ventricle on the proximal aorta. The rationale is that β-blocker therapy reduces the force and velocity of aortic ejection on the

Thoracic aortic aneurysm

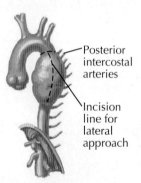

Posterior intercostal arteries

Incision line for lateral approach

Typically, repair is deferred until risk of rupture outweighs potential complications of repair. Of paramount concern is decreased spinal cord perfusion (due to damage to posterior intercostal arteries) and paraplegia.

Prosthetic graft sewn into position

Aneurysm wall (oversewn after graft)

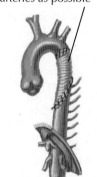

Oblique graft may be utilized to maintain perfusion in as many posterior intercostal arteries as possible

Completed aortic graft

weakened tissue of the aorta and thus slows the progression of aortic dilation. Nondihydropyridine calcium channel antagonists may give similar results.

Surgical therapy of Marfan syndrome is considered when the risk of aortic dissection is apparent with progressive enlargement of the aortic root (see Plate 6.48). Two methods are used. With the traditional method, the surgeon replaces the aorta with a graft and the aortic valve with a mechanical valve. With the valve-sparing method, the ascending aorta is replaced with a graft and the valve reimplanted (see also Plate 6.55).

SURGICAL MANAGEMENT OF ABDOMINAL AND THORACIC AORTIC DISSECTION AND ANEURYSMS

Surgical management of other types of aortic dissections and aneurysms is typically deferred until risk of rupture outweighs the risk of repair. Currently, endovascular therapy of dissection or aneurysm repair is often used by vascular surgeons or cardiac surgeons to treat an abdominal or thoracic aortic aneurysm or dissection. With this procedure, a large stent is introduced into the aorta percutaneously.

Plate 6.50

Acquired Heart Disease

SYPHILITIC AORTIC DISEASE

Syphilis of the aorta is a classic cause of aortic valve regurgitation. In rheumatic heart disease or infective endocarditis, changes in the valve cusps represent the primary causes of valvular incompetence. In syphilis, aortic insufficiency results primarily from changes in the aortic wall rather than in the cusps. Moreover, syphilitic heart disease has another manifestation; this relates to coronary artery obstruction because this is an *aortic vasculitis*.

The primary affected site is the media of the thoracic aorta, which shows many microscopic foci where tissue has been lost and replaced by delicate *stellate scars*. Lymphocytes and plasma cells may be present in the scars. In addition, alterations may occur within the adventitial and intimal layers. The adventitia shows fibrous thickening and lymphocytic and plasma cell infiltration. Also, the vasa vasorum may show nonspecific fibrous proliferation of the intima, with corresponding degrees of narrowing of the lumen. This change has led investigators to determine whether the medial change of syphilis is an effect of direct infection of the media or a result of faulty aortic nutrition, secondary to the alterations in the vasa vasorum.

Certain gross characteristics are displayed by the aorta, which is the end organ in syphilitic disease. Clinical identification of these features provides circumstantial evidence for a syphilitic background in the patient with aortic regurgitation.

The combination of two features of syphilitic heart disease—widening of the affected portion of the aorta and localization to the thoracic portion of the vessel—results in a characteristic appearance of the syphilitic aorta. Beginning at the root of the aorta and extending for a variable distance along the thoracic portion, the vessel is widened. In the classic example, widening extends to the level of the diaphragm, where because of a lack of dilation of the abdominal portion, the descending aorta assumes a funnel shape as it becomes continuous with the abdominal segment. Grossly, another feature usually becomes apparent: a strong tendency for the involved portion to show *diffuse atherosclerosis*. This lesion may display focal calcification and may be ulcerated. Calcification in the secondary atherosclerotic lesion of the thoracic aorta involving the ascending aorta may be observed in chest radiographs. This process, together with evidence of dilation of the ascending aorta, presents strong but not specific evidence of *syphilitic aortitis*. The complicating process of atherosclerosis may result in one of the classic features of syphilitic aortic disease, *narrowing of the coronary arterial ostia*. The same process in the aorta may also compromise the lumen of the branches arising from the arch.

In addition to the effects of secondary atherosclerosis, the syphilitic aorta may show complications of the medial disease beyond simple uniform dilation. These include formation of saccular aneurysms in any segment of the thoracic aorta, except in the wall of the aortic sinuses of Valsalva, which appears to be spared any significant effect. Rupture of the thoracic aorta into a serous cavity or an adjacent vessel, such as the superior vena cava or pulmonary artery, may be a complication of a saccular aneurysm or simple dilation.

In the specific area of the ascending aorta, the process of widening may be responsible for aortic regurgitation. As the aorta widens, each aortic valve cusp may

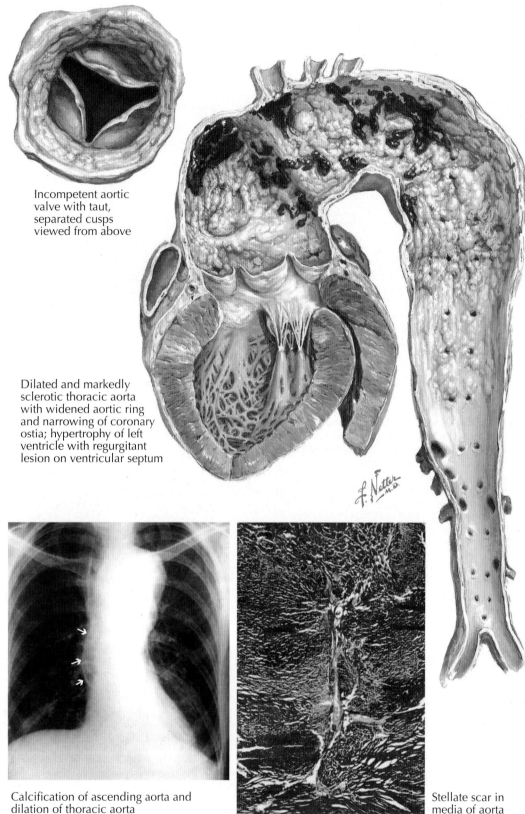

Incompetent aortic valve with taut, separated cusps viewed from above

Dilated and markedly sclerotic thoracic aorta with widened aortic ring and narrowing of coronary ostia; hypertrophy of left ventricle with regurgitant lesion on ventricular septum

Calcification of ascending aorta and dilation of thoracic aorta

Stellate scar in media of aorta

be pulled away from its neighbor at the commissure, resulting in the classic feature of commissural separation. More important, as related to complicating aortic regurgitation, the widening of the aorta causes undue tension on the individual cusps. The cusps become bowed, and their length shortens relative to the size of the aortic orifice. A triangular deficiency in the aortic valve appears, and aortic regurgitation ensues. Once the valve becomes incompetent, secondary fibrotic changes may occur in the free extremities of the cusps. The *aortic valve incompetence* causes LV hypertrophy. Also, at the impact site of the regurgitant stream, the LV outflow area may show regurgitant jet lesions.

Syphilitic aortic disease has become a rare disease in developed countries since the advent of penicillin use after World War II.

Plate 6.51

Cardiovascular System: VOLUME 8

PROSTHETIC VALVE SURGERY: FIRST AND SECOND GENERATION

SURGERY FOR ACQUIRED HEART DISEASE

Effective surgery for acquired heart disease began about 1897 when Rehn first successfully sutured a wound of the heart. Surgical procedures for acquired valvular disease were initiated with Cutler's pioneering effort (1920), which converted mitral stenosis into mitral insufficiency by using a valvulotome inserted transventricularly. Souttar had an early success (1925) with a transatrial *mitral commissurotomy* for mitral stenosis. Contributions by Bailey and Harken to closed mitral operations aided in the meteoric development and popularization of cardiac surgery.

A true breakthrough in curative efforts was achieved when the techniques of cardiopulmonary bypass were introduced in 1954, when a direct surgical approach to all cardiac valves first became feasible. These benefits and advantages are so demonstrably sound that, although closed mitral commissurotomy still is suitable in some patients, open-heart techniques are preferable for the correction of valvular pathology in most patients.

With the introduction of direct-vision procedures, it was hoped that restoration of valvular function could be accomplished with the natural valvular structures. Therefore for both calcific aortic and mitral stenoses, debridement and mobilization of fixed valve cusps were attempted. Unfortunately, success was usually incomplete and transient. Somewhat better results have been obtained following plication of a dilated insufficient valvular annulus of the type present in some cases of mitral or tricuspid insufficiency. Also, plication of valve cusps, in the management of certain forms of ruptured chordae tendineae, has functioned acceptably. The overall immediate and long-term accomplishments of procedures for acquired valve disease were substantially amplified by the introduction and (shortly thereafter) ready availability of prosthetic devices, which permitted total valvular replacement. To be realistic, however, it must be emphasized that none of the presently available prosthetic valves achieve the physiologic and mechanical features of a normal human heart valve.

FIRST-GENERATION PROSTHETIC VALVES

First-generation prosthetic heart valves were designed as mechanical occluders (Plate 6.51). Second-generation prosthetic valves were either mechanical or bioprosthetic. The mechanical valves were initially pivoting hingeless, and somewhat later, hinged leaflet valves were developed. Bioprosthetic valves are either porcine or human valves and valves made from pericardium (porcine or bovine). First-generation prosthetic valves were free floating (e.g., caged disks or balls). In 1952 Hufnagel designed and implanted the Hufnagel valve, a ball valve that moves up and down inserted in the descending aorta, primarily used to prevent blood from returning back into the heart of patients with severe aortic regurgitation.

In 1960, Albert Starr implanted the Starr-Edwards valve, a free-floating ball in a cage. Until early this century, the Starr-Edwards valve was used often in patients with aortic and mitral disease who needed replacement. Anticoagulation was needed whether the valve was placed in the aorta or mitral position. Introduced in 1964, the Smeloff-Cutter valve, a mechanical valve prosthesis, was hemodynamically similar to the Starr-Edwards prosthesis. The Smeloff-Cutter valve was a double cage-ball prosthesis and represented a major

design difference from the Starr-Edwards valve. The Smeloff-Cutter was used in the aortic position with less risk of thrombosis than the Starr-Edwards, particularly in select patients who could not be anticoagulated. Both mechanical valves allowed many patients to lead long and useful lives and could be implanted in the aortic or mitral position. These valves were discontinued as evolution of valve technology resulted in other mechanical valves.

Arthur Beall invented a free-floating disc valve with a very low profile (Beall valve) that could be used in the mitral position, particularly in patients with a small LV cavity (Plate 6.51). The low profile seemed to be an advantage of the Beall valve. The free-floating disc valve evolved between 1960 and 1962 primarily for the atrioventricular position. Initially it uniformly produced essentially normal hemodynamics and excellent clinical results, without embolization. It does not impinge on

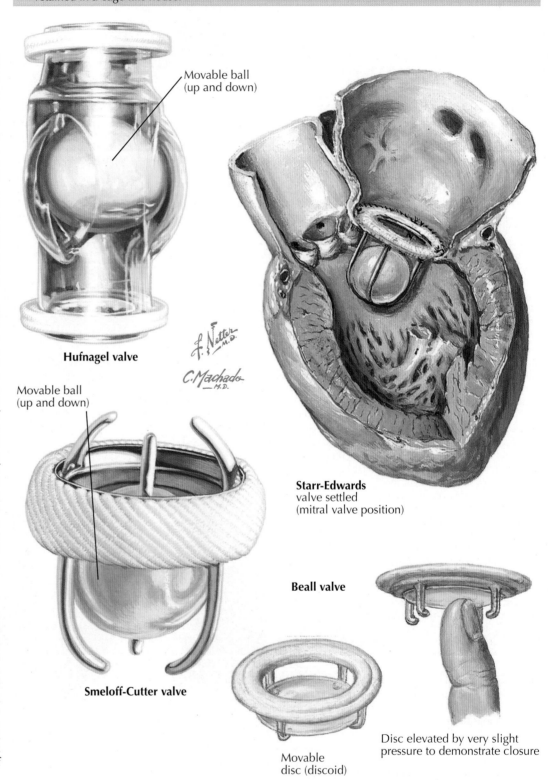

FIRST GENERATION OF SYNTHETIC PROSTHETIC VALVES

The first generation of clinically useful synthetic valves had a free-floating ball or disc occluder retained in a cage-like house.

Movable ball (up and down)

Hufnagel valve

Movable ball (up and down)

Smeloff-Cutter valve

Starr-Edwards valve settled (mitral valve position)

Beall valve

Movable disc (discoid)

Disc elevated by very slight pressure to demonstrate closure

Plate 6.52

Acquired Heart Disease

PROSTHETIC VALVE SURGERY: FIRST AND SECOND GENERATION (Continued)

the ventricular septum or obstruct the LV outflow tract. The extremely lightweight polypropylene disc allows for a rapid response with minimal pressure variations. Closure of the valve is complete on initiation of systole.

The replacement of mitral and tricuspid valves presented a particularly difficult problem because of several factors: (1) low pressure in the atrium and the resultant tendency toward thrombus formation with systemic embolization; (2) overgrowth of tissue on the metallic or plastic parts, which results in valvular dysfunction, necrosis of tissue, and embolization; (3) inertia of the valvular mechanism; (4) occlusion of a portion of the mechanism, with regurgitation before complete closure and dislodgement of the sewing ring produced by the large mass striking the areas of suture; (5) incomplete ventricular filling because of the large size of the occluding portion of the mechanism, thus requiring use of a valve of small orifice size; and (6) obstruction to the LV outflow area because of the angulation.

The Beall valve was used extensively worldwide from 1965 to 1970 but was replaced by other mechanical valves, such as pivoting hingeless valves.

SECOND-GENERATION PROSTHETIC VALVES

Second-generation mechanical prosthetic valves were initially pivoting, hingeless, tilting-disc valves (e.g., Medtronic-Hall, Björk-Shiley) that could be used in the aortic or mitral position (Plate 6.52). These valves consisted of a circular occluder with excursion limited by metal struts. The disc provided two orifices, one large and one somewhat smaller, when in the open position. Both valves do require anticoagulation.

The tilting-disc valves were used for many years until mechanical hinged leaflet valves were developed (St. Jude and Carbometrics bileaflet valves). This type of bileaflet mechanical valve replaced all the previous mechanical valves and is now the most favored type of mechanical valve. These valves have struts attached to the valve ring that contain two semicircular leaflets. The bileaflet valves provide more blood flow than either cage-ball or tilting-disc mechanical valves. In fact, the bileaflet valves have almost a square centimeter opening greater than other mechanical valves. Thrombogenicity remains a problem, but these valves are less thrombogenic than previous versions of mechanical valves. The bileaflet valves do require chronic anticoagulation, but these valves can last 20 years or longer, provided that the patient adheres to a rigid anticoagulation protocol, principally with warfarin. Patients must also be aware that these valves can also cause hemolysis, but that is not a common problem.

A new mechanical valve under development is the ONYX bileaflet valve made of Pyrolite carbon. This valve may require less anticoagulation than previous mechanical valves. Long-term results compared with other bileaflet valves will be needed for further evaluation.

BIOLOGIC VALVES

Bioprosthetic or biologic valves (tissue valves) are made from animal aortic valves (e.g., porcine aortic valves) or biologic tissue (e.g., bovine or equine pericardium). These types of biologic valve are called *xenografts*. When used to form the valve leaflets, pericardium is

SECOND GENERATION OF SYNTHETIC PROSTHETIC VALVES AND BIOLOGIC VALVES

Second-generation synthetic prosthetic valves were hingeless pivoting disk valves and hinged bileaflet valves.

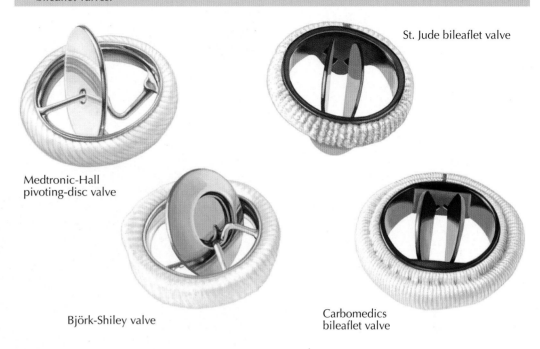

Medtronic-Hall pivoting-disc valve

St. Jude bileaflet valve

Björk-Shiley valve

Carbomedics bileaflet valve

Tissue valves made of porcine aortic valves, pericardium, or cadaver homografts are also important in valve replacement surgical therapy.

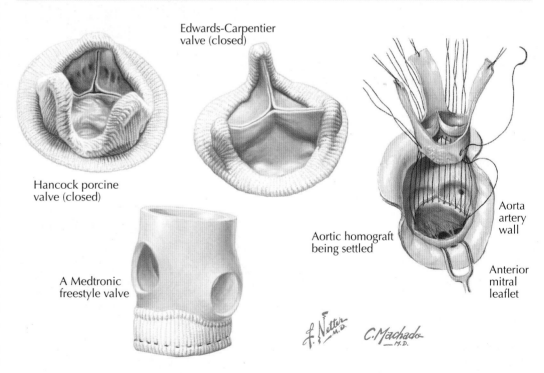

Edwards-Carpentier valve (closed)

Hancock porcine valve (closed)

A Medtronic freestyle valve

Aortic homograft being settled

Aorta artery wall

Anterior mitral leaflet

sewn into a circular metal frame. The valve leaflets are extremely flexible, and patients do not need lifelong anticoagulation with warfarin. These bioprostheses include the Edwards Laboratories Magna bovine pericardial valve, the Mosaic-Medtronic porcine aortic valve, the Medtronic freestyle valve, the Hancock porcine valve, and the Edwards-Carpentier valve (Plate 6.52).

Human valves, called *homografts,* are obtained from human cadavers, usually within 12 hours after death of the donor. The normal aortic valve is removed with

its own support structure in place. The valves are sterilized by the freeze-irradiation method. When implanted in patients, homografts require no anticoagulation. Human valves have minimal residual gradient across the valve and the best hemodynamic performance for the patient. The human valve is often used in patients whose aortic valve is damaged by infective endocarditis. Long-term results are excellent, and replacement of the valve because of deterioration at 10 years is about 10%.

Plate 6.53

Cardiovascular System: VOLUME 8

MITRAL VALVE REPLACEMENT

Right anterolateral thoracotomy

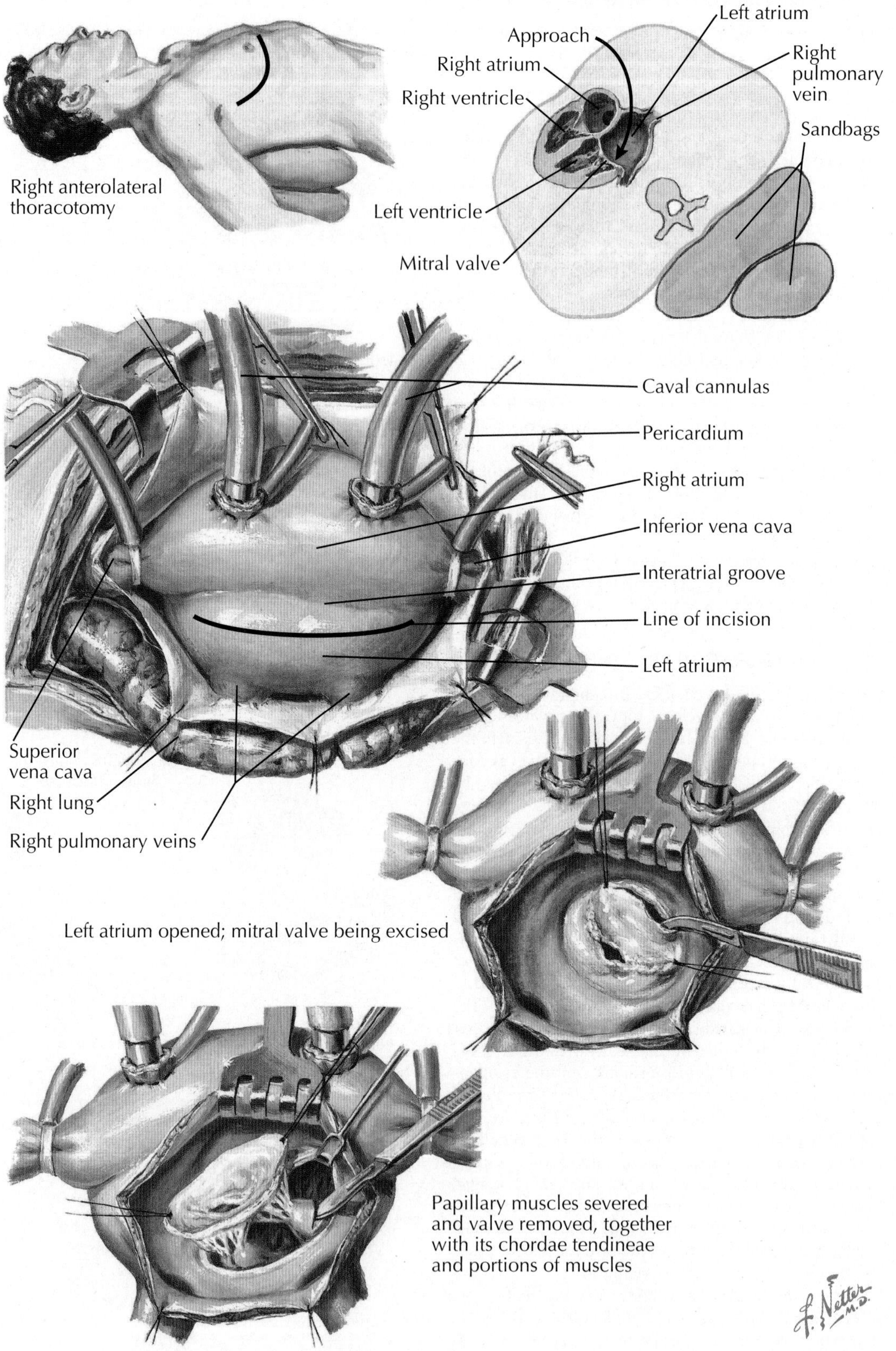

Approach

Left atrium

Right atrium

Right ventricle

Right pulmonary vein

Sandbags

Left ventricle

Mitral valve

Caval cannulas

Pericardium

Right atrium

Inferior vena cava

Interatrial groove

Line of incision

Left atrium

Superior vena cava

Right lung

Right pulmonary veins

Left atrium opened; mitral valve being excised

Papillary muscles severed and valve removed, together with its chordae tendineae and portions of muscles

SURGERY FOR ACQUIRED HEART DISEASE (VALVAR REPLACEMENT)

See previous discussion, "Surgery for Acquired Heart Disease," in Plate 6.51.

Critical goals for improved prosthetic heart valve design are superior flow characteristics, development of prosthetic materials that arouse less adverse reactions in soft tissues or blood, and the elimination of mechanical breakdown. The cage-ball valve of Starr and Edwards was used in the aortic, mitral, and tricuspid areas.

MITRAL VALVE REPLACEMENT

Acquired calcific mitral stenosis is the most common valvular lesion resulting from rheumatic fever and four times more common in females than in males. Patients in New York Heart Association (NYHA) classes II and III are appropriate candidates for surgical relief of mitral stenosis (Plate 6.53). Those in NYHA Class IV, although operable, clearly have a higher surgical risk. Mitral commissurotomy (balloon valvuloplasty or surgery) is still indicated for patients with pure mitral stenosis who have pliable mitral valves detected by physical examination and cardiac ultrasound. Coexisting heart failure is treated, whenever possible, until compensation has been achieved. However, a few patients with severe right-sided heart failure, acute pulmonary edema, or severe hemoptysis may not respond to all forms of medical management and may require emergency mitral valvotomy. Rheumatic activity and bacterial endocarditis are relative temporal contraindications for surgery. On the other

hand, neither pregnancy nor older age represents an absolute contraindication.

When surgery is indicated, a mitral valve procedure under direct vision is the method of choice for managing significant mitral insufficiency, whether alone or with mitral stenosis. Cardiopulmonary bypass (CPB) is also the best technique if the mitral valve is heavily

calcified or mitral disease coexists with aortic or tricuspid valve problems. Also, CPB should be used primarily in most patients with a history of peripheral embolization. Certain patients in NYHA class II, and virtually all in NYHA III and IV are candidates, with less risk for patients in classes II and III. Preferably, all patients will come to operation restored to cardiac compensation by

Plate 6.54

Acquired Heart Disease

AORTIC VALVE REPLACEMENT

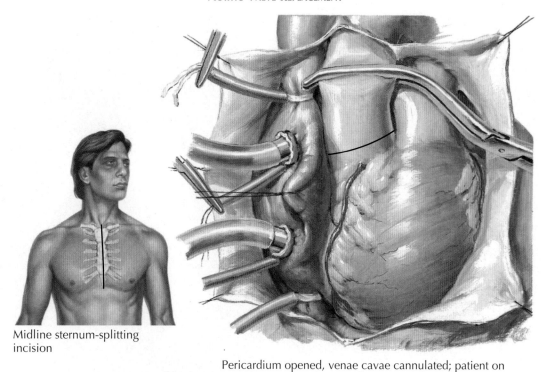

Midline sternum-splitting incision

Pericardium opened, venae cavae cannulated; patient on complete cardiopulmonary bypass with hypothermia; aorta clamped (transverse aortotomy line indicated)

Coronary arteries cannulated and perfused with cold blood; calcified stenotic or incompetent valve excised

Aortotomy sutured: aortic clamp removed before last stitch, allowing air and blood to escape; closure then oversewn with continuous suture

SURGERY FOR ACQUIRED HEART DISEASE (VALVAR REPLACEMENT) (Continued)

an adequate period of appropriate treatment. However, in isolated patients in NYHA class IV, mitral valve replacement may represent the sole remaining resource, and therefore the operation must be undertaken, despite residual cardiac failure.

Prosthetic valve replacement is almost always necessary in severely calcific mitral stenosis. This is not necessarily true for most patients with acquired mitral insufficiency who should have mitral valve repair. An exceptional case of ruptured papillary muscles or chordae tendineae can be realistically corrected by suture approximation of the cusps. Pericardial patch closure of a perforated valve cusp, secondary to bacterial endocarditis, does not require prosthetic replacement. Ring annuloplasty of the mitral annulus, to reduce the size of the valve's orifice and improve the approximation of the cusps, usually accompanies mitral valve repair in patients with mitral regurgitation.

AORTIC VALVE REPLACEMENT

Prosthetic aortic valve replacement has an increasingly significant role in the management of patients with aortic stenosis or insufficiency in whom clinical manifestations of cardiac decompensation, syncope, and angina regularly affect their life activities. This role prevails because patients with hemodynamic evidence of a serious compromise of cardiac function, particularly those with significantly elevated LVEDP, are unlikely to be benefited long

by procedures other than aortic valve replacement. All potential candidates should undergo right- and left-sided heart catheterization (and angiography of the aorta and left ventricle) to evaluate hemodynamic function more precisely. The diseased valve cusps are carefully excised, and calcium is removed from the valve's annulus or even from the LV outflow area, preserving a small valvular

remnant on the wall. Particular care must be exercised to ensure that the upper rim of the valvular prosthesis lies well below the coronary ostia (Plate 6.54).

Aortic Valve Regurgitation

Aortic valve regurgitation can result from not only intrinsic aortic valve disease but also lesions of the

Plate 6.55

Cardiovascular System: VOLUME 8

EXCISION OF AORTIC ANEURYSM AND REPLACEMENT OF AORTIC VALVE FOR CYSTIC MEDIAL NECROSIS

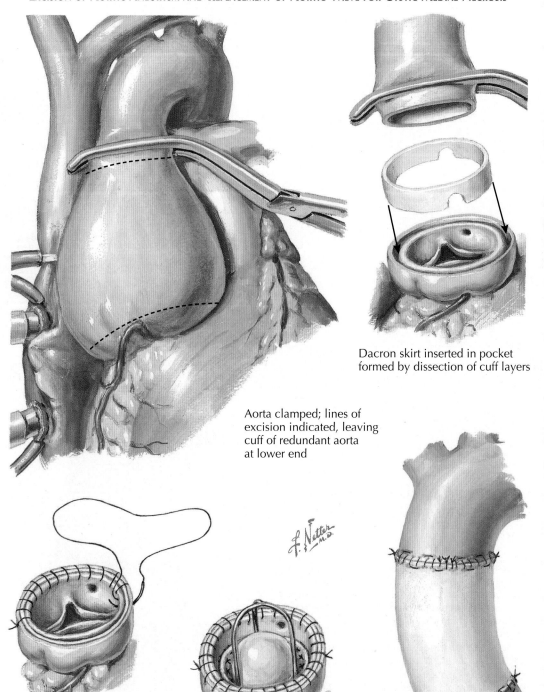

Aorta clamped; lines of excision indicated, leaving cuff of redundant aorta at lower end

Dacron skirt inserted in pocket formed by dissection of cuff layers

Dacron skirt sutured in place by continuous stitch passing through aortic wall, Dacron skirt, and outer layer of cuff, thus reinforcing site of proximal aortic suture line

Aortic valve excised and prosthetic valve sutured in place below coronary orifices

Aortic defect bridged by Dacron graft

SURGERY FOR ACQUIRED HEART DISEASE (VALVAR REPLACEMENT) (Continued)

ascending aorta. Syphilitic aortic disease, aortic dissection, weakness of aortic media (Marfan syndrome), senile or idiopathic aortic dilation, and traumatic nonspecific inflammatory aortic disease may lead to aortic regurgitation because of dilation of the aortic annulus or structural fatigue of the tissue supporting the aortic cusps. Regurgitation may be associated with idiopathic cystic medial necrosis, producing aneurysmal dilation of the ascending aorta (Plate 6.55). The aortic valve is usually tricuspid and contains no calcifications. Aortic regurgitation is secondary to dilation of the annulus, thereby increasing the area of the valvular orifice. The cusps are thinned out, and the free edges of the valve cusps may be rolled. The ascending aortic wall proper is dilated and thinned. Disruption and fragmentation of the elastic fibers occur. At times, early aortic dissection with limited extravasations within the media is observed. These patients may exhibit classic signs and symptoms of aortic regurgitation. Simple anteroposterior and lateral chest radiographs show marked dilation of the ascending aorta. Left-sided heart catheterization and angiocardiography usually confirm the evidence for the diagnosis of massive aortic regurgitation in the presence of a widely dilated ascending aorta.

Surgical Technique

After clinical, ultrasound, and hemodynamic evaluation, surgical correction of the aortic lesion includes prosthetic valvular replacement, resection of the ascending aortic aneurysm, and replacement with a prosthetic graft (Plate 6.55). Through a midline sternotomy, the patient is placed on CPB and moderate systemic hypothermia induced. The aorta is cross-clamped distal to its point of dilation, usually immediately proximal to the takeoff of the innominate artery. The proximal line of resection is about 1 cm above the level of the coronary arterial takeoffs. The aneurysm is completely excised, and the coronary arteries are cannulated and perfused continuously throughout the procedure. Dissecting hematoma within the proximal aortic cuff may be encountered. To obliterate this and particularly to ensure a firmer base for suturing the graft to the diseased and thinned aortic wall, a synthetic polyester (Dacron) skirt is fashioned and positioned within the split residual aortic root. This Dacron cylinder is sutured in place by

Plate 6.56

Acquired Heart Disease

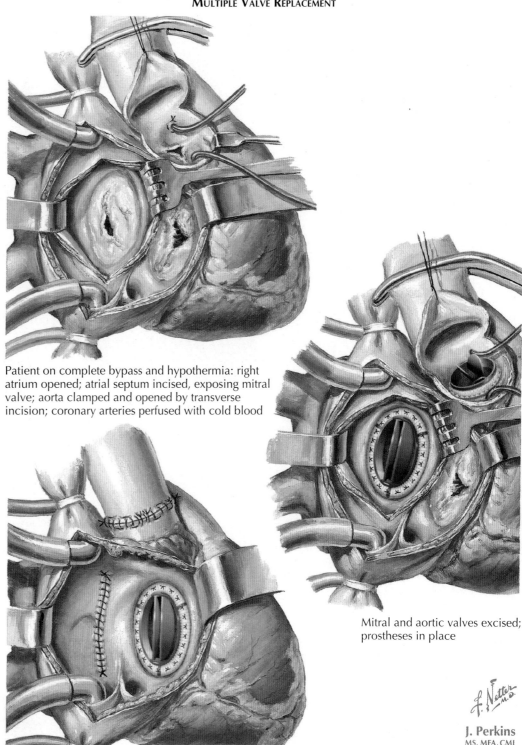

MULTIPLE VALVE REPLACEMENT

Patient on complete bypass and hypothermia: right atrium opened; atrial septum incised, exposing mitral valve; aorta clamped and opened by transverse incision; coronary arteries perfused with cold blood

Mitral and aortic valves excised; prostheses in place

J. Perkins
MS, MFA, CMI

Atrial septum closed: aorta sutured and clamp removed; tricuspid valve replaced as patient is rewarmed

SURGERY FOR ACQUIRED HEART DISEASE (VALVAR REPLACEMENT) (Continued)

continuous stitches, passing successively through the inner aortic wall, the polyester skirt, and the outer aortic layer. This procedure reinforces the proximal aorta. Once this has been accomplished, the aortic valve is resected and replaced by a prosthesis, which may be a composite conduit and valve. Prosthetic valvular replacement is necessary because these secondarily deformed aortic valves are usually not suitable candidates for reconstructive procedures.

MULTIPLE-VALVE REPLACEMENT

Significant involvement of more than one cardiac valve is more complicated to evaluate quantitatively and to manage surgically (Plate 6.56). Aortic and mitral valve disease is the most common combination and requires particularly careful study. The best decision in the more complex cases is based on the physical findings, cardiac ultrasound, left- and right-sided catheterization, and angiocardiographic findings. These data usually provide appropriate qualitative and quantitative estimations of the overall state of valvular disease.

Decisions involving the tricuspid valve are less precisely based on derivable data. In general, however, when serious organic involvement of the tricuspid valve is present, prosthetic replacement is required. On the other hand, functional tricuspid insufficiency, most often in mitral stenosis, usually improves after correction of the primary problem. In many patients the tricuspid

valve can be restored to competency with a ring valvuloplasty, especially if no structural valve damage is present. Thus experience can only partly resolve the dilemma of whether to intervene surgically. Patients who show little or no improvement in signs and symptoms of tricuspid valve disease, despite prolonged intense medical treatment for multivalve-induced cardiac failure, usually require prosthetic tricuspid replacement. The same holds true for patients who, in the presence of normal or near-normal pulmonary artery pressure

(at catheterization), have significant structural damage to the tricuspid valve resulting in tricuspid regurgitation. Surgery provides an additional opportunity for evaluating tricuspid valve function, using intraoperative transesophageal ultrasound while the heart is beating, as well as direct inspection within the atrium after instituting CPB. In general, if the tricuspid valve seems to be structurally damaged, it should be replaced rather than repaired, or a semirigid valvuloplasty ring should be used.

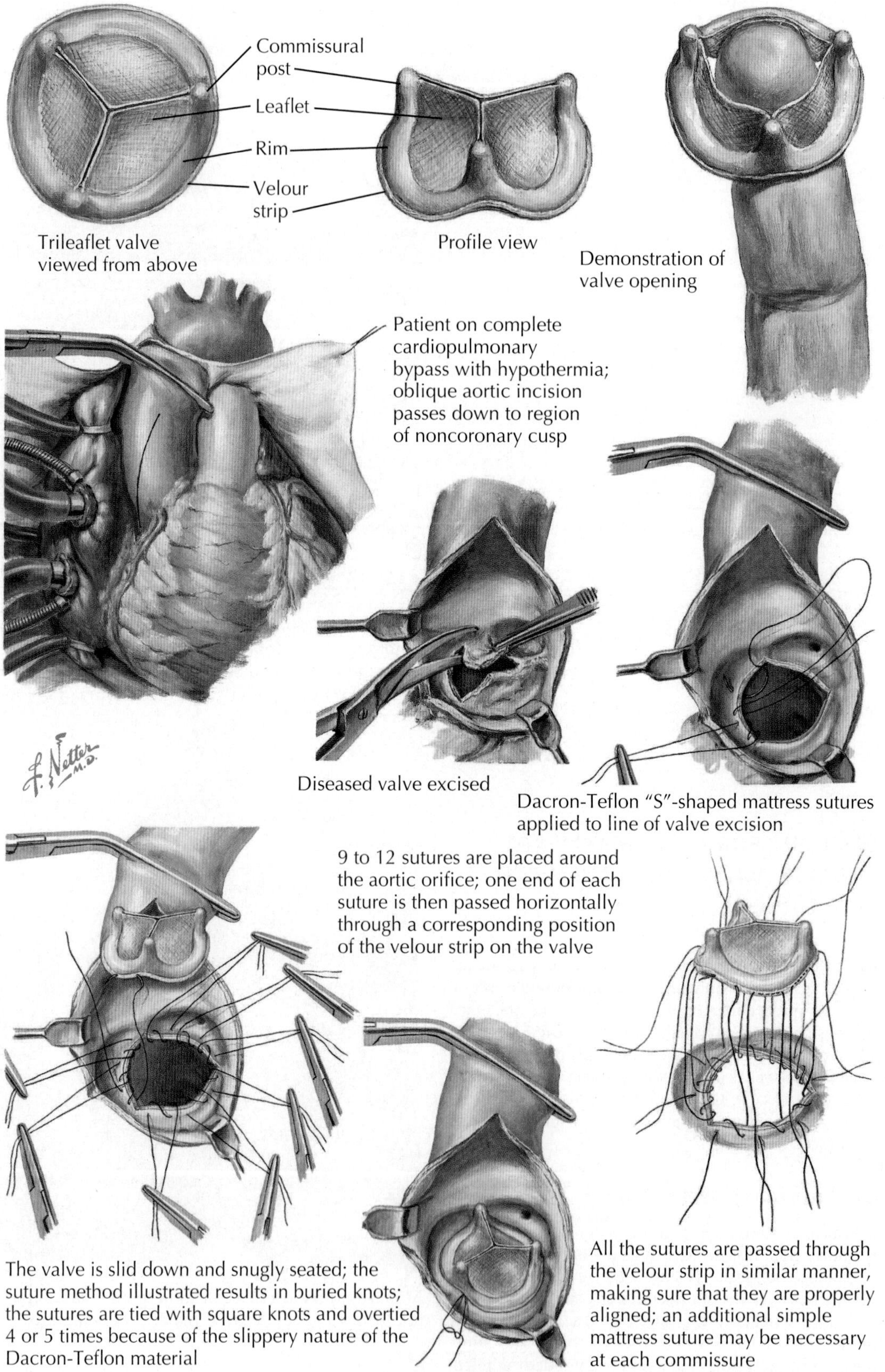

Plate 6.57

Cardiovascular System: VOLUME 8

Commissural post

Leaflet

Rim

Velour strip

Trileaflet valve viewed from above

Profile view

Demonstration of valve opening

Patient on complete cardiopulmonary bypass with hypothermia; oblique aortic incision passes down to region of noncoronary cusp

Diseased valve excised

Dacron-Teflon "S"-shaped mattress sutures applied to line of valve excision

9 to 12 sutures are placed around the aortic orifice; one end of each suture is then passed horizontally through a corresponding position of the velour strip on the valve

Insertion of Trileaflet Aortic Valve

The basic concept of an artificial valvular mechanism that would function permanently and reliably in the human body was first introduced in 1952. Since that time, many variations of the original ball valve have been evolved. The free-floating discoid valve was a later type, first used clinically in 1962. Although all of these variations produced progressively better results, all had an inherent problem as well: the central space was occupied by the occlusive portion of the valve mechanism. All such valves produced an alteration in the direction of blood flow, introduced a resistance imposed by the ball or disc in this area of high-pressure and high-velocity flow, and depended on availability of a marginal or restricted space at the periphery of the occlusive part of the mechanism in the plane of maximum travel.

The *trileaflet tissue valve* embodies the principle of self-suspended flexible leaflets (cusps) and has certain features not previously used in mechanical prosthetic valves. The first leaflet valves were made of polypropylene covered with silicone rubber. Polypropylene is extremely resistant to flexion fatigue, and no other currently available plastic material approaches it in flex life. The three leaflets were suspended from the base within the aortic sinuses, without attachment to the aortic wall at their commissure. This makes closure independent of changes in the aortic diameter and configuration because these may vary widely from individual to individual and under different physiologic conditions. The leaflets are very pliable, and the valve has an extremely low opening pressure. Subsequent trileaflet valves are biologic tissue, either a porcine or bovine valve or an equine pericardial valve.

The proximal orifice of the trileaflet aortic valve is equal to the size of the ventricular outflow area. The profile is sufficiently low to permit the entire valve to lie within the sinuses of Valsalva. The base of the valve follows a scalloped contour that duplicates the configuration of the normal aortic cusp attachments to the aortic root. This was the first valve requiring only secure attachment of its base to the aortic annulus; once this was achieved, valve opening and closure were ensured. Trileaflet aortic valves are lightweight, and

The valve is slid down and snugly seated; the suture method illustrated results in buried knots; the sutures are tied with square knots and overtied 4 or 5 times because of the slippery nature of the Dacron-Teflon material

All the sutures are passed through the velour strip in similar manner, making sure that they are properly aligned; an additional simple mattress suture may be necessary at each commissure

their low resistance to blood flow permits fixation with minimal technical difficulty. Accumulation of clots with subsequent embolism has been a serious problem in previous types of mechanical valvular prostheses and remains so in current mechanical valves that require chronic anticoagulation.

Trileaflet valve sizes must be selected appropriate to the aortic root. Because of the wide valve orifice and the low resistance to flow, care should be taken not to attempt the insertion of an oversized valve; even the smaller trileaflet valves provide an orifice approaching normal. Accurate sizing simplifies insertion.

Plate 6.58

Acquired Heart Disease

AORTIC VALVE BIOLOGIC GRAFTS

Aortic valve replacement using homograft or hetero-graft valves has been evaluated clinically over many years. The advantages of these nonviable tissue grafts are the absence of late peripheral arterial emboli and elimination of postoperative long-term anticoagulation therapy.

The technique of harvesting, preparing, sterilizing, and storing these homograft valves has an influence on their structure and function. Laboratory tests have shown that the freeze-irradiation method of steriliza-tion and storage of the aortic valve homografts causes the least change in their gross morphology and tensile strength. The principal feature of this technique is irradiation of the graft in the frozen state to bactericidal energy levels of 2 to 2.2 megarads in a 5- to 6-second exposure. The packaged sterilized valve (available from valve bank) uses a discolored *quartz bead* as an indica-tor of radiation exposure (Plate 6.58, *A*). The aortic valves are obtained unsterile from autopsy specimens less than 12 hours after death. All valves are trimmed of fat and cardiac muscle to reduce the bulk of muscle that may become interposed between the graft and the host. Careful dissection of the aortic root is required to pre-serve the aortic sinuses. The internal diameter of the valve is measured and recorded before packaging and freezing the graft to −50° C.

A graft is selected equal in size to the internal diam-eter of the patient's aortic root following excision of the diseased aortic valve (Plate 6.58, *B*). The 2- to 3-mm wall thickness of the graft ensures a replacement that is somewhat greater in diameter than the aortic root implant site. The valve selected is reconstituted in warm saline solution under sterile conditions (Plate 6.58, *C*). Excess muscle and mitral valve tissue are trimmed from the homograft valve, leaving a 2-mm rim below the si-nuses of Valsalva. Parts of the homograft aortic wall are excised into the sinuses to accommodate the host's coronary artery orifices. The struts of the aortic wall remaining on the homograft valve will be used later, during implantation, to provide added support for the cusp commissures.

The graft is positioned so that the mitral valve rem-nant lies below the left coronary orifice to reduce bulk and to ensure placement *well below the lumen* of the coronary artery. Sutures are then passed through the base of the homograft from inside out, thus placing the suture line between the host aorta and the graft (Plate 6.58, *D–F*).

The technique of biologic valve implantation is more precise and time-consuming than that required for the artificial prosthesis. Correct positioning and suturing of these grafts are essential for proper valve function postoperatively. The operative mortality and clinical results of aortic homograft valve replacement compare favorably with those reported after insertion of the ball-valve prosthesis. The absence of late peripheral arterial emboli and lack of the need for postoperative anticoagulation therapy are the strongest arguments for the use of the homografts. Postoperative aortic diastolic murmurs have been reported, usually not of hemodynamic significance.

A satisfactory size relationship must exist between the host aortic root and the homograft, and the homograft

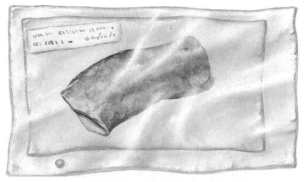

A. Homografts are sterilized by radiation, stored frozen in sealed double-plastic envelopes, and cataloged by size; quartz bead that turns brown on radiation is sterilization control

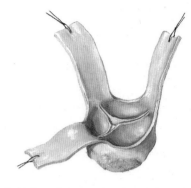

C. Valve of proper size reconstituted in warm saline, trimmed, and shaped

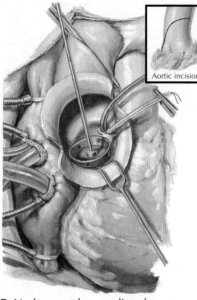

Aortic incision

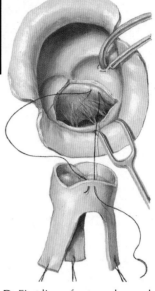

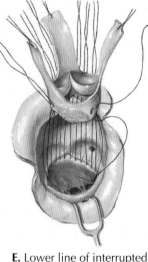

B. Under complete cardiopulmonary bypass and hypothermia, aorta opened by curved incision passing down to noncoronary cusp; diseased valve excised and orifice size determined by calibrated measuring cup

D. First line of sutures begun by a stitch well down in aortic root beneath left coronary orifice and passing outward through lower edge of homograft

E. Lower line of interrupted sutures is continued completely around graft; when homograft is settled into position, knots will be buried between graft and aortic wall

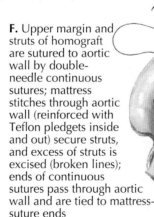

F. Upper margin and struts of homograft are sutured to aortic wall by double-needle continuous sutures; mattress stitches through aortic wall (reinforced with Teflon pledgets inside and out) secure struts, and excess of struts is excised (broken lines); ends of continuous sutures pass through aortic wall and are tied to mattress-suture ends

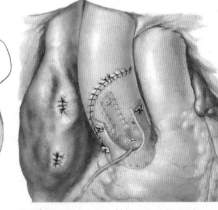

G. Phantom view of homograft in place

valve selected must be large enough in diameter to remain sufficient when the aortic ring is distended by systemic pressure. The graft size selected is based on the internal diameter of the aortic root of the recipient; thus the wall thickness of the graft, 2 to 3 mm, represents the excess area available when the aortic root dilates. Tailor-ing the aortic root helps reduce the diameter of large aortic bases to accommodate the homograft.

Clinical follow-up indicates the aortic homograft valve functions satisfactorily, with no evidence of break-down or restenosis. Late peripheral arterial emboli are rare, and, again, no postoperative anticoagulation is re-quired. Although changes in the design of artificial prostheses will ultimately solve the thromboembolism problem, at present the aortic homograft remains far superior in this regard.

Plate 6.59

Cardiovascular System: VOLUME 8

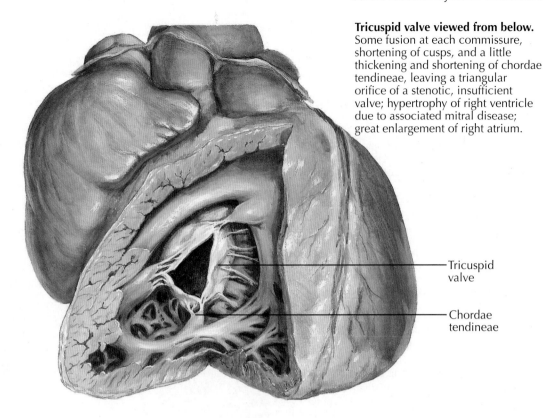

Tricuspid valve viewed from below. Some fusion at each commissure, shortening of cusps, and a little thickening and shortening of chordae tendineae, leaving a triangular orifice of a stenotic, insufficient valve; hypertrophy of right ventricle due to associated mitral disease; great enlargement of right atrium.

Tricuspid valve

Chordae tendineae

Pulmonary valve

Aortic valve

Multivalvular disease viewed from above. Aortic valve stenotic and incompetent from fusion of all three commissures; mitral valve has only a slit-like stenotic orifice; tricuspid valve a triangular, fixed, stenotic, and incompetent orifice; pulmonary valve normal.

Mitral valve

Tricuspid valve

TRICUSPID STENOSIS AND REGURGITATION AND MULTIVALVULAR DISEASE

STENOSIS AND REGURGITATION OF TRICUSPID VALVE

Rheumatic deformity of the tricuspid valve is characterized principally by fusion at each of the commissures and shortening of the cusps; chordal changes are usually minimal. These changes are responsible for reduced caliber of the orifice and incompetence of the valve. The usual coexistence of stenosis and insufficiency in the rheumatic tricuspid valve contrasts with involvement of the mitral valve, often manifested as stenosis *or* insufficiency. One characteristic effect of rheumatic tricuspid valve disease is an enlarged right atrium (Plate 6.59). Chronic rheumatic involvement of the tricuspid valve is rarely if ever an isolated phenomenon; the mitral valve is also involved and, in some cases, the aortic valve as well.

In patients with mitral stenosis and evidence of tricuspid regurgitation, it remains to be determined whether the regurgitation represents intrinsic involvement of the tricuspid valve or is secondary to the mitral stenosis promoting right ventricular failure. Certain features favor secondary tricuspid insufficiency in the patient with known mitral stenosis; congestive heart failure is usually evident. In *intrinsic* rheumatic disease of the tricuspid valve, stenosis and insufficiency usually coexist, whereas in *secondary* tricuspid insufficiency, stenosis is absent. Therefore patients with no signs of tricuspid stenosis must be seen as having secondary rather than primary insufficiency.

MULTIVALVULAR DISEASE

Involvement of more than one valve by deforming rheumatic disease generally consists of disease of the mitral and aortic valves while the tricuspid valve is essentially unaffected. The combination of aortic and mitral disease usually takes the form of predominant mitral stenosis and predominant aortic regurgitation but some aortic stenosis. Both severe primary aortic

Plate 6.60

Acquired Heart Disease

TRICUSPID STENOSIS AND/OR INSUFFICIENCY

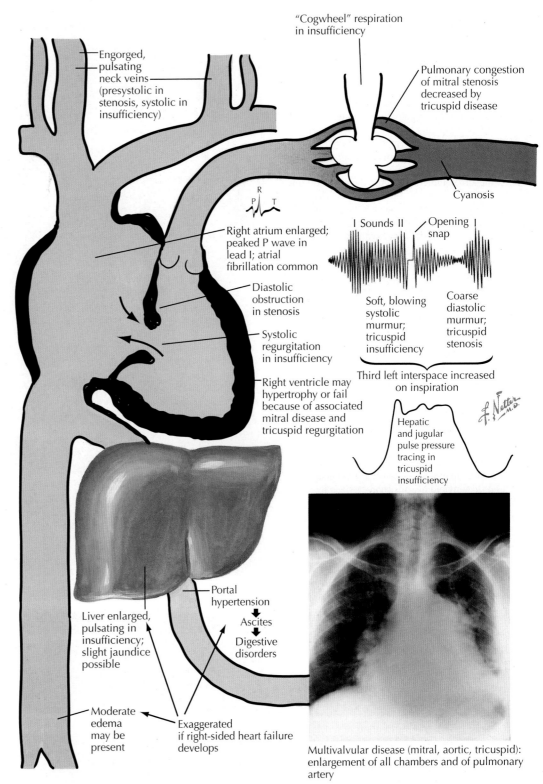

"Cogwheel" respiration in insufficiency

Engorged, pulsating neck veins (presystolic in stenosis, systolic in insufficiency)

Pulmonary congestion of mitral stenosis decreased by tricuspid disease

Cyanosis

Right atrium enlarged; peaked P wave in lead I; atrial fibrillation common

Diastolic obstruction in stenosis

Systolic regurgitation in insufficiency

Right ventricle may hypertrophy or fail because of associated mitral disease and tricuspid regurgitation

I Sounds II   Opening snap

Soft, blowing systolic murmur; tricuspid insufficiency

Coarse diastolic murmur; tricuspid stenosis

Third left interspace increased on inspiration

Hepatic and jugular pulse pressure tracing in tricuspid insufficiency

Portal hypertension
↓
Ascites
↓
Digestive disorders

Liver enlarged, pulsating in insufficiency; slight jaundice possible

Moderate edema may be present

Exaggerated if right-sided heart failure develops

Multivalvular disease (mitral, aortic, tricuspid): enlargement of all chambers and of pulmonary artery

TRICUSPID STENOSIS AND REGURGITATION AND MULTIVALVULAR DISEASE (Continued)

regurgitation and severe primary mitral regurgitation are rarely seen together, possibly because their coexistence tends to be a lethal combination.

When three valves are involved, the pulmonary valve is usually spared of major disease, but the tricuspid valve is affected. In trivalvular rheumatic disease, the lesions of the aortic and mitral valves are generally similar to those observed when only the left-sided heart valves are affected. The tricuspid valve shows the characteristic features of intrinsic rheumatic disease (see Plate 6.59). When multiple valves are involved, the effects on the chambers vary with both the state of compensation of the heart and the dominance of the disease in the various valves. Involvement of the tricuspid valve is universally associated with enlargement of the right atrium. The mitral valvular disease results in right ventricular hypertrophy. When congestive heart failure is present, regardless of the state of the tricuspid valve, the right ventricle is enlarged. In the compensated heart with mitral valve disease and a normal tricuspid valve,

the right ventricle may be of normal size. The pulmonary artery and the left atrium are enlarged because of the high pressure in the left atrium (and thus the pulmonary artery) secondary to the mitral disease.

In patients with multivalvular disease in whom the aortic valve also participates with the mitral valve,

the left ventricle is hypertrophied, but considerably less than observed in patients with isolated aortic valvular disease. The mitral valve disease tends to be associated with a low cardiac output, so the effects of aortic valvular disease, especially aortic stenosis, are minimized.

Plate 6.61

Cardiovascular System: VOLUME 8

AMYLOIDOSIS

Accumulation of insoluble amyloid results in a restrictive infiltrative cardiomyopathy that may occur under four circumstances: (1) as part of primary systemic amyloidosis, (2) as part of amyloidosis complicating multiple myeloma, (3) as part of secondary systemic amyloidosis, and (4) as a localized phenomenon in elderly persons. In *primary systemic amyloidosis*, the liver, spleen, and kidneys are usually found without amyloid deposits. Of 99 patients with primary amyloidosis, 92 showed severe involvement of the heart. Patients with multiple myeloma often develop amyloidosis of the heart.

The clinician should consider the diagnosis of amyloidosis of the heart when chronic, intractable heart failure develops in a patient aged 50 years or older, particularly if the heart failure remains unexplained, even in the presence of the usual symptoms and signs. The heart typically is enlarged, but hypertension is absent. The excursions of the heart are slow, and noncharacteristic murmurs may be heard. Murmurs typical of valvular disease can be detected only if the valves are affected by depositions of amyloid. The ECG indicates a low voltage (Plate 6.61). Disturbances of the atrioventricular conduction may be caused by amyloidosis of the bundle of His and the bundle branches. Cardiac ultrasound with Doppler imaging often reveals a restrictive cardiomyopathy. Cardiac muscle also may "sparkle" on the echocardiogram. Cardiac biopsy and staining with Congo red confirm the diagnosis of amyloidosis of the heart by demonstrating apple-green birefringence under polarized light. Electron microscopic studies of homogeneous amyloid demonstrate delicate fibers thought to be responsible for the effect of the green birefringence. Biopsies of the skin, rectal mucosa, or myocardium may help establish the diagnosis. On ultrasound the amyloid heart is characterized by biventricular thickening, biatrial enlargement, restrictive hemodynamics, and a small cavity with a relatively preserved ejection fraction.

On cardiac biopsy, microscopic homogeneous deposits of amyloid are translucent and refract the light strongly (Plate 6.61). Sections of myocardium stained with Congo red exhibit a network of homogeneous bands surrounding the bundles of myocardial fibers and separating them. The myocardial fibers are compressed and often are atrophied to very flat fibers with pin-like nuclei. The interstices are diffusely widened but not infiltrated by inflammatory cells. The pseudomyocardial hypertrophy explains the insufficiency of both heart chambers. Rarely, as a result of obstruction of a coronary artery by nodular deposits of amyloid, infarction or disseminated necroses of the myocardium may occur. When amyloidosis complicates multiple myeloma (20% of cases), the distribution of amyloidosis resembles that in primary systemic amyloidosis. Cardiac involvement is common.

Secondary typical or *systemic amyloidosis* occurs in diseases with chronic inflammation and severe tissue necrosis, especially chronic tuberculosis of the lungs or other organs. Other primary underlying diseases are bronchiectasis, empyema of the pleural cavities, chronic osteomyelitis, and tumors, as well as leprosy, syphilis, and echinococcosis (hydatid disease). The incidence of secondary amyloidosis has decreased as a result of antibiotic therapy. In systemic amyloidosis, the liver, spleen, and kidneys are affected predominantly, but the heart also may be involved. The depositions of amyloid are much less extensive than in primary systemic amyloidosis of

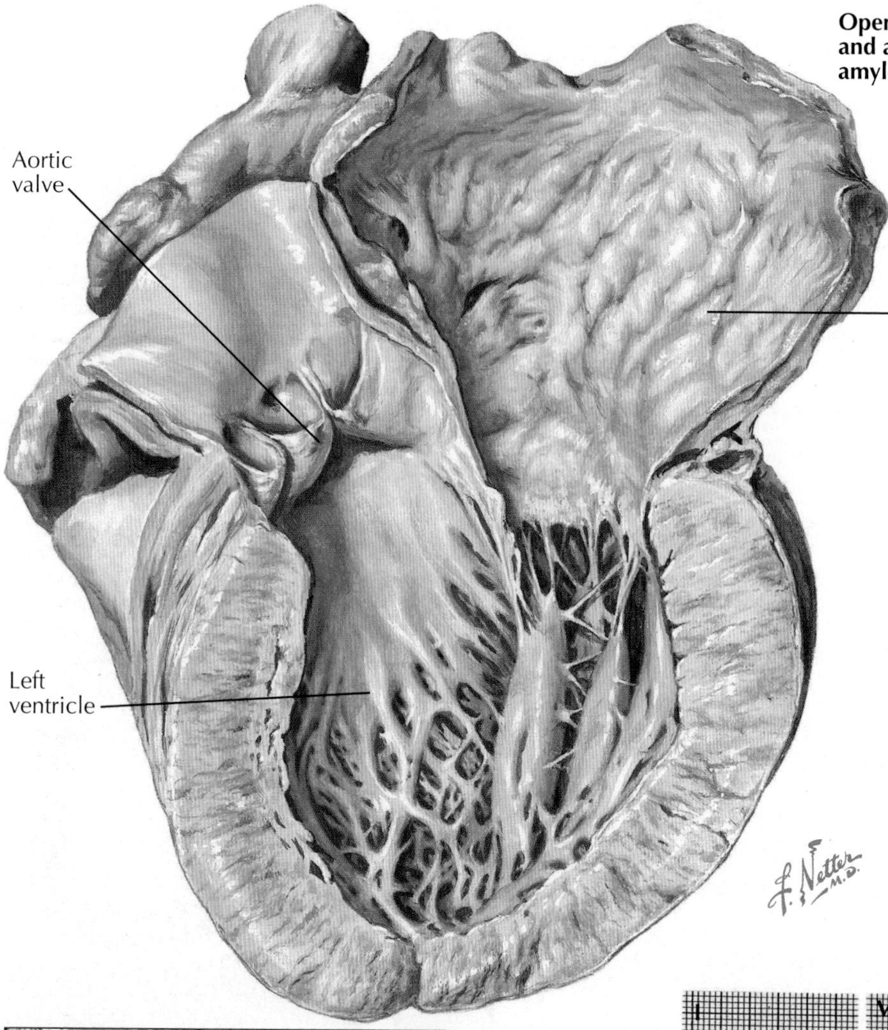

Opened left ventricle and atrium showing amyloid deposits

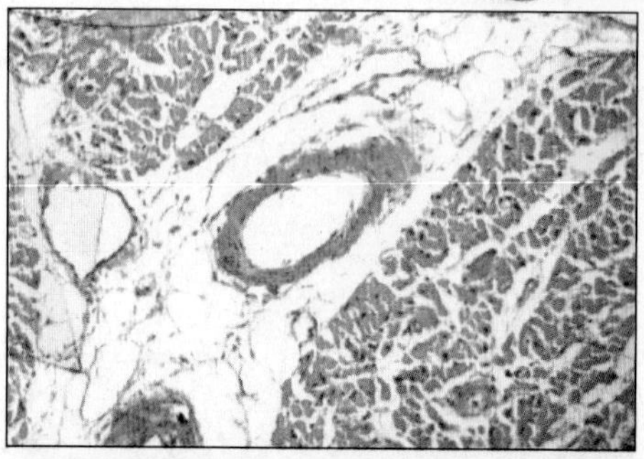

Aortic valve

Left atrium with deposits

Left ventricle

Perivascular amyloid deposits in myocardium

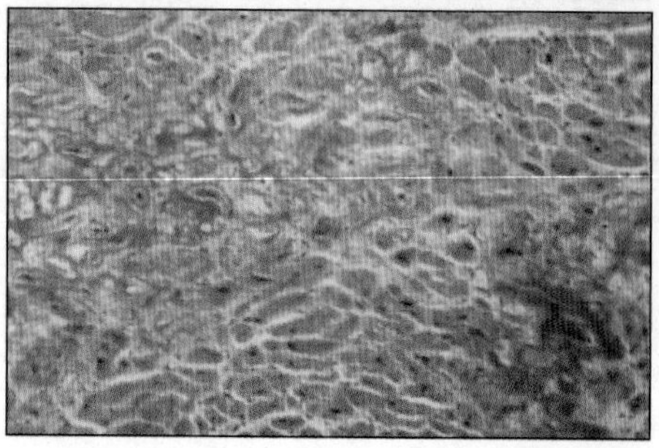

Focal deposition of amyloid around muscle cells of heart with dead myocardial fibers

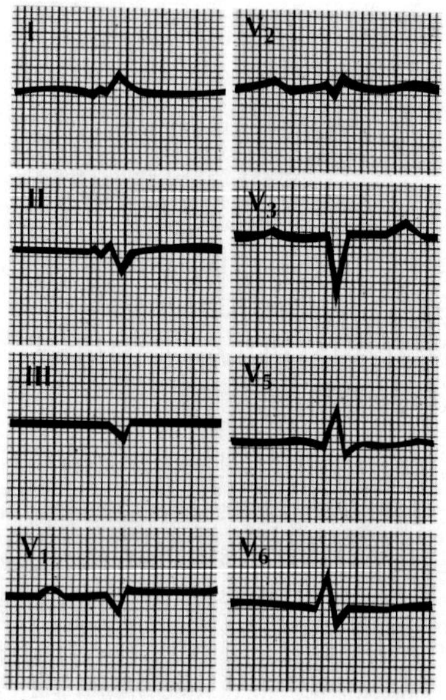

Electrocardiogram in primary amyloidosis of heart, showing extremely low voltage

the heart and demonstrate a different pattern. Amyloid is usually deposited in the media of the arteries and veins and in the capillaries between the endothelial cells and the basement membrane. The lumen of the capillaries remains patent, as in the arteries and veins, and thus the complications are not so serious as in primary systemic amyloidosis of the heart.

Deposits of amyloid may be found in the blood vessels and in relation to myocardial fibers of the myocardium of elderly persons without underlying disease. The incidence of *presenile* or *senile amyloidosis*, which also may involve the brain, is low in patients younger than 60 years. However, the heart can be affected in patients older than 80 years.

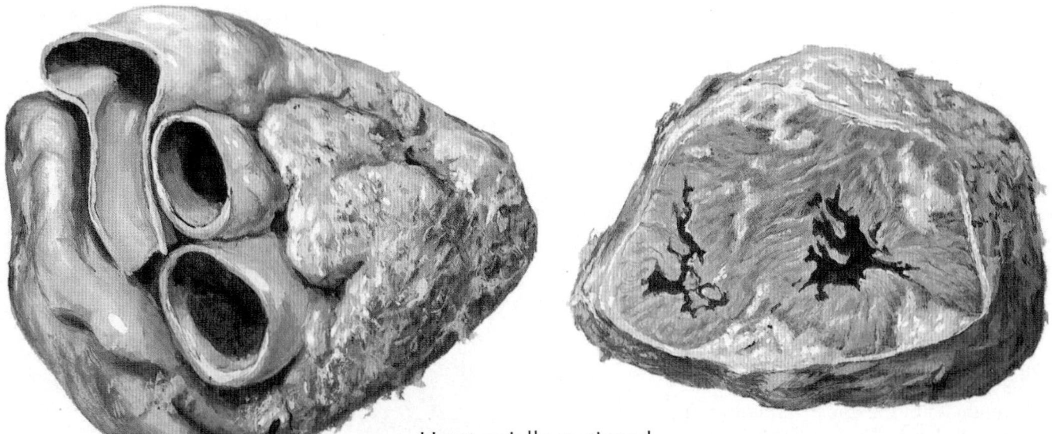

Plate 6.62

Acquired Heart Disease

Heart serially sectioned, revealing multiple intramural and subepicardial abscesses with pericarditis

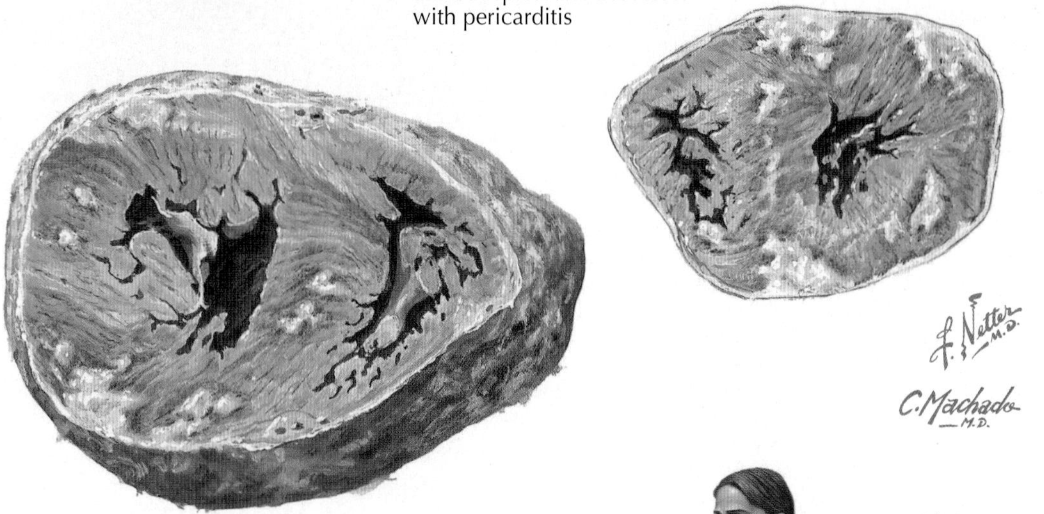

SEPTIC MYOCARDITIS

Septic or suppurative myocarditis can lead to myocardial abscesses and other complications, but it is rarely seen since the introduction of antibiotics, not disappearing completely because of the development of antibiotic-resistant strains of bacteria. The number of known major foci permitting the spread of infection by bacteremia (which precedes suppurative myocarditis) increases with the use of new diagnostic and therapeutic methods, such as indwelling intravascular catheters.

Any virulent bacterium is capable of causing acute septic myocarditis. Newborns, nursing mothers, and patients with previous viral infection are predisposed, as are diabetic and severely burned patients. In some patients the process is associated with or a complication of bacterial endocarditis; in others the valves are not affected. The first nonspecific signs of myocarditis in septicemia are fever, leukocytosis, and shock. Circumscribed areas of necrotic and damaged myocardium may lead to ECG changes. Murmurs can be heard only in patients who have developed endocarditis or pericarditis. Frequently, in the patient with acute bacteremia, no macroscopic changes are visible in the heart because the rapid course of the septicemia does not allow the tissues to react against the spreading bacteria. Clinically, signs of sepsis predominate (e.g., shock).

Diagnosis and treatment of septic myocarditis depend on culture of the myocardial strains. Dense colonies of bacteria within the dilated capillaries and veins are the earliest detectable finding in microscopic sections of the myocardium (Plate 6.62). In later stages these are small abscesses showing abundant bacteria in their centers, with a circular wall of numerous PMNs. The surrounding myocardial fibers can reveal homogeneous cytoplasm with unstained or pyknotic nuclei. The entire focus is surrounded by a hemorrhagic marginal zone.

When the heart is sectioned at autopsy, myocardial abscesses are often visible as small yellow points or stripes, measuring 1 or 2 mm, beneath the thin endocardium of the right ventricle (Plate 6.62). The irregular and bizarre formation of the abscesses is usually determined by the anatomic course of the muscle bundles.

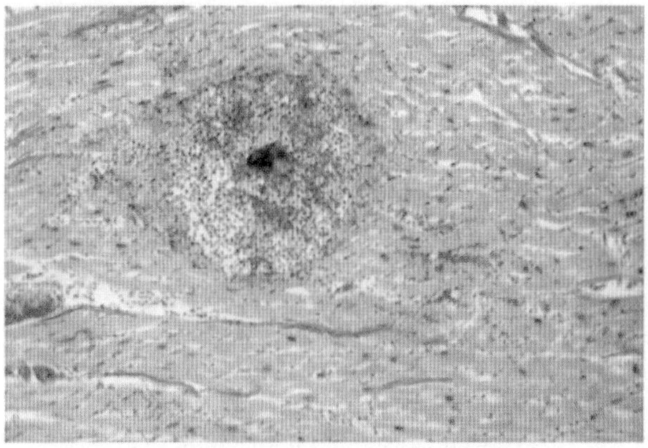

Abscess in heart muscle. Central mass of bacteria surrounded by leukocytes, destroyed muscle, and dilated blood vessels

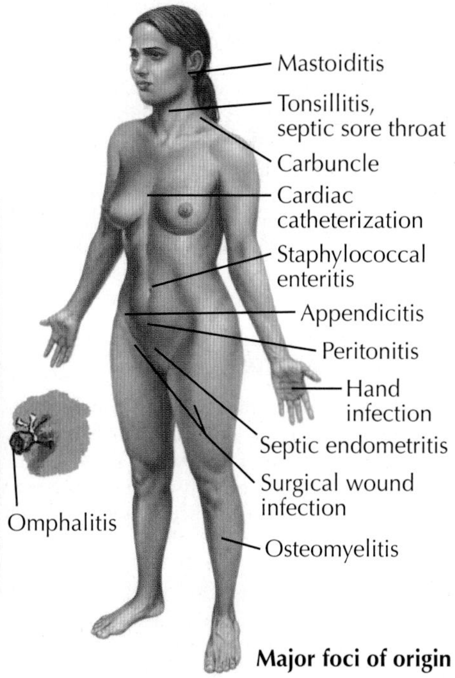

Omphalitis

- Mastoiditis
- Tonsillitis, septic sore throat
- Carbuncle
- Cardiac catheterization
- Staphylococcal enteritis
- Appendicitis
- Peritonitis
- Hand infection
- Septic endometritis
- Surgical wound infection
- Osteomyelitis

Major foci of origin

Subendocardially located abscesses can perforate into the ventricular lumen and cause bacterial endocarditis. Subepicardial abscesses can involve the pericardium as well. Frequently, the focus often can be detected easily, such as after perforation into the pericardial sac, but in a few cases it may be impossible to find. Therefore primary hematogenous spread cannot always be ruled out with certainty.

Microorganisms (viruses, rickettsiae, bacteria, protozoa) or their toxins can produce myocarditis. The morphologic findings alone do not clarify the etiology of myocarditis. Focal or diffuse myocarditis may develop without clinical manifestations. Therefore, to diagnose myocarditis, all clinical information and bacteriologic and virologic examination results should be evaluated together.

Plate 6.63   Cardiovascular System: VOLUME 8

DIPHTHERITIC AND VIRAL MYOCARDITIS

DIPHTHERITIC MYOCARDITIS

In diphtheria of the upper respiratory tract or the result of wound diphtheria, myocarditis is caused by the powerful exotoxins of *Corynebacterium diphtheriae* (Klebs-Löffler bacillus). This type of toxic myocarditis occurred frequently before the introduction of active immunization, and even now small epidemics may occur outside the United States.

In acute diphtheria the heart is flabby, and the myocardial fibers have a boiled appearance. Both ventricles are dilated, and small mural thrombi may be found between the trabeculae (Plate 6.63). The left ventricle, particularly the apex, may be filled with large ball thrombi. Decreasing blood pressure, arrhythmias, and complete heart block may precede acute heart failure. Microscopically, the myocardial fibers are swollen and demonstrate a dust-like fatty degeneration. The interstices are edematous. In subacute cases the myocardial fibers show granular or hyaline necrosis. PMNs and mobilized histiocytes are distributed throughout the interstitial connective tissues.

The secondary inflammatory reactions are frequently arranged focally but also may be diffuse. In the surrounding areas of *toxic necrosis,* circulatory disturbances also may develop, leading to further necrosis. The protracted shock finally affects the coronary blood supply in such a manner that additional disseminated *hypoxic necrosis* occurs. After several weeks the necrotic myocardial fibers will be organized and replaced by fine reticular fibrosis. The extent of such diffuse fibrosis can often be determined only by quantitative methods, measuring the components of connective tissue and myocardial fibers. Fibrosis and even scarring can be so severe that death results from chronic heart failure.

VIRAL MYOCARDITIS

The incidence of viral myocarditis has increased. Known causative organisms in humans are coxsackievirus group, adenovirus, parvovirus, echovirus, Epstein-Barr virus, German measles, and human immunodeficiency virus. The etiology can be ascertained only if virologic examination is successful. Epidemiologic studies can provide only hints about the possible organism. Newborns, infants, children, and adolescents are predisposed. Myocarditis can be preceded by meningitis, encephalitis, pleurisy, hepatitis, and pericarditis, as well as gastrointestinal symptoms. After 3 to 10 days, fever, tachycardia, cyanosis, and, finally, signs of cardiac failure may develop. The ECG reveals severe changes suggesting damaged myocardium (e.g., increased troponin T) or alterations of the conduction system. Radiography shows an enlarged heart. Cardiac ultrasound usually reveals diminished global or regional ventricular function.

Except for dilation of both ventricles, the myocardium appears macroscopically unchanged. Several tissue blocks should be sampled for microscopic examination because viral myocarditis affects the myocardium *focally,* and

Diphtheritic myocarditis

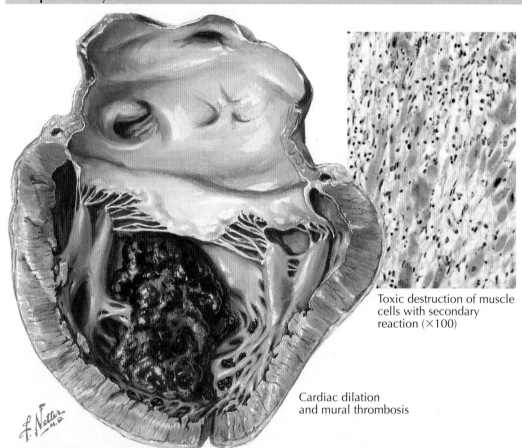

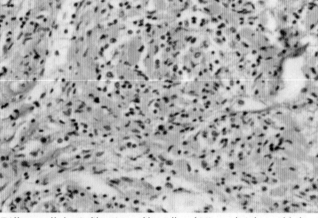

Toxic destruction of muscle cells with secondary reaction (×100)

Cardiac dilation and mural thrombosis

Viral myocarditis

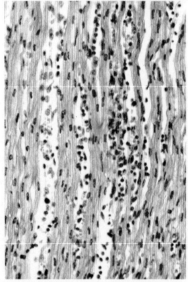

Coxsackievirus group B infection.
Diffuse and patchy interstitial edema; cellular infiltration with only moderate muscle fiber destruction (×100).

Diffuse cellular infiltration of bundle of His and right and left bundle branches (×100)

large areas of the heart may be spared. The histologic findings also depend largely on the stage of the inflammatory process. The first stage of viral invasion into the myocardial fiber can only be studied experimentally. During the next stage, disturbances of cell metabolism, a few or several myocardial fibers may undergo *necrosis.* In the third stage, interstitial accumulations of lymphocytes,

plasma cells, and histiocytes are the predominant features. These third-stage changes are observed most frequently in sections of the myocardium and the conduction system at autopsy. The *diffuse* interstitial fibrosis of the fourth stage does not differ from the fibrosis caused by toxic myocarditis. The extensive scarring may cause chronic congestive heart failure.

Plate 6.64

Acquired Heart Disease

Sarcoidosis

- Brain + (15%)
- Eyes ++ (20%)
- Nasal and pharyngeal mucosa, tonsils + (10%)
- Salivary glands + (1%)
- Lymph nodes ++++ (80%)
- Lungs ++++ (80%)
- Heart ++ (20%)
- Liver ++++ (70%)
- Spleen ++++ (70%)
- Skin ++ (30%)
- Bones ++ (30%)

Relative frequency of organ involvement in sarcoidosis

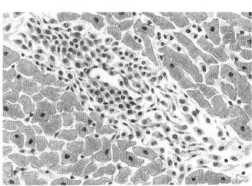

Perivascular infiltration, chiefly of histiocytes in cardiac interstitium

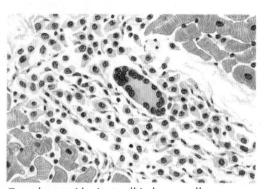

Granuloma with giant cell in heart wall

MYOCARDITIS IN SARCOIDOSIS AND SCLERODERMA

SARCOIDOSIS

Among the forms of interstitial myocarditis, *sarcoidosis* (Besnier-Boeck-Schaumann disease) is second in incidence to rheumatic myocarditis. In sarcoidosis, the lungs, liver, spleen, and lymph nodes are involved much more frequently and extensively than the heart (Plate 6.64). However, the heart may be affected in 20% of all cases, and death may result from myocarditis in 6%. Sarcoidosis of the lungs can lead to pulmonary hypertension and thus right-sided heart failure and cor pulmonale without myocarditic changes.

Myocarditic granulomas are found particularly in the LV myocardium but may also be present in other areas of the heart. Some granulomas measure up to 4 mm in diameter and are recognizable grossly. Granulomas of the right atrium may cause arrhythmias and sinus tachycardia. Granulomas involving the bundle of His and the AV node can lead to abnormalities in atrioventricular conduction (sarcoid of AV node), including complete AV block. Therefore death may occur during Morgagni-Adams-Stokes attacks. At first the myocarditic foci consist of perivascular accumulations of histiocytes. Later, granulomas develop and demonstrate a few Langhans giant cells (Plate 6.64). Finally, granulomas may be replaced by hyaline scars. The recurrent course of the disease may result in diffuse fibrosis of the myocardium. However, the granulomatous lesions are nonspecific. Similar changes can occur in tuberculosis, brucellosis, and tularemia. Therefore the histologic findings can be interpreted only within the context of the clinical situation.

The etiology of sarcoidosis is unknown. Some experts hypothesize that cardiac sarcoid is related to an abnormal immune response to environmental factors (e.g., pine pollen) or infectious agents (e.g., mycobacterium) in a genetically susceptible individual. Sarcoidosis shows a special predilection for Black patients of African descent. More than one case of sarcoidosis can be observed in families or in siblings, for reasons still undetermined.

SCLERODERMA

An interstitial myocarditis can also occur in scleroderma. Myocardial fibrosis may be caused by impaired

Scleroderma

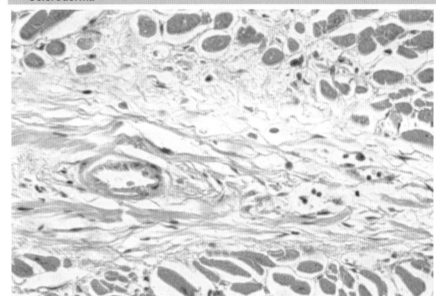

Extensive fibrosis between and around cardiac muscle fibers and in arterial wall, with only moderate lymphocytic and histiocytic infiltration

perfusion secondary to arteriolar and microvascular disease. The focal myocardial lesions consist mainly of lymphocytes and histiocytes (Plate 6.64). In later stages, perivascular interstitial fibrosis progresses, and scarring extends diffusely throughout the myocardium. Similar changes are seen in systemic lupus erythematosus (SLE) and dermatomyositis. Therefore the diagnosis

can be made only after a review of all clinical data. The etiology of scleroderma (*systemic sclerosis*) is unknown. Initially, the disease is characterized by edema and erythema of the skin, followed by hardening and atrophy. In addition to cardiac involvement, other internal organs are often affected, including the lungs, kidneys, and alimentary tract.

Plate 6.65

Cardiovascular System: VOLUME 8

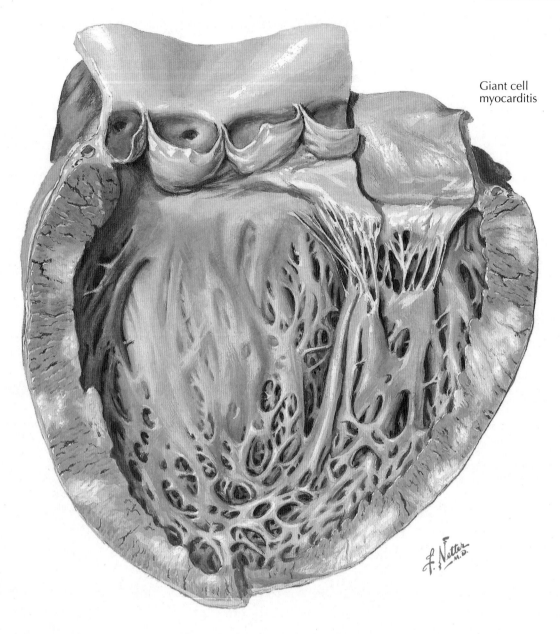

Giant cell
myocarditis

IDIOPATHIC MYOCARDITIS

GIANT CELL MYOCARDITIS

Among the isolated forms of myocarditis of unknown origin, *granulomatous myocarditis with giant cells* should be distinguished. However, giant cell myocarditis can only be diagnosed by endomyocardial biopsy. Animal studies suggest that the disease is mediated by T lymphocytes.

In granulomatous myocarditis the enlarged heart shows dilation of both ventricles and atria and usually weighs 500 g or more. The cut surface of the myocardium has a dim, gray, patchy appearance. The focal lesions are not surrounded by hemorrhagic marginal zones. The coronary arteries are delicate. The typical gross findings often facilitate the diagnosis. Microscopically, the focal granulomatous lesions are composed of dense infiltrates of lymphocytes, plasma cells, and histiocytes, together with giant cells of the Langerhans type. As remnants of

myocardial fibers, giant cells with numerous nuclei may also be present. Other areas of the myocardium show fibrosis. Some cases of giant cell myocarditis also reveal granulomas in other organs, suggesting an association with sarcoidosis. However, as long as the etiology of granulomatous myocarditis with giant cells remains unclear, final classification is still unresolved, although the disease is thought to be caused by T lymphocytes.

The diagnosis of giant cell myocarditis often can be made at cardiac biopsy and at autopsy. Clinical examination reveals an enlarged heart, with passive congestion of the lungs and abdominal organs. Usually the body temperature is not elevated, but in a few cases it may reach septic levels. The ECG shows abnormalities indicating myocardial damage or conduction system disturbances. A diagnosis of giant cell myocarditis is justified only if other causes of cardiac failure (e.g., rheumatic heart disease, idiopathic cardiac hypertrophy, amyloidosis) can be excluded.

ACUTE ISOLATED (FIEDLER) MYOCARDITIS

Isolated eosinophilic myocarditis (Fiedler myocarditis) reveals necroses of myocardial fibers associated with dense interstitial infiltrates of eosinophilic leukocytes, as well as a few lymphocytes and plasma cells. Some believe that viruses cause acute isolated (idiopathic) myocarditis, and others that certain features suggest allergic reactions in the etiology. However, etiology and pathogenesis remain unknown. *Parietal thromboses* may develop over foci located directly beneath the endocardium and may spread as extensively, as in parietal fibroplastic endocarditis. Some patients with eosinophilic myocarditis also develop vascular lesions, as in pericarditis.

Idiopathic myocarditis usually takes a rapid, fatal course and often is called *pernicious myocarditis*. Thus endomyocardial biopsy should be performed urgently and, if positive, high-dose steroids should be administered.

Plate 6.66

Acquired Heart Disease

Endomyocardial Fibrosis

Endomyocardial fibrosis is common in many tropical countries, although cases are seen in temperate regions as well. The pathologic lesion is a scar replacing the endocardium and subjacent myocardium, which is confined to the ventricular inflow areas. A raised, firm ridge marks the junction of the inflow and outflow areas, best seen in the left ventricle. The unscarred part of the endocardium may show a mild opacification from elastomyofibrosis. Lesions may be focally distributed in the inflow area, and the areas of preference are the apex and the site behind the posterior cusp of the AV valve; the cusp adheres to the mural endocardium. In more severe cases, the posterior cusp is lost in a mass of fibrous tissue extending from atrium to apex and partly up the septal and anterior walls, engulfing the papillary muscle and rendering the AV valve incompetent. The AV valves exhibit no specific lesions, and the semilunar valves are entirely unaffected.

On the right side, the ventricular configuration results in filling and obliterating the ventricular cavity with a mass of thrombus and organizing fibrous tissue. This can be recognized externally by a severe recession of the right apex or less often by a recession higher on the ventricular wall. The effective cavity is reduced to a shallow saucer, and fibrous tissue extends upward toward the pulmonary valve; the endocardium immediately below the valve is normal or opacified by elastomyofibrosis. The right atrium may be enormously dilated, similar to a rubber balloon.

In both ventricles the endocardium may be covered by thrombi. Although it may detach and produce a massive embolus in rare cases, the thrombus is usually firmly attached and does not loosen, so infarctions are uncommon. Beneath the thickened endocardium, there are small blood lagoons—dilated thebesian veins—and from these and the endocardial scar tissue, tongues of fibrous tissue extend into the inner third or half of the myocardium but never involve its full thickness. The major coronary vessels are normal; no changes are seen in the minor vessels except for an occasional small focus of inflammatory cells and, in late stages when fibrosis is severe, an obliterative arteritis. Severe calcification may develop in the valve or mural endocardium, which is important radiologically, indicating that the constriction is endocardial, not pericardial, although a large pericardial effusion may be present. No constant extracardiac lesions are seen except for those of congestion. The heart weight may be increased but is often reduced, and despite the voluminous atria, the ventricles often are small and shrunken.

The cause of endocardial myofibrosis is unknown, and the early lesions have not yet been identified. Most cases are seen only when endocardial scarring is advanced. The disease may be biventricular, and the clinical manifestations may change depending on which ventricle is most diseased. If the left ventricle alone is affected, myofibrosis runs a rapid course with severe pulmonary hypertension. If the right side alone is involved, progress is much slower. Patients have high central venous pressure and may show exophthalmos. They have no peripheral edema but severe, extremely

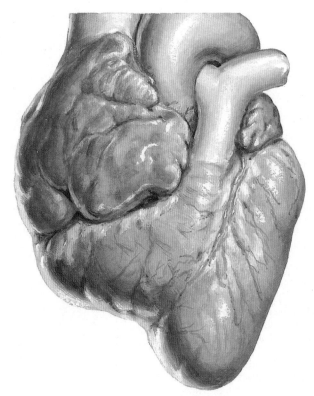

Characteristic recession of right apex, forming bizarre notch: enlargement of right atrium

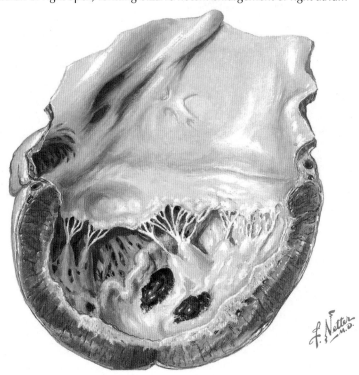

Dense collagen layer lining left ventricle, involving posterior papillary muscle and chordae tendineae, demarcated by a ridge, sparing outflow tract; posterior mitral cusp adherent to wall; mural thrombi

tense ascites with high-protein fluid. The liver is exceptionally large.

Differentiation from constrictive pericarditis may be extremely difficult in some cases, but diagnosis of endomyocardial fibrosis has been greatly facilitated by cardiac ultrasound and angiocardiography. The posterior AV valve cusp is severely damaged regardless of the ventricle affected, with resulting mitral and tricuspid incompetence and usually stenosis. The early lesion

may be a pyrexial form of carditis, followed shortly by evidence of progressive cardiac damage. Whatever the cause, the pathogenesis is destruction of the endocardium and underlying myocardium of the ventricular inflow areas, with the formation of scar tissue. Elastic tissue in the affected areas is almost entirely lost, and elastosis is infrequently seen, except at the edges of the scar. No significant diagnostic blood changes have been found.

Plate 6.67

Cardiovascular System: VOLUME 8

Brain

Multiple embolic infarcts
(lung, brain, spleen, kidney)
and diffuse arteriolitis

Heart
enlarged

Liver
enlarged

Ascites

Edema

Leukocytosis,
eosinophilia

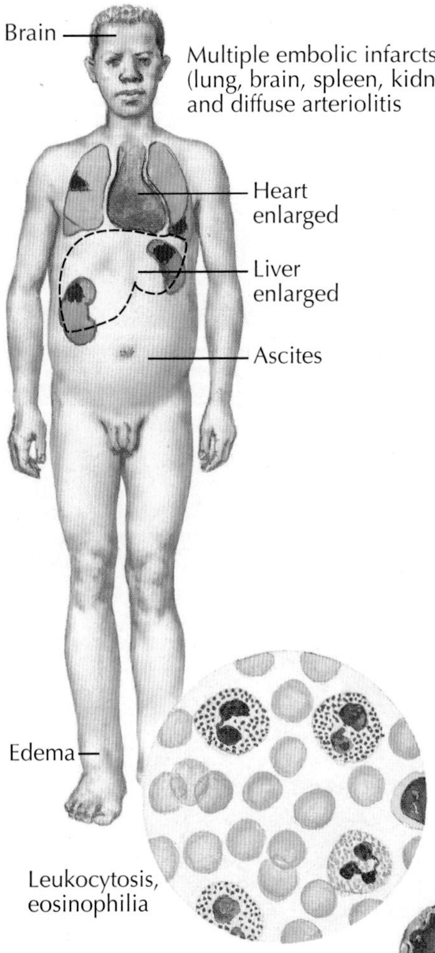

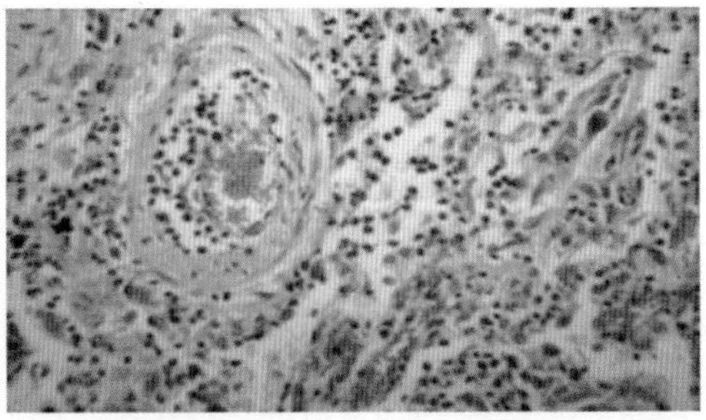

Acute eosinophilic endarteritis in lung; similar lesions
occur in small vessels of brain, kidney, and other organs.

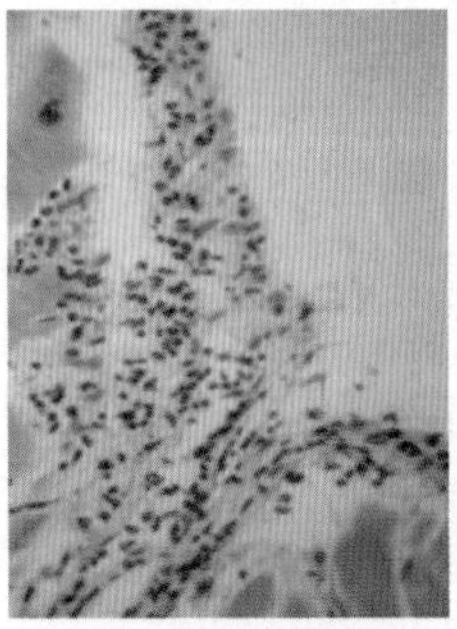

Acute eosinophilic and
neutrophilic infiltration
of subendocardium

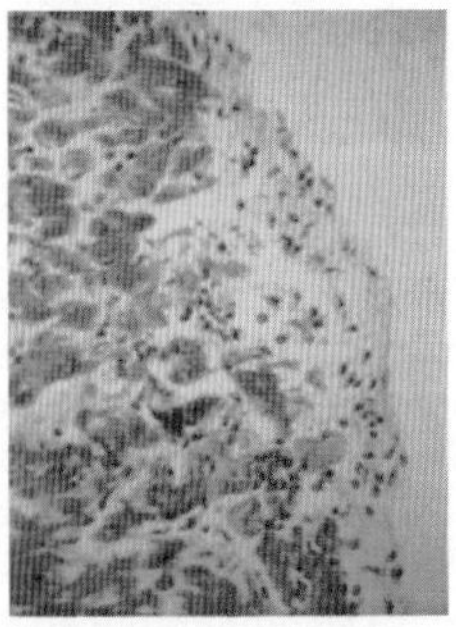

Eosinophilic infiltration
and early myocardial
damage

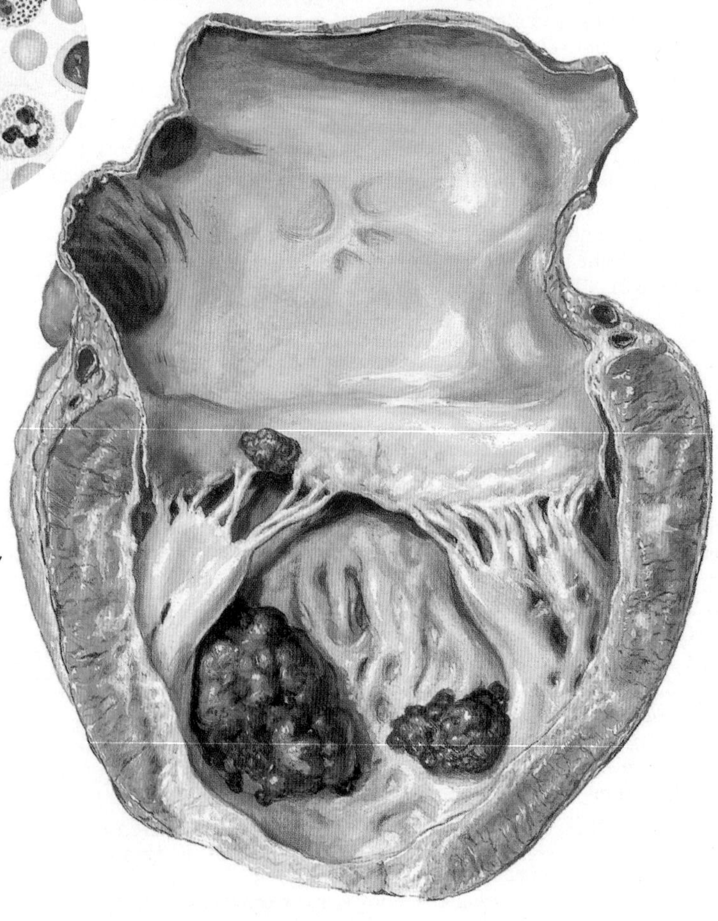

LOEFFLER ENDOCARDITIS

Loeffler endocarditis, or *eosinophilic endomyocardial disease*, is an uncommon but distinctive form of disease in which the heart is the organ mainly affected by eosinophilic arteritis, probably allergic. Males are affected most often, and the disease occurs between ages 7 and 65 years. The disease has worldwide distribution, and no specific cause of Loeffler endocarditis is known. At autopsy the changes of congestive heart failure are seen, usually with considerable effusion into the serous cavities. Fresh or older infarcts are often found in the brain, kidneys, and other organs. The heart may be of normal size but is usually enlarged, either generally or only on one side, most often the left. In acute cases, minimal change may be observed, except marked pallor of the endocardium and subjacent myocardium. However, electron microscopy shows swelling and necrosis of the endothelial cells, an eosinophilic infiltration of both the endocardium and the thebesian veins, focal necrosis of myocardial fibers with an eosinophilic infiltration, and an eosinophilic arteritis of the small coronary arteries with an occasional focus of fibrinoid necrosis. A similar eosinophilic arteritis is found in the small arteries of the brain, kidneys, lungs, and striated muscle, but the main coronary arteries are not involved.

More advanced cases will show extensive lesions. The endocardium is thickened and scarred, gray-white in color, and covered with mural thrombi, both atrial and ventricular, in varying stages of organization and attachment. Scar tissue may cover the papillary muscle and shorten and thicken the chordae tendineae, thus distorting the AV valve, which itself usually exhibits valvulitis with vegetations. The semilunar valves may also show these lesions. The myocardium has areas of necrosis, sometimes with frank hemorrhage, organization, and scarring; the lesions often involve the full thickness of the ventricular myocardium. Between the myocardium and the thickened endocardium, small blood lagoons may be detected in dilated thebesian veins. A great eosinophilic infiltration usually is present in the necrotic and fibrosing areas of the myocardium. The cells are also abundant in the thickened endocardium. The original endocardium is largely destroyed, replaced by scar tissue with some elastosis. In more chronic cases, tissue eosinophilia may diminish or disappear, the arteries show only an obliterative arteritis, and severe endomyocardial scarring is found, usually maximal at the apex and spreading to involve the endocardial inflow and outflow tracts.

The basic arteritis may result in cerebral, abdominal, or renal manifestations initially or arthralgias, muscle pains, and, in some cases, polyneuritis. The symptoms may present acutely with a fulminant course or slowly with a progressive evolution. In a special patient subgroup, the endocarditis develops after several years of attacks of respiratory disease with bronchospasm. Cardiac decompensation develops, often with major embolic accidents. Pyrexia is common. Radiology may demonstrate cardiac enlargement, and ECG evidence

Greatly enlarged heart: extensive
fibrosis of endocardium and
subendocardial myocardium
with extension through entire
thickness of heart wall and
involvement of papillary muscles,
chordae tendineae, and valve
cusps; mural thrombi

may suggest necrosis, especially of the subendocardial myocardium, and probably confirmed by cardiac MRI. Mitral insufficiency may develop. High blood eosinophil count is most important in diagnosis, with levels as high as 130,000 cells/mm³ reported. The eosinophilia may not be marked or even present at the onset, and it frequently diminishes and may disappear terminally or in the chronic stages, when the disease may closely mimic all the signs and symptoms of a constrictive pericarditis.

The important points in distinguishing Loeffler endocarditis are blood and tissue eosinophilia (in the endocardium and myocardium particularly), eosinophilic arteritis, endocardial scarring which may involve the inflow or outflow areas, valvulitis, and involvement of the whole thickness of the ventricular myocardium.

Plate 6.68

Acquired Heart Disease

BECKER DISEASE

Becker disease occurs in all races in South Africa but is found in other areas as well. It appears to be a specific type of heart disease; the basic lesion is a form of *verrucous angiitis* that especially affects the subendocardial blood vessels. The lesions found at autopsy reflect the acuteness or chronicity of Becker disease. At any stage that death occurs, severe lesions of congestive heart failure with large effusions in the serous cavities are found, as well as multiple infarctions in the lungs and often in the brain, spleen, kidneys, and other organs as well. The heart is greatly dilated and usually considerably heavier. Mural thrombi are present in the ventricles and may be small or may cover two-thirds of the mural endocardium, interfering mechanically with AV valve function. The heart valves show no specific lesions, and the main coronary arteries are normal. In acute cases, the endocardium not covered by thrombus is neither thickened nor opaque, although a fine surface deposition of fibrin may be seen. Small, dark spots may be visible, representing hemorrhagic polyps on the endocardial surface. In acute cases, pallor of the myocardium under the mural thrombi is seen, and in the later stages, small areas of granulation tissue and streaks of fibrous tissue are visible in the inner third of the myocardium. In more chronic cases, irregular plaques of fibroelastotic endocardial thickening are found, scattered irregularly over the inflow and outflow tracts but most evident at the apex. The hearts often are stiff and rubbery with a curious tan or yellowish color.

Microscopically, progressive changes are recognizable. In the acute stage of Becker disease, the endocardium is thickened with a serous and mucinous edema, and it may be acellular or infiltrated with inflammatory cells, wholly polymorphonuclear or mixed in type. Fibrin is diffusely or focally deposited on the endocardial surface, and, where damage is severe, the thrombus accretes. The focal fibrin deposits may form polyps, and hemorrhaging polyps may produce the black spots. The deposited fibrin and elastic tissue proliferation organize into the fibroelastotic plaques of the late stages. A verrucous angiitis of the subendocardial vessels commences with ectatic dilation and deposits of fibrin on the walls. These may develop into narrow-stalked polyps, which break loose and produce microembolic lesions, or the fibrin deposits may be organized into a fibrinofibrous cushion, rich in capillary tissue, to one side of the vessel or occasionally occluding it. Similar changes are found in pulmonary blood vessels. In the acute stages, the myofibers show little change, and the loss of striation, nuclear hyperchromatism, and fragmentation appear to be anoxic. Interstitial edema may be marked, and the changes are confined to the inner third of the myocardium. In the chronic stages, some interstitial fibrosis may develop. Small perivascular inflammatory cell infiltrates may be seen, but usually minimal myocardial inflammatory cell infiltration is seen.

The cause of Becker disease is unknown. It may develop acutely, with severe congestive heart failure, and the serous effusions are typically out of proportion to the severity of the cardiac failure. Abdominal pain from acute liver congestion may be intense. There is often a fever with PMN leukocytosis but no eosinophilia with tachycardia or cardiomegaly. Radiology reveals only an enlarged and flaccid

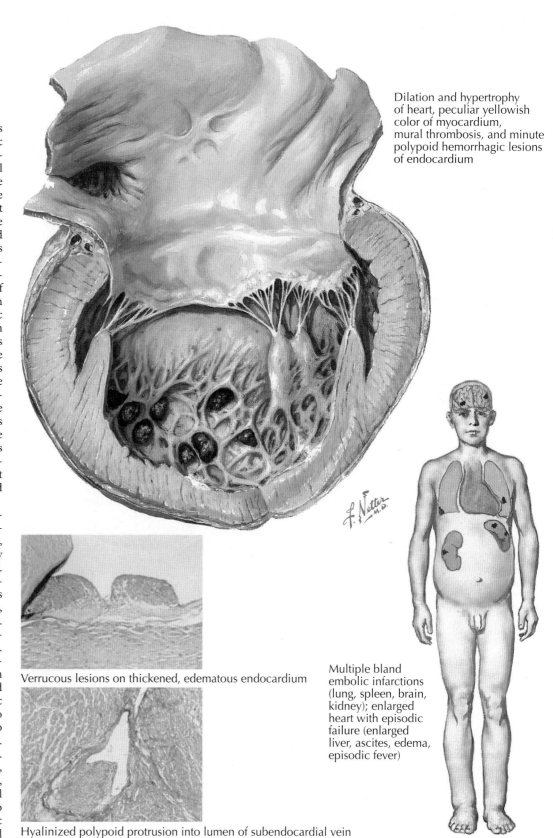

Dilation and hypertrophy of heart, peculiar yellowish color of myocardium, mural thrombosis, and minute polypoid hemorrhagic lesions of endocardium

Verrucous lesions on thickened, edematous endocardium

Hyalinized polypoid protrusion into lumen of subendocardial vein

Multiple bland embolic infarctions (lung, spleen, brain, kidney); enlarged heart with episodic failure (enlarged liver, ascites, edema, episodic fever)

heart. ECG changes are not distinctive, and low-voltage patterns are usual. Embolic episodes, large or small, are common. The patient may progress to death in cardiac failure, unresponsive to all treatment, or may recover completely. After a variable interval, relapse occurs, which may result in recovery or death. The episodes may be repeated over many months, with the intervals of improvement progressively shorter and periods of congestive failure progressively protracted. Treatment at all stages is disappointing because Becker disease is refractory to all therapy. Ultimately, death occurs, often rapidly, in a final episode of heart failure.

Pathologically, the cardiac lesions in Becker disease can be recognized by the enlargement and stiffness of the heart, the fibroelastotic patches, and the distinctive verrucous angiitis of the subendocardial blood vessels.

Plate 6.69

Cardiovascular System: VOLUME 8

BERIBERI

The term *beriberi* should be confined to the lesions that result from a dietary deficiency of thiamine. *Cardiovascular beriberi* is seen as a fulminant disease of small, breast-fed infants, reflecting severe thiamine deficiency in the mothers. It has a seasonal incidence, as does adult cardiovascular beriberi, in regions where the disease is caused by a diet deficient in a simple staple such as husked rice. Small epidemics may occur in prisons, camps, and fishing boats. Beriberi is sometimes seen as an acute disease in alcoholic patients with a restricted diet. The crucial feature of all these types is that they respond to adequate thiamine quickly, except in the most severe terminal cases. The response is rapid and dramatic.

The circulatory rate in cardiovascular beriberi is extremely rapid, with bounding pulse and increased blood pressure. "Pistol shot" sounds are heard over the extremities, and the hands and feet are warm despite peripheral edema of rapid onset; ascites may occur, possibly with polyneuritis. The heart must increase its workload to meet the demand of this hyperkinetic circulation, and the rapid return of blood to the heart leads to disproportionate right-sided dilation and hypertrophy. The basic change apparently is in the peripheral circulation, with a great opening of arteriovenous anastomoses, especially in striated muscles. The initial effect of thiamine seems to be on the peripheral circulation; the workload on the heart is abruptly diminished, and rapid alteration in heart size and rate results. These changes are so rapid that thiamine administration can be used as a therapeutic test for cardiovascular beriberi. When terminal, death results from the sudden failure of the heart to meet the sustained call for high output. The terminal failure may be sudden, with severe pulmonary edema.

It has been impossible thus far to define specific changes caused by thiamine deficiency in human hearts with cardiovascular beriberi. The hearts invariably exhibit a degree of right-sided dilation and hypertrophy, but the microscopic findings may show only myofiber hypertrophy, with enlargement and hyperchromatism of the nuclei, which are cigar shaped or blunt ended. Watery vacuolation of the myofibers and interstitial edema have often been recorded, along with fatty infiltration and varying degrees of myocardial fibrosis. These changes seem to reflect the patient's general nutritional status rather than specific lesions of thiamine deficiency. These lesions do not resemble those found in animal models of thiamine deficiency. The animals die suddenly, showing focal patchy necrosis of muscle cells with an inflammatory infiltrate. Lesions of this type are not reported in humans. The lesions seen in animals are similar to those induced by extreme potassium deficiency, but a combination of thiamine and potassium deficiency does not produce the lesions.

In Western countries, a high-output cardiovascular disease seen in patients with alcoholism may respond completely to thiamine administration. Some patients taking thiamine may have their status changed from high-output failure to low-output failure, in all probability the result of an alcoholic cardiomyopathy.

Nutritional deficiencies in humans only rarely are caused by lack of a single essential dietary element. Thiamine deficiency may occur in otherwise well-nourished individuals; most patients have diets typically low in protein and fat but high in carbohydrates, thus developing multiple deficiencies. Because its administration is so effective in cardiovascular beriberi, thiamine should be given as quickly as possible. If improvement does not follow, or if only some cardiovascular modifications are altered, the remaining cardiovascular lesions are from some cause other than thiamine deficiency. In light of current views on the metabolic derangements in thiamine deficiency, it seems unlikely that a state of chronic beriberi heart disease could exist.

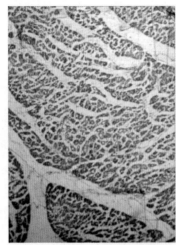

Vacuolation of cardiac muscle with interstitial edema (chiefly on right side)

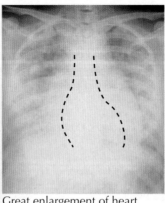

Great enlargement of heart (broken line indicates return to normal after thiamine administration)

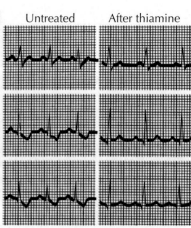

Untreated   After thiamine

Tachycardia, low voltage, ST-segment and T-wave abnormalities; return to normal after thiamine

Pulmonary circulation

Right heart failure, enlarged

Left heart tachycardia, increased output

Liver congested, enlarged

Hypertension

Increased venous pressure

Portal circulation ascites

Blood decreased colloid osmotic tension

Systemic circulation edema

Plate 6.70

Acquired Heart Disease

CARDIAC MYOPATHIES POSSIBLY DUE TO VARIOUS METABOLIC CAUSES

CARDIOMYOPATHIES

In any cardiac clinic, an occasional patient is seen who exhibits evidence of cardiac disease, typically with a greatly enlarged heart but with no evidence of valvular disorder, coronary artery disease, or hypertension. The term *nonischemic cardiomyopathy* is often used with these patients. Clues to the cause and nature of the disease may be found in the family history, a past episode of infections, or evidence of accompanying endocrine disturbance, a generalized vasculitis, or some form of systemic disease. Hemochromatosis, amyloidosis, glycogen storage disease, and nervous system disorders must be excluded and evidence of a persisting or past episode of bacterial, viral, or protozoal disease evaluated.

The cause of the cardiomegaly is still obscure in some patients, including females later in pregnancy or in the postpartum state, called *peripartum cardiomyopathy*. There is a sizable group of patients worldwide with "idiopathic cardiomegaly." Many are suspected to have malnutrition or a history of alcoholism (often difficult to elicit in detail), which indicates thiamine deficiency, but administration often produces no improvement. Some patients may recover spontaneously, only to relapse later with a later pregnancy. In some the cardiomyopathy may progress rapidly and relentlessly, or slow deterioration may occur. Physicians should be alert to epidemics, particularly with *beer drinker's cardiomyopathy*. In many cases, alcohol is the most important factor, although similar conditions also affect those who do not drink alcohol.

Radiologic and ultrasonic examination is usually unhelpful other than in demonstrating a grossly enlarged heart, which typically continues to increase in size. The ECG usually is abnormal, but the abnormalities are nonspecific (e.g., left bundle branch block, T-wave changes). Cardiac ultrasound and MRI confirm the poor contraction. Ultrasound can easily define chamber dilation and decreased ejection fraction. Unfortunately, if the cause was not found in life, it cannot be satisfactorily established at autopsy. Evidence of congestive heart failure is found with an enlarged heart, compounded by varying degrees of hypertrophy and dilation. Some degree of coronary arteriosclerosis may be found, especially in communities where beriberi is common, but this is usually insufficient to explain the ventricular derangement. The coronary vessels are often normal or may be widely patent. The myocardium is often soft and flabby or may be stiffer than normal and exhibit pallor, with evidence of myocardial fibrosis. The endocardium may be normal or covered in part by mural thrombi or may be patchily thickened and opaque.

The histologic changes in cardiomyopathy may also be indeterminate, and some patients may show only hypertrophy of myocardial fibers, with enlarged, hyperchromatic, blunt-ended or cigar-shaped nuclei. Watery vacuolation of myofibers may occur, perhaps with some accumulation of lipid droplets. The myofibers may be separated by interstitial edema. Diffuse fibrosis or focal scars may be present. Cellular infiltration of variable intensity is seen; the cell types vary but typically include

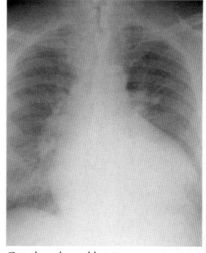

Greatly enlarged heart

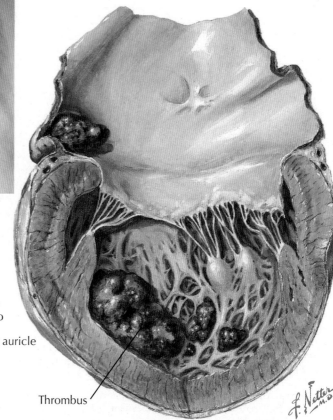

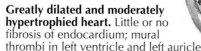

Greatly dilated and moderately hypertrophied heart. Little or no fibrosis of endocardium; mural thrombi in left ventricle and left auricle

Thrombus

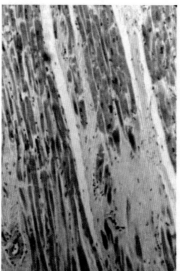

Diffuse foci or irregular fibrosis, replacing cardiac muscle fibers

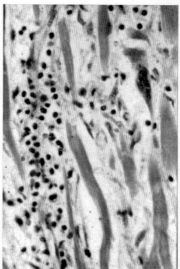

Infiltration of cardiac muscle with lymphocytes and monocytes; edema and occasional giant cell

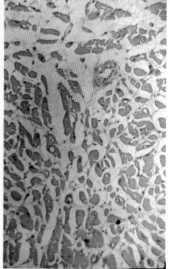

Vacuolation of myocardial fibers and interstitial edema similar to that seen in beriberi

an infiltrate of lymphocytes and monocytes and occasionally a giant cell. Histochemical studies may show greatly diminished numbers of oxidative enzymes.

Study of the endocardial lesions, especially areas of endocardial thickening, may help elucidate the pathogenetic mechanisms in cardiomyopathy. Considerable endocardial smooth muscle hypertrophy indicates previous acute cardiac dilation. Pathologic study should

include carefully oriented blocks and exact mapping of lesions, as well as careful correlation with any extracardiac lesions, to identify the causes of these presumed metabolic cardiomyopathies. However, meticulous clinical history taking into the patient's background and circumstances surrounding onset of cardiomyopathy is most important. As a rule, only symptomatic relief can be given.

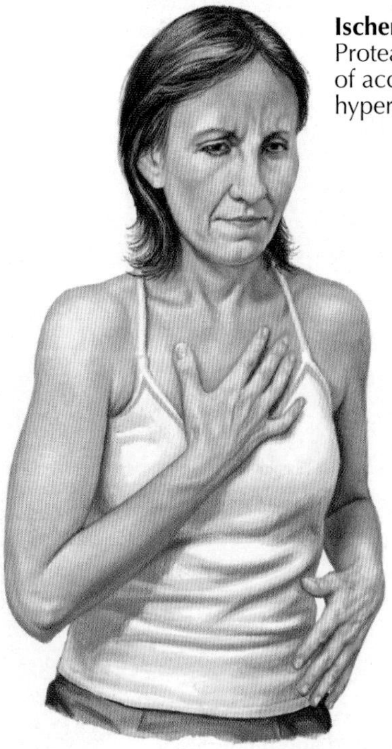

Plate 6.71

Cardiovascular System: VOLUME 8

CARDIAC MANIFESTATIONS OF AIDS

Ischemic cardiovascular disease in patients who are HIV positive. Protease inhibitors (PIs) may be associated with the development of accelerated atherosclerosis by inducing insulin resistance, hypertension, and dyslipidemia in patients with HIV.

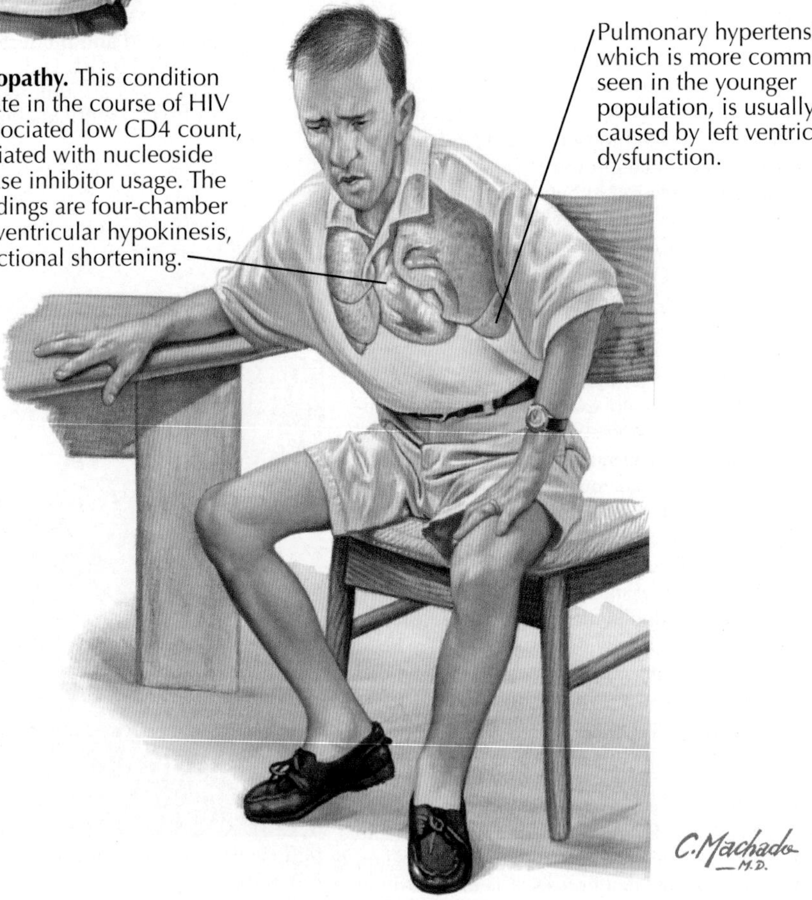

ACQUIRED IMMUNODEFICIENCY SYNDROME AND THE HEART

Patients with human immunodeficiency virus (HIV) are living much longer because of highly active antiretroviral therapy. As a result of the chronicity of HIV infection, however, patients can develop multiple cardiovascular manifestations, including hypertension, pericarditis, cancer (rare), endocarditis, and pulmonary hypertension. An estimated 20% or more of patients with HIV infection at autopsy have some evidence of heart disease (Plate 6.71).

Drugs used to treat HIV infection (e.g., protease inhibitors) can increase the risk for coronary artery disease and development of accelerated coronary atherosclerosis. The mechanism probably relates to the induction of insulin resistance as well the development of systemic hypertension and hypercholesterolemia. Patients who develop heart disease should have treatment based on the pathogenesis and etiology, similar to patients without HIV infection, although drug interactions in patients with HIV may require adjustments in therapy. Despite this caveat, any modifiable risk factor (e.g., lipid abnormalities, hypertension, smoking, diabetes, heart failure) need aggressive therapy. In any patient with HIV, opportunistic infections such as tuberculosis can complicate cardiac management, and thus prophylaxis must be considered based on the patient's level of immunity.

Other conditions such as dilated cardiomyopathy can occur, usually late in the disease course. HIV infection can directly affect the myocardium, and the decreased immunity makes the heart more susceptible to infection than in the patient without HIV. The heart failure caused by cardiomyopathy is usually associated with a low CD4 count and may be associated with reverse transcriptase inhibitor use. The typical cardiac findings in these heart failure patients are marked LV dysfunction, manifested by global hypokinesis and decreased ejection fraction. Drug use (cocaine, amphetamines) can contribute to the cardiac failure of patients with HIV who have cardiomyopathy. Pulmonary hypertension can result from the elevated LVEDP in these heart failure patients.

In the modern era of highly active antiretroviral therapy, patients with HIV are living longer, and cardiac

Dilated cardiomyopathy. This condition typically occurs late in the course of HIV infection, with associated low CD4 count, and may be associated with nucleoside reverse transcriptase inhibitor usage. The most common findings are four-chamber enlargement, left ventricular hypokinesis, and decreased fractional shortening.

Pulmonary hypertension, which is more commonly seen in the younger population, is usually caused by left ventricular dysfunction.

disease has become a growing problem; pericarditis, pericardial effusions from tuberculosis, Kaposi sarcoma, or lymphoma can occur. The pericardial effusions can be readily detected by cardiac ultrasound and other noninvasive modalities. Rarely, cardiac tamponade can occur. Cardiac cancers, infective endocarditis, and ischemic heart disease are also relatively rare complications of HIV. Infections, however, including fungal (e.g.,

Candida, histoplasmosis, cryptococcosis, aspergillosis), viral (e.g., herpes simplex, cytomegalovirus), bacterial (e.g., tuberculosis), and parasitic (e.g., toxoplasmosis), can cause myocarditis in patients with HIV. Conduction disturbance can result from lymphomatous infiltration. The cardiologist and infectious disease specialist must work together to meet the therapeutic challenge of cardiovascular disease in patients with HIV.

Plate 6.72

Acquired Heart Disease

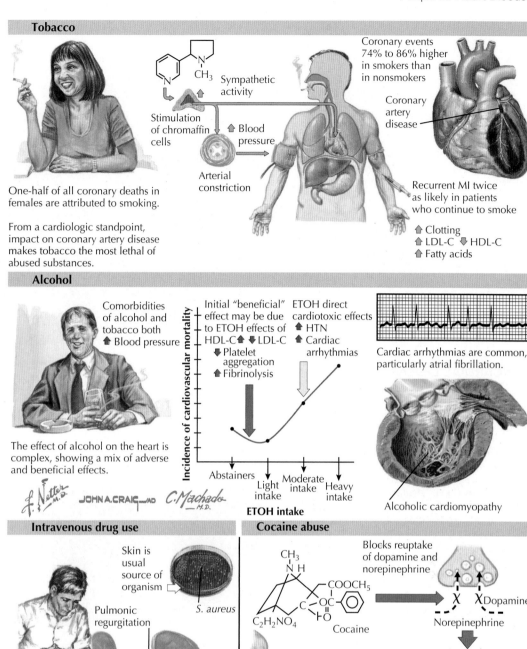

Tobacco

Sympathetic activity

Stimulation of chromaffin cells

Blood pressure

Arterial constriction

Coronary events 74% to 86% higher in smokers than in nonsmokers

Coronary artery disease

Recurrent MI twice as likely in patients who continue to smoke

⬆ Clotting
⬆ LDL-C ⬇ HDL-C
⬆ Fatty acids

One-half of all coronary deaths in females are attributed to smoking.

From a cardiologic standpoint, impact on coronary artery disease makes tobacco the most lethal of abused substances.

Alcohol

Comorbidities of alcohol and tobacco both
⬆ Blood pressure

Initial "beneficial" effect may be due to ETOH effects of
HDL-C ⬆ ⬇ LDL-C
⬇ Platelet aggregation
⬆ Fibrinolysis

ETOH direct cardiotoxic effects
⬆ HTN
⬆ Cardiac arrhythmias

Incidence of cardiovascular mortality

Abstainers | Light intake | Moderate intake | Heavy intake

ETOH intake

The effect of alcohol on the heart is complex, showing a mix of adverse and beneficial effects.

Cardiac arrhythmias are common, particularly atrial fibrillation.

Alcoholic cardiomyopathy

Substance Abuse and the Heart

The combination of addiction and physical harm makes *IV heroin* probably the most dangerous abused drug, followed by cocaine, barbiturates, and amphetamines. Any use of injected drugs can transmit bacteria (most often *Staphylococcus aureus*) from the skin into the bloodstream. This can result in septic emboli to the lung, pneumonia, and infective endocarditis of any valve, especially tricuspid and pulmonary.

TOBACCO AND ALCOHOL

Tobacco and alcohol are extremely addicting but usually less harmful in the short term than heroin and cocaine. Half of all coronary deaths in females are attributed to cigarette smoking. Coronary events, such as myocardial infarction, are approximately 80% higher in tobacco smokers than in nonsmokers. Recurrent MI is twice as likely to occur in patients who continue to smoke than in those who stop. Tobacco smoking increases sympathetic activity and catecholamines, constricts blood vessels, and increases blood pressure.

The effect of alcohol on the heart has been shown to have adverse and beneficial effects. Alcohol and smoking can both raise blood pressure. The initial beneficial effect may be related to increased HDL cholesterol, decreased LDL cholesterol (LDL-C), decreased platelet aggregation, and increased fibrinolysis. However, alcohol has direct cardiotoxic effects (e.g., alcoholic cardiomyopathy) because it can increase blood pressure and increase cardiac arrhythmias; for example atrial fibrillation (Plate 6.72; *HTN,* hypertension). Although there is some evidence that light intake of alcohol is beneficial, it is not recommended that a person who does not drink alcohol should start, because even low levels of alcohol may increase blood pressure.

Cannabis is less addicting than tobacco or alcohol, although it may be harmful related to judgment errors. In the United States, as of March 2023, the use of cannabis for medical purposes is legal in 38 states, four out of five permanently inhabited US territories, and the District of Columbia.

COCAINE

As with amphetamines, cocaine (a common illegal drug) acts by multiple mechanisms on brain catecholaminergic neurons; its reinforcing effects may involve inhibition of dopamine uptake. By blocking the reuptake of dopamine and norepinephrine, the latter increases sympathetic

Intravenous drug use

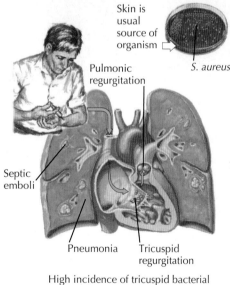

Skin is usual source of organism

S. aureus

Pulmonic regurgitation

Septic emboli

Pneumonia

Tricuspid regurgitation

High incidence of tricuspid bacterial endocarditis with IV drug use

Cocaine abuse

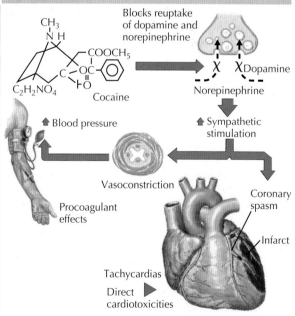

Blocks reuptake of dopamine and norepinephrine

Dopamine

Norepinephrine

CH_3
N H
COOCH$_5$
C
OC
HO
$C_2H_2NO_4$ Cocaine

⬆ Blood pressure

⬆ Sympathetic stimulation

Vasoconstriction

Procoagulant effects

Coronary spasm

Infarct

Tachycardias

Direct cardiotoxicities

stimulation of blood vessels, increases blood pressure, has procoagulant effects, and may induce tachycardias and coronary artery spasm, which may lead to MI. Cocaine also has direct cardiotoxicity; in the United States, 15,000 people die directly from cocaine use or from judgment errors (e.g., motor vehicle crashes). Several cardiovascular complications are closely related

to cocaine use. Chest pain syndromes may result in MI. Other adverse cardiac events are related to hypertension and include aortic dissection, stroke, nonfatal arrhythmias such as atrial fibrillation, and fatal dysrhythmias such as ventricular tachycardia and fibrillation. On occasion, patients present with heart failure symptoms related to pulmonary edema.

Plate 6.73

Cardiovascular System: VOLUME 8

PRESENTATION AND TREATMENT OF PERICARDITIS

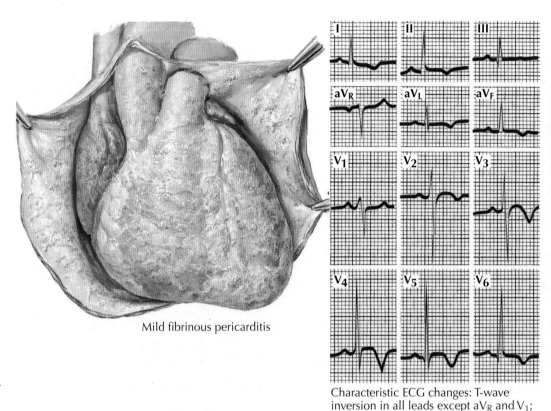

Mild fibrinous pericarditis

Characteristic ECG changes: T-wave inversion in all leads except aV_R and V_1; isoelectric in lead III

Pericardial effusion (loculated on right side)

Pericardial effusion; pleuropericardial window being created and biopsy specimen taken via incision in 5th left intercostal space

PERICARDIAL DISEASE

Pericarditis can be acute, subacute, or chronic inflammation of the pericardium. Identifying the cause of pericarditis is important because therapy depends on the underlying process; thus the best way to classify pericarditis is by etiology. Pericarditis can result from infection (viral, bacterial, parasitic), systemic autoimmune diseases (lupus, rheumatoid arthritis), immune processes (rheumatic fever, post-MI), myocardial disease (acute MI, myocarditis), metabolic disorders (uremia, myxedema), trauma, direct injury (penetrating thoracic/esophageal perforation, cardiac perforation from device), blunt trauma to chest (steering wheel injury), mediastinal radiation, and cancer (primary tumors, secondary metastases/melanoma).

The incidence of pericarditis depends on several factors, including flu-like epidemics (viral pericarditis), areas of the world in which trauma is common (war zones, etc.), and areas of the world in which infectious disease or rheumatic fever is still prevalent (Africa, India, etc.). Benign *viral* or *idiopathic* pericarditis tends to recur. Bacteriologic studies show a viral origin in some patients; however, many cases are not caused by a viral infection but probably result from an autoimmune reaction, because recurrences can be suppressed by therapy with nonsteroidal antiinflammatory drugs, aspirin, and colchicine.

ACUTE PERICARDITIS

Acute pericarditis may occur as serous, serosanguineous, purulent, and bloody forms. *Serous* pericarditis is the type usually seen in rheumatic fever and benign nonspecific or viral pericarditis. *Purulent* pericarditis usually results from bacterial infection with such organisms as pneumococcus, staphylococcus, or streptococcus, but any bacterium can be infective. *Serosanguineous* pericarditis must be distinguished from hemorrhage into the pericardium and is most often noted when the etiology is a malignancy or pericardial injury. *Adhesive* pericarditis may develop, rarely after the acute serous or serosanguineous forms and more likely after purulent or bloody pericarditis (Plate 6.75). The chronic effusive adhesive form is also seen in *tuberculous* pericarditis, often with pericardial

thickening. Constriction of one or both cardiac tracts (inflow and outflow) can result from chronic adhesive pericarditis and may require pericardiectomy.

The onset of pericarditis usually is accompanied by chest pains, although pain is not a prominent symptom and may even be absent in some cases, especially when pericardial effusion appears early, which probably prevents the parietal and visceral pericardia from rubbing

together. The pain usually is substernal and may radiate to the left shoulder and arm or the neck. The character of the pain may closely simulate that of the onset of acute MI, thus presenting a difficult diagnostic problem. Classically, the pain of pericarditis is relieved by sitting up. If there is pleural involvement, the pain may be increased by deep inspiration. With the development of effusion, dyspnea becomes the more prominent symptom (see

Plate 6.74

Acquired Heart Disease

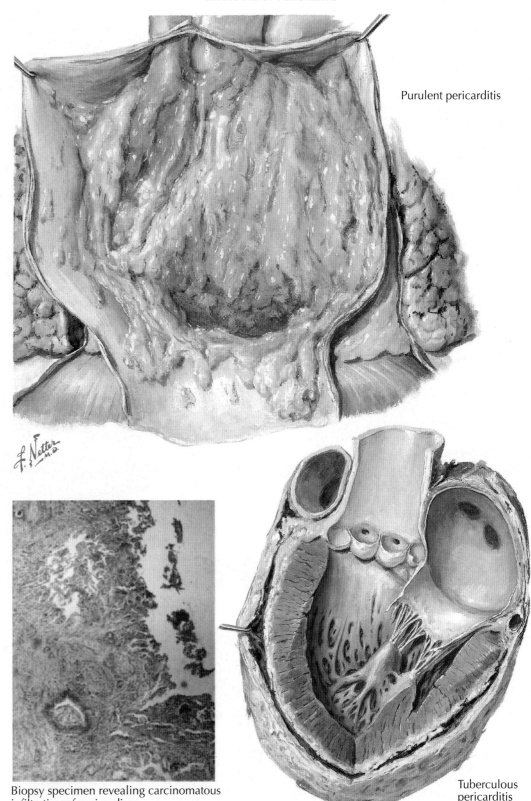

ETIOLOGIES OF PERICARDITIS

Purulent pericarditis

Biopsy specimen revealing carcinomatous infiltration of pericardium

Tuberculous pericarditis

PERICARDIAL DISEASE (Continued)

Plate 6.73). This is probably caused by mechanical pressure on the lungs, compressing not only the alveolar structure but also the smaller bronchial branches. If cardiac tamponade occurs, physiologic changes include distention of neck veins from increased right atrial pressure. Associated symptoms depend on the etiology of pericarditis. In acute inflammatory conditions, chills, fever, and sweating often are present.

The most important physical sign of acute pericarditis is a pericardial *friction rub,* usually heard best just to the left of the sternum and fairly well localized. This to-and-fro scratching sound seems to be closer to the ear than other cardiac sounds or murmurs. In pericarditis caused by inflammatory conditions or MI, the rub may be heard for only a short time, but it is usually persistent when pericarditis results from neoplasm or uremia. The friction rub may be heard in the presence of considerable pericardial effusion, even as much as 1 L, because of the uneven accumulation of fluid in the pericardium.

In the presence of significant effusion, the heart sounds will diminish in intensity, and on percussion the area of cardiac dullness will be increased. An area of dullness with bronchial breathing may be noted below the angle of the left scapula (Ewart sign). Occasionally, there may be so much pericardial fluid that by greatly increasing intrapericardial pressure, it interferes with cardiac function (cardiac tamponade). Venous pressure rises, heart rate increases, pulse slows, and pulse amplitude may decrease during inspiration (paradoxical pulse). Blood pressure may fall as much as 20 mm Hg at the end of inspiration, an exaggeration of the normal drop in blood pressure. The rapid formation of pericardial effusion is important in determining whether tamponade will occur. A small, rapidly developing effusion may cause tamponade, whereas a large effusion developing over several weeks, as in tuberculous pericardial effusion, or effusion related to hypothyroidism, will not cause tamponade.

Serial chest radiographs in particular demonstrate an enlarging cardiac silhouette suggesting pericardial effusion. However, the fluid volume must be at least 250 mL before a significant change in the cardiac shadow permits a definitive diagnosis. The cardiac silhouette, depending on the amount of fluid present, will assume a pear-shaped or "water bottle" form.

The ECG is important in the diagnosis of pericarditis, which may be confused with acute myocardial infarction (see Plate 6.73). Classically, elevation of the ST segment usually occurs in most of the 12 leads, whereas in MI, depending on the location of the infarction, the precordial leads or inferior leads show changes (ST elevation). The shape of the ST segment may also be similar to that seen in MI. In pericarditis, the PR segments may be depressed in lead II and elevated in lead aVR. The most common ECG abnormality is nonspecific T-wave changes. The ECG changes probably reflect inflammation of the epimyocardium because the pericardium itself is electrically inert. Two-dimensional

Plate 6.75

Cardiovascular System: VOLUME 8

CONSTRICTIVE PERICARDITIS

Adhesive pericarditis

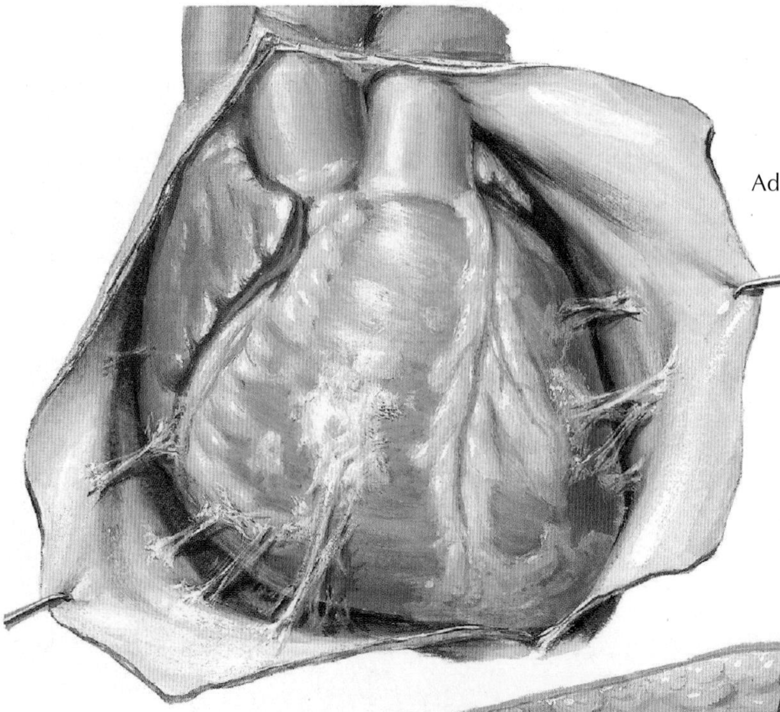

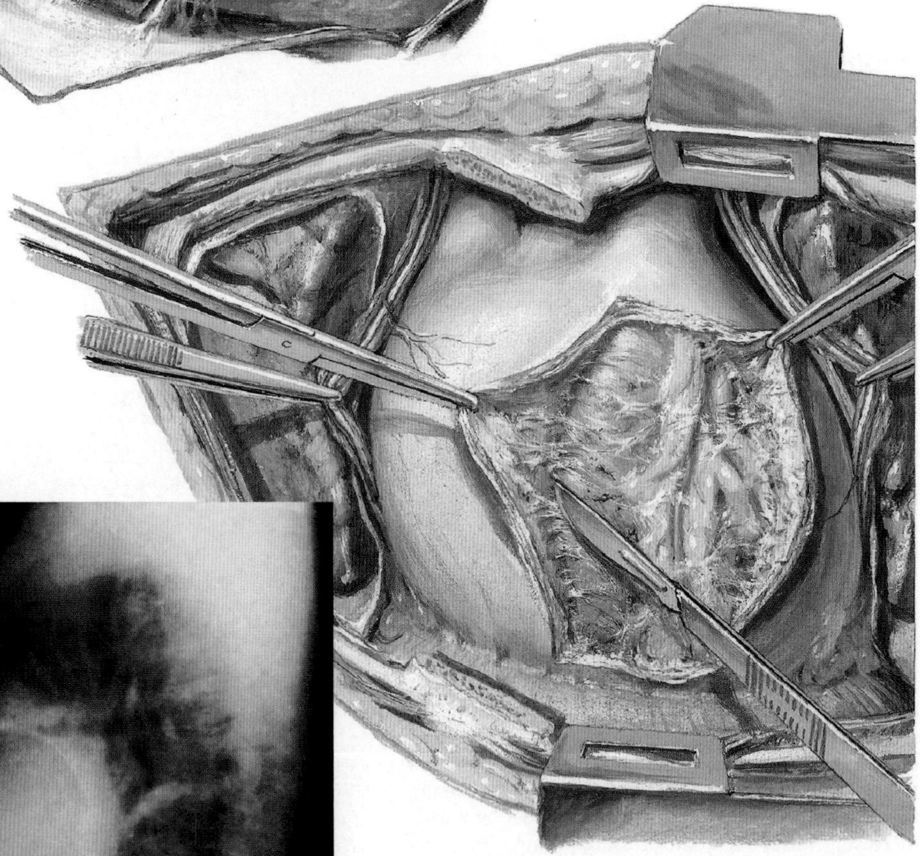

Excision of constrictive pericardium via transsternal incision: phrenic nerves and accompanying vessels preserved

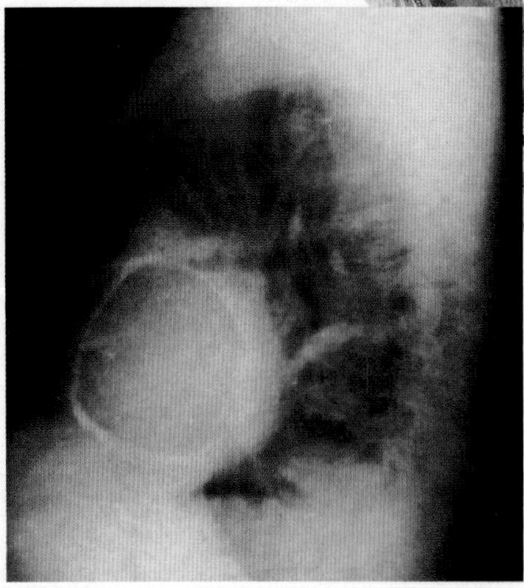

Calcified constrictive pericarditis

PERICARDIAL DISEASE
(Continued)

cardiac ultrasound readily determines the presence and location of pericardial effusion and is required if pericardiocentesis is planned.

PURULENT PERICARDITIS

Purulent pericarditis may not be recognized because of being part of the general disease (see Plate 6.74). However, ECG changes suggesting pericarditis (and epimyocarditis), cardiac ultrasound evidence of pericardial effusion, or ultrasonic evidence of diminished cardiac pulsations may call attention to the purulent condition. A pericardial rub is also helpful, but it is *not* diagnostic for purulent pericarditis. Antibiotics and early drainage by pericardiocentesis or surgery are indicated, and when used early, these measures substantially reduce mortality, which is otherwise close to 100%.

TUBERCULOUS PERICARDITIS

Tuberculous pericarditis is a complication usually resulting from extension of a contiguous tuberculous process in the lungs or the lymph nodes (see Plate 6.74). It starts as a fibrinous reaction, with or without effusion (see Plate 6.73), and then the pericardium thickens as a result of tubercles, caseation, and fibrosis. The thickened, adherent pericardium assumes a "shaggy" appearance. *Constrictive* effusive pericarditis may occur in this early period, or later if pericardial calcification results. Treatment in the early stages before constriction is by conventional long-term antitubercular therapy (as determined by tuberculosis specialist). When constrictive physiology is present, pericardiectomy is required (Plate 6.75).

NONSPECIFIC PERICARDITIS

The recurrent nonspecific type of pericarditis, such as associated with autoimmune reactions, postcommissurotomy pericarditis, and post-MI pericarditis, is often benefited by antiinflammatory therapy (steroids, nonsteroidal antiinflammatory drugs, aspirin, colchicine).

Such treatment merely suppresses the signs and symptoms and therefore is usually continued indefinitely.

In the patient with pericardial effusion, pericardiocentesis is required only when tamponade threatens, or for diagnostic purposes, as in suspected malignancy or bacterial infection. A surgical approach removes fluid through a "pericardial window" into the

left pleural space, and pericardial biopsy can be obtained (see Plate 6.73). When a pericardial window is created, fluid in the pericardial space passes into the left pleural cavity, from where it is absorbed. Alternatively, a catheter can be inserted into the pericardial space to facilitate pericardial drainage to a collecting system.

Plate 6.76

Acquired Heart Disease

Acute Cor Pulmonale and Pulmonary Embolism

In the field of cardiovascular disease, the interdependence of the heart and lungs as a unit is most apparent in *cor pulmonale*—heart disease caused by hypertension in the pulmonary circulation—which in turn results from an abnormal resistance to blood flow and lung perfusion by blood flow from the right ventricle. The classic symptoms of *pulmonary emboli* are tachypnea and tachycardia. Chest pain is not a classic symptom unless pulmonary infarction is evident; these patients usually have heart failure. *Acute* cor pulmonale most often results from pulmonary embolism caused by a clot dislodged in the venous system, or from a mural thrombus in the right side of the heart. The embolus may arise in an area of thrombophlebitis, perhaps with some prior warning. More often, however, silent phlebothrombosis occurs in the large veins of the legs (e.g., femoral, pelvic), and the ensuing clinical syndrome is determined chiefly by the size and number of the pulmonary arteries obstructed.

Pulmonary emboli are related to other forms of heart disease and may precipitate or aggravate existing congestive heart failure or produce a clinical picture simulating acute myocardial infarction. Bed-bound patients, especially those who have heart failure, malignant disease, polycythemia, or venous disease; who have recently had pelvic orthopedic or prostate surgery; or who who are obese or of advanced age, are predisposed to embolism. These patients often receive prophylactic anticoagulation to prevent pulmonary emboli. Emboli occasionally arise from the right side of the heart from mural thrombosis caused by injury to the right atrium or ventricle or with long-standing right-sided heart failure combined with atrial fibrillation.

Pulmonary emboli occasionally consist of tumor fragments from a carcinomatous invasion of the large abdominal veins. Fat emboli may be initiated by soft tissue trauma. Amniotic fluid emboli after delivery may cause obstruction to the pulmonary arteries or the right ventricle itself, as can, occasionally, air bubbles introduced into the veins during surgical procedures (e.g., cannulation of internal jugular vein).

Although it is well known that a 50% reduction in the cross-sectional area of the pulmonary circulation (as after pneumonectomy) does not increase resting pulmonary artery (PA) pressure, pronounced pulmonary hypertension may occur after pulmonary embolism; this can later be shown to have obstructed only a small proportion of the PA circulation. Therefore pulmonary vasoconstriction may contribute to the demonstrated rise in PA pressure. Oxygen administration to a patient with acute pulmonary embolism may significantly lower PA pressure, reducing vasoconstriction, thus indicating the presence of a significant reflex vasoconstriction as a cause of symptoms.

MASSIVE EMBOLIZATION

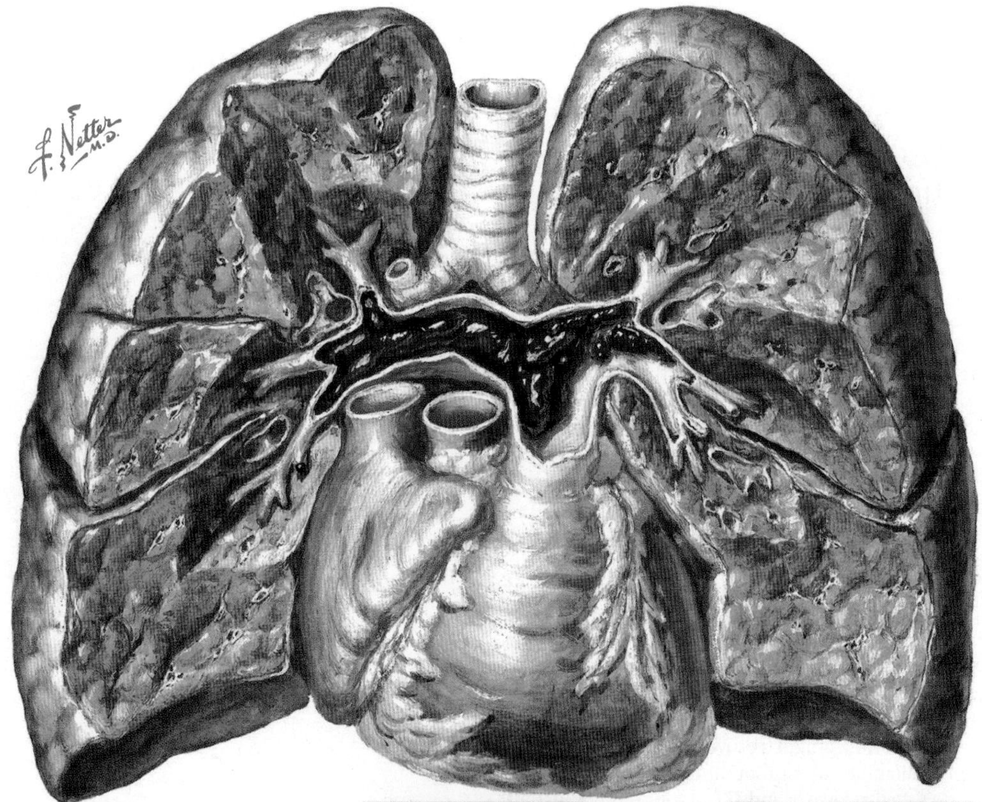

In embolization of the pulmonary arteries, because of the increased resistance to pulmonary blood flow, cardiac output is significantly decreased, with an associated fall in systemic blood pressure. In addition, PA pressure rises, compromising right ventricular (RV) function. Massive pulmonary embolism may result in

MASSIVE EMBOLIZATION

Saddle embolus completely occluding right pulmonary artery and partially obstructing main and left arteries

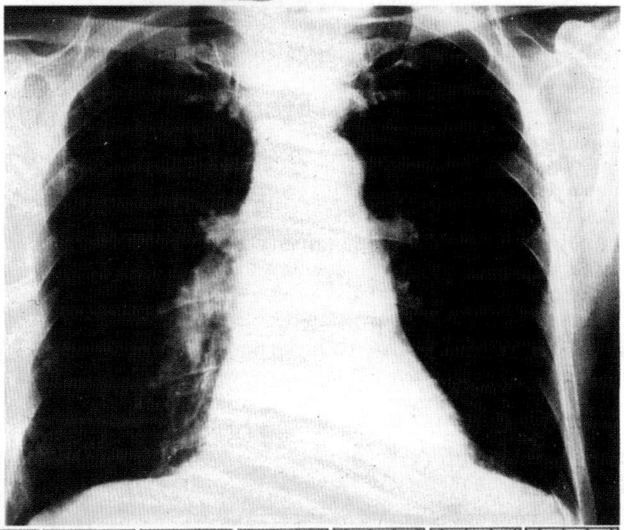

Radiograph showing dense shadow of right pulmonary artery with increased luminescence of peripheral lung fields

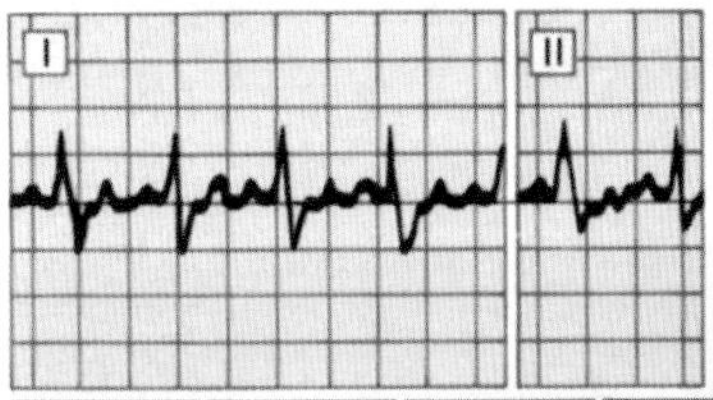

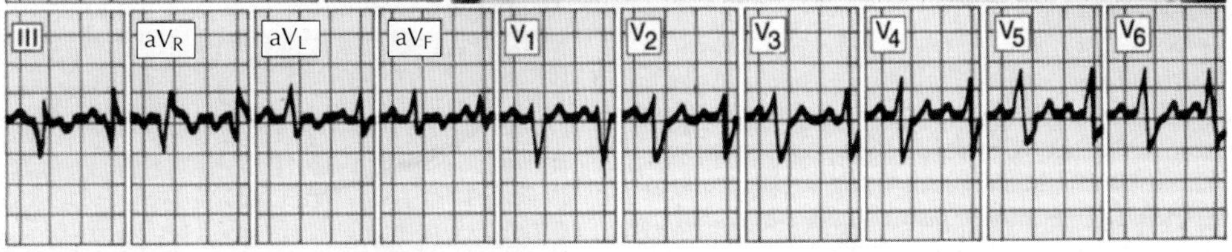

Characteristic electrocardiographic findings in acute pulmonary embolism. Deep S_1; prominent Q_3 with inversion of T_3; depression of ST segment in lead II (often also in lead I) with staircase ascent of ST_2; T_2 diphasic or inverted; right axis deviation; tachycardia.

myocardial ischemia or even cardiogenic shock because of the resulting fall in coronary blood flow, which may be further aggravated by reflex coronary constriction mediated by the vagus nerves. If RV pressure is greatly increased, theoretically the thebesian venous drainage of the heart may be impaired as well (Plate 6.76).

Bronchospasm may occur and may be caused by the release of thromboxane from platelets in the vicinity of

or in the clot itself. Both experimental animal data and human observations confirm the classic symptoms of hyperventilation and tachypnea. Reduced arterial O_2 content results from venous admixture, and decreased alveolar-arterial CO_2 tension difference is presumably caused by underperfused but still-ventilated segments of the lung. The typical picture of massive pulmonary embolization is characterized by the sudden onset of

Plate 6.77

Cardiovascular System: VOLUME 8

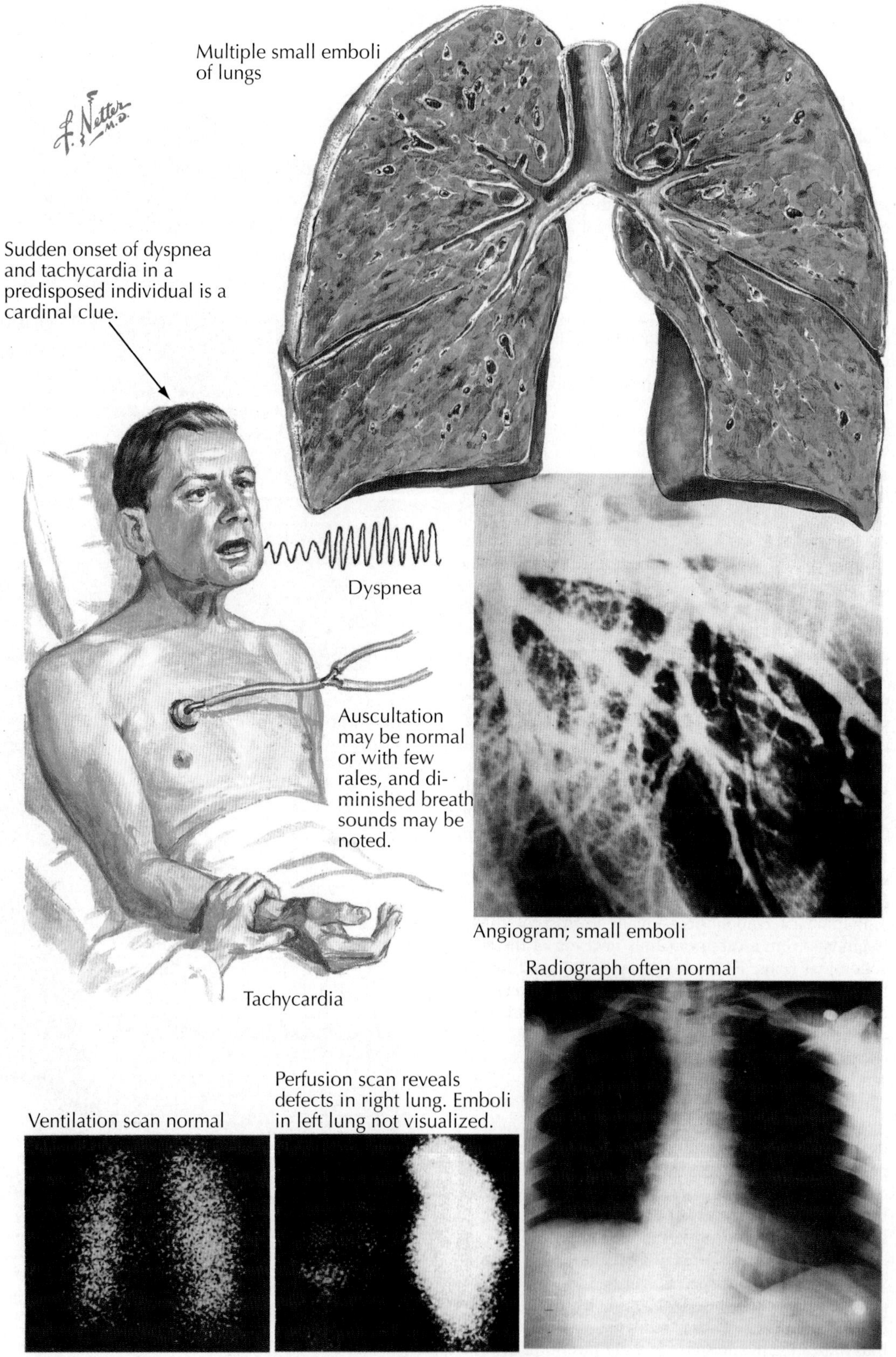

ACUTE COR PULMONALE AND PULMONARY EMBOLISM (Continued)

dyspnea, tachycardia, substernal discomfort, and possibly systemic hypotension. Clinical evidence of right ventricular dysfunction and failure may develop rapidly and should be suspected when increasing prominence of the pulmonic component (P_2) of the second heart sound (S_2) is detected, together with RV presystolic gallop (S_4) along the right sternal border and distention of the cervical veins, as confirmed by ultrasound. The ECG may be the most useful diagnostic aid available. The typical pattern includes a prominent S wave, with a depressed ST segment in lead I and perhaps lead II, and a deep Q (S_1–Q_3 pattern) and a late inversion of T in lead III. There usually are prominent precordial P waves and an inversion of precordial T waves of variable degree and distribution.

Occasionally with massive embolization, it must be decided quickly whether surgical embolectomy or thrombolytic therapy is indicated in a critically ill patient who possibly might recover spontaneously. The prompt availability of cardiopulmonary bypass facilities, a qualified surgeon, and CT angiography must all be considered, with many reports of successful pulmonary embolectomy. Thrombolytic therapy is also considered in a patient who is not bleeding.

SMALLER EMBOLI

Pulmonary embolism of less massive proportions may be associated with dyspnea, hyperventilation, cyanosis, restlessness, chest discomfort of a pleuritic nature, especially if there is pulmonary infarction and, in some patients, syncope. Evidence of RV overload may develop, followed later by hemoptysis, fever, chest radiographic evidence of pulmonary consolidation, pleural friction rub, and jaundice. A CT angiogram with contrast can provide confirmatory anatomic evidence of pulmonary embolus, whereas radionuclide pulmonary perfusion studies provide confirmatory evidence of perfusion deficits in the lung (Plate 6.77).

Most patients who have normal hearts and lungs before pulmonary embolism show a striking ability to reabsorb emboli. Study of right-sided heart pressures, even with pulmonary angiography and nuclear perfusion tests, shows no significant abnormality. However, such recovery depends on the prevention and avoidance of recurrent thromboembolism using heparin anticoagulation and sometimes implantation of a device in the inferior vena cava to prevent movement of clot from below the inferior vena cava (IVC) to the lung. This is done particularly if recurrent pulmonary embolus occurs while the patient is anticoagulated.

In the acute stage of pulmonary embolism, heparin is recommended both as an anticoagulant and as an antiserotonin factor in the reduction of bronchospasm with its attendant respiratory disturbance. Inotropic and vasodilatory therapy is indicated if there is evidence of RV failure. Symptomatic relief with narcotics, nitrates, atropine, and vasopressors should be considered according to the indications of the individual patient.

Although recurrent, small pulmonary emboli may often go unrecognized; the alert clinician should have a high index of suspicion when finding unexplained transient increases in pulse rate and tachypnea, chronic fatigue, and especially the unexplained appearance of RV hypertrophy on ECG or ultrasound without evidence of intrinsic pulmonary disease. This clinical syndrome may be avoided largely by (1) early ambulation of postoperative patients, (2) administering prophylactic low-dose subcutaneous heparin or increasing venous return from the lower extremity with devices that gently massage the legs in bed-bound patients, and (3) identifying the problem, especially in persons with malignant disease, congestive heart failure, polycythemia, varices of the lower extremities, recent pelvic trauma, splenectomy, or previous venous thrombosis.

EMBOLISM OF LESSER DEGREE WITHOUT INFARCTION

Multiple small emboli of lungs

Sudden onset of dyspnea and tachycardia in a predisposed individual is a cardinal clue.

Dyspnea

Auscultation may be normal or with few rales, and diminished breath sounds may be noted.

Tachycardia

Angiogram; small emboli

Radiograph often normal

Ventilation scan normal

Perfusion scan reveals defects in right lung. Emboli in left lung not visualized.

Plate 6.78

Acquired Heart Disease

CHRONIC COR PULMONALE AND DEEP VEIN THROMBOSIS

CHRONIC COR PULMONALE

Although chronic pulmonary hypertension occurs in disorders of the left side of the heart, such as left ventricular failure and mitral stenosis, or left-to-right shunts in congenital cardiac lesions, the term *cor pulmonale* is usually applied to heart disease caused by *intrinsic* disorders of the lungs and pulmonary circulation.

Whereas the normal pulmonary circuit is characterized by low pressure, low resistance, and a large distensible vascular bed, notable changes in these features may occur in pulmonary disorders with anatomic restriction of the pulmonary parenchyma and vascular structures or vasoconstriction in the arterial circulation from associated pulmonary dysfunction. Studies of lung function in diseases that cause pulmonary hypertension may show altered ventilation (as in chronic obstructive pulmonary disease [COPD]), disturbed ventilation-perfusion relationships, or reduced diffusing capacity (as in alveolocapillary block syndromes). All of these functional disturbances are marked by *hypoxia,* affecting either the pulmonary capillary and venous blood or the alveolar gas itself. Hypoxia is capable of producing vasoconstriction of the pulmonary bed, thus contributing to an increase in pulmonary vascular resistance.

Clinically, four general categories of pulmonary diseases result in cor pulmonale: COPD, pulmonary fibrosis, musculoskeletal thoracic disorders, and primary pulmonary hypertension (Plate 6.78). COPD causes 85% to 90% of cor pulmonale seen worldwide. COPD includes cases of chronic *bronchial asthma,* with widespread intermittent narrowing of the airways, and obstructive *emphysema,* with loss of elasticity, increased residual volume, decreased lung compliance, and especially fewer and smaller alveolar capillaries. Some chronic bronchitis is usually present, with many disturbances in pulmonary function but mainly *ventilatory insufficiency* and the principal symptom of *dyspnea.*

Pulmonary fibrosis of various types, sometimes associated secondarily with emphysema, also comprises a large group of pulmonary disorders that typically lead to hypertension and cor pulmonale. Tuberculosis, bronchiectasis, and other pulmonary infections have been associated with cor pulmonale less frequently in recent years, probably because of the widespread use of antibiotics and antimicrobial agents. Pulmonary hypertension may result from some pneumoconioses because of inhalation of foreign substances, particularly silicon, bauxite, diatomaceous earth, and beryllium, possibly only in patients hyperreactive to these agents. Sarcoidosis, scleroderma, and fibrosing interstitial pneumonitis (Hamman-Rich syndrome) may likewise result in severe reduction of the pulmonary vascular bed, with

LESIONS THAT MAY CAUSE PULMONARY HYPERTENSION AND CHRONIC COR PULMONALE

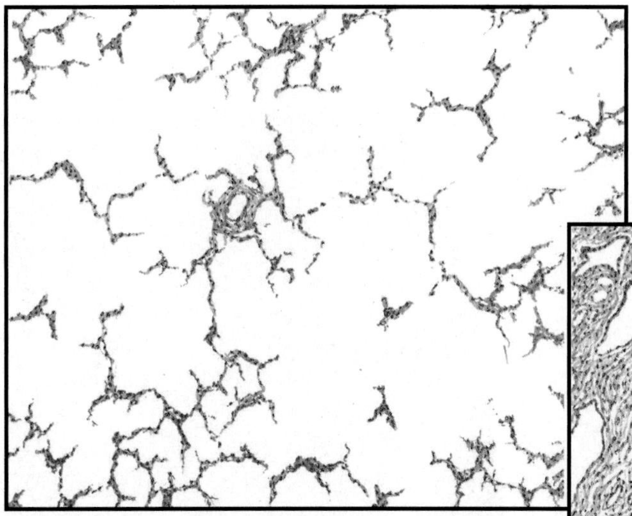

Emphysema, the most common cause of cor pulmonale

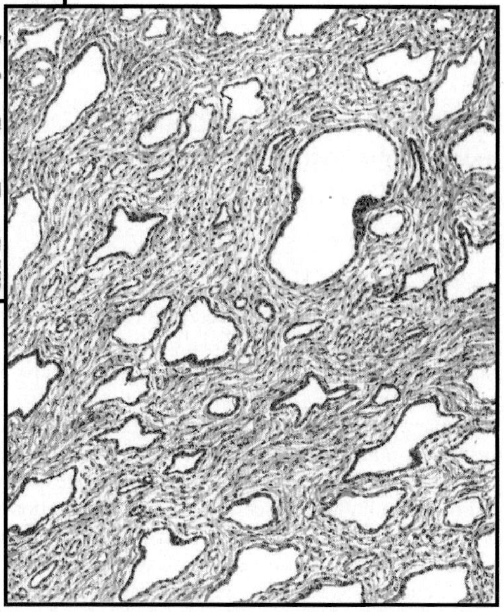

Pulmonary fibrosis: may be secondary to silicosis, asbestosis, hemosiderosis, tuberculosis, blastomycosis, fibrocystic disease of the pancreas, schistosomiasis, radiography of breast; possibly primary

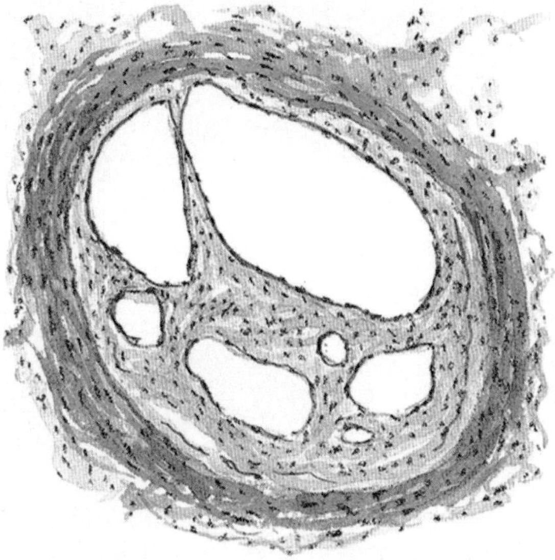

Organized and canalized thrombus in a small pulmonary vessel

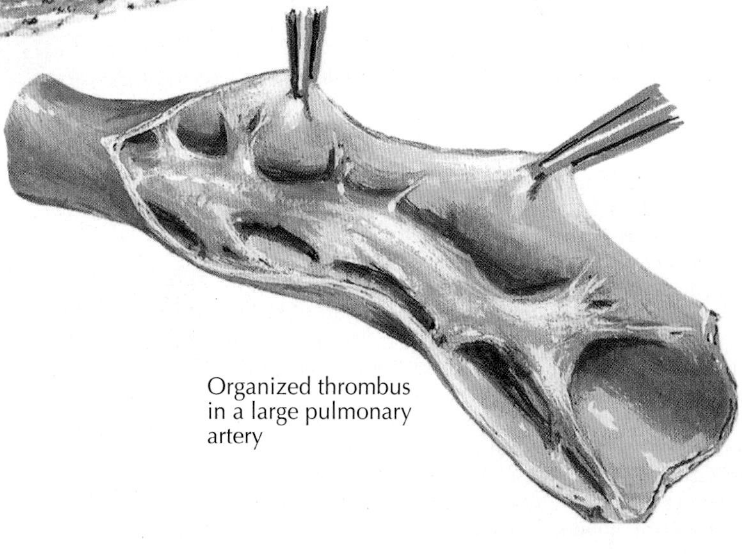

Organized thrombus in a large pulmonary artery

altered alveolocapillary membrane and impaired oxygen diffusion as well as impaired lung compliance and distorted ventilation-perfusion. *Hypoxia* is prominent, with its attendant hyperventilation and cyanosis, which are more marked clinical features than dyspnea.

Musculoskeletal or mechanical disorders of the thoracic cage, as in kyphoscoliosis, thoracoplasty, poliomyelitis, and muscular dystrophy, may cause pulmonary

dysfunction to the extent of causing cor pulmonale. All of these disorders share an uneven ventilation-perfusion relationship, with regional emphysema combined with fibrosis in other parts of the lungs. Regional alveolar hypoventilation with right-to-left shunting of unaerated blood develops, resulting in hypoxic pulmonary vasoconstriction and anatomic restriction of the capillary bed. Alveolar hypoventilation resulting from extreme obesity

Plate 6.79

Cardiovascular System: VOLUME 8

CHRONIC COR PULMONALE

Trachea   Aorta

Pulmonary trunk

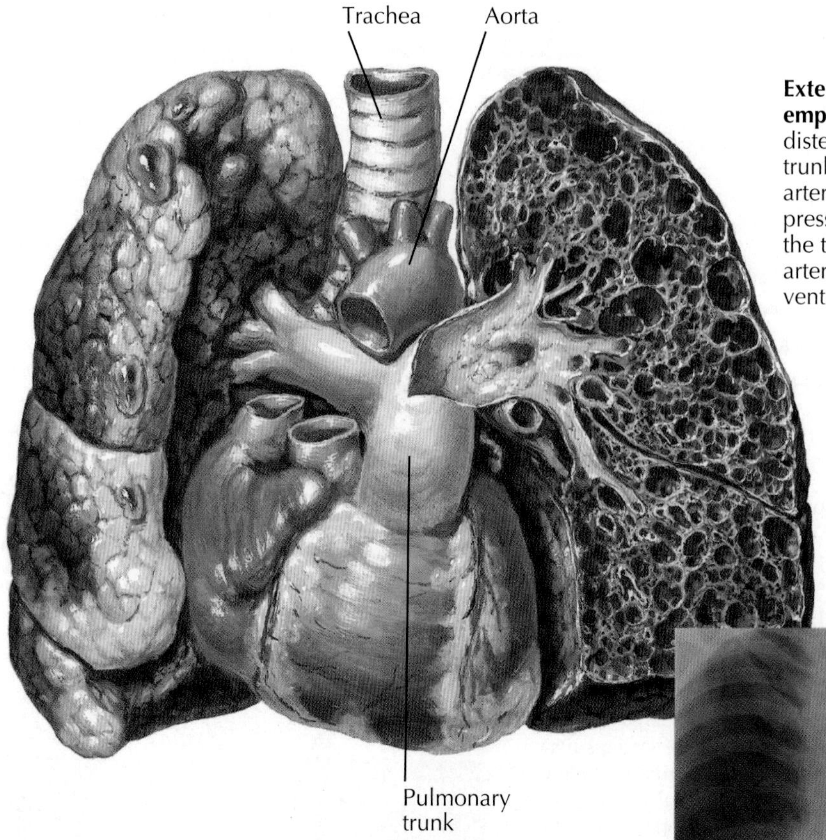

Extensive pulmonary emphysema. With great distention of pulmonary trunk and main pulmonary arteries, which have pressed the aorta against the trachea: pulmonary arteriosclerosis and right ventricular hypertrophy

CHRONIC COR PULMONALE AND DEEP VEIN THROMBOSIS (Continued)

or occasionally intrinsic hyposensitivity of the respiratory center to carbon dioxide, infrequently results in hypoxic pulmonary vasoconstriction and a functional form of cor pulmonale, which is completely reversible when the underlying disorder is promptly recognized and treated.

Primary disease of the pulmonary vessels themselves *(primary pulmonary hypertension)* comprises the fourth important group of causes, distinguished by the absence of intrinsic pulmonary disease or other apparent etiologic factors. In some patients, widespread organization of apparent pulmonary thrombosis of various ages is discovered at autopsy, and no history of pulmonary embolism can be found in retrospect. The lesions at the arteriolar and capillary levels are often indistinguishable in cases of so-called primary pulmonary hypertension in which there is no suspicion of multiple emboli. In both cases there are variable degrees of intimal hyperplasia, vascular occlusion, and recanalization, with medial hypertrophy of the muscular arteries and atherosclerosis of the larger vessels. These microscopic changes may be either the cause or the result of hypertension in the pulmonary circuit, and controversy surrounds the pathogenesis. At times the disorder seems familial, occurring more often in females than in males. A history of complicated pregnancy may suggest amniotic fluid embolization as an initial factor (see Plate 6.78).

The clinical diagnosis of chronic cor pulmonale requires a high index of suspicion in regard to the patient with chronic lung disease of any type known to increase resistance in the pulmonary circulation. Usually, the initial symptoms are those of the underlying pulmonary disorder; therefore cough and dyspnea are prominent even before detectable cardiac involvement, suspected if the pulmonic component (P_2) of the second heart sound (S_2) is prominent, along with cyanosis, finger clubbing, increased cervical venous pressure, or left parasternal heave. P_2 may be absent in many patients with obstructive lung disease with increased anteroposterior chest diameter, in whom epigastric pulsation may be prominent. Atrial and ventricular gallop sounds may appear along with the murmurs of tricuspid or pulmonic insufficiency. These signs are accentuated on inspiration and decreased on expiration, in contrast to the similar physical signs in left ventricular failure.

With the advancing decompensation of cor pulmonale, the usual findings of dependent edema, ascites, cyanosis, and hepatomegaly may appear. Chest radiography is often unremarkable, usually showing a normal cardiac silhouette or simply the changes caused by the underlying lung disease. Sometimes, dilation of the pulmonary artery and its branches is evident, but

Atrioventricular septum

Left ventricle

Right ventricle

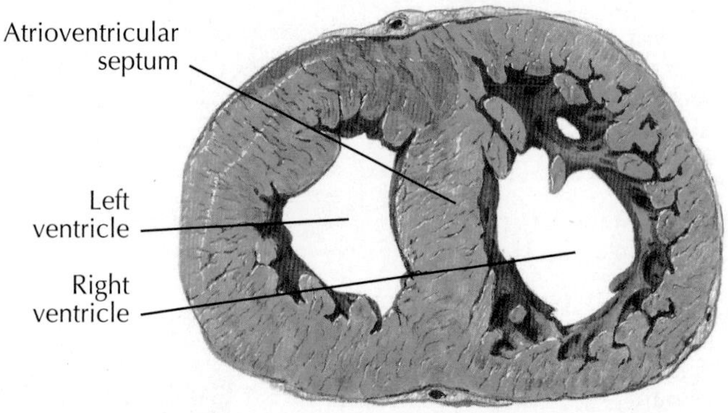

Hypertrophy and dilation of right ventricle. Seen in coronal section of heart.

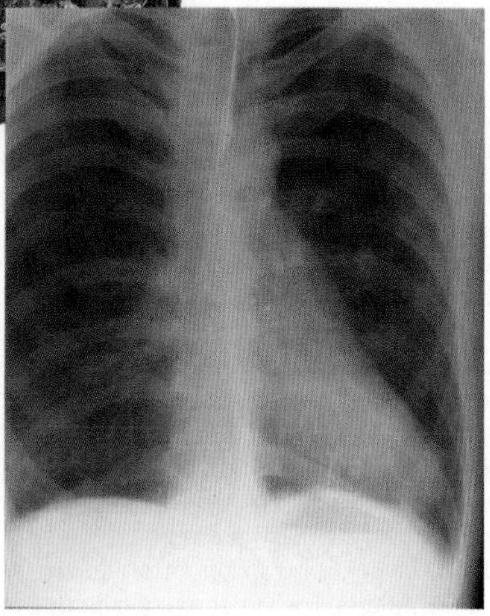

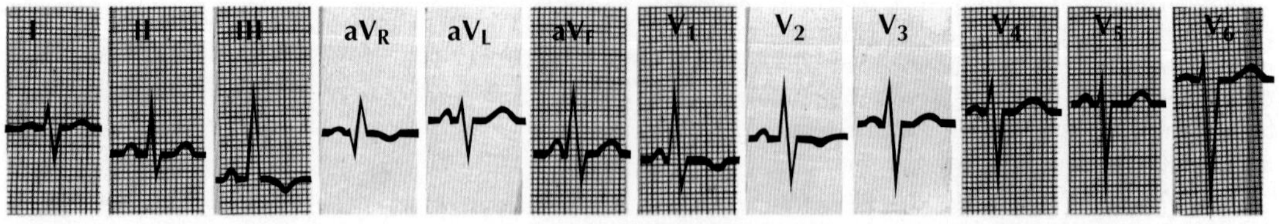

Radiograph: Chronic obstructive emphysema with cor pulmonale

R waves. In leads V_1 and V_2 as well as S, waves in leads I, V_4, V_5, and V_6 are indicative of right ventricular hypertrophy. Prominent P waves in leads II, III, aVF, V_1, and V_2 suggest right atrial enlargement.

enlargement of the right ventricle is difficult to demonstrate, except when evaluated with cardiac ultrasound or computed tomographic angiography. Some prominence or increased convexity of the right ventricular outflow tract may be seen on the right on the posteroanterior projection.

The ECG of chronic cor pulmonale may remain within normal limits until mean pulmonary pressure is

fixed at more than twice normal. Patients with chronic lung disease frequently have a vertical electrical position with clockwise rotation, which is responsible for ECG changes attributed to right ventricular hypertrophy. One of the first reliable signs of cor pulmonale, however, is that of right atrial enlargement, with prominence and peaking of the P waves in leads II and III and a relative increase in the initial component of P in

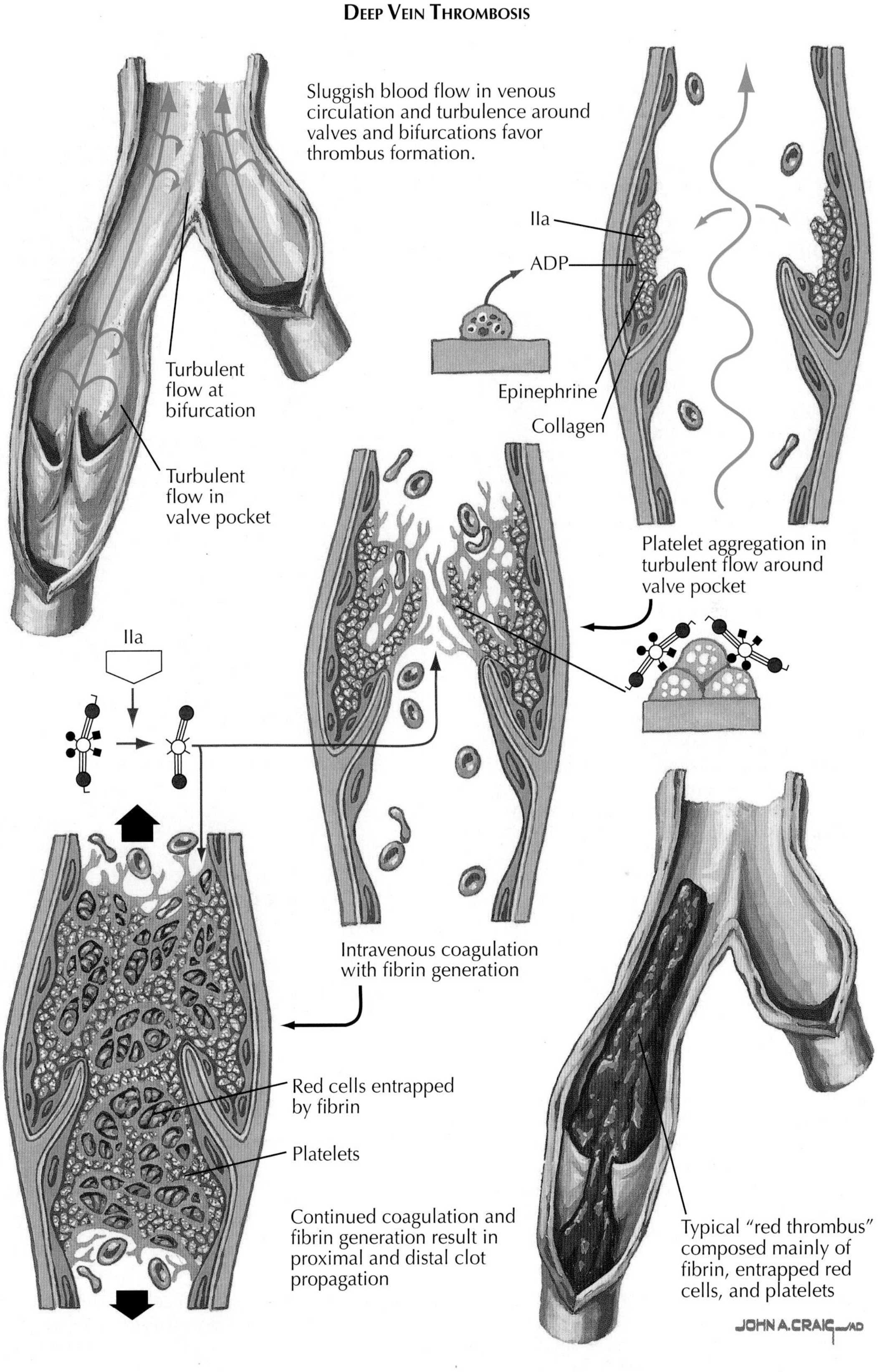

Plate 6.80

Acquired Heart Disease

CHRONIC COR PULMONALE AND DEEP VEIN THROMBOSIS (Continued)

V_1. When RV hypertrophy develops, right-axis deviation occurs in the frontal plane, with increased amplitude of the R waves in V_1. The precordial QRS electrical transition zone shifts to the left, and the rSR pattern of incomplete or complete right bundle branch block may appear. In early cor pulmonale, absence of ECG abnormality does not exclude pulmonary hypertension (see Plate 6.79).

The technique of right-sided heart catheterization provides the only reliable method of measuring the PA and RV pressures, which may occasionally reach systemic levels. Cardiac ultrasound can estimate RV (and thus PA pressure). When RV failure is present, there is a characteristic elevation of RV end-diastolic pressure (RVEDP), together with a reduction in cardiac output compared with normal values, but much less reduction than with other forms of heart failure. Cardiac catheterization has also proved the reversibility of pulmonary hypertension, which depends somewhat on its underlying cause, but justifies a vigorous therapeutic program for these patients to modify their formerly poor prognosis.

The treatment of chronic cor pulmonale depends primarily on the management of the underlying pulmonary disease. In the most common form of bronchopulmonary disorder associated with obstructive lung disease, antibacterial agents to control infection, as well as bronchodilator agents, are crucial. Corticosteroids are occasionally justified. Intermittent positive pressure breathing therapy also allows the administration of oxygen in a relatively safe manner, because increased ventilation is provided simultaneously, and the paradoxical respiratory depression, with CO_2 retention in patients with emphysema, can be avoided.

Tracheostomy, sometimes permanent, assists most in improving alveolar ventilation, particularly in patients with severe hypercapnia. Tracheostomy is occasionally indicated as an emergency measure if the patient is comatose or acidotic when first examined.

Cardiac measures recommended in the treatment of decompensated cor pulmonale include inotropic support, which improves cardiac output, although PA pressure initially may rise as a result of increased stroke volume. Sodium restriction and diuretic medications are indicated, as in other forms of congestive failure. General supportive measures include adequate rest and avoidance of excessive exertion, as in other forms of cardiac failure, and the functional state of many patients improves. Drugs to treat pulmonary hypertension include prostaglandins, endothelin receptor antagonists, and phosphodiesterase type 5 inhibitors. Digitalis preparations may reduce symptoms in some patients.

DEEP VEIN THROMBOSIS

Sluggish blood flow in venous circulation and turbulence around valves and bifurcations favor thrombus formation.

Turbulent flow at bifurcation

Turbulent flow in valve pocket

IIa

ADP

Epinephrine

Collagen

Platelet aggregation in turbulent flow around valve pocket

IIa

Intravenous coagulation with fibrin generation

Red cells entrapped by fibrin

Platelets

Continued coagulation and fibrin generation result in proximal and distal clot propagation

Typical "red thrombus" composed mainly of fibrin, entrapped red cells, and platelets

JOHN A. CRAIG—AD

DEEP VEIN THROMBOSIS

The most serious complication of deep vein thrombosis (DVT) is pulmonary embolus (Plate 6.80). DVT occurs in about 1 in 1000 adults per year and may result from venous stasis, damage to blood vessels, and hypercoagulable states. DVTs are often found in the calf vessels, but the most dangerous location is the femoral circulation, where thrombi are most prone to embolize to the pulmonary circulation. Cancer, trauma, surgery, and antiphospholipid syndrome increase the risk of DVT, along with age, immobilization, oral contraceptives (particularly with cigarette smoking), and pregnancy. Vascular ultrasound can establish the diagnosis. Treatment for DVT is anticoagulation. If PA embolization occurs after appropriate anticoagulation, placement of a vena cava filter should be considered.

Plate 6.81

Cardiovascular System: VOLUME 8

INFECTIVE ENDOCARDITIS: PORTALS OF ENTRY AND PREDISPOSING LESIONS

Infective endocarditis is a bacterial or fungal infection of the endocardium. Classically, the heart valves are involved primarily, but the endocardium of a cardiac chamber or the intima of a great vessel may also be infected, yielding a clinical picture similar to classic valvular infective endocarditis.

Infective endocarditis requires that two conditions be met: a *portal of entry* for the organism into the bloodstream to establish bacteremia and a site susceptible to infection. The site may be identifiable as a lesion existing before infection (e.g., rheumatic valvulitis or disease), but in patients with highly virulent bacteria, no predisposing lesion need be identifiable for infection to occur. A portal of entry cannot always be recognized, but the important sites include the mouth (most common), skin, and upper respiratory and male genital tracts. The various infectious lesions associated with the gums and teeth may deliver *Streptococcus viridans* to the bloodstream. The male genital tract is a source of *Streptococcus faecalis,* with entry into the bloodstream usually following manipulation within the urethra, such as a prostatectomy. Gonococcal urethritis may be followed by bacteremia that may cause infective endocarditis. The skin, especially in infants with eczematous lesions, may permit entry of highly virulent staphylococci. From infection of the upper respiratory tract, β-hemolytic streptococci occasionally cause infective endocarditis. Pulmonary infections are important sources of bacteremia, most often with pneumococci.

Just as a portal of entry is not always recognized in patients with infective endocarditis, so too is a predisposing lesion not always identified, especially if the infection is fulminating. When identified, a predisposing lesion is usually associated with trauma to valvular or vascular cardiac lining. Fibrous thickening of freely movable cusps permits these structures to traumatize each other. A narrow stream of blood passing through a narrow opening, of high velocity because of the pressure difference across the opening, is a basis for trauma. At the site of impact by such a stream, the lining of the vessel or endocardium involved is susceptible to infection (e.g., ventricular septal defect [VSD], patent ductus arteriosus [PDA]).

The most common sites of infective endocarditis involve the mitral and aortic valves. Predisposing lesions of the mitral valve are usually rheumatic, but normal and prosthetic valves can be attacked as well. The degree of valvular involvement by the rheumatic process is inadequate to cause significant hemodynamic changes, and the patient is often unaware of underlying cardiac disease. Characteristically, the changes are represented by mild fibrous thickening of the cusps along the line of closure. Chordal changes usually are minor, and commissural fusion is insignificant, if present. Vascularization of the anterior mitral cusp is often present as a sign of antecedent rheumatic carditis. A valve affected as described displays free motion of its cusps, but endothelium may be denuded in relation to

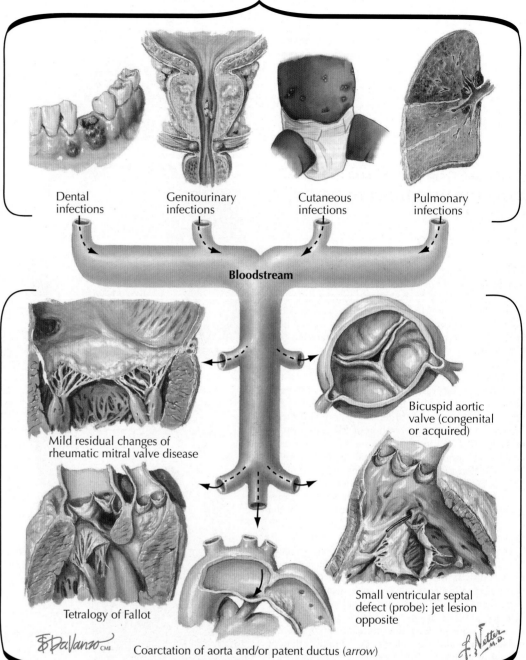

Common Portals of Bacterial Entry in Bacterial Endocarditis

Dental infections · Genitourinary infections · Cutaneous infections · Pulmonary infections

Bloodstream

Mild residual changes of rheumatic mitral valve disease

Bicuspid aortic valve (congenital or acquired)

Tetralogy of Fallot

Small ventricular septal defect (probe): jet lesion opposite

Coarctation of aorta and/or patent ductus (*arrow*)

Common Predisposing Lesions

the areas of fibrous thickening. Such areas are susceptible if infectious bacteria are circulating. In the aortic valve, a common valve susceptible to endocarditis is the bicuspid valve. The bicuspid aortic valve is usually of congenital origin but can be an acquired condition resulting from rheumatic endocarditis. Bacterial endocarditis may also occur in patients with significant aortic stenosis, of any etiology.

Bacterial endocarditis on the right side of the heart occurs under two circumstances: (1) a highly infectious organism (staphylococcus, β-hemolytic streptococcus, pneumococcus, gonococcus) infects previously normal valves or (2) an underlying condition is present, which is more common and generally congenital. The malformation is usually responsible for forcing a high-pressure,

high-velocity stream of blood through a narrow opening. Thus in tetralogy of Fallot, the RV infundibulum of the right ventricle is susceptible, as is the tricuspid valve or the right ventricular wall (jet lesion) in instances of small VSD. In PDA, a similar condition exists because part of the pulmonary artery opposite the ductus, struck by the stream of blood flowing through the ductus, is "fertile soil" for infection (Plate 6.81).

Peripheral blood vessels are also subject to infection, including the aorta (1) beyond a site of coarctation, (2) at an atheroma, or (3) within a saccular aneurysm, the latter usually of the abdominal segment of the vessel. In more peripheral vessels, arteriovenous fistulas predispose to infection.

Plate 6.82

Acquired Heart Disease

EARLY LESIONS OF INFECTIVE ENDOCARDITIS

Cardiac valves and sites within blood vessels that become infected may exhibit preexisting lesions that predispose areas to trauma. The traumatic stimulus causes endothelial denudation, and fibrin and platelets are deposited at the site of erosion. Such deposits have a particular affinity for the arrest of circulating bacteria and for the nutrition of organisms caught in the adhesive material. Organisms meshed in fibrin and platelets multiply and invade the underlying tissue.

Although the role of a preexisting lesion in predisposing an area to infection seems clear, the basis for localization of infection is less evident when no recognizable lesion is present. The clinician cannot easily ascertain whether a preexisting lesion was present in some patients because it may be impossible to distinguish fibrous lesions as resulting from infective endocarditis or as representing a preexisting lesion. Regardless of the presence or absence of a preexisting lesion, the early established lesion is similar, characterized by bacterial invasion and later by a reactive healing process. In the early lesion, bacteria invade the tissues as bacterial multiplication, edema, tissue destruction, and leukocytic infiltration occur within the tissues. Granulation tissue, evidenced by proliferation of the capillaries and fibroblasts, may occur in later stages.

At the same time on the infected surface, a vegetation forms, characterized by platelet and fibrin deposits and bacterial proliferation and so extensive in some cases as to form colonies. Fragmentation of vegetative material maintains the bacteremia and causes secondary occlusive effects in the peripheral circulation. The most distinctive gross feature of the early lesion of endocarditis is the vegetation at the site of primary infection. Because of its basic content, the vegetation fundamentally appears tan, but if erythrocytes become enmeshed in the fibrin, it may become purple. An important gross characteristic of the vegetation is its friable nature. Gross appearance of these vegetations vary greatly, ranging from barely visible flat plaques to verrucous masses. Characteristically, the vegetations are deposited focally. Even in some early lesions, one or several vegetations may occur. Regardless of this detail, however, it is classic that the cusps are affected only in part. In the aortic valve, which often is bicuspid, the early vegetation tends to involve either the fused commissure of an acquired bicuspid valve or the region related to the raphe of a congenital bicuspid valve. In the mitral valve, vegetations are first deposited on the atrial surface, along the *contact line* of closure of the cusp (Plate 6.82).

Soon after the establishment of the primary site of infection, there may be evidence of secondary lesions on the same valve. These are derived from bacterial contamination of initially uninvolved segments of the valve that make contact with the site of primary infection. Secondary foci of infection so derived are called *contact* or "kissing" lesions. Once established, the secondary lesion appears similar to the primary focus, and thus determination of primary versus secondary sites of

infection is not always possible. In addition to contact lesions, an early lesion may show a tendency to spread, a feature exemplified by early extension of vegetations from the atrial surface of an atrioventricular valve onto its underlying chordae tendineae.

Grossly, the vegetations of bacterial endocarditis must be distinguished from other conditions that characteristically show vegetative deposits on the valves, including active rheumatic endocarditis, endocardial

lesions of SLE, and marantic (marasmic) vegetations. The focal nature of the vegetations of bacterial endocarditis readily distinguishes them from the small, uniform rheumatic vegetations. In SLE and marantic lesions, the focal nature of the vegetations makes gross distinction less simple. The general nature of the problem is an aid, but a specific diagnosis depends on the presence of bacteria only in the vegetations of bacterial endocarditis.

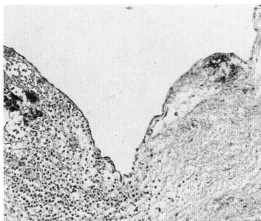

Deposit of platelets and organisms (stained dark), edema, and leukocytic infiltration in very early bacterial endocarditis of aortic valve

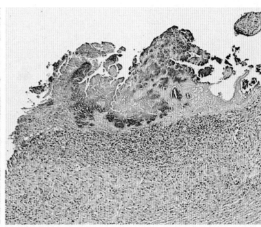

Development of vegetations containing clumps of bacteria on tricuspid valve

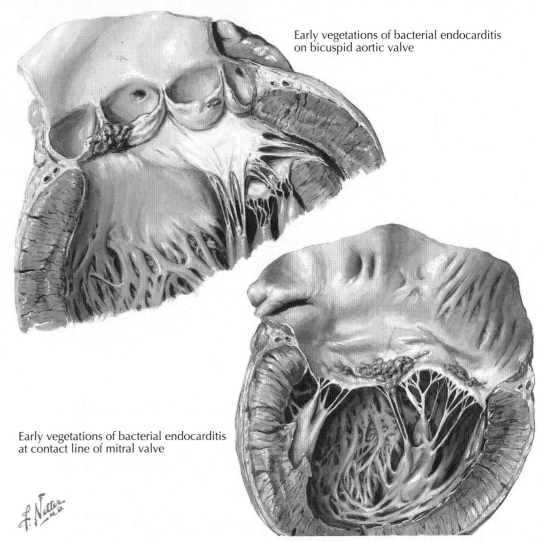

Early vegetations of bacterial endocarditis on bicuspid aortic valve

Early vegetations of bacterial endocarditis at contact line of mitral valve

Plate 6.83

Cardiovascular System: VOLUME 8

ADVANCED LESIONS OF INFECTIVE ENDOCARDITIS

As bacterial endocarditis becomes advanced, it becomes a systemic disease that can affect each organ, including the myocardium. If the disease is not arrested in an early stage, heart changes become more advanced, leading to greater involvement of the valve primarily affected as well as other valves. Spread from one valve to another may occur as a manifestation of *forward infection;* the aortic valve, contiguous with the mitral valve, becomes secondarily involved with primary mitral valve disease, or the reverse may occur. This "reverse" infection depends on the development of *incompetence* of the primarily involved valve, which arises in three main ways. Most simply, bulky vegetations prevent proper apposition of cusps, causing incompetence. More serious is the phenomenon characterized by destruction of valvular substance, as well as chordae tendineae in the mitral valve, resulting in perforation and erosion of valve tissue. A third route is the contiguous spread of the infection from one valve to another. When the aortic valve is primarily involved, incompetence during the active infection leads to infection of those sites against which regurgitant streams become impacted. This may cause either mural infection of the LV outflow area or infection of mitral valve components.

The anterior mitral cusp lies directly subjacent to the aortic valve and is particularly vulnerable to secondary infection, in contrast to the posterior mitral cusp. Such a process is represented first by vegetations on the ventricular surface of the cusp. Destruction of tissue beneath such vegetations may lead to focal weakness, with aneurysm formation in the cusp, or to perforation, with or without the intermediary stage of aneurysm formation. Perforation of a mitral cusp leads to mitral insufficiency, as does rupture of mitral chordae tendineae. If the regurgitant stream from the incompetent aortic valve is directed inferiorly, mitral chordae tendineae may become sites of infection. On the basis of anatomic orientation, chordae tendineae inserting into the anterior mitral cusp are more likely to be involved than those inserting into the posterior cusp, although the latter are not totally protected from this problem. Infected chordae tendineae may rupture, leading to inadequate support of a mitral cusp and mitral regurgitation (Plate 6.83).

Direct spread from the aortic valve may involve structures other than the mitral valve. Extending inferiorly along the contact surface of the involved aortic cusps, the infection may attack the region of the ventricular septum. From here, the destruction may cause an aneurysm of the ventricular septum, which in turn presents either into the right ventricle or the right atrium. Extension of infection from an aortic cusp may advance into an aortic sinus, which may cause an acquired type of aortic sinus aneurysm. If the secondary infection involves the aortic valve above the level of the sinus and penetrates the aortic wall, it may lead to the rare complication of *suppurative pericarditis.* When the mitral valve is primarily involved, regurgitation of blood may result in mural infection of the left atrium at sites struck by regurgitant streams of infected blood.

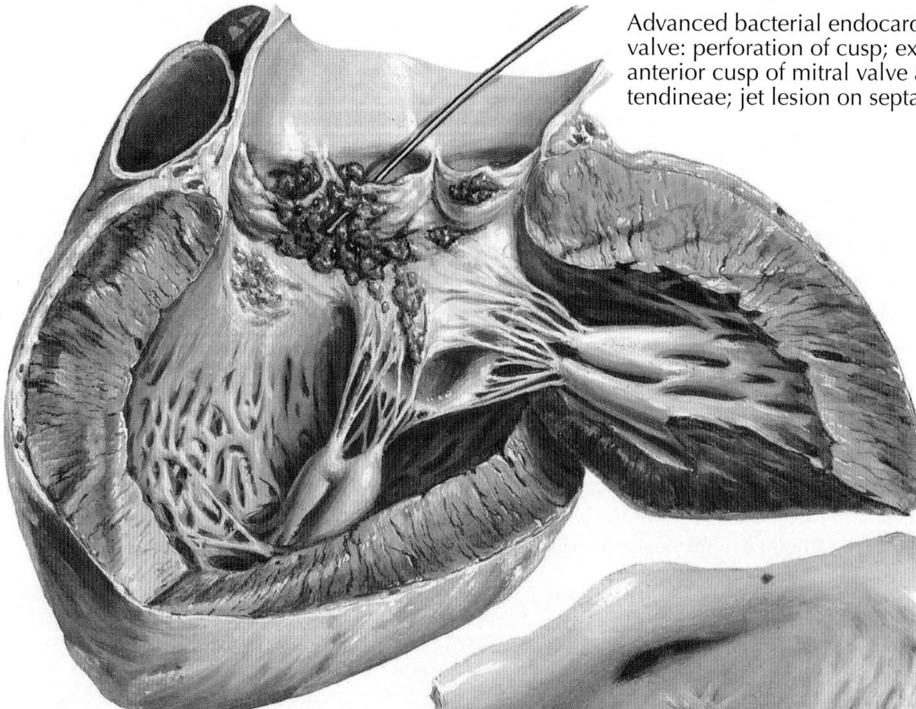

Advanced bacterial endocarditis of aortic valve: perforation of cusp; extension to anterior cusp of mitral valve and chordae tendineae; jet lesion on septal wall

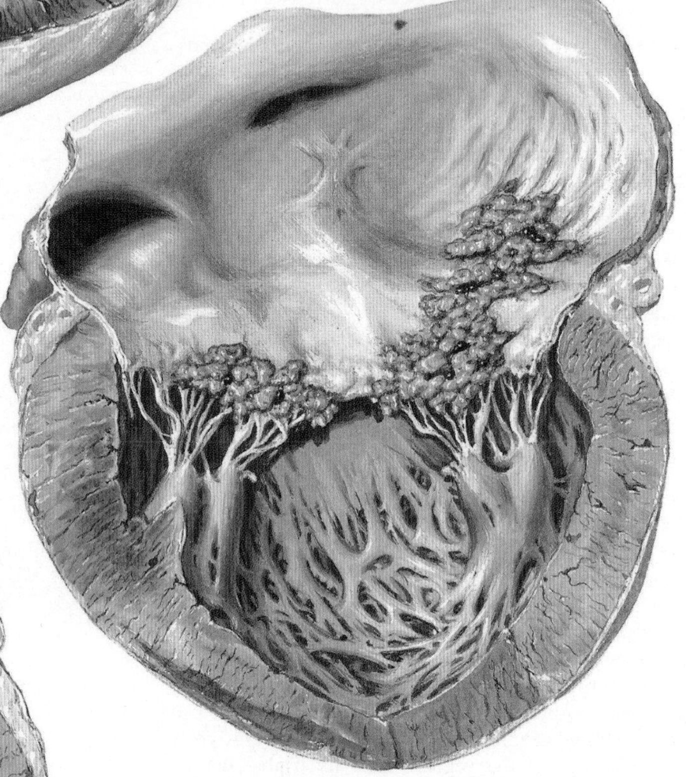

Advanced lesion of mitral valve: vegetations extending onto chordae tendineae with rupture of two chordae; also extension to atrial wall and contact lesion on opposite cusp

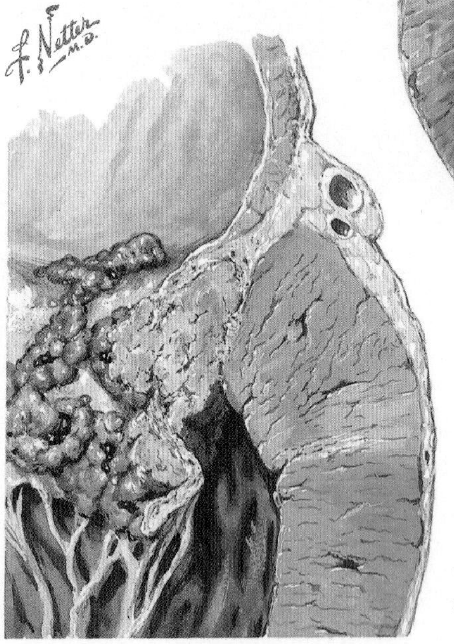

Vegetations of bacterial endocarditis on underside as well as on atrial surface of mitral valve

Another advanced lesion involving the valves is infection of the posterior mitral cusp and the adjacent left ventricular mural endocardium in the angle formed by these two structures. Although the infection characteristically starts on the contact aspect of the cusps, it rapidly extends through the full thickness of the cusp. In the case of the posterior mitral cusp, vegetations may then form on its ventricular aspect. Organisms in this material may secondarily infect adjacent structures, including the LV wall and the wedge of epicardium that extends to the nearby mitral ring.

Much different from the various types of intracardiac infectious spread that characterize advanced lesions, the destructive effects of the infection represent a common problem. Excavation of valvular tissue tends to cause loss of support and prolapse of valvular tissue. Perforations of cusps and rupture of chordae tendineae on valves primarily or secondarily involved are additional important causes of valvular incompetence.

Plate 6.84

Acquired Heart Disease

RIGHT-SIDED HEART INVOLVEMENT IN INFECTIVE ENDOCARDITIS

Infective endocarditis involving the right side of the heart and pulmonary artery system is much less common than primary involvement of the left side. The most common type of right-sided bacterial endocarditis complicates classic patent ductus arteriosus. In this form of PDA, aortic pressure is not fully transmitted into the pulmonary arteries, but velocity is transmitted because of the relative narrowness of the ductus. The stream of blood entering the PA system through the shunt strikes the PA wall opposite the ductus. Here a jet lesion is set up, predisposing this area to infection. While in the clinical state of "infected ductus arteriosus," the ductus itself may be involved, and more often the primary site of infection is in the pulmonary trunk or left pulmonary artery. The ductus itself may become secondarily involved.

A second anatomic situation leading to right-sided bacterial endocarditis is ventricular septal defect. As in PDA, infection usually occurs when systemic arterial pressure is diminished but high velocity is transmitted through the VSD. Thus bacterial endocarditis is uncommon in patients with "large" VSD, in which RV and PA hypertension is present. On the contrary, the "small" VSD, in which the RV pressure is near normal, is particularly vulnerable to endocarditis. Also as in PDA, the primary infection is at the site of impact of the shunted stream. Therefore it tends to occur either on the anterior wall of the right ventricle or on the septal cusp of the tricuspid valve, because these structures lie opposite the VSD. Infection of the defect's edges occurs in some patients. When a left-side structure such as the aortic valve is involved, it usually follows infectious spread from the right-side structures through the defect.

Several types of congenital pulmonary stenosis, including the classic tetralogy of Fallot, isolated right ventricular infundibular stenosis, and pulmonary valve stenosis, constitute the usual additional congenital conditions in which bacterial endocarditis may develop. In each, RV pressure is elevated, increasing velocity and trauma to the tricuspid valve. In all of these conditions, primary tricuspid bacterial endocarditis may occur. More frequently, however, infection involves the compartment beyond the obstructive lesion. In tetralogy and isolated infundibular stenosis, the RV infundibulum is susceptible. In pulmonary valve stenosis, the region predisposed to infection, in addition to the valve itself, is at the bifurcation of the pulmonary trunk, the area struck by the high-velocity stream passing through the stenotic pulmonary valve.

The gross appearance of the lesions is essentially that seen in left-sided bacterial endocarditis. In the primary infection, vegetations vary considerably, from flat, barely detectable aggregations to bulky masses. When a major pulmonary artery is infected, the destructive process may lead to formation of a mycotic aneurysm. In fact, more than half of the localized saccular aneurysms of major pulmonary arteries are of mycotic origin.

Whether right-sided bacterial endocarditis starts in a normal heart or in one with a congenital malformation,

the clinical picture differs from left-sided endocarditis. Petechiae of the skin and mucous membranes and embolic phenomena in organs supplied by the systemic circulation are absent. The concentration of manifestations is in the lungs, as a result of embolism of vegetative material from the primary infection into many small branches of the pulmonary arteries. Classically, this causes widely distributed peripheral infarcts of the lungs. A pleural reaction characteristically fibrinous in nature occurs over these lesions, leading to clinical

evidence of pleurisy. When the organisms are virulent, the pulmonary infarcts suppurate and the picture, both clinically and radiographically, is of widely distributed pulmonary infiltrates.

In protracted right-sided bacterial endocarditis with pulmonary complications, heavy concentrations of organisms are fed through the pulmonary veins into the left side of the heart. This in turn may establish secondary foci of infection on either or both of the left-side cardiac valves.

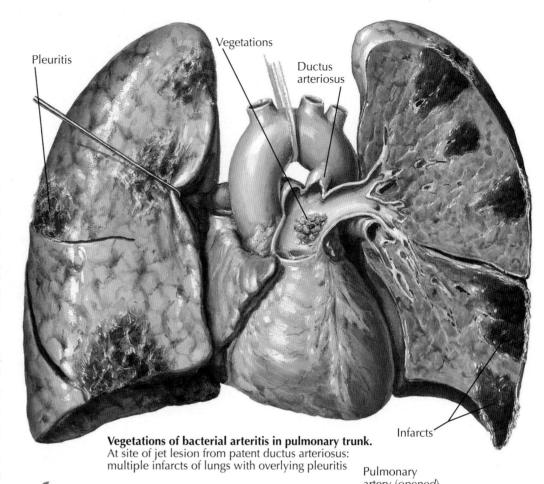

Vegetations of bacterial arteritis in pulmonary trunk.
At site of jet lesion from patent ductus arteriosus: multiple infarcts of lungs with overlying pleuritis

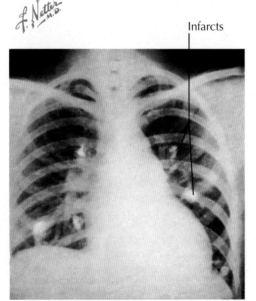

Radiograph: Multiple pulmonary infarcts. Resulting from pulmonary arteritis in patent ductus arteriosus

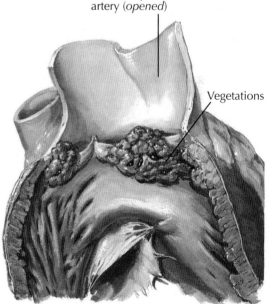

Vegetations on pulmonary valve and outflow tract of right ventricle

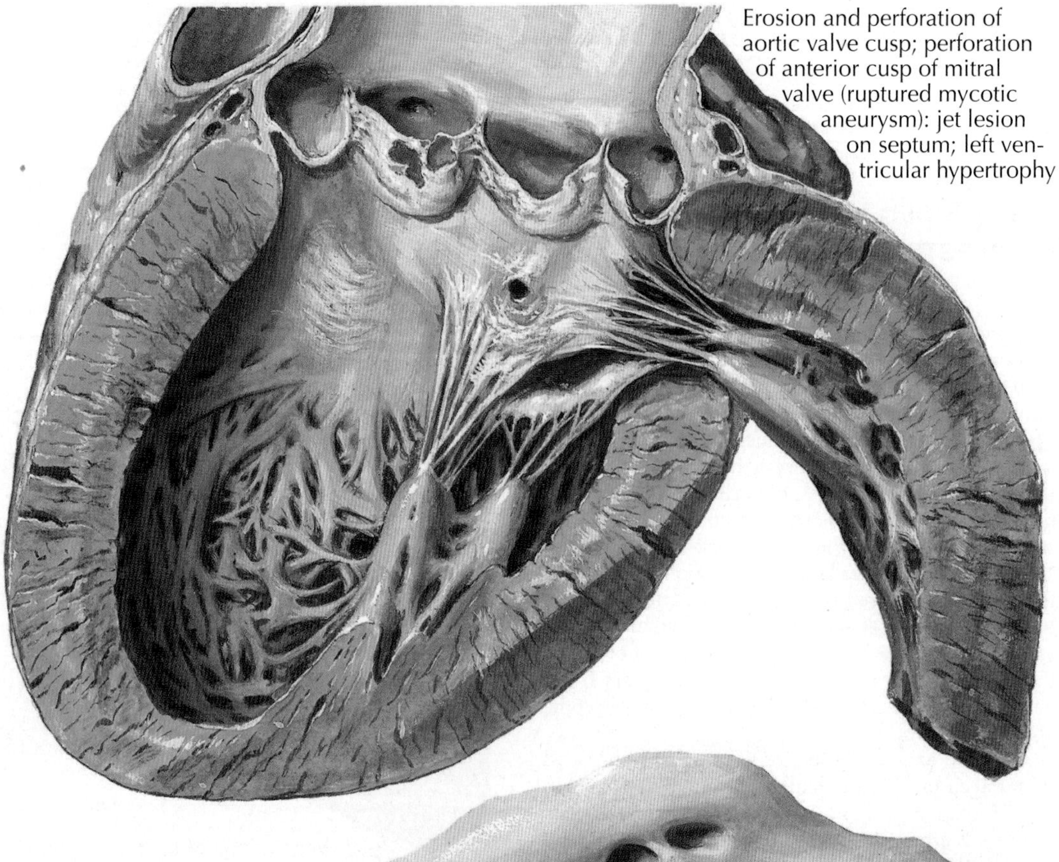

Plate 6.85

Cardiovascular System: VOLUME 8

Erosion and perforation of aortic valve cusp; perforation of anterior cusp of mitral valve (ruptured mycotic aneurysm): jet lesion on septum; left ventricular hypertrophy

CARDIAC SEQUELAE OF INFECTIVE ENDOCARDITIS

Cardiac sequelae of bacterial endocarditis tend to fall into two groups: (1) sequelae with residual changes that cause little functional disturbance of the valve and (2) those attended by a severe degree of anatomic change, usually manifested as valvular insufficiency. Infective endocarditis, even though not recognized clinically, may heal. In some patients this may be spontaneous; in others, antibiotics administered for an undiagnosed condition may heal unsuspected bacterial endocarditis. Healed lesions that have caused minimal disturbance are the end result of inflammation of the valve with surface deposits of vegetation. The sites of valvulitis are characterized by vascularization and varying degrees of fibrous thickening. The vegetation is replaced by fibrous tissue and by foci of calcification. Focal thickening is seen on contact surfaces of cusps, representing not only the primary vegetation but also similar fibrous "kissing" lesions.

Healed lesions responsible for valvular dysfunction typically are characterized by tissue destruction. The various forms include mural fibrous plaques in the left atrium or ventricle, observed as the residua of focal mural endocarditis present during the active infection. Lesions of the aortic valve, responsible for hemodynamic disturbance from bacterial endocarditis, may be characterized by focal erosion leading to a serrated free edge of the involved cusp(s), perforation of the cusps, and destruction of the part of the cusp that attaches to the aortic wall, with resulting prolapse of the involved cusp. These lesions are responsible for aortic insufficiency and in some patients may be associated with mitral insufficiency. This form of aortic insufficiency causes secondary LV changes similar to those resulting from other etiologic types of aortic insufficiency. These changes include massive enlargement of the LV cavity and an increase in its muscle mass. The hypertrophy often is severe, leading to cardiomegaly of a degree not seen with conditions other than aortic insufficiency.

Jet lesions resulting from the impact of the regurgitant stream may be observed in the endocardium of the LV outflow area or on the ventricular surface of the anterior mitral cusp.

Mitral insufficiency following bacterial endocarditis of the aortic valve may occur in several ways. When major LV enlargement results from aortic insufficiency, mechanical interference in the mitral valve mechanism may cause valvular insufficiency. In other patients, mitral insufficiency follows the destruction of mitral valve elements or mitral chordae tendineae as a result of aortic regurgitation during stages of active aortic valve endocarditis. Through concomitant insufficiency, active

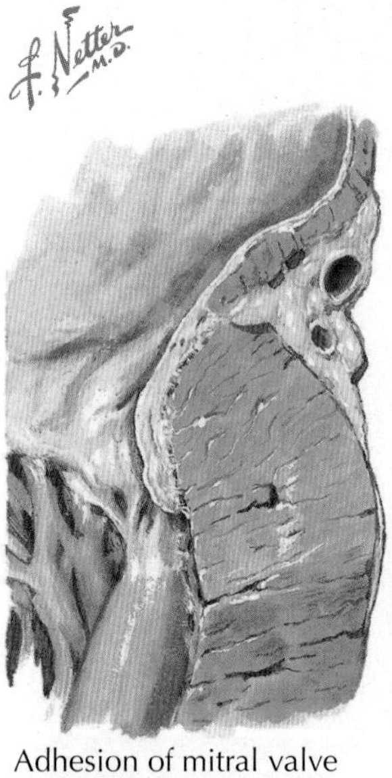

Adhesion of mitral valve cusp to ventricular wall resulting from vegetations on undersurface of valve

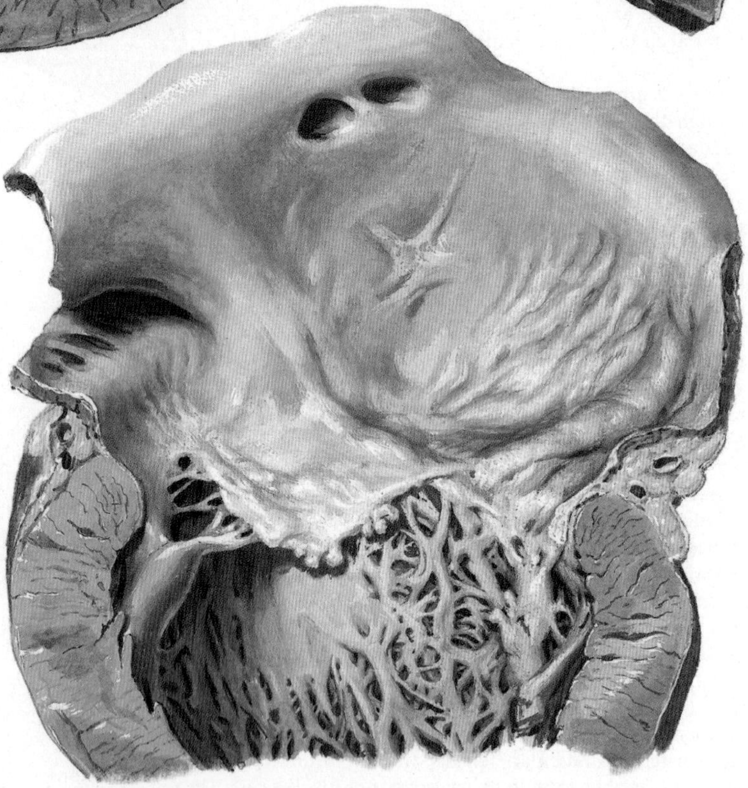

Thickening and erosion of mitral valve with stumps of ruptured chordae tendineae: enlargement of left atrium

aortic endocarditis could cause either mitral valve anterior cusp or mitral chordae tendineae infection. The end effect is mitral insufficiency from perforation of the anterior mitral cusp or rupture of chordae tendineae, with inadequate support of the cusps.

Primary mitral valve endocarditis leading to mitral insufficiency may result from destruction of cusp tissue (e.g., inflammation or myxomatous degeneration), rupture of chordae tendineae, or adhesion of the posterior mitral cusp to the LV wall. The last process follows

fibrous replacement of vegetations that were deposited in the angle between the posterior mitral cusp and LV wall during active disease. Because of this adhesion, the posterior mitral cusp ceases to function as a flap of valvular tissue. When mitral insufficiency ensues from bacterial endocarditis, the visual secondary effects of mitral insufficiency are present, including left atrial enlargement and right ventricular hypertrophy. LV hypertrophy is also present but to a lesser degree than from aortic insufficiency.

Plate 6.86

Acquired Heart Disease

MYCOTIC ANEURYSMS AND EMBOLI IN THE HEART

The manifestations of infective endocarditis range from localized valvular lesions to involvement of organs remote from the heart. Within this complex are secondary lesions at the origin of the aorta and a variety of embolic lesions within the myocardium. Involvement of the aortic origin may come from infection of the mitral or more often the aortic valve. Infection of the aortic origin from aortic valve endocarditis may occur in one of three ways. The first is direct extension from the infected valve to the *aortic sinus* and the adjacent aortic wall. Second, during systole, infected vegetation on an aortic cusp may make contact with the aortic wall, leading to bacterial deposit there. The third way is in effect embolic, as blood containing a high concentration of bacteria flows against the aortic wall.

MYCOTIC ANEURYSMS

Infection of the aortic origin starts in the intima and progresses through the underlying wall. Just as it is to valves, the infection is destructive to the aorta. The resulting weakened aorta may allow an aneurysm to form at the site of infection. Such aneurysms are usually called *mycotic aneurysms,* regardless of the specific organism characterizing the infection. The ultimate effect of an aneurysm depends primarily on whether it ruptures. Unruptured aneurysms are usually silent. The major part of the aortic origin is intracardiac, and thus aneurysms involving this part do not alter the contour of the cardiovascular shadow in chest radiographs. The only exception is an aneurysm involving the aorta near the origin of the left coronary artery. This part of the aorta lies against the epicardium, where an aneurysm may create a silhouette immediately superior to that of the left atrial appendage.

When a mycotic aneurysm of the aortic origin ruptures, the manifestations depend primarily on the site of the aneurysm. Plate 6.86 shows the diverse anatomic relationships of the aortic origin and several structures into which aneurysms rupture. Mycotic aneurysms are derived from a destructive infectious process; thus, although certain anatomic rules apply as to the potential for rupture, variations occur as the infection progresses. Also, *congenital* aneurysms of the aortic sinuses (Valsalva) may become infected after rupturing into a cardiac chamber, and using pathologic examination to determine whether a given aneurysm was primarily bland and secondarily infected, or, conversely, primarily mycotic may be difficult.

Mycotic aneurysms of the *posterior* (noncoronary) aortic sinus tend to rupture into the right atrium and rarely into the left atrium. Because the right aortic sinus is closely related to the infundibulum of the right ventricle, an aneurysm involving this sinus usually leads to the right ventricle but rarely through the ventricular septum into the left ventricle. Because the left aortic sinus is related to the epicardium and to the pulmonary trunk, an aneurysm of this sinus may either lead to suppurative pericarditis or rupture into the pulmonary trunk.

CARDIAC EMBOLI

Embolism into the coronary arterial system is common in left-sided bacterial endocarditis. Usually,

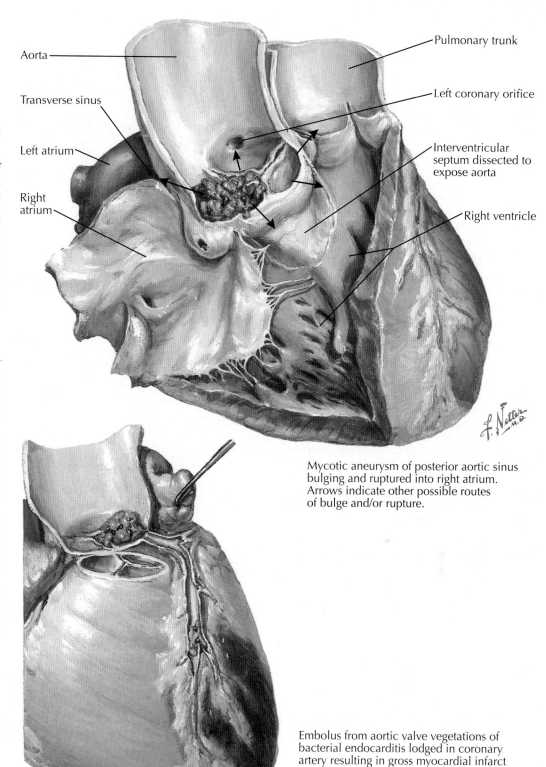

Mycotic aneurysm of posterior aortic sinus bulging and ruptured into right atrium. Arrows indicate other possible routes of bulge and/or rupture.

Embolus from aortic valve vegetations of bacterial endocarditis lodged in coronary artery resulting in gross myocardial infarct

this takes the form of multiple small particles delivered into many intramyocardial ramifications of the coronary arteries. The consequences depend on the virulence of the organism involved in the valvular infection. The organism usually is of relatively low virulence; numerous small, seemingly bland *microinfarcts* are seen in the myocardium. With highly virulent organisms, such as β-hemolytic streptococci or staphylococci, the embolic process causes *microabscesses* of the myocardium.

An embolus lodged in an epicardial branch of a coronary artery is a serious complication and may lead rapidly to death from acute extensive myocardial ischemia. If the patient survives such an event, the effects may be apparent both in the involved artery and in the myocardium supplied by it. The myocardium may show typical gross myocardial infarction, whereas a mycotic aneurysm may form in the affected artery. A rare occurrence is rupture of a coronary artery mycotic aneurysm, leading to hemopericardium.

Plate 6.87

Cardiovascular System: VOLUME 8

REMOTE EMBOLIC EFFECTS OF INFECTIVE ENDOCARDITIS

An important characteristic of bacterial endocarditis is its *tendency for embolism,* which dictates the varied effects of the disease and depends on which side of the heart is involved. In right-sided bacterial endocarditis the lungs become involved, usually dominating the clinical picture. In left-sided infective endocarditis the potential embolic effects are more disseminated because any organ or tissue supplied by the systemic arterial circulation may be affected. Important consequences are lesions of the brain, myocardium, or kidney. Involvement of other body areas may have significant sequelae, representing important features that lead to clinical suspicion of the underlying disease.

Embolic lesions of the brain, as in the myocardium, vary depending on the size of the obstructed artery and the virulence of the organism; an especially dramatic effect results from obstruction of an element in the circle of Willis or one of its branches. Characteristically, the resulting lesion is an infarct. Initially a pale avascular lesion, the *cerebral infarct* may ultimately become hemorrhagic, and determining whether the hemorrhage is a primary lesion or derived indirectly through infarction may be impossible. *Primary* brain hemorrhages result from rupture of arteries infected from bacteria in an impacted embolus. Such hemorrhages may be single and massive or multiple and small (Plate 6.87). More common than gross infarcts or hemorrhages of the brain are widespread *microinfarcts.* These may be silent or may cause variable signs or symptoms, often transient, including headache, focal paresis, aphasia, loss of memory, and confusion.

Just as highly virulent organisms may be responsible for multiple microabscesses in other organs, such lesions may also occur in the brain, causing the same types of cerebral disturbance as with disseminated microinfarcts. Petechial lesions may form in any organ or tissue supplied by the systemic circulation. Whether these result from infection of small arterial vessels (with rupture) or from microinfarction (with secondary hemorrhage in the affected tissues) is debatable. However, *petechiae* often occur and help alert the physician to the possible bacterial endocarditis. Petechiae may be readily observed in the retina, skin, and mucous membranes; when present, a subungual location also is common (Plate 6.87).

Patients may have clubbing of the fingers and toes, especially those with bacterial endocarditis following a protracted course.

The kidney may be affected in its major arteries or parenchyma. The classic renal lesion is focal embolic *glomerulonephritis.* Grossly, the picture is that of the "flea-bitten" kidney, with widespread petechiae in the cortex. Histologically, the process is characterized by focal infarction of glomerular tufts and by glomerular and tubular hemorrhages. An uncommon parenchymal lesion is diffuse glomerulonephritis. Microabscesses generally disseminate if the infecting organism is highly virulent. Embolism to renal arteries is common, leading to infarction of parts of the renal substance, with attendant hematuria. The embolism's episodic nature is evidenced by *renal infarcts* of various ages often being

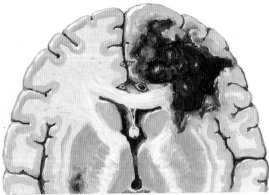

Infarct of brain with secondary hemorrhage from embolism to right anterior cerebral artery; also small infarct in left basal ganglia

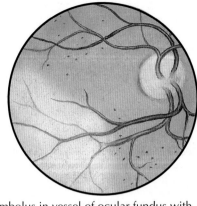

Embolus in vessel of ocular fundus with retinal infarction; petechiae

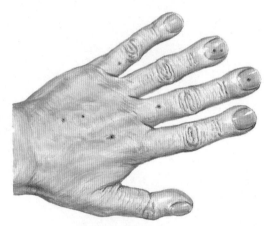

Multiple petechiae of skin and clubbing of fingers

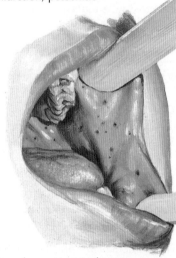

Petechiae of mucous membranes

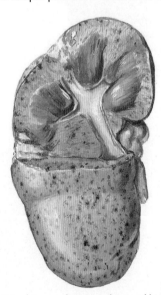

Petechiae and gross infarcts of kidney

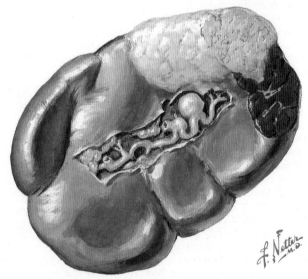

Mycotic aneurysms of splenic arteries and infarct of spleen; splenomegaly

found. Mycotic aneurysms of a renal artery or one of its smaller branches typify the involvement of major branches in this organ.

The *spleen* plays a prominent role in bacterial endocarditis; *splenomegaly* is an important clinical sign. In addition, the spleen may be the site of mycotic aneurysm, and infarction is common, as in the kidney. The splenic infarction may be marked by left upper abdominal pain. Usually, the infarcts are relatively bland but rarely may suppurate and rupture, leading to subdiaphragmatic abscess.

In the gastrointestinal tract the most common phenomenon is petechiae. Less often, intestinal infarction or the formation of mycotic aneurysms of mesenteric arteries may result from embolism of gross vegetative particles. Mycotic aneurysms also are occasionally observed in the extremities, with or without surrounding cellulitis or abscess formation.

Plate 6.88

Acquired Heart Disease

NONBACTERIAL THROMBOTIC (MARANTIC) ENDOCARDITIS

Among the various forms of so-called verrucous or vegetative endocarditis is nonbacterial thrombotic endocarditis (NBTE), also called marantic endocarditis. Rheumatic endocarditis and SLE endocarditis also are nonbacterial forms. "Marantic" is derived similar to "marasmus" and was originally applied as a condition seen in wasting diseases. Although this feature still applies, marantic endocarditis may also be seen in individuals who do not exhibit wasting, for any reason, but who harbor *malignant tumors*. In some patients the complication of NBTE, in the form of embolism to systemic arteries, may represent the primary evidence of a malignant tumor not yet apparent, particularly with a relatively occult, primary tumor in the body or tail of the pancreas (Plate 6.88).

Marantic vegetations may occur on any valve but typically affect the left-sided valves. Both the mitral and aortic valves may be involved simultaneously. The gross appearance is friable, brown-to-gray material attached focally to the contact surface of the valve cusps. Marantic vegetations are focal in distribution and vary in size and thus do not resemble the fine, regularly deposited vegetations of acute rheumatic endocarditis. On the other hand, vegetations in NBTE may be confused grossly with those of bacterial endocarditis or SLE, although other distinguishing features are present. In contrast to bacterial endocarditis, marantic vegetations are not associated with destructive lesions of the valve cusps or chordae tendineae. Moreover, vegetations in NBTE are sterile, failing to contain bacteria, as determined by histologic examination. In SLE the vegetations are deposited not only on the contact surface of the valve cusps, as in the case of marantic vegetations, but also on the mural endocardium of the chambers. Also, vegetations may be present in the angle between the posterior mitral cusp and the left ventricular wall. Histologically, lupus endocarditis, as characterized by nonbacterial inflammation of the valve cusp, involves a heavy leukocytic infiltration. In contrast, the valve cusp beneath NBTE vegetation shows little if any leukocytic infiltration (Plate 6.88).

Some controversy surrounds whether NBTE is in fact a disease of the cusp or merely of vegetative material deposited on a normal cusp. The exhaustive study by Allen provided evidence that the primary process is in the substance of the cusp. In essence, this shows focal swelling of collagen and secondary microrupture of the overlying portion of the cusp. On such areas, products derived from the blood, platelets, and fibrin are deposited, constituting marantic vegetations.

Marantic vegetations do not cause significant deformity of the valve, and the only serious potential complication is embolism. Most of these vegetations occur on left-sided heart valves, so embolism may involve any organ except the lung. Depending on the sites of lodgment of marantic vegetations, the embolism may cause infarction of the brain, kidney, spleen, or other organs. Embolism from marantic vegetations is known to cause systemic arterial occlusion in patients with malignant tumors. Also in such a patient, however, metastases infrequently may be deposited in the left side of the heart. Either the mural endocardium or the valves may be involved, the valves requiring histologic examination to distinguish from NBTE vegetations. When metastases are present in the left side of the heart, systemic embolism may result from fragmentation of neoplastic nodules or thrombotic material deposited on intracavitary foci of secondary tumors.

Among patients with malignant tumors, *systemic venous thrombosis* is more common than NBTE. The primary effect of venous thrombosis is pulmonary embolism, yielding clinicopathologic features unlike those of marantic vegetations. In an unusual situation of pulmonary embolism, however, paradoxical embolism to the left side of the heart may occur, usually through a patent foramen ovale. Paradoxical embolism in turn may lead to systemic arterial occlusion and infarction of organs. In this regard, systemic venous thrombosis and nonbacterial thrombotic (marantic) endocarditis may share key features.

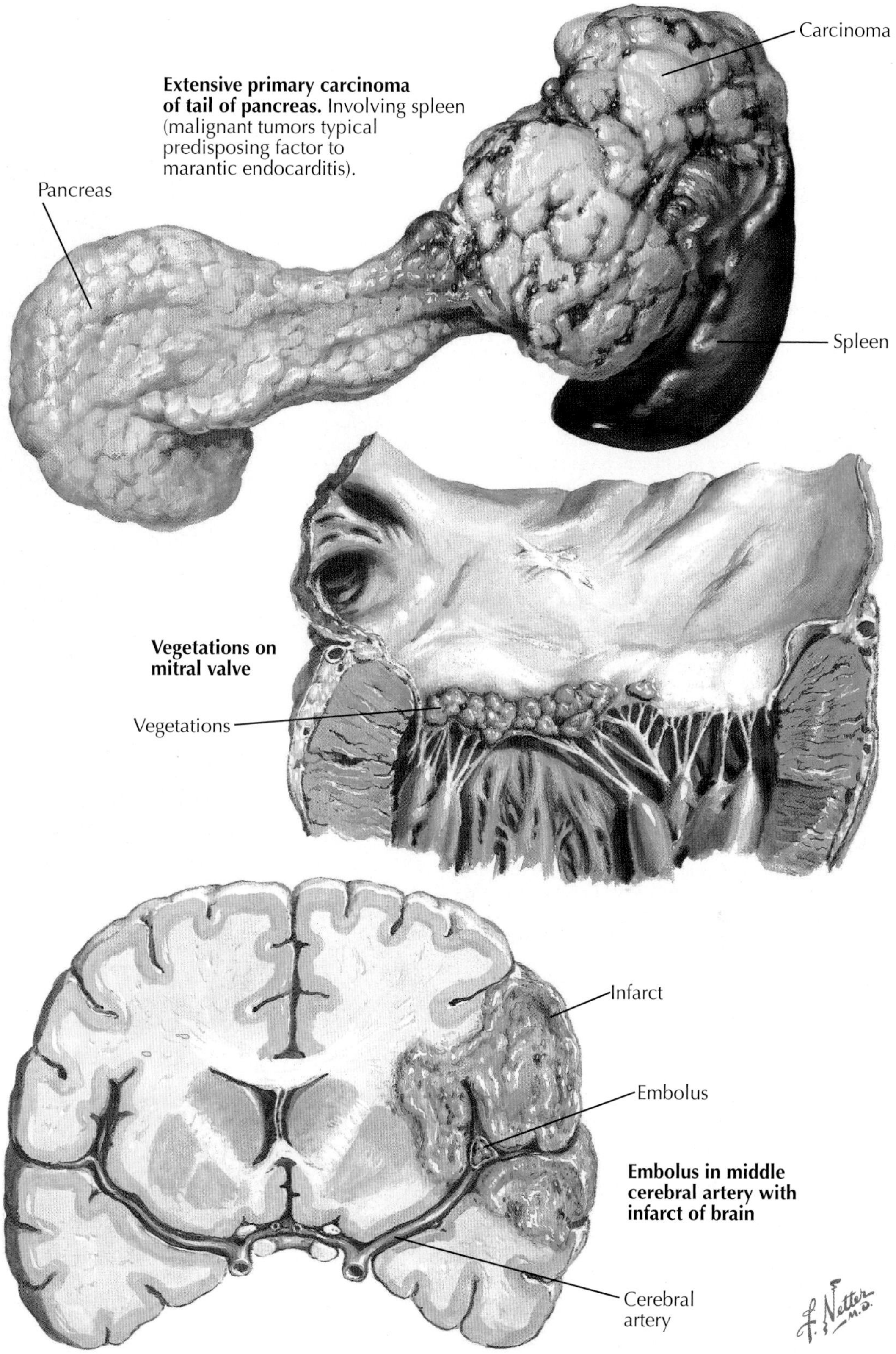

Extensive primary carcinoma of tail of pancreas. Involving spleen (malignant tumors typical predisposing factor to marantic endocarditis).

Carcinoma

Pancreas

Spleen

Vegetations on mitral valve

Vegetations

Infarct

Embolus

Embolus in middle cerebral artery with infarct of brain

Cerebral artery

Plate 6.89

Cardiovascular System: VOLUME 8

CARDIOPULMONARY RESUSCITATION AND HYPOTHERMIA THERAPY

EXTERNAL RESUSCITATION

Cardiopulmonary arrest, or sudden death, is the immediate and unexpected cessation of spontaneous circulation and respiration. It may occur in drowning, in asphyxia from any other cause (e.g., adverse reaction to drugs or anesthesia), in sudden and complete heart block, in electrocution, or after excessive vagal stimulation. The etiology of cardiopulmonary arrest primarily may involve ventilatory insufficiency—as in conditions caused by asphyxia, with cardiac arrest resulting from the myocardial anoxia—or it may include cardiac malfunction such as a mechanically ineffective arrhythmia (ventricular tachycardia/fibrillation, asystole) after myocardial infarction.

The three types of ECG patterns in cardiopulmonary arrest are (1) *cardiac asystole,* with a straight-line tracing; (2) ventricular fibrillation with an irregular, uncoordinated ECG pattern, resulting from asynchronous contraction of the various myocardial fibrils; and (3) pulseless electrical activity (PEA), in which a coordinated electrical discharge may be recorded, but with no resultant effective mechanical action of the myocardium. Asystole usually results from some generalized cardiac hypoxia secondary to respiratory insufficiency or arrest. PEA may also occur after sudden and complete atrioventricular dissociation, profound drug overdose, or marked vagal stimulation. Ventricular fibrillation is usually secondary to irritability of the ventricular myocardium, most often related to ischemic heart disease. PEA may result from generalized myocardial depression or ischemia.

In treatment, emergency measures are directed toward artificial reinstitution of the circulation of blood oxygenated by artificial ventilation. The brain is the body tissue most sensitive to anoxia and can sustain irreversible cellular damage in 4 to 6 minutes, depending on the antecedent physiologic conditions. Emergency measures must be instituted within this brief period. After artificial reestablishment of the circulation of oxygenated blood, definitive measures are made to reestablish the spontaneity of both ventilation and circulation as well. These measures include (1) use of drugs to stimulate the myocardium and improve the artificial circulation; (2) ECG determination of cardiac activity; (3) defibrillation from ventricular fibrillation or other arrhythmias, if present; and (4) further use of cardiac stimulatory drugs or, if necessary, depressants. After successful reactivation of ventilation and circulation, the central nervous system must be protected from further insult by prevention of cerebral edema. Currently, *hypothermia* is employed in resuscitated cardiac arrest patient who remain unconscious.

Cardiopulmonary Resuscitation

The 2013 guidelines for cardiopulmonary resuscitation (CPR) emphasize doing chest compressions first. The previous "ABC" method (airway, breathing, and compressions) caused delays in chest compressions, which are critical to perfusion of the brain and other vital organs.

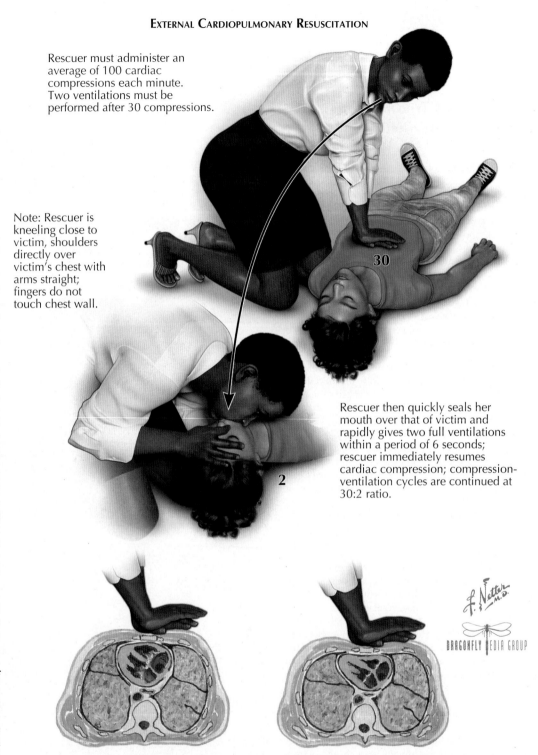

EXTERNAL CARDIOPULMONARY RESUSCITATION

Rescuer must administer an average of 100 cardiac compressions each minute. Two ventilations must be performed after 30 compressions.

Note: Rescuer is kneeling close to victim, shoulders directly over victim's chest with arms straight; fingers do not touch chest wall.

Rescuer then quickly seals her mouth over that of victim and rapidly gives two full ventilations within a period of 6 seconds; rescuer immediately resumes cardiac compression; compression-ventilation cycles are continued at 30:2 ratio.

Heart intermittently compressed between sternum and vertebrae

Out-of-hospital CPR is now done in the following sequence (Plate 6.89).

1. Call 911 immediately on discovering the patient.
2. If the person is comatose, roll them on their back.
3. Start chest compressions.
4. Compress the chest 2 inches 100 times per minute.
5. Open airway with a head tilt and chin lift.
6. Pinch nose of patient and provide two 1-second mouth-to-mouth breaths.
7. Continue cycle of 30 compressions, two breaths.
8. Defibrillate as quickly as possible if defibrillator (or automatic external defibrillator) is available.

Internal Cardiac Massage

The recognition by mid–19th-century physicians that sudden circulatory (cardiac) arrests were occurring in patients because of an idiosyncratic reaction to anesthetics led to experimental investigation and eventually effective CPR. In 1881 Niehaus reported the first but unsuccessful resuscitation in humans using the open-chest cardiac compression (Schiff) technique, first successfully used in 1901. In 1885, however, Koenig described *external* cardiac compression, successfully applied twice by Maass in 1891. External CPR, however, essentially remained unused until its rediscovery by

Plate 6.90

Acquired Heart Disease

CARDIOPULMONARY RESUSCITATION AND HYPOTHERMIA THERAPY (Continued)

Kouwenhoven and use by Jude and Knickerbocker in 1960. *Internal* (open chest), or *direct,* cardiac massage, the prevailing procedure for cardiac arrest from 1901 to 1960, is still often used and specifically when the cause of the sudden cardiac arrest may be within the thorax, such as after a crushing or penetrating chest wound. Internal massage also is mandatory if external cardiac compression is impossible in a large patient. When the chest already is open, as during a thoracic procedure, and sudden cardiac arrest occurs, internal cardiac massage is the proper method (Plate 6.90).

In an emergency, a left anterior thoracotomy is rapidly done under unsterile conditions, opening the chest in the fourth or fifth intercostal space. The ribs are pulled apart manually, the left hand is introduced, and the heart is grasped, initially through the pericardium with the palm of the hand toward the apex of the ventricles. A milking motion squeezes the heart from the apex toward the base, and blood is pumped into both the pulmonary and the systemic circulation. The compression is held for one-third to one-half of a second and then totally released, to allow venous filling, and repeated 80 to 100 times per minute. The pericardium is opened anterior to the phrenic nerve as soon as forceps and scissors are available. A better grasp of the heart and better cardiac compression can be provided once the pericardium is open.

As soon as available, a rib spreader is inserted, and more sterile conditions are undertaken. Simultaneously with the artificial circulation, the lungs must be ventilated by intubation of the trachea and positive-pressure insufflation with a self-expanding bag. The expired-air methods of ventilation are less effective with the chest open but can be used.

With internal cardiac massage (compression) the status of heart action is readily identified. Asystole is recognized by a totally quiet heart. Ventricular fibrillation is identified by a diffuse, irregular twitching or waving motion of the heart without coordinated contraction and by PEA. Weak ventricular contractions are not expelling blood. Ventricular defibrillation may be ineffective in this patient, but inotropic therapy may succeed.

With external cardiopulmonary resuscitation, the initial cardiotonic and vasopressor drugs are administered even before the type of cardiac arrest is known, because they are equally applicable in all situations. In general, with internal cardiac massage, the same agents are employed immediately. *Epinephrine* is given directly into the bloodstream, by intracardiac injection or IV. This dose of epinephrine is repeated as necessary for continuous stimulation of the heart and peripheral vasoconstriction, causing more blood to be pumped to the brain and myocardium. Sodium bicarbonate (or another alkalizing agent) is also administered intravenously, to prevent development of severe metabolic acidosis. In general, for patients in cardiopulmonary arrest, use of external massage techniques along with cardiotonic vasopressor agents will result in reinstitution of cardiac activity from asystole or profound

INTERNAL CARDIAC MASSAGE

Position of the hand on the heart for direct cardiac compression massage

Thorax opened in left 4th or 5th intercostal space; heart grasped and intermittently compressed by left hand as vasopressor cardiotonic agent is injected into heart

cardiovascular collapse. Ventricular fibrillation requires defibrillation as soon as possible.

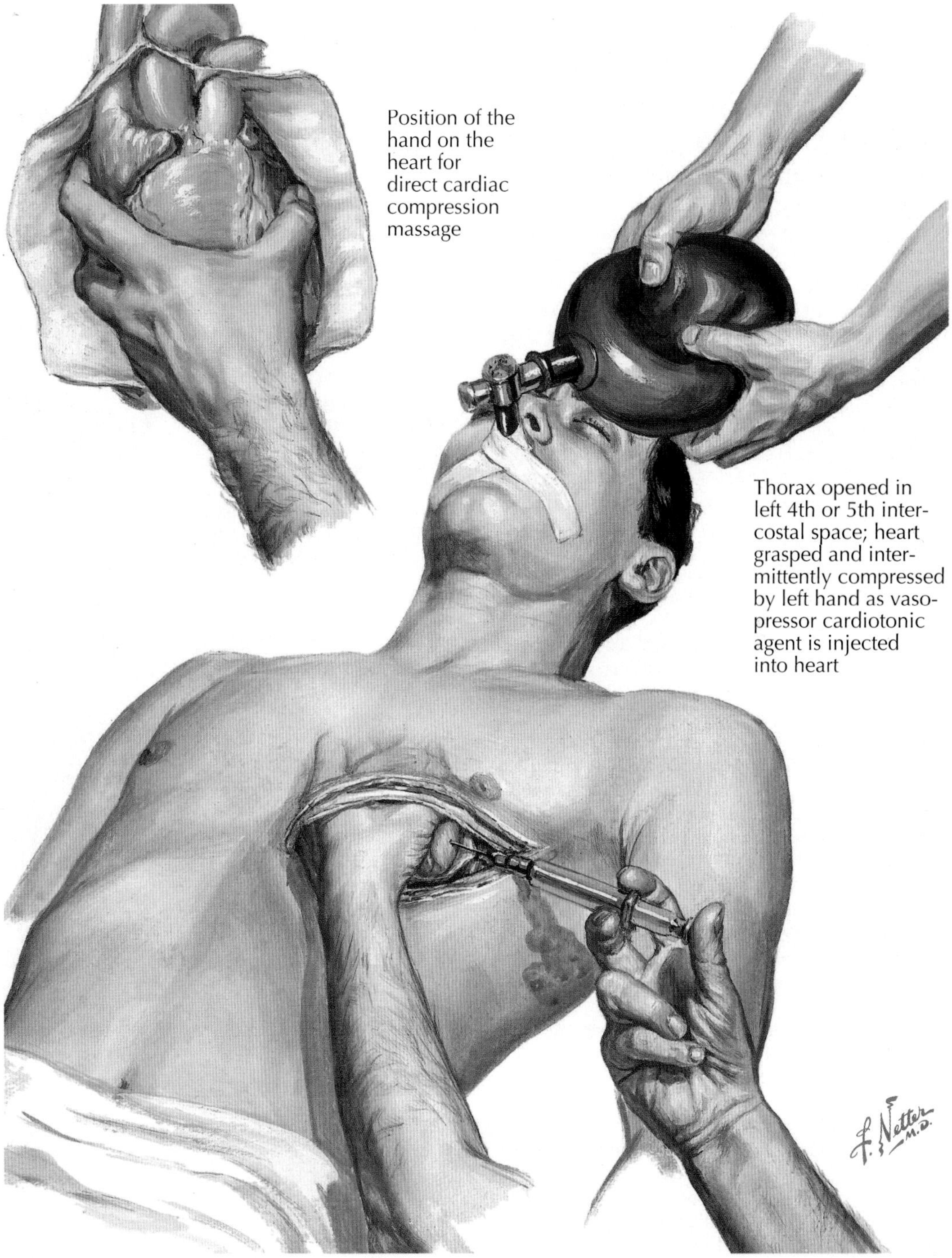

DEFIBRILLATION

Ventricular fibrillation is the incoordination of contractions of the heart muscle caused by an independent discharge of the electrical potential of the myocardial fibrils. It rarely reverts spontaneously to a sinus rhythm. In 1889 Prevost and Battelli investigated electrical methods to terminate the fibrillation and reinstitute spontaneous sinus rhythm, with follow-up studies by Hooker, Kouwenhoven, and Langworthy from 1928 to 1932, and first successful application—using direct-contact electric shock—by Beck in 1947. In the mid-1950s, Kouwenhoven and Zoll independently developed a

closed-chest electrical defibrillator, revolutionizing the use of electricity in treatment of cardiac arrhythmias. Presently, the direct-current defibrillator can convert not only the dangerous ventricular fibrillations and tachycardias into a coordinated sinus rhythm, but also can convert the less serious atrial flutter, atrial fibrillation, and other supraventricular rhythms.

In external (closed-chest) defibrillation of the heart, for either ventricular or supraventricular arrhythmias, large insulated paddle electrodes are placed on the chest wall, one over the apex of the heart (just below the left nipple) and the other over the base of the heart (in the first right intercostal space). In using the direct-current defibrillator, 120 to 200 J on a biphasic defibrillator or 360 J using a monophasic defibrillator is selected and current applied with a switch on an electrode handle but only

Plate 6.91

Cardiovascular System: VOLUME 8

CARDIOPULMONARY RESUSCITATION AND HYPOTHERMIA THERAPY (Continued)

after all other personnel have broken contact with the patient. If the ECG shows the initial shock is not successful in defibrillating the heart, repeated shocks are necessary, possibly at a higher joule setting (Plate 6.91).

Internal or open-chest defibrillation is carried out through a left anterior thoracotomy. The pericardium must be opened. The electrode paddles, a special type with a concave surface, are wrapped in gauze and soaked in saline. One paddle is placed over the right atrium and the other over the left ventricle. Between 10 and 60 J is then administered through the heart, again after all others have broken contact. The shock must be given under the control of the physician holding the paddles.

To obtain permanent defibrillation of the ventricle, it may be necessary to administer cardiac drugs such as lidocaine or amiodarone intravenously as a 300-mg bolus and then repeated with 150 mg in 3 to 5 minutes. In external (closed-chest) defibrillation, status of the heart is interpreted from the ECG, whereas with open-chest defibrillation the status can be determined by direct observation.

The quality of the myocardial fibrillations must be vigorous and coarse enough that spontaneous coordinated discharge can occur after complete depolarization of the myocardium by massive electric shock. In the unoxygenated myocardium, and when the fibrillations are of poor quality, defibrillation may not be possible. IV epinephrine will strengthen myocardial action and allow greater ease of defibrillation, but one must remember that too much epinephrine may be cardiotoxic and result in an epinephrine-induced cardiomyopathy.

Once spontaneous cardiac action has been resumed, cardiac function is supported by vasopressor drugs, as necessary. Endotracheal intubation and ventilation are continued until good spontaneous ventilations are present.

After open-chest cardiac compression, the patient must be taken to the operating room for closure of the thorax. The pleural space and pericardium are irrigated with saline, and the pericardium is closed loosely. The ribs are approximated, and the chest wall is closed in layers. Wide-spectrum antibiotics are left in the pleural space, and the patient is given large doses of IV antibiotics for 1 week. Surprisingly, the infection rate is quite low, even though emergency cardiac open-chest massage is done under unsterile conditions.

With external CPR, no special surgical procedure is necessary, but the patient should be admitted to a cardiac care unit for close observation of any evidence of decreased cerebral flow deficits.

HYPOTHERMIA FOR CARDIAC ARREST

Increased brain temperature can exacerbate brain injury after cardiac arrest. After 10 minutes of brain anoxia, without defibrillation, about 10% of patients will survive and leave the hospital, many with residual cognitive impairment. This occurs despite modern efforts to improve survival with emergency medical services,

automatic external defibrillators, and bystander CPR. Prompt defibrillation in any patient with cardiac arrest from ventricular fibrillation is the treatment of choice. In a patient who has been defibrillated and is unconscious, prompt defibrillation followed by hypothermia may help preserve brain function by reducing ischemic injury related to decreased blood flow to the brain. Current resuscitation recommendations support the use of hypothermia protocols after defibrillation, and evidence supports its benefit in patients with ventricular fibrillation as the initial rhythm.

Accomplishing hypothermia in these patients requires an organized approach by emergency department physicians and the cardiologists responsible for care of these critically compromised patients on

hospital admission. Protocols to lower body temperature must be rapidly implemented and maintained for approximately 24 hours. Some patients who have had ST-elevated MI need emergent revascularization before or concurrent with hypothermia. If the patient remains unconscious after revascularization, the hypothermia protocol should be instituted. Neurologic consultation should assess the comatose patient's status before, during, and after the hypothermia treatment. Patient temperature should be reduced to a goal 32°C to 34°C (~90°F) and drugs to control shivering administered. These agents (e.g., propofol) should sedate and paralyze the patient. After 24 hours the patient should be rewarmed slowly, to avoid complications such as hypotension and hyperkalemia.

DEFIBRILLATION

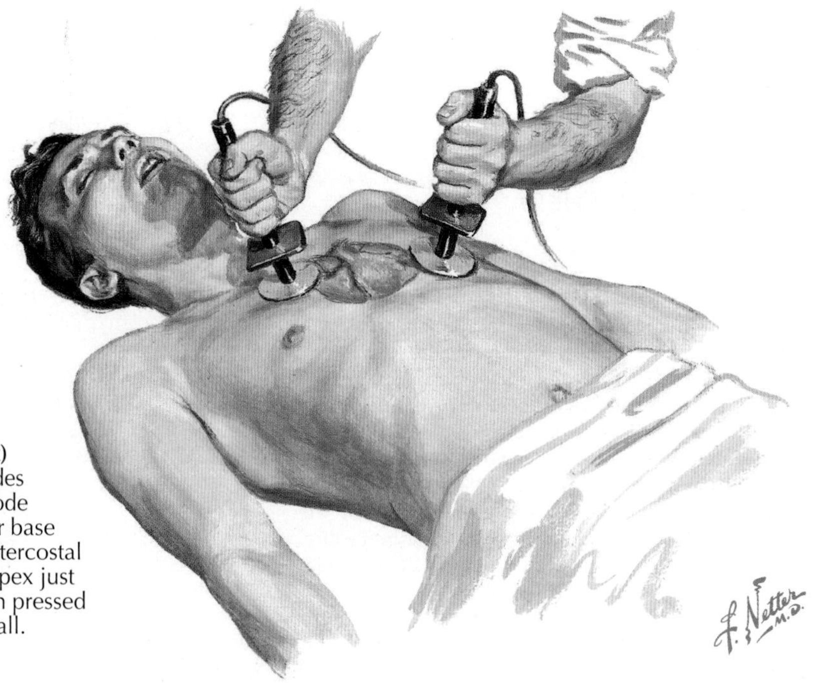

External (closed-chest) defibrillation. Electrodes lubricated with electrode paste; one placed over base of heart at first right intercostal space, and one over apex just below left nipple; both pressed firmly against chest wall.

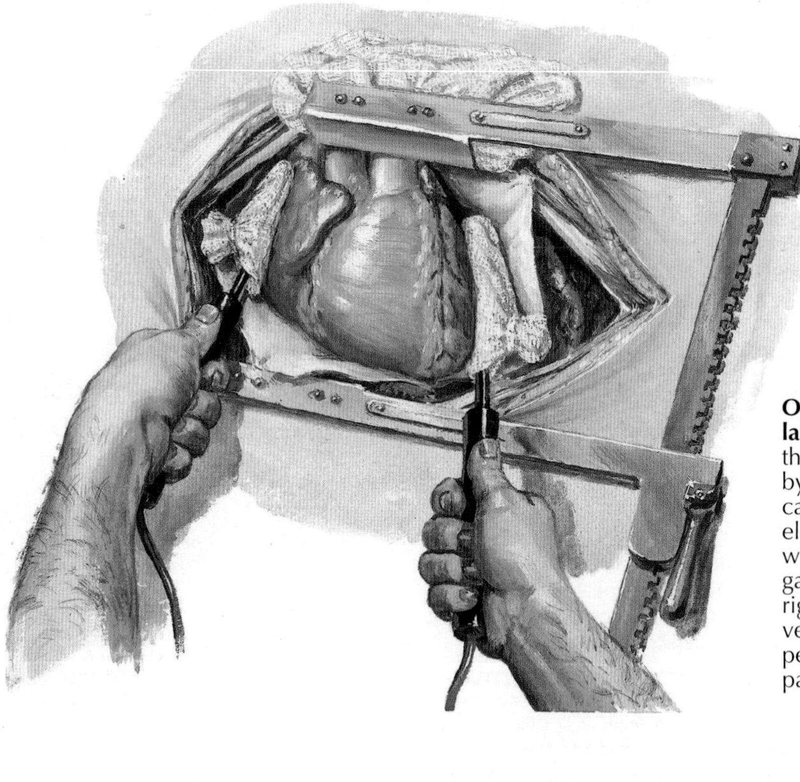

Open-chest defibrillation. Left anterior thoracotomy held open by rib spreader, pericardium opened, electrodes wrapped with saline-soaked gauze applied over right atrium and left ventricle. No other personnel may touch patient or bed.

Plate 6.92

Acquired Heart Disease

EXTRAARTICULAR MANIFESTATIONS IN RHEUMATOID ARTHRITIS

Nodular episcleritis with scleromalacia

Affected hand with subcutaneous nodules over knuckles, swan-neck deformity of middle finger, ulnar deviation of fingers, and muscle atrophy

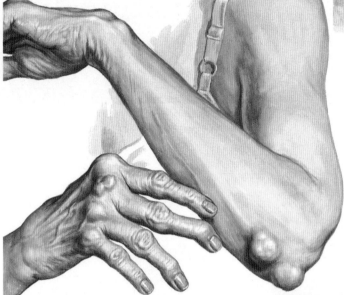

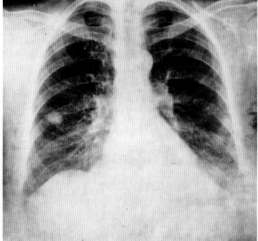

Subcutaneous nodule just distal to olecranon process and another in olecranon bursa

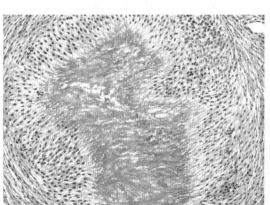

RHEUMATOID ARTHRITIS

Because humans are living longer, aging patients with rheumatoid arthritis (RA) are subject to the same risk of cardiovascular disease as anyone. In addition to longer life span, another factor in the increasing prevalence of cardiovascular disease in older patients with RA is the common use of sophisticated noninvasive detection technology, including CT, ultrasound with Doppler, peripheral vascular imaging (carotid arteries, aorta; renal, iliac, and femoral arteries), coronary flow reserve studies to detect microcirculatory changes, and ECG and electrophysiologic studies to detect conduction disease. The chronic inflammatory state of patients with RA—an autoimmune disease more often affecting females—is thought to contribute to the development and progression of atherosclerotic disease, including coronary artery and carotid disease. Mortality of aging patients with RA is usually related to ischemic heart disease and vascular disease (e.g., MI, cerebrovascular accident).

Currently, most patients with RA are treated with antiinflammatory agents to slow development and progression of atherosclerotic disease in the heart and vasculature (carotid and coronary arteries, other peripheral vascular sites). Methotrexate is often used to

Section of rheumatoid nodule. Central area of fibrinoid necrosis surrounded by zone of palisading mesenchymal cells and peripheral fibrous tissue capsule containing chronic inflammatory cells.

Radiograph shows rheumatoid nodule in right lung. Lesion may be misdiagnosed as carcinoma until identified by biopsy or postsurgical pathologic analysis.

treat patients with RA. Low-dose methotrexate is being tested with patients with ischemic heart disease to assess the efficacy and safety of using an antiinflammatory agent to decrease major adverse cardiovascular events.

Other cardiovascular manifestations of RA include vasculitis (uncommon), pericarditis and pericardial effusion (usually not clinically significant), and myocardial disease (may lead to heart failure secondary to

diastolic dysfunction). Valvular disease is a common finding (e.g., mitral valve prolapse, mitral regurgitation) and usually detected by cardiac ultrasound but not clinically significant. The most frequent cardiac manifestations involve valvular heart disease, with aortic and mitral valve regurgitation and aortic root dilation occurring most often. These abnormalities rarely are symptomatic. Less common cardiac manifestations are myocarditis and arrhythmias.

Plate 6.93

Cardiovascular System: VOLUME 8

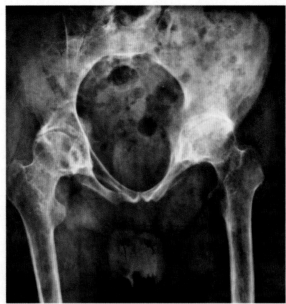

Radiograph shows complete bony ankylosis of both sacroiliac joints in late stage of disease.

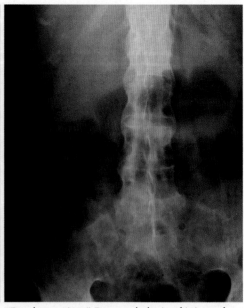

"Bamboo spine." Bony ankylosis of joints of lumbar spine. Ossification exaggerates bulges of intervertebral discs.

Complications

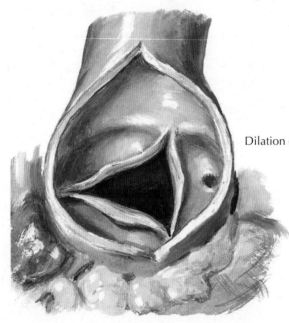

Iridocyclitis with irregular pupil due to synechiae

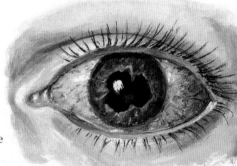

Dilation of aortic ring with valvular insufficiency

ANKYLOSING SPONDYLITIS

The cardiac manifestations of ankylosing spondylitis (AS) are valvular lesions and particularly *aortitis*, which may result in aortic regurgitation. Transesophageal cardiac ultrasound can identify these abnormalities (one or more) in approximately 80% of patients. Pericarditis and myocarditis can occur but are less common than aortitis and valvulitis. AS is a systemic inflammatory disorder that involves the entire spine and sacroiliac joints (spondyloarthropathy). AS is a disease that predominately affects males; onset usually begins in young adulthood. AS can involve the peripheral joints but much less than seen in the classic patient with RA. If musculoskeletal disease is present, the tendons and ligaments that attach to bone are involved. The cause of AS is unknown, but infection in a genetically predisposed host is a current working hypothesis.

The hallmark cardiovascular manifestations of AS are aortic disease and aortic regurgitation. Distinctive features at autopsy include thickening of the aortic wall caused by adventitial scarring, as well as intimal proliferation limited to the aortic root (ascending aorta) but extending into the membranous ventricular septum. Aortic valve leaflets are diffusely thickened and shortened and thus incompetent. These findings of aortic root and valve thickening are easily seen using transthoracic and transesophageal ultrasound, which shows mild aortic regurgitation in most patients with AS. In some, ultrasonic detection of aortic regurgitation may precede development of joint manifestations. Mild aortic root dilation in AS may be caused by aortitis. Confirmation by cardiac ultrasound is difficult, and the aortic root dilation could result from aortic regurgitation. Also at autopsy, conduction system disease can be seen, caused by inflammation and fibrous scarring of

the interventricular septum. First-degree atrioventricular block is the most common conduction system disease, although more serious AV blocks as well as right and left bundle branch blocks can occur as well.

Using cardiac ultrasound, abnormal diastolic filling patterns have been detected in patients with AS. However, it is unclear whether this is related to myocardial fibrosis or degree of aortic regurgitation. Other, noncardiac manifestations of AS include ankylosis of

sacroiliac joints, bony ankylosis of lumbar spine joints (bamboo spine), uveitis, lung lesions, and amyloidosis (Plate 6.93).

Treatment of patients with ankylosing spondylitis is generally received poorly, although tumor necrosis factor-α antagonists may have a role. Death of patients with AS is usually not related to ischemic heart disease, and carotid intimal medial thickness is not increased as it may be in patients with RA.

Plate 6.94

Acquired Heart Disease

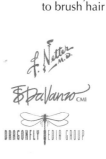

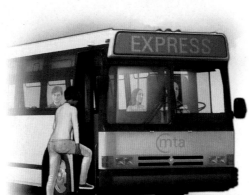

Difficulty in arising from chair, often early symptom

Difficulty in raising arm to brush hair

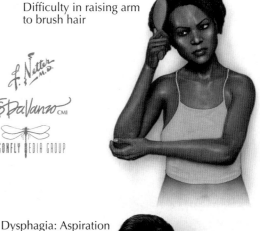

Dysphagia: Aspiration of food may cause pneumonia.

Difficulty in stepping into bus or in climbing stairs

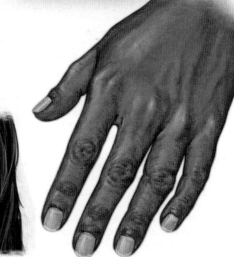

Edema and heliotrope discoloration around eyes a classic sign. More widespread erythematous rash may also be present.

Erythema and/or scaly, papular eruption around fingernails and on dorsum of interphalangeal joints

POLYMYOSITIS AND DERMATOMYOSITIS

Polymyositis and dermatomyositis are both characterized by chronic inflammation of skeletal muscle. The inflammatory cellular infiltrates are typically composed of T cells and macrophages. The histopathology of patients with myocarditis resembles the inflammation in the skeletal muscle with mononuclear inflammatory cell infiltrates. Histopathologic changes similar to those in the myocardium can be found in the conducting system and include lymphocytic infiltration and fibrosis of the sinoatrial node.

Polymyositis and dermatomyositis present clinically as muscle weakness and fatigue (Plate 6.94). Before steroids were available, more than half of myositis patients died of disease complications within 5 years; a large percentage of patients now survive beyond 5 years. Cardiac involvement is associated with worse prognosis for survival, and cardiovascular manifestations (heart failure, arrhythmia, cardiac arrest, MI) are the most common causes of death.

In the modern era, noninvasive assessments (e.g., CK level, MRI) have increased detection of cardiac involvement, which is clinically important in patients with polymyositis or dermatomyositis, although the actual frequency can only be determined by large-scale epidemiologic studies. Cardiac manifestations occur in more than 70% of patients, but only a small percentage are symptomatic. With myocardial involvement, arrhythmias occur, and pericardial effusions can be found by ultrasound in as many as 25% of patients. The most common cardiac manifestations are conduction abnormalities and arrhythmias detected by 12-lead or ambulatory ECG monitoring. ECG abnormalities include atrial and ventricular arrhythmias, bundle branch block, AV blocks, high-grade heart block, prolongation of PR intervals, ventricular premature beats, left atrial abnormality, and abnormal Q waves as well as nonspecific ST-T wave changes. Conduction abnormalities may lead to symptomatic bradycardia caused by complete heart block. Coronary artery disease is found in these patients but is not the major cardiac manifestation as in rheumatoid arthritis. Coronary artery manifestations more often involve the microcirculation rather than the epicardial arteries. The most frequently reported cardiac problem is congestive heart failure, usually concurrent with active skeletal muscle involvement. The most common cardiac problems in patients

with myositis are impaired LV function and arrhythmias, which could also be secondary to vascular changes in the heart.

Gadolinium-enhanced MRI in the patient with polymyositis and congestive heart failure is highly sensitive to myocardial inflammatory areas compatible with myocarditis. Endomyocardial biopsies can confirm myocardial inflammation in patients with myositis, although they are rarely used in clinical practice. Troponin is the most sensitive and reliable serum marker

to detect myocardial damage in patients with inflammatory muscle disease or acute MI. A CK-MB/total CK ratio greater than 3% is the threshold for myocardial damage.

Treatment for the patient with polymyositis or dermatomyositis is based on corticosteroids in high doses over a long time in combination with other immunosuppressive drugs such as azathioprine or methotrexate. In addition, there is a role for exercise in the treatment regimen in combination with the immunosuppressives.

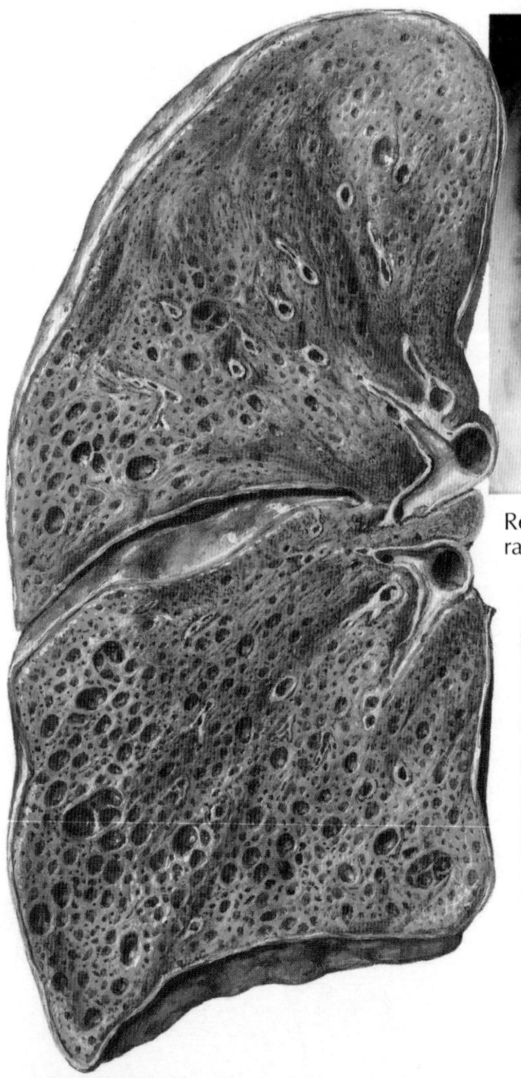

Plate 6.95

Cardiovascular System: VOLUME 8

SCLERODERMA (PROGRESSIVE SYSTEMIC SCLEROSIS)

Progressive systemic sclerosis (scleroderma) is a rare autoimmune disorder of unknown etiology occurring predominantly in females and is characterized by tissue fibrosis due to excess accumulation of collagen and other extracellular matrix proteins. Inflammation and fibrosis cause changes in multiple organs, including lungs, skin, blood vessels, kidney, and gastrointestinal tract. The most specific autoantibodies found in patients with systemic sclerosis are antinuclear antibodies. The cardiac manifestations are cardiomyopathy, microvascular dysfunction (myocardial Raynaud phenomenon), arrhythmias, pulmonary hypertension, and rarely pericarditis. Scleroderma is a symmetric thickening, tightening, and induration of the skin of the fingers and the skin proximal to the metacarpophalangeal or metatarsophalangeal joints (sclerodactyly). The face (pinched facies), neck, and trunk may also be involved. Digital pitting scars, loss of substance in the finger pad, and pulmonary fibrosis of the lung bases are part of the clinical picture (Plate 6.95).

Visceral involvement, particularly the heart, substantially increases mortality. Myocardial disease in systemic sclerosis may be multifactorial, related to associated pulmonary or renal involvement or hypertension. At autopsy the heart often shows focal areas of contraction band necrosis, a reperfusion lesion, and fibrosis in both ventricles despite patent epicardial and normal intramural coronary arteries and no evidence for Raynaud phenomenon or renal disease. These findings likely were related to the development of congestive heart failure, conduction abnormalities, ventricular arrhythmias, and cardiovascular death. It is speculated that intermittent vasoconstriction of the intramyocardial arteries might be responsible for the myocardial abnormalities. Thus left ventricular regional wall motion abnormalities and impaired coronary flow reserve in patients without epicardial coronary stenoses can occur. When microvascular disease, especially spasm, is present, the calcium antagonist nifedipine can be effective therapy, as in patients with Raynaud phenomenon.

Right ventricular dysfunction can occur in patients with scleroderma even in the absence of pulmonary hypertension. Abnormal stiffness of large arteries (e.g., carotid) can occur, but no evidence indicates that carotid intimal medial thickness is present. Patients with scleroderma can have conduction abnormalities and arrhythmias related to fibrosis of the sinus node and bundle branches (pathology) and diffuse conduction abnormalities and arrhythmias on ambulatory ECG and electrophysiology studies. These electrophysiologic abnormalities could be related to fibrosis or myocardial

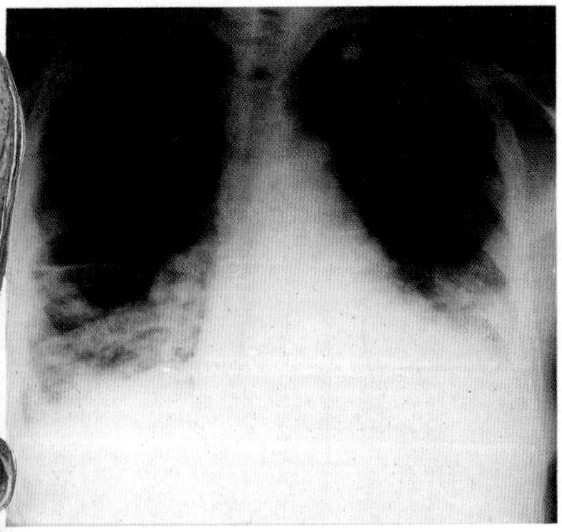

Reticular opacification in both lungs with small radiolucencies interspersed

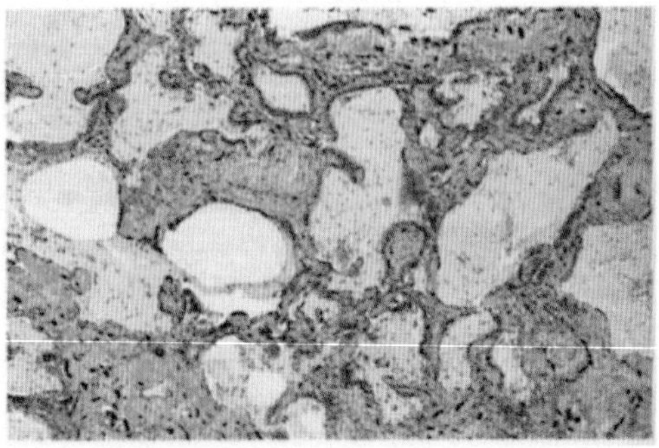

Microscopic section of lung. Fibrosis with formation of microcysts, many of which represent dilated bronchioles

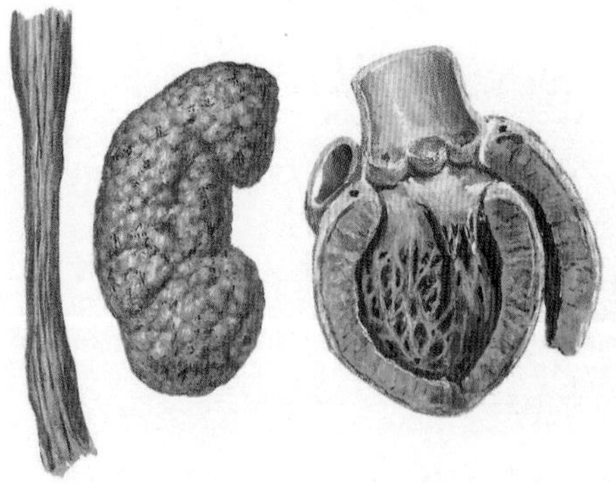

Grossly sectioned lung. Extensive fibrosis and multitudinous small cysts. Visceral pleura thickened but not adherent to chest wall.

Esophagus, kidneys, heart, skin, and other organs, as well as joints, may also be affected.

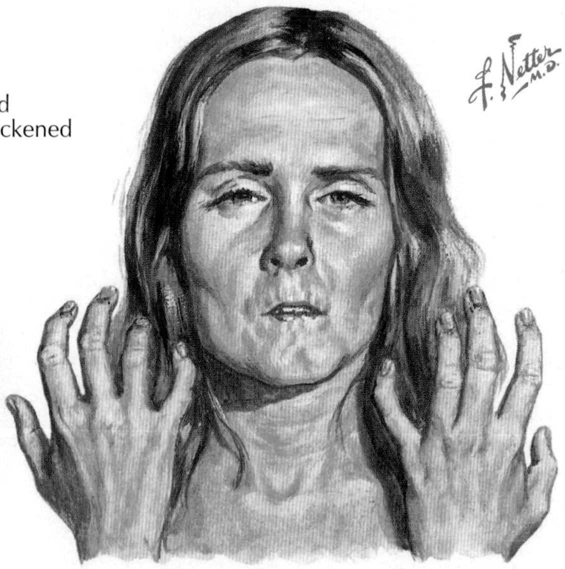

Rigid, pinched facies and sclerodactyly

ischemia secondary to microvascular disease. Patients with scleroderma typically do not have clinically important pericardial disease, although inflammatory changes may be seen at autopsy. Echocardiography shows small pericardial effusions in some patients.

Common cardiovascular abnormalities associated with systemic sclerosis are microvascular perfusion abnormalities of the ventricular myocardium resulting in ischemia, fibrosis (may occur independent of ischemia),

systolic/diastolic dysfunction, and conduction system disease. Inflammation and microvascular disease result in stiffening of the conduit arteries. Prognosis in systemic sclerosis is worsened by the presence of cardiac involvement. Nifedipine therapy may improve myocardial digital perfusion in patients with Raynaud phenomenon. Therapy generally is poorly received in patients limited by cardiovascular complications of systemic sclerosis.

Plate 6.96

Acquired Heart Disease

SYSTEMIC LUPUS ERYTHEMATOSUS

Systemic lupus erythematosus primarily involves the vascular system. Renal glomeruli, the vascular structures most susceptible to the injurious effects of the circulating agents, are frequently damaged during the course of SLE. Multiple visceral organs may be affected, with cardiac involvement a prominent feature of this syndrome. The cardiac lesions may be considered in relation to damage involving the valves and endocardium, blood vessels, connective tissue of the myocardium, and the pericardium. Pericarditis is the earliest and most common signs of SLE. Noninfective endocarditis may be associated with systolic or diastolic murmurs. The vegetations do not embolize. Myocarditis may be difficult to recognize because clinical effects are usually mild and do not lead to cardiac dilation or failure, although MRI may reveal subtle disease.

Nonbacterial endocarditis, described by Libman and Sacks, was found originally in many hearts of patients with SLE. Since the advent of steroid therapy, cardiac lesions found at autopsy have diminished. The mitral and tricuspid valves are most frequently affected by single or mulberry-shaped excrescences 1 to 4 millimicrons in size and occur randomly, both on and away from the line of closure and on both surfaces of the valve as well as on the chordae tendineae, papillary muscles, and mural endocardium, usually at the base of the ventricles. Microscopically, the excrescences have a superficial layer of partially hyalinized platelet and fibrin thrombi. Deeper layers may show evidence of eosinophilic collagen degeneration and necrosis, with a variable infiltrate of neutrophilic and mononuclear cells (Plate 6.96, A). Bacteria have not been demonstrated. Some patients have fibrous thickening of the valve indicative of previous episodes of endocarditis. In the region of the valve ring, the base of the valve and valve pocket proliferation of endothelial cells and myocytes may be prominent. Hematoxylin bodies may be seen in areas of endocardial inflammation.

Fibrinoid necrosis of the small and medium-sized arterioles may be associated with myocarditis. Endothelial proliferative and granular plugs of fibrin occlude the lumen of small vessels, showing necrosis of the wall. Infiltrations of neutrophils in the acute stage and mononuclear cells in the older lesions are prominent. Fluorescent antibody assay demonstrates deposits of gamma globulin and the C3 complement in the acute vascular lesion (Plate 6.96, B). In the late stages of vessel involvement, endothelial proliferation, thickening, and partial occlusion may be found.

Foci of myocardial inflammation associated with interstitial edema and eosinophilic degeneration of collagen may be prominent (Plate 6.96, C). Lymphocytes, plasma cells, and large histiocytes form the infiltrate. Hematoxylin bodies are also found in interstitial areas of inflammation. Degenerative changes in the myocardial fibers usually do not occur, and the myocarditis evident in SLE is usually not extensive, although areas of fibrosis may result.

Organizing fibrinous pericarditis occurs in up to 60% of patients with SLE (detected by ultrasound) not associated with uremia, and fibrinoid necrosis of the pericardial connective tissue has also been observed. Serosanguineous effusions may accompany the pericarditis. Although fibrous adhesions may be seen,

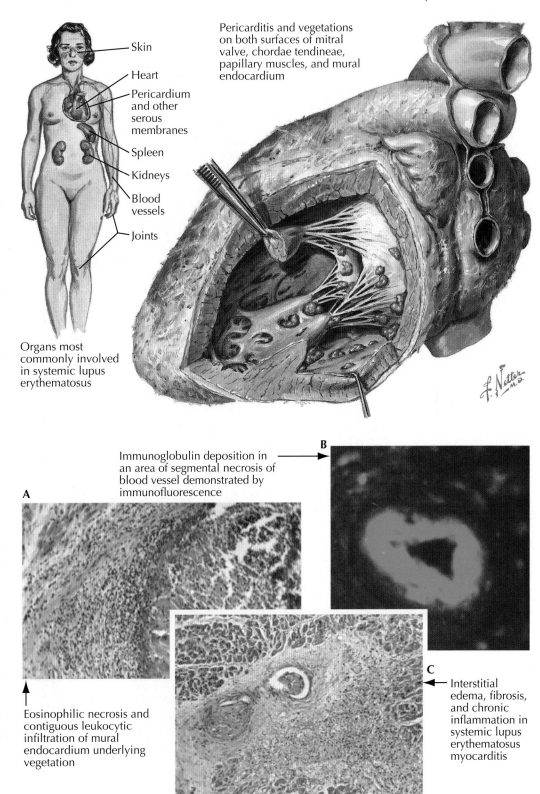

Organs most commonly involved in systemic lupus erythematosus

Pericarditis and vegetations on both surfaces of mitral valve, chordae tendineae, papillary muscles, and mural endocardium

Immunoglobulin deposition in an area of segmental necrosis of blood vessel demonstrated by immunofluorescence

Eosinophilic necrosis and contiguous leukocytic infiltration of mural endocardium underlying vegetation

Interstitial edema, fibrosis, and chronic inflammation in systemic lupus erythematosus myocarditis

constrictive pericarditis does not occur. Cardiac manifestations of SLE are often mild and asymptomatic. Because pericarditis is the most frequent manifestation of SLE, patients should have periodic ultrasound to detect pericardial effusions.

Vasculitis or antiphospholipid antibodies associated with SLE can result in occlusive vascular disease. However, premature atherosclerosis is the most frequent cause of coronary artery disease in SLE patients, and modification of traditional risk factors should be vigorously pursued.

The cardiac valvular lesions of SLE must be differentiated from those of rheumatic fever. Rheumatic vegetations occur on the atrial surface of the valve and are less prone to necrosis. The characteristic Aschoff nodule is absent in SLE. As in RA, SLE results in premature development of atherosclerosis, MI, and arterial stiffening. LV hypertrophy develops in SLE unrelated to traditional stimuli and may be caused by inflammatory arterial stiffening. Pericardial disease is common, and clinically significant valvular disease caused by SLE develops in a minority of patients.

Plate 6.97

Cardiovascular System: VOLUME 8

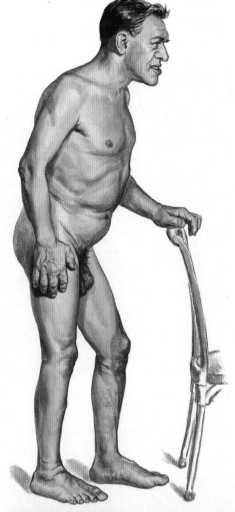

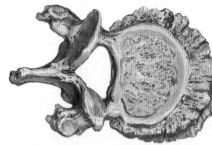

Thoracic vertebra in acromegaly: Hyperostosis, especially marked on anterior aspect

The effects of the chronic GH excess include acral and soft tissue overgrowth, coarsening of facial features, prognathism, frontal bossing, and progressive dental malocclusion (underbite).

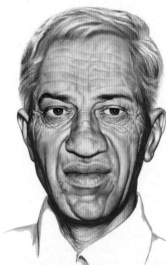

ACROMEGALY

Acromegaly is a rare disease with slow onset often unnoticed by the patient. Eventually, acromegalic changes are recognized by friends, spouses, and the patient's physician, often over several years. The clinical picture of acromegaly is related to excessive secretion of human growth hormone (GH) from an overfunctioning pituitary adenoma. When this adenoma secretes GH, the liver responds by secreting insulin-like growth factor 1 (IGF-1). IGF is responsible for many phenotypic and other clinical manifestations in acromegalic patients, including excessive growth of skin, connective tissue, cartilage, bone, viscera, and many epithelial tissues.

The cardiac manifestations of acromegaly include hypertension, concentric left ventricular hypertrophy, valve dysfunction, and systolic/diastolic ventricular dysfunction (Plate 6.97). Cardiomyopathy can result in heart failure symptoms and arrhythmias. Diabetes is a common coexisting disease. Coronary artery disease is probably associated with the high incidence of hypertension and diabetes in acromegalic patients and may be unrelated to hormonal abnormalities. As the pituitary adenoma expands, patients with acromegaly often experience headache and abnormalities related to cranial nerve defects, such as pressure on the optic chiasm resulting in a bitemporal hemianopsia or other visual field defects. Cardiovascular disease is the primary cause of death in patients with acromegaly; this risk is reduced when acromegaly is successfully treated.

The myocardium of the patient with acromegaly is directly affected by GH/IGF-1 and responds by enlarging. The hypertrophy is concentric and involves both right and left ventricles. The restructured heart is

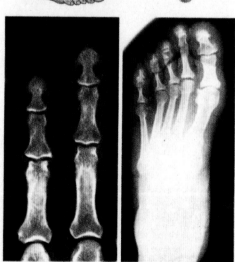

Tufting of phalanges in hands and narrowing of phalanges in feet

Radiograph of skull in acromegaly: enlargement of sella turcica, with occipital protuberance, thickening of cranial bones, enlargement of sinuses and of mandible

further affected by systemic hypertension stimulated by GH and IGF-1. Initially the enlarged heart is hyperkinetic, with increased heart rate and cardiac output. Ventricular hypertrophy may result in diastolic dysfunction, leading to heart failure symptoms with preserved ejection fraction. Mitral and aortic valve regurgitation often occur in the late stages of acromegaly, mainly determined by ultrasound with Doppler imaging. The unclear etiology of the valve disease probably is related to morphologic changes.

Patients with acromegaly may have an increased potential for arrhythmias, including ectopic beats, paroxysmal atrial fibrillation, paroxysmal supraventricular tachycardia, sick sinus syndrome, ventricular tachycardia, and bundle branch blocks. Treatment reduces or eliminates GH production using surgery, medication (e.g., somatostatin analogs, dopamine agonists), and/or radiation. Radiation therapy reduces GH levels slowly and may take years to improve symptoms.

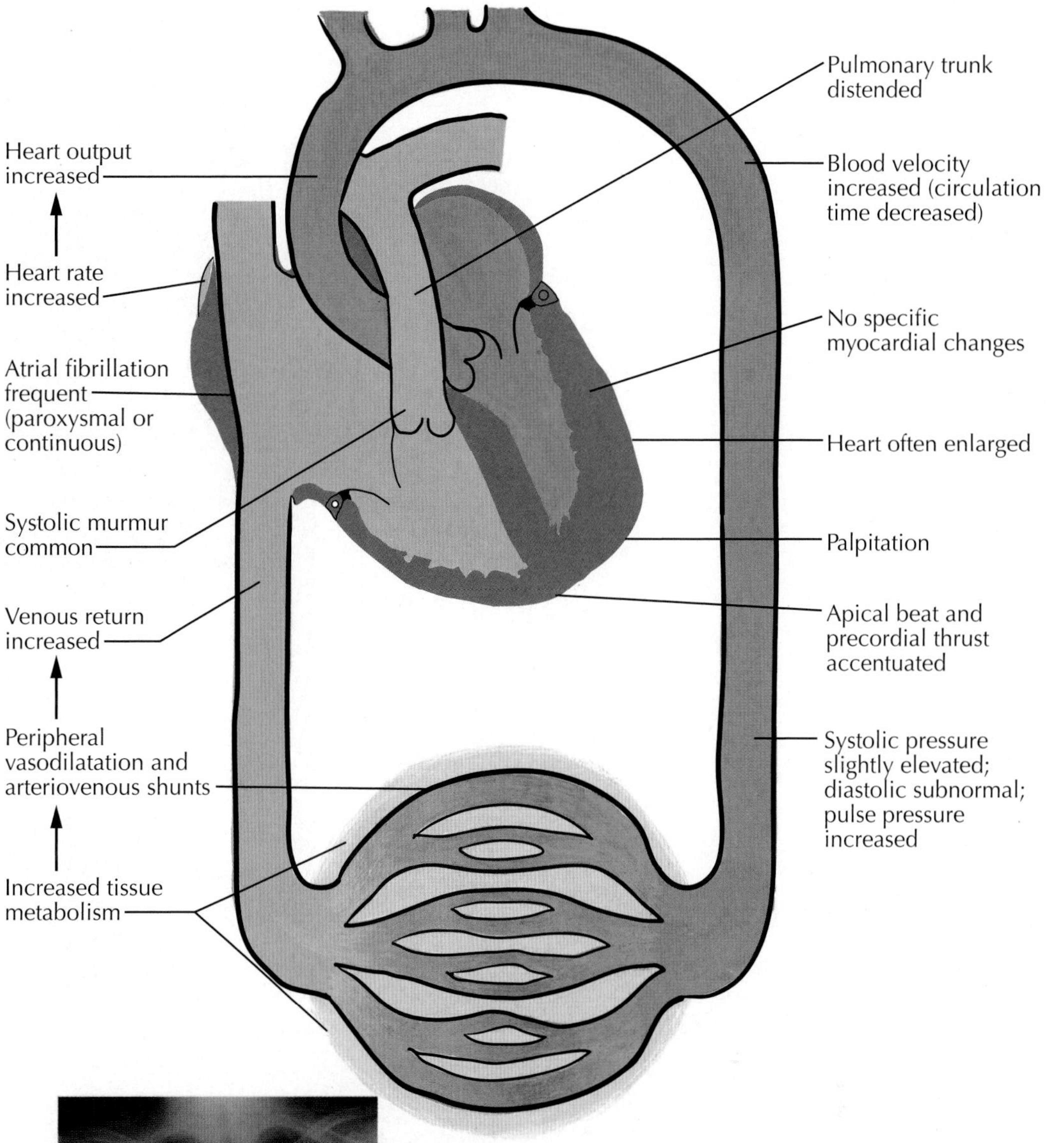

Plate 6.98

Acquired Heart Disease

Hyperthyroidism: Thyrotoxicosis

The striking relationship between thyrotoxicosis and the circulation was recognized as early as 1786 by Parry, who described "enlargement of the thyroid gland in connection with enlargement or palpitation of the heart." In response to increased metabolism, the circulation becomes *hyperdynamic*. Vasodilation makes the skin flushed, warm, and moist. Systolic blood pressure often rises, diastolic pressure drops, and pulse pressure increases. The pulse is vigorous, rapid, and (sometimes) irregular. The cardiac impulse is dynamic and may be displaced to the left. The heart sounds are forceful; velocity of blood flow is increased. Systolic ejection murmurs and edema of the lower extremities are common.

The combination of dyspnea, tachycardia, arrhythmia, murmurs, and edema may suggest cardiac decompensation, although these also accompany thyrotoxicosis. The ECG changes include sinus tachycardia, atrial fibrillation, prolongation of PR interval, generalized ST-T changes, and shortening of the QTc interval. Atrial fibrillation, often paroxysmal, is particularly common in patients older than 40 years (Plate 6.98). Chest radiographs may show moderate cardiac enlargement and a prominent pulmonary artery. The hemodynamic changes in thyrotoxic patients result from the general increase in metabolic rate, greater sensitivity to catecholamines, and direct effect of thyroid hormones on the heart. The velocity of muscle shortening and the rate of tension development are augmented, and duration of the active or contractile state of cardiac muscle is decreased.

Early in hyperthyroidism, while compensation persists, the cardiac output is augmented often greater than the increase in body oxygen consumption; arteriovenous oxygen difference may be decreased. The enhanced cardiac index results from accelerated heart rate and increased stroke volume. The response to exercise is a further increase in heart rate and cardiac output. The hemodynamic changes occur without a significant variation in pressure in the right atrium or the pulmonary artery. Of particular importance is the distribution of the greater cardiac output. Flow to the skin and muscles improves but with no increase in cerebral or splanchnic flow. The additional renal blood flow parallels the general increase in oxygen consumption. Coronary blood flow is augmented but constitutes a normal fraction of the increased CO.

The patient with previous coronary artery disease may develop angina pectoris under the burden of this cardiac workload. Similarly, with rheumatic valvular deformity, congestive heart failure may supervene. The normal heart may eventually fail as the result of increased cardiac work of long duration (tachycardia-induced cardiomyopathy). Pathologic examination reveals no characteristic lesion, although prolonged hyperthyroidism results in cardiac hypertrophy in animal and human studies. When the heart fails in thyrotoxicosis, cardiac output decreases, not to absolute low levels but low in relation to body oxygen consumption.

Heart output increased

Heart rate increased

Atrial fibrillation frequent (paroxysmal or continuous)

Systolic murmur common

Venous return increased

Peripheral vasodilatation and arteriovenous shunts

Increased tissue metabolism

Pulmonary trunk distended

Blood velocity increased (circulation time decreased)

No specific myocardial changes

Heart often enlarged

Palpitation

Apical beat and precordial thrust accentuated

Systolic pressure slightly elevated; diastolic subnormal; pulse pressure increased

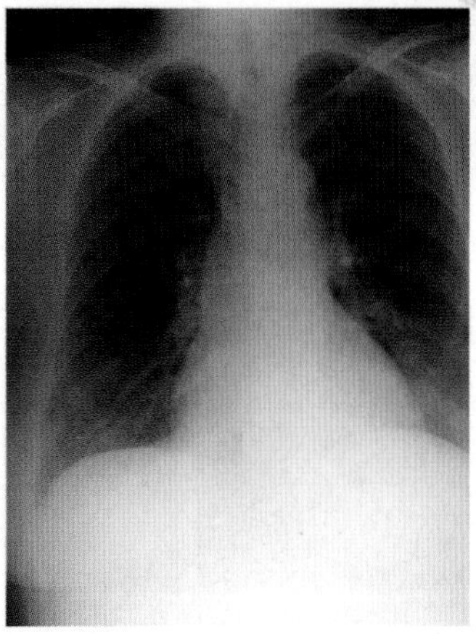

Radiograph: heart moderately enlarged, pulmonary artery prominent

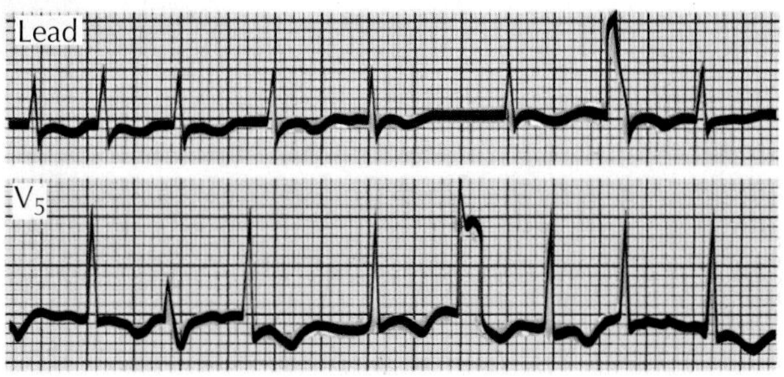

Lead

V_5

ECG: atrial fibrillation

The stroke index falls, the response to exercise is poor, and right atrial and pulmonary artery pressures are elevated.

The response of the hyperthyroid patient to therapy is dramatic. β-Blockers can slow the heart but do not treat the underlying condition. Antithyroid therapy decreases the velocity of blood flow, and peripheral vascular resistance rises. As heart rate falls, cardiac output and right and left ventricular work decrease, and the myocardial oxygen consumption returns to normal.

Patients with angina pectoris and heart failure may show striking improvement. Even in the absence of recognizable heart disease, however, evidence of congestive heart failure may persist or recur, despite the euthyroid state. The same is true of atrial fibrillation. After return to normal thyroid function, sinus rhythm may recur spontaneously or in response to antiarrhythmic therapy, although atrial fibrillation may persist in a substantial group of patients, particularly those with congestive heart failure.

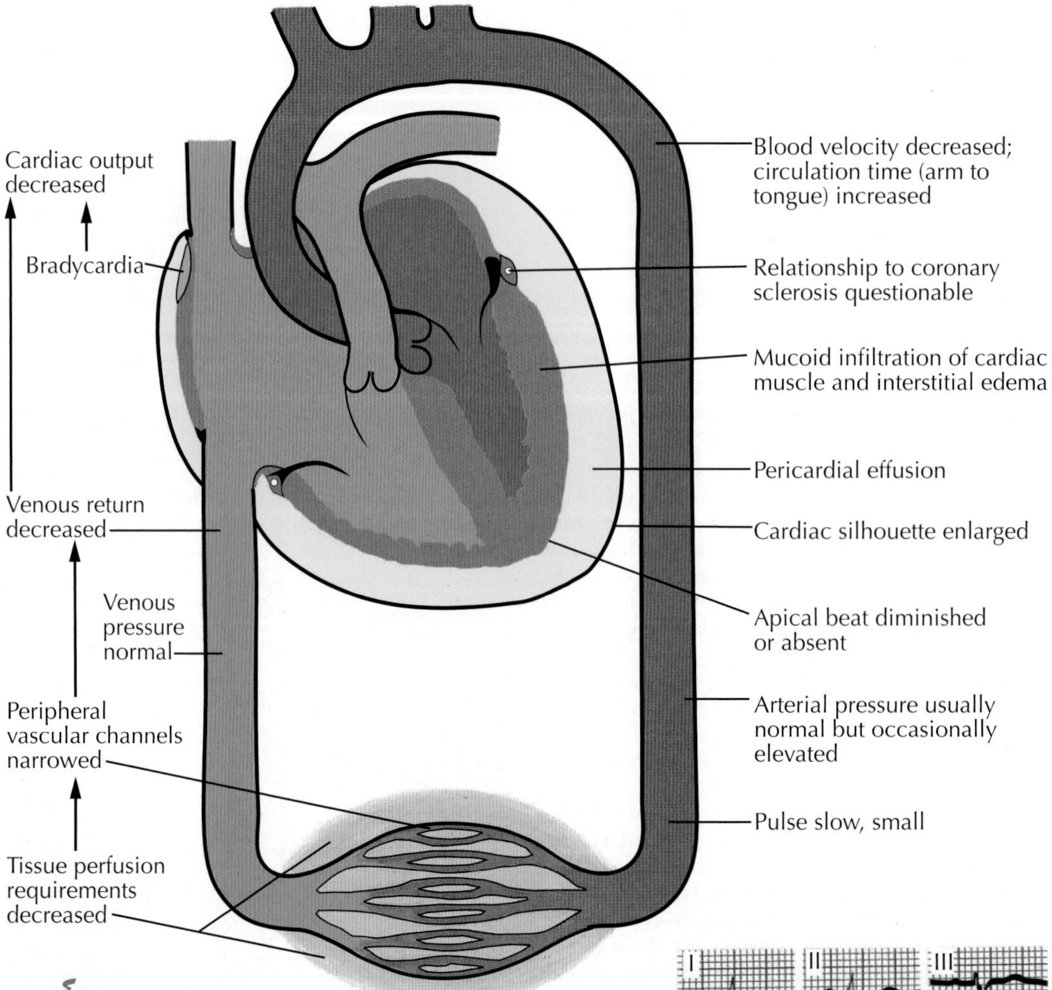

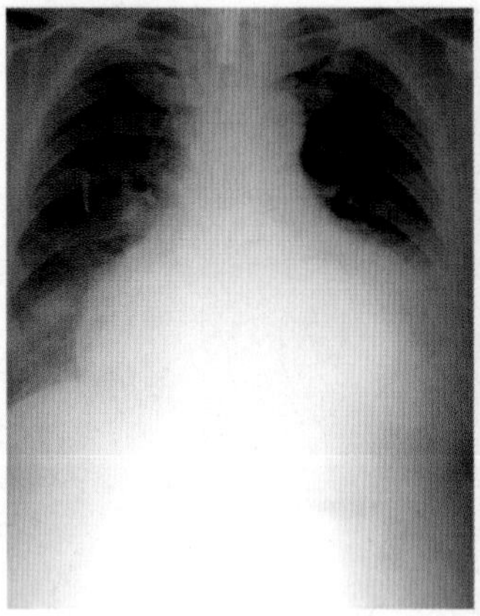

Plate 6.99

Cardiovascular System: VOLUME 8

Cardiac output
decreased

Bradycardia

Venous return
decreased

Venous
pressure
normal

Peripheral
vascular channels
narrowed

Tissue perfusion
requirements
decreased

Blood velocity decreased;
circulation time (arm to
tongue) increased

Relationship to coronary
sclerosis questionable

Mucoid infiltration of cardiac
muscle and interstitial edema

Pericardial effusion

Cardiac silhouette enlarged

Apical beat diminished
or absent

Arterial pressure usually
normal but occasionally
elevated

Pulse slow, small

HYPOTHYROIDISM: MYXEDEMA

In myxedema the circulation can be considered *hypo-dynamic* but adequate for the diminished flow requirements and decreased body oxygen consumption of this condition. The patient's skin is cool and thickened, reflecting changes not only in the skin but also of peripheral vasoconstriction and impaired velocity of flow. The neck veins are not distended. The cardiac impulse is sluggish and feeble, the pulse is slow, and the heart sounds are muffled. The blood pressure is usually normal but may be elevated. The ECG often contains characteristic (but not diagnostic) changes, including low voltage, flattening or inversion of the T waves, and increased PR interval (Plate 6.99). On chest radiographs, size of the cardiac silhouette is increased, largely because of pericardial effusion; actual heart size is normal without effusion.

The level of thyroid function profoundly affects the contractile state of cardiac muscle. Muscles from hypothyroid animals develop tension at a slower rate, but this is compensated for by a prolonged period of contraction. Cardiac output decreases because of the slow rate and a small stroke volume. On the other hand, the ratio of cardiac output to total oxygen consumption is normal. Right atrial and pulmonary artery pressures generally are normal. In response to exercise, cardiac output, rate, and stroke volume may increase. The low output of the myxedematous heart is in contrast with that of cardiac decompensation, in which output is low and not proportional to oxygen consumption, right atrial pressure is high, and the heart responds to exercise with an inadequate increase in cardiac output and marked elevation of atrial pressure.

Pathologic data in patients with untreated hypothyroidism are sparse regarding the state of the heart, described as "flabby," pale, and dilated. Fibrous tissue

Radiograph before therapy: greatly enlarged cardiac silhouette due to pericardial effusion

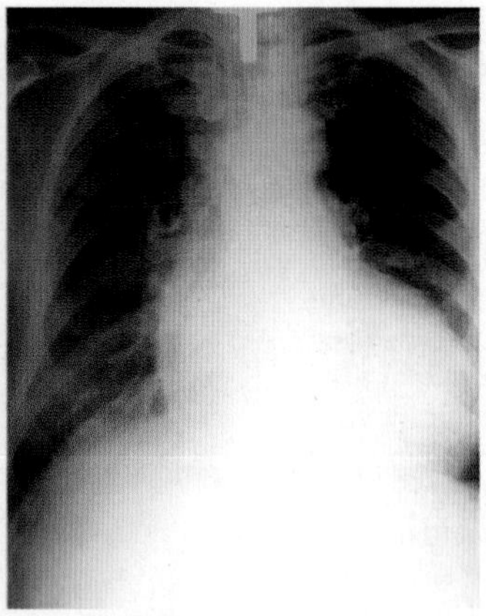

After thyroid therapy: effusion resorbed; heart enlarged due to coexisting hypertension

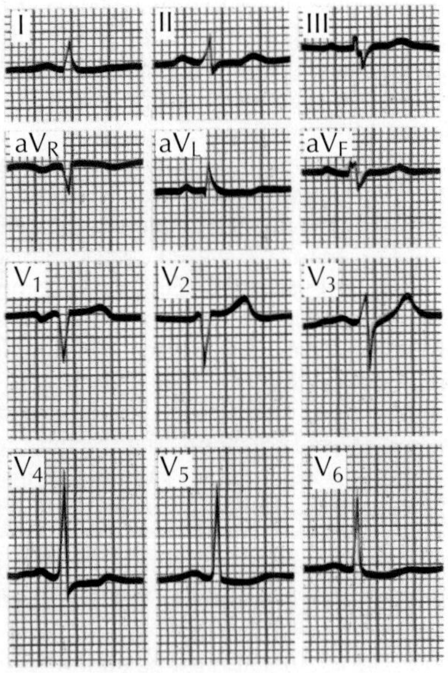

ECG in myxedema: low voltage and ST-segment depressions

replacement and infiltration are described. Microscopic changes include swelling of muscle cells, degeneration of muscle fibers, fatty infiltration, and interstitial edema with accumulation of mucinous interstitial fluid with high protein and nitrogen content. These conditions are difficult to evaluate because they also occur in the normal changes of aging. Hypercholesterolemia is often seen in patients with myxedema and may lead to an increased incidence of atherosclerosis.

The changes in the circulation in myxedema are reversed by thyroid substitution therapy. The heart size shrinks, cardiac output rises, ECGs normalize, velocity of blood flow increases, peripheral flow becomes greater, and elevated blood pressure may fall. Because primary myxedema is a disease of later life, when coronary artery disease may also be present, therapy should be undertaken cautiously to avoid the risk of precipitating myocardial ischemia with thyroid medication.

Plate 6.100

Acquired Heart Disease

Causes of Cushing syndrome

Clinical features

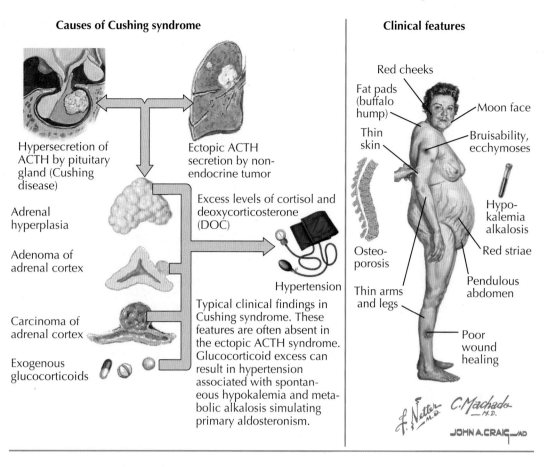

Hypersecretion of ACTH by pituitary gland (Cushing disease)

Ectopic ACTH secretion by non-endocrine tumor

Adrenal hyperplasia

Adenoma of adrenal cortex

Carcinoma of adrenal cortex

Exogenous glucocorticoids

Excess levels of cortisol and deoxycorticosterone (DOC)

Hypertension

Typical clinical findings in Cushing syndrome. These features are often absent in the ectopic ACTH syndrome. Glucocorticoid excess can result in hypertension associated with spontaneous hypokalemia and metabolic alkalosis simulating primary aldosteronism.

Red cheeks

Fat pads (buffalo hump)

Thin skin

Osteoporosis

Thin arms and legs

Moon face

Bruisability, ecchymoses

Hypokalemia alkalosis

Red striae

Pendulous abdomen

Poor wound healing

CUSHING SYNDROME

Classic Cushing syndrome is caused by hypersecretion of adrenocorticotropic hormone from any tumor (pituitary, adrenal, ectopic) or treatment for any condition with exogenous glucocorticoids. Typical features of Cushing syndrome include the classic "buffalo hump" (related to fat pads), red cheeks, moon face, hypokalemic alkalosis, red abdominal striae, pendulous abdomen, thin arms and legs, poor wound healing, and osteoporosis. Chronic cortisol hypersecretion causes a metabolic syndrome of central obesity, hypertension, glucose intolerance, insulin resistance, dyslipidemia, and prothrombotic state. The increased cardiovascular risk results not only from metabolic complications but also from vascular and cardiac alterations caused by atherosclerosis, which in turn can lead to myocardial infarction, peripheral vascular disease with limb loss, and stroke.

Hypertension is a common manifestation of Cushing syndrome. Possible mechanisms associated with glucocorticoid excess include increased production of vasoconstrictor agents such as angiotensinogen, endothelin, and adrenergics, combined with decreased production of vasodilator agents such as nitric oxide, prostaglandins, and atrial natriuretic peptide. This combination results in vasoconstriction and increased peripheral vascular resistance. In addition, sodium retention and increased water reabsorption result in increased plasma volume and increased cardiac output. The final common path leads to systemic hypertension (Plate 6.100).

In the clinical management of these patients, therapy must include global treatment of all cardiovascular risk factors during the active phase of the disease as well as long after risk factors are controlled (i.e., for life). Long-term management of patients with Cushing syndrome should focus on identifying the global cardiovascular risk to control not only hypertension but also other

Possible mechanisms of hypertension associated with glucocorticoid excess

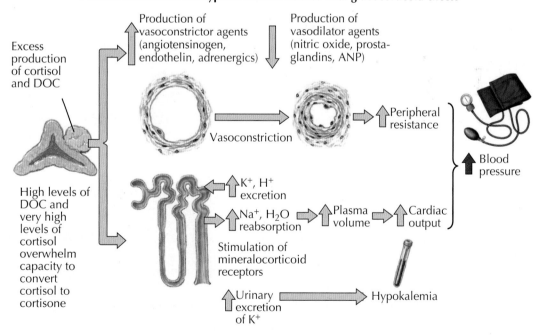

Excess production of cortisol and DOC

Production of vasoconstrictor agents (angiotensinogen, endothelin, adrenergics)

Production of vasodilator agents (nitric oxide, prostaglandins, ANP)

Vasoconstriction

Peripheral resistance

Blood pressure

High levels of DOC and very high levels of cortisol overwhelm capacity to convert cortisol to cortisone

K^+, H^+ excretion

Na^+, H_2O reabsorption

Plasma volume

Cardiac output

Stimulation of mineralocorticoid receptors

Urinary excretion of K^+

Hypokalemia

associated risk factors, such as obesity (weight loss, exercise), glucose intolerance, insulin resistance, dyslipidemia (statins, other lipid-lowering agents), endothelial dysfunction, and the prothrombotic state (aspirin, other antiplatelet agents). Clinical remission from hypercortisolism may be difficult to achieve, and thus the cardiovascular risk can persist even during disease remission. Therefore care and control of all cardiovascular risk factors should be a primary goal during patient follow-up. As would be expected, mortality from cardiovascular disease in Cushing syndrome is higher than in a normal population.

Cardiomyopathies are usually associated with left ventricular hypertrophy, although this occurs infrequently because most patients are treated well before a cardiomyopathy evolves. Dilated cardiomyopathy is even less common. However, in patients with known cardiomyopathy of any etiology who develop Cushing syndrome, heart failure can be precipitated by salt retention as a result of increased mineralocorticoids.

Plate 6.101

Cardiovascular System: VOLUME 8

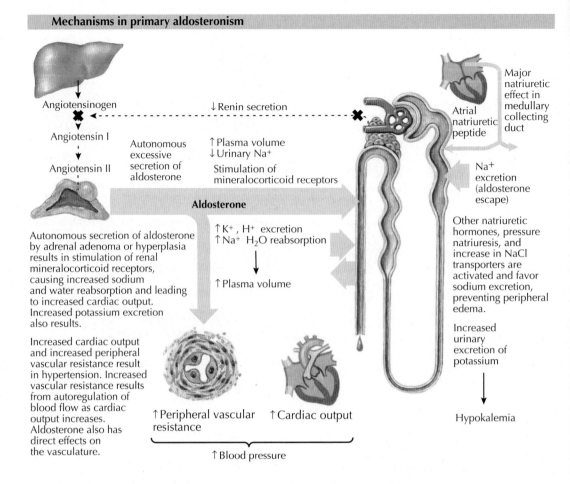

Mechanisms in primary aldosteronism

Angiotensinogen

↓Renin secretion

Major natriuretic effect in medullary collecting duct

Atrial natriuretic peptide

Angiotensin I

Angiotensin II

Autonomous excessive secretion of aldosterone

↑Plasma volume
↓Urinary Na⁺

Stimulation of mineralocorticoid receptors

Na⁺ excretion (aldosterone escape)

Aldosterone

Autonomous secretion of aldosterone by adrenal adenoma or hyperplasia results in stimulation of renal mineralocorticoid receptors, causing increased sodium and water reabsorption and leading to increased cardiac output. Increased potassium excretion also results.

↑K^+, H^+ excretion
↑Na^+ H_2O reabsorption

↑Plasma volume

Other natriuretic hormones, pressure natriuresis, and increase in NaCl transporters are activated and favor sodium excretion, preventing peripheral edema.

Increased cardiac output and increased peripheral vascular resistance result in hypertension. Increased vascular resistance results from autoregulation of blood flow as cardiac output increases. Aldosterone also has direct effects on the vasculature.

Increased urinary excretion of potassium

↑Peripheral vascular resistance   ↑Cardiac output

Hypokalemia

↑Blood pressure

Primary Hyperaldosteronism: Mineralocorticoid Hypertension

Primary hyperaldosteronism (Conn syndrome) results from autonomous secretion of aldosterone caused by a benign cortical adenoma or bilateral adrenal hyperplasia. Both diseases cause oversecretion of the salt-retaining hormone aldosterone. Conn syndrome is an uncommon disorder. Primary hyperaldosteronism accounts for less than 1% of all cases of hypertension. It is more common in females and can occur at any age but most often in young adulthood. Aldosterone stimulates renal mineralocorticoid receptors, increasing sodium and water reabsorption as well as plasma volume, which leads to increased cardiac output and potassium secretion. Increased potassium may result in hypokalemia, in turn causing hypokalemic alkalosis and clinical signs (Chvostek, Trousseau), probably related to hypokalemic alkalosis, hyperventilation, and calcium shifts. Increased peripheral vascular resistance results from autoregulation of blood flow as cardiac output increases. Aldosterone may also have direct effects on the vasculature. The increased output and resistance can result in hypertension.

Secondary causes of hyperaldosteronism include any condition that decreases blood flow to the kidney, including dehydration, renal artery constriction, cardiac failure, shock, liver disease, pregnancy, and renin-secreting kidney tumors.

Patients typically have mild to moderate hypertension but may be poorly responsive to antihypertensive therapy. The few patients reported with heart failure

Clinical features

Hypokalemic alkalosis may cause Chvostek and Trousseau signs

↑Blood pressure

↑Muscle weakness and cramps

↑Plasma aldosterone concentration (PAC)

↓Plasma renin activity (PRA)

↑Polyuria and nocturia

JOHN A.CRAIG—MD
with
E. Hatton

Primary aldosteronism
PAC >10 ng/dL
+
PRA <1 ng/mL/hr

Confirmatory testing

Subtype testing

CT (axial image) shows a 1-cm aldosterone-producing adenoma (*arrow*) in the lateral aspect of the right adrenal gland.

may have underlying myocardial dysfunction and hypertension. Primary hyperaldosteronism can be distinguished from "essential" hypertension by blood and urine tests to assess high aldosterone levels; hypernatremia, hypokalemia, hyperkaluria, and high alkalinity are the electrolyte abnormalities. CT or MRI can detect tumors that secrete aldosterone (Plate 6.101). Symptoms include muscle weakness, frequent urination, nighttime urination, headache, excessive thirst, visual

disturbances, temporary paralysis, muscle twitching, and cramps. The severity of these symptoms varies and depends on the degree of electrolyte abnormality.

Secondary hyperaldosteronism caused by kidney enlargement or heart disease is usually treated with medical therapy. Primary hyperaldosteronism resulting from a tumor is usually treated by adrenalectomy. Patients with bilateral hyperplasia receive potassium-sparing diuretics such as spironolactone.

Plate 6.102

Acquired Heart Disease

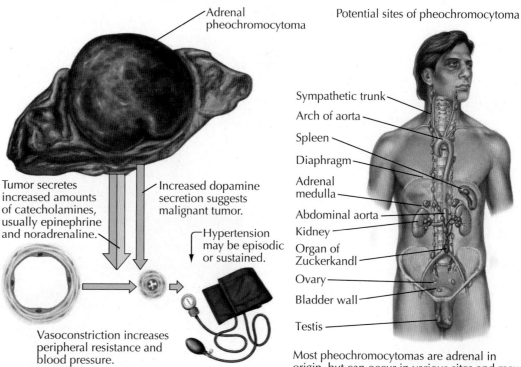

Adrenal pheochromocytoma

Potential sites of pheochromocytoma

Tumor secretes increased amounts of catecholamines, usually epinephrine and noradrenaline.

Increased dopamine secretion suggests malignant tumor.

Hypertension may be episodic or sustained.

Vasoconstriction increases peripheral resistance and blood pressure.

Pheochromocytoma is a chromaffin cell tumor secreting excessive catecholamines, resulting in increased peripheral vascular resistance and hypertension.

Sympathetic trunk
Arch of aorta
Spleen
Diaphragm
Adrenal medulla
Abdominal aorta
Kidney
Organ of Zuckerkandl
Ovary
Bladder wall
Testis

Most pheochromocytomas are adrenal in origin, but can occur in various sites and may be associated with multiple endocrine neoplasia (MEN) syndromes. Most are sporadic, but some are hereditary.

Clinical features of pheochromocytoma

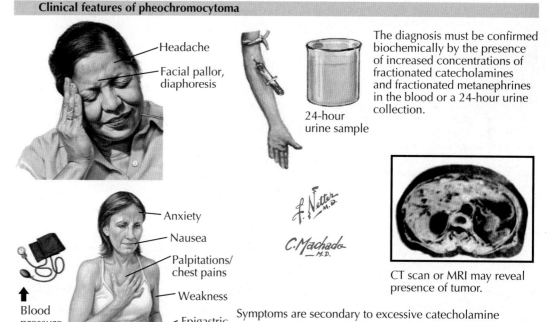

Headache
Facial pallor, diaphoresis

24-hour urine sample

The diagnosis must be confirmed biochemically by the presence of increased concentrations of fractionated catecholamines and fractionated metanephrines in the blood or a 24-hour urine collection.

Anxiety
Nausea
Palpitations/ chest pains
Weakness
Blood pressure
Epigastric pain
Tremor

CT scan or MRI may reveal presence of tumor.

Symptoms are secondary to excessive catecholamine secretion and are usually paroxysmal. However, because of the increased use of CT imaging and familial testing, pheochromocytoma is diagnosed in more than 60% of patients before any symptoms develop.

PHEOCHROMOCYTOMA

A pheochromocytoma is a rare chromaffin cell tumor of the adrenal medulla marked by excessive and uncontrolled catecholamine secretion, resulting in vasoconstriction and increased peripheral vascular resistance. The most common symptom is hypertension, which can be sustained or episodic. Some tumors are hereditary, but most are sporadic. "Catecholamine surges" can result in hypertensive encephalopathy, stroke, or MI and perhaps myocardial stunning, resulting in apical ballooning of the left ventricle.

Pheochromocytoma may present with ventricular wall motion abnormalities and biventricular dilation. These are common in *catecholamine cardiomyopathy*, which may be caused by coronary vasospasm, increased vascular resistance, persistent tachycardia, or direct catecholamine-mediated myocyte injury. Injury can stimulate myocardial remodeling secondary to onset of hypertension. Rapid cardiac deterioration with recovery in a few weeks has been documented clinically and echocardiographically in iatrogenically induced catecholamine cardiomyopathy, in which development is not necessarily related to catecholamine dose and may be associated with the variable susceptibility of the ventricular muscle.

Long-term constant secretion of catecholamine excess may result in a catecholamine cardiomyopathy similar to that reported in patients taking methamphetamines. The tumor usually secretes epinephrine or norepinephrine and occasionally dopamine, which suggests a malignant tumor. Most pheochromocytomas originate in the adrenal medulla. Other sites of pheochromocytoma

are called *paragangliomas* and may be associated with multiple endocrine neoplasia (MEN) syndromes. These paragangliomas include the sympathetic trunk, aortic arch, diaphragm, spleen, abdominal aorta, kidney, Zuckerkandl body, ovary, bladder, and testes.

The clinical features of pheochromocytoma include headache, sweating, flushing, anxiety with panic attack symptoms, nausea, palpitations, chest discomfort, weakness, epigastric pain, and tremor. These features are

secondary to excessive catecholamine secretion and are usually paroxysmal. Diagnosis can be made by urine assay (24-hour sample) for metanephrine and free catecholamines. CT or MRI may reveal the presence of a tumor with a distinctive appearance (Plate 6.102). The treatment of choice is surgical removal of the tumor, with the patient first receiving 10 to 14 days of α-blocker therapy to prevent excessive catecholamine production at surgery.

Plate 6.103

Cardiovascular System: VOLUME 8

MYXOMA AND RHABDOMYOMAS

Myxoma. Characteristically originating from interatrial septum and almost filling left atrium; right ventricular hypertrophy

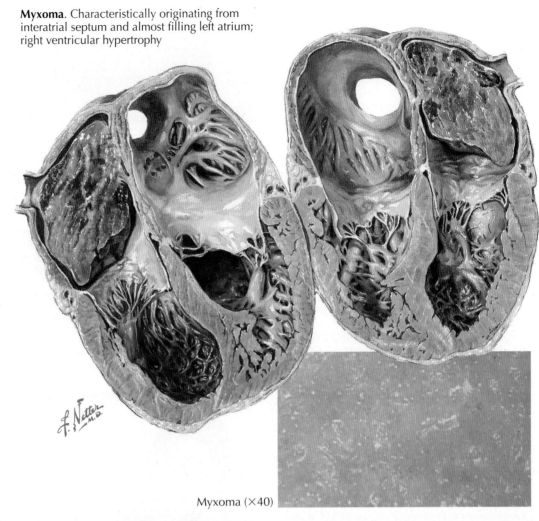

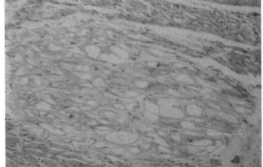
Myxoma (×40)

HEART TUMORS

MYXOMAS

Primary tumors of the heart are rare. There are fibromas, lipomas, angiomas, and sarcomas, but more than 50% of the observed cases are *myxomas,* arising from the endocardium of the left atrium (rarely the right atrium) and other cardiac chambers. Myxomas most often occur between ages 30 and 60 and more frequently in females. Often, they develop in the region of the fossa ovalis and have a thin pedicle. The tumors are sometimes small and bean-like but may grow to large, smooth, ball-shaped or villous structures filling the atria almost entirely but leaving the rest of the endocardium and myocardium unchanged. On a cut surface the myxomas are gelatinous and often show patchy hemorrhagic areas (Plate 6.103).

Microscopically, myxomas of the atria demonstrate large stellate cells embedded in a myxomatous ground substance, resembling Wharton jelly. In other areas, collagen and elastic fibers and numerous small blood vessels may be present. Therefore some tumors may be called a myxofibroma, elastomyxoma, or fibroangiomyxoma. Because of the delicate vessels, hemorrhages can easily occur, demonstrated as iron deposits. Secondary parietal thromboses may organize and fuse with the surrounding endocardium. In such thrombosed and organized structures, the original primary tumor may be difficult to assess.

Clinically, patients with left atrial myxoma may experience fainting when the tumor transiently obstructs the mitral valve. In some patients, peripheral vascular disorders may be noted, associated with trophic changes in the nails and skin. The left atrial tumor may produce chronic passive congestion of the lungs,

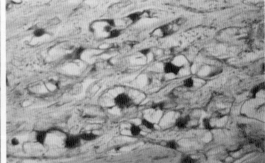
Rhabdomyoma (×40)   Rhabdomyosarcoma (×40)

similar to that seen in mitral stenosis. Tumors of the right atrium may lead to early congestion of the abdominal organs. Cardiac ultrasound, CT, and MR and contrast angiocardiography can help differentiate mitral stenosis and left atrial tumor. Surgical removal of the myxoma is usually indicated, requiring open heart surgery with cardiopulmonary bypass.

RHABDOMYOMAS

Rhabdomyoma, a congenital nodular glycogenic degeneration of myocardial fibers, may be found as single or

multiple nodules, especially in the hearts of infants or children. Rhabdomyomas are often observed in patients with tuberous sclerosis or other malformations of the heart, blood vessels, and kidneys. Some of the nodules are so small that they can be discovered only by *microscopic* examination; others may be as large as chestnuts. Rhabdomyomas are localized and are separated from uninvolved myocardium. Sometimes a fibrous capsule may exist. The cells of rhabdomyomas are arranged irregularly; size of the nuclei varies only slightly, but the cytoplasm is engorged with glycogen (Plate 6.103).

Plate 6.104

Acquired Heart Disease

METASTATIC TUMORS OF THE HEART

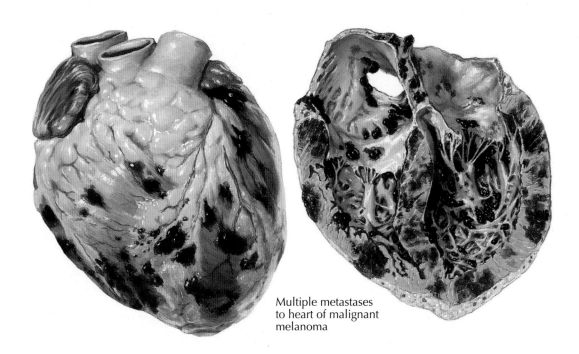

Multiple metastases
to heart of malignant
melanoma

HEART TUMORS (Continued)

Rhabdomyosarcoma, a malignant variant of the rhabdomyoma, grows invasively and may perforate into the lumen of the cardiac chambers and metastasize. Size of the nuclei varies considerably, in contrast to rhabdomyoma. The rhabdomyosarcoma has giant nuclei with large nucleoli and "spider cells" with reduced, string-like cytoplasm. All remaining spaces of the cells are filled with glycogen.

Rhabdomyoma is considered a tissue malformation, resulting from a localized disorder of glycogen metabolism caused by an enzyme defect. Clinical manifestations depend on the size and localization of the tumor-like nodules.

METASTATIC HEART TUMORS

Metastatic tumors of the heart may be present in 6% of all autopsies revealing malignant neoplasms. Among carcinomas, *bronchiogenic carcinoma* is the most frequent primary tumor metastasizing to the heart. Some metastases may be discovered only by microscopic examination, but others may be so large that the entire wall of one chamber or the septum is involved. The spread of carcinoma from the lung may be hematogenous, lymphangial, or by direct extension. The metastases involve the pericardium and myocardium, and, rarely, the endocardium may also be involved (Plate 6.104).

Besides bronchiogenic carcinoma, metastases to the heart are found in patients with carcinoma of the breast and carcinoma of the thyroid gland. In addition, almost every other carcinoma may metastasize to the heart. Sarcomas may also metastasize to the heart. In 44% of

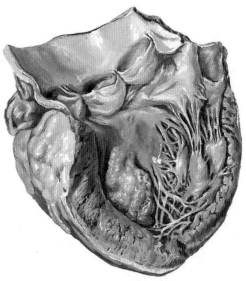

Metastasis of bronchial carcinoma
to heart wall

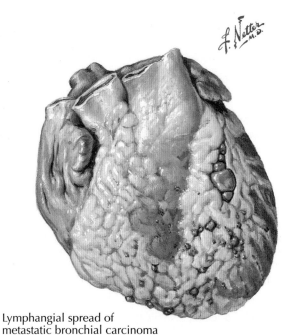

Lymphangial spread of
metastatic bronchial carcinoma

malignant melanomas, metastases to the heart and pericardium can be found. The epicardium, myocardium, and endocardium may be dotted by pigmented metastases. Even if large areas of the myocardium are affected by metastases, no clinical symptoms may be observed. Also, retrospective analyses of the clinical data and autopsy findings can correlate only about 10% of the clinical signs and anatomic changes.

Heart failure from metastases rarely develops. Secondary tumor nodules involving the conduction

system can cause abnormalities in the atrioventricular conduction, as demonstrated on ECG. Involvement of the pericardium by metastatic carcinoma may lead to inflow stasis, either through pericardial effusion (at times, hemorrhagic) or less often through constriction of the heart by an encasing layer of tumor. Metastases that reach the endocardium of the ventricles or the atria can initiate parietal thromboses. Within the embolic material of such thrombi, tumor cells occasionally may be found.

Plate 6.105

Cardiovascular System: VOLUME 8

INTERDEPENDENT AND INTERACTING FACTORS IN BLOOD PRESSURE REGULATION

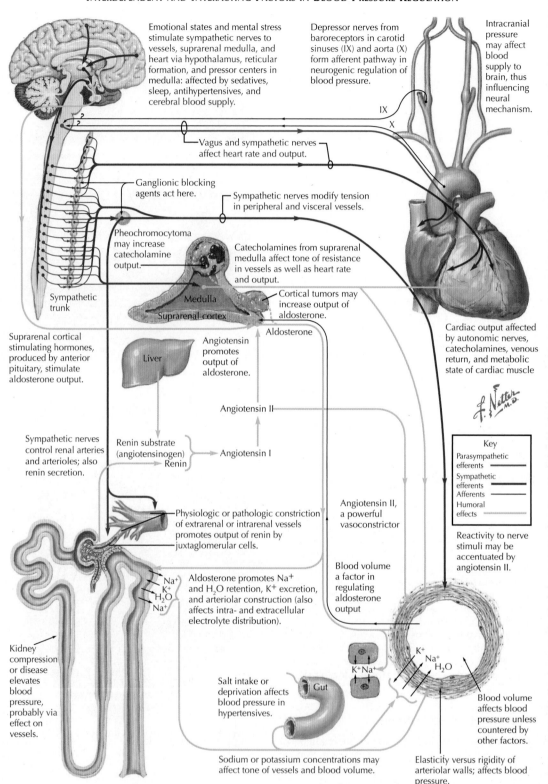

Emotional states and mental stress stimulate sympathetic nerves to vessels, suprarenal medulla, and heart via hypothalamus, reticular formation, and pressor centers in medulla: affected by sedatives, sleep, antihypertensives, and cerebral blood supply.

Depressor nerves from baroreceptors in carotid sinuses (IX) and aorta (X) form afferent pathway in neurogenic regulation of blood pressure.

Intracranial pressure may affect blood supply to brain, thus influencing neural mechanism.

IX
X

Vagus and sympathetic nerves affect heart rate and output.

Ganglionic blocking agents act here.

Sympathetic nerves modify tension in peripheral and visceral vessels.

Pheochromocytoma may increase catecholamine output.

Catecholamines from suprarenal medulla affect tone of resistance in vessels as well as heart rate and output.

Sympathetic trunk

Medulla

Suprarenal cortex

Cortical tumors may increase output of aldosterone.

Suprarenal cortical stimulating hormones, produced by anterior pituitary, stimulate aldosterone output.

Aldosterone

Liver

Angiotensin promotes output of aldosterone.

Cardiac output affected by autonomic nerves, catecholamines, venous return, and metabolic state of cardiac muscle

Angiotensin II

Sympathetic nerves control renal arteries and arterioles; also renin secretion.

Renin substrate (angiotensinogen)
Renin

Angiotensin I

Physiologic or pathologic constriction of extrarenal or intrarenal vessels promotes output of renin by juxtaglomerular cells.

Angiotensin II, a powerful vasoconstrictor

Key
Parasympathetic efferents
Sympathetic efferents
Afferents
Humoral effects

Reactivity to nerve stimuli may be accentuated by angiotensin II.

Blood volume a factor in regulating aldosterone output

Kidney compression or disease elevates blood pressure, probably via effect on vessels.

Na^+
K^+
H_2O
Na^+

Aldosterone promotes Na^+ and H_2O retention, K^+ excretion, and arteriolar construction (also affects intra- and extracellular electrolyte distribution).

K^+ Na^+
K^+Na^+

Salt intake or deprivation affects blood pressure in hypertensives.

Gut

K^+ Na^+
H_2O

Blood volume affects blood pressure unless countered by other factors.

Sodium or potassium concentrations may affect tone of vessels and blood volume.

Elasticity versus rigidity of arteriolar walls; affects blood pressure.

HYPERTENSION: A DISEASE OF REGULATION

Arterial blood pressure is only one of the functions that perfuses tissues. Because organs require different amounts of blood at different times, blood must be withdrawn from one part of the body and transferred to the part in need, in the correct amount and at the appropriate time. To solve this hemodynamic problem, the body has many interworking regulatory devices. The concept of the interrelated and equilibrated system is called the "mosaic theory" of hypertension (Plate 6.105).

Understanding the many factors that control arterial blood pressure depends on the physiology and biochemistry of these mechanisms and does apply to diagnosis, treatment, and prognosis. The regulatory mechanisms may be divided into renal, endocrine, neural, and cardiovascular factors, although all are interdependent and maintain self-equilibrium. Several mechanisms are of the feedback type, sensing the need for blood and for its orderly delivery, to avoid depriving an essential organ such as the brain of blood because of the demand of other, less essential tissues (Plate 6.106).

CHEMICAL MECHANISMS IN BLOOD PRESSURE CONTROL

Renal Factors

The enzyme *renin* is contained in the juxtaglomerular cells surrounding the afferent arterioles in the kidneys. Renin secretion is under the influence of mean arteriolar pressure, sodium content of the tubular fluid, and neural innervation of the juxtaglomerular cells. Released into the bloodstream, renin splits renin substrate (angiotensinogen) to produce angiotensin I, which in turn is split by converting enzymes to angiotensin II, a polypeptide containing eight amino acids. Angiotensin II is a powerful pressor substance, a powerful regulator of aldosterone secretion, and actively involved in renovascular hypertension.

Plate 6.106

Acquired Heart Disease

ETIOLOGY OF HYPERTENSION

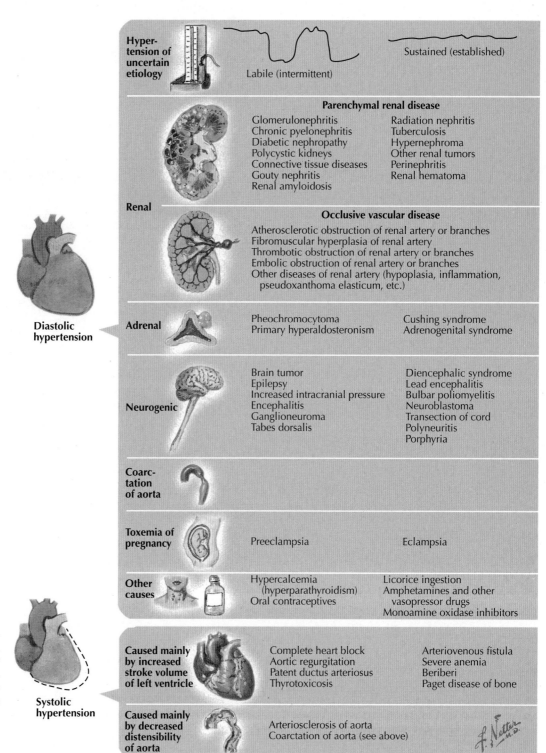

Hypertension of uncertain etiology — Labile (intermittent) — Sustained (established)

Renal

Parenchymal renal disease

Glomerulonephritis	Radiation nephritis
Chronic pyelonephritis	Tuberculosis
Diabetic nephropathy	Hypernephroma
Polycystic kidneys	Other renal tumors
Connective tissue diseases	Perinephritis
Gouty nephritis	Renal hematoma
Renal amyloidosis	

Occlusive vascular disease

Atherosclerotic obstruction of renal artery or branches
Fibromuscular hyperplasia of renal artery
Thrombotic obstruction of renal artery or branches
Embolic obstruction of renal artery or branches
Other diseases of renal artery (hypoplasia, inflammation, pseudoxanthoma elasticum, etc.)

Adrenal

Pheochromocytoma	Cushing syndrome
Primary hyperaldosteronism	Adrenogenital syndrome

Neurogenic

Brain tumor	Diencephalic syndrome
Epilepsy	Lead encephalitis
Increased intracranial pressure	Bulbar poliomyelitis
Encephalitis	Neuroblastoma
Ganglioneuroma	Transection of cord
Tabes dorsalis	Polyneuritis
	Porphyria

Coarctation of aorta

Toxemia of pregnancy — Preeclampsia — Eclampsia

Other causes

Hypercalcemia (hyperparathyroidism)	Licorice ingestion
Oral contraceptives	Amphetamines and other vasopressor drugs
	Monoamine oxidase inhibitors

Diastolic hypertension

Caused mainly by increased stroke volume of left ventricle

Complete heart block	Arteriovenous fistula
Aortic regurgitation	Severe anemia
Patent ductus arteriosus	Beriberi
Thyrotoxicosis	Paget disease of bone

Caused mainly by decreased distensibility of aorta

Arteriosclerosis of aorta
Coarctation of aorta (see above)

Systolic hypertension

HYPERTENSION: A DISEASE OF REGULATION (Continued)

Angiotensin has become the focal point of the proposed mechanisms responsible for renal hypertension. It is believed that obstructive lesions of the renal artery cause hypertension by the large release of renin, with formation of angiotensin. Several clinical methods are used to determine blood levels of angiotensin and renin; none has proved simple in application. Plate 6.107 summarizes the pathophysiology of the renin-angiotensin-aldosterone system effect on blood pressure.

Angiotensin is a vasoconstrictor and increases sodium reabsorption in proximal tubules. When angiotensin rises to easily detectable levels, overt arterial hypertension occurs. Many effects of angiotensin suggest that it acts with other humoral agents in control of tissue perfusion. For example, minute amounts of angiotensin injected into the blood supply of the suprarenal gland cause excessive secretion of catecholamines. Instead of the trivial rise in blood pressure expected from a tiny amount of angiotensin, a preternaturally large increase occurs. Angiotensin II receptor blockers, ACE inhibitors, and aldosterone receptor blockers (ARBs; spironolactone) are used to treat hypertension and heart failure and to reverse cardiac hypertrophy.

The kidney has other methods of regulating blood pressure, such as control of salt and water metabolism. Low-salt diets reduce blood pressure, and diuretics are used to treat hypertension. Salt causes water retention, which raises blood volume, which increases blood pressure. This phenomenon is seen clearly, especially when both kidneys are removed from a patient preparatory to renal transplantation. As salt and water are retained, blood volume rises, as does arterial pressure. If the salt is dialyzed, pressure usually returns to normal.

Human renal hypertension has multiple causes, some of which are correctable by surgery or drugs. Detection of obstructive lesions in the renal arteries by renal angiography has greatly aided the surgeon and interventional cardiologist in their removal, resulting in a reasonably high cure rate. Treatment of pyelonephritis may also

Plate 6.107

Cardiovascular System: VOLUME 8

RENIN-ANGIOTENSIN SYSTEM

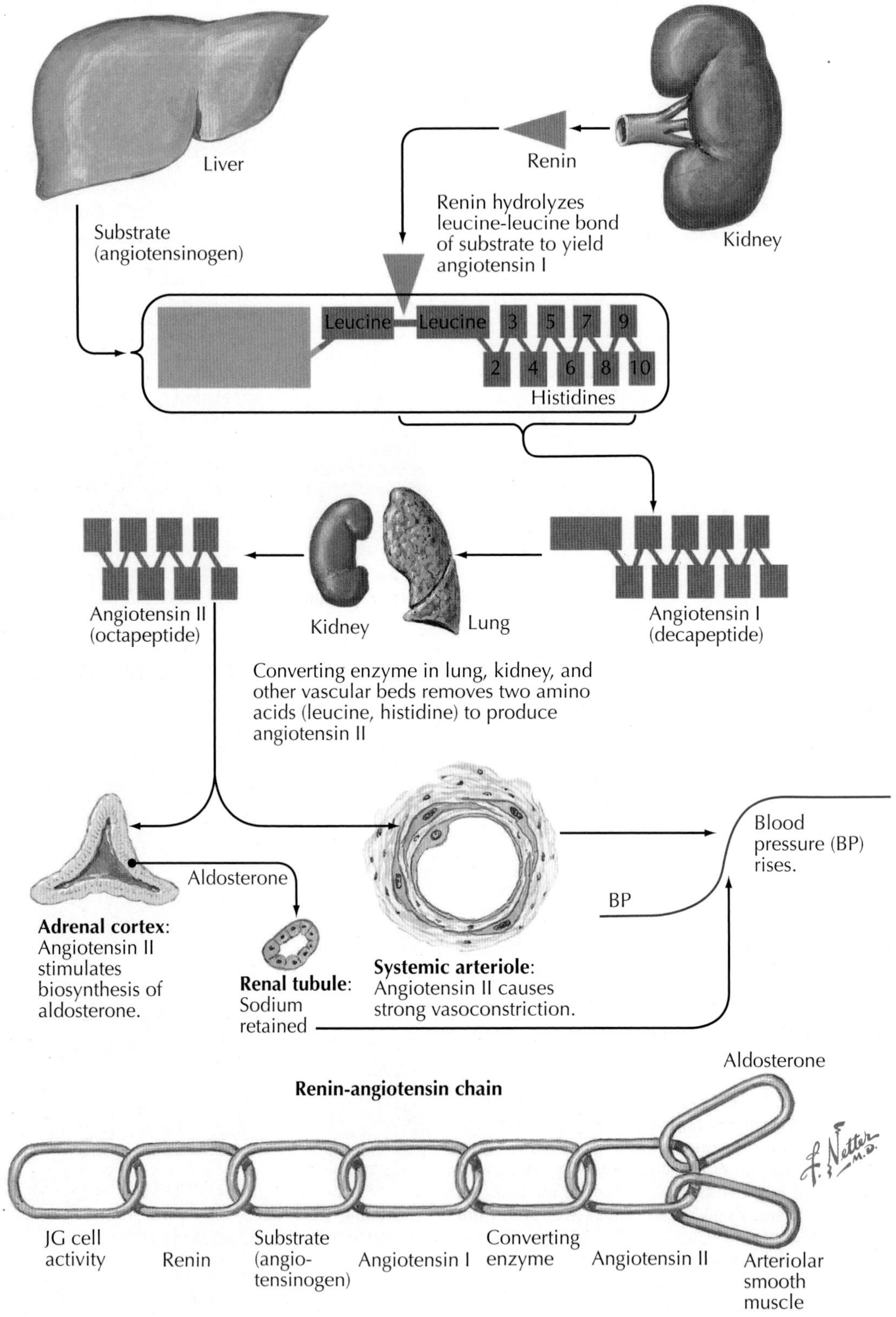

Liver

Substrate (angiotensinogen)

Renin

Renin hydrolyzes leucine-leucine bond of substrate to yield angiotensin I

Kidney

Leucine — Leucine 3 5 7 9
2 4 6 8 10
Histidines

Angiotensin II (octapeptide)

Kidney   Lung

Angiotensin I (decapeptide)

Converting enzyme in lung, kidney, and other vascular beds removes two amino acids (leucine, histidine) to produce angiotensin II

Blood pressure (BP) rises.

BP

Aldosterone

Adrenal cortex: Angiotensin II stimulates biosynthesis of aldosterone.

Renal tubule: Sodium retained

Systemic arteriole: Angiotensin II causes strong vasoconstriction.

Aldosterone

Renin-angiotensin chain

JG cell activity   Renin   Substrate (angiotensinogen)   Angiotensin I   Converting enzyme   Angiotensin II   Arteriolar smooth muscle

HYPERTENSION: A DISEASE OF REGULATION (Continued)

lower the blood pressure, provided that the renal parenchyma is not too badly damaged.

Endocrine Factors

Tumors of the suprarenal medulla produce paroxysmal types of hypertension, and those of the renal cortex cause a more moderate but sustained hypertension. These are illustrated by pheochromocytoma and primary aldosteronism (see Plates 6.101 and 6.102). Because angiotensin has a strong controlling influence on aldosterone secretion, which results in salt retention, this retention of salt and water is one of the important mechanisms of hypertension. Another possible mechanism is the stimulation by angiotensin of the release of catecholamines from the adrenal medulla.

Recent discussion has focused on whether many patients with a diagnosis of hypertension of uncertain etiology do not have primary aldosteronism, many of them being normokalemic. Decreased tolerance to carbohydrate is believed to be a characteristic of hypertension, with adrenocortical adenomas in some patients used as further evidence.

Aldosterone antagonists are beneficial when the patient is losing large amounts of potassium as a part of secondary hyperaldosteronism.

OTHER MECHANISMS OF BLOOD PRESSURE CONTROL

Neural Factors

The neural network regulating blood pressure is vast and complicated (Plate 6.105). A mental component, characterized chiefly by emotions of hostility, may play some part in the mechanisms of hypertension. The sympathetic nervous system and the parasympathetic system actively participate in vascular regulation. Probably the most powerful regulatory device is the *carotid-sinus baroreceptor*. The central integrating areas for vasomotor control are widely scattered in the brain but occur especially in the midbrain and medulla. The efferent pathways end on the blood vessels, heart, adrenal medulla, and juxtaglomerular cells.

Plate 6.108

Acquired Heart Disease

WAVE REFLECTION AND ISOLATED SYSTOLIC HYPERTENSION

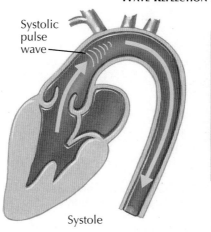

Systolic pulse wave

Systole

Pulse wave generation

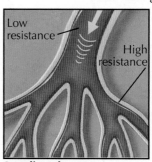

Low resistance

High resistance

Systolic pulse wave

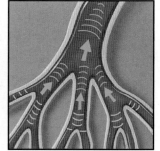

Reflected pulse wave

Systolic pulse wave reflected at transition from low- and high-resistance vessels and returned centrally as secondary pulse wave

Normal diastolic return

Reflected (secondary) pulse wave

Pulse wave velocity

Abnormal systolic return

Summation of systolic and reflected pulse waves

Pulse wave velocity

ECG

200
180
160
140
120
100
80
60

Systolic pulse wave

Secondary pulse wave

Brachial artery

Ascending aorta

Amplitude of reflected wave greatest in periphery, accounting for higher systolic pressures in extremities than in aorta. Diastolic return of reflected wave to heart increases coronary perfusion and decreases afterload.

ECG

200
180
160
140
120
100
80
60

Arterial pressure (mm Hg)

Systolic hypertension

Brachial artery

Ascending aorta

Stiffening of arterial wall increases pulse wave velocity and results in systolic return of reflected wave with increase in systolic pressure (isolated systolic hypertension), decreased diastolic pressure, increased afterload, and left ventricular hypertrophy.

HYPERTENSION: A DISEASE OF REGULATION (Continued)

The neural component exhibits the phenomenon of negative feedback and baroreceptor resetting. When arterial pressure rises in the carotid sinus, the vasomotor activity (especially of medulla oblongata) is inhibited and peripheral resistance falls, and vice versa. Normal average blood-pressure levels are thus maintained. If the elevated arterial pressure is persistent, however, resetting of the barostat occurs, and now the carotid-sinus regulatory mechanism tries to maintain the elevated pressure. In short, inhibition does not occur until the preternaturally high pressure has been further exceeded. The normal level has now been reset upward, which is why blood pressure must be maintained persistently at lower levels with drugs to maximize treatment effectiveness. The same type of resetting phenomenon apparently controls renin release by the kidneys. Catheter-based *radiofrequency ablation* of renal sympathetic nerves that carry both efferent sympathetic and afferent sensory fibers greatly reduces norepinephrine spillover from the kidney, decreasing systemic blood pressure.

Cardiovascular Factors

Arteries and arterioles have an inherent *tone* that responds with change to tissue needs (autoregulatory). Also, the anatomy of the blood vessels is so tailored to the particular needs of an organ that it helps regulate blood supply. Responsiveness of blood vessels to various stimuli may change. For example, blood vessels may constrict 10 times as powerfully in response to the same stimulus, a phenomenon called *cardiovascular reactivity*. Caffeine, cigarette smoking, and even "white coat hypertension" can be caused by vasoconstriction. Again, blood vessels exhibit *autoregulation,* the ability to adjust their caliber to the needs of the tissue with a changing blood pressure. Thus kidneys need not become ischemic when arterial pressure falls. This powerful regulatory force seems inherent in the function of smooth muscle of blood vessels.

Plate 6.108 summarizes the relationship of systolic and diastolic pulse wave velocity to systolic hypertension.

Plate 6.109

Cardiovascular System: VOLUME 8

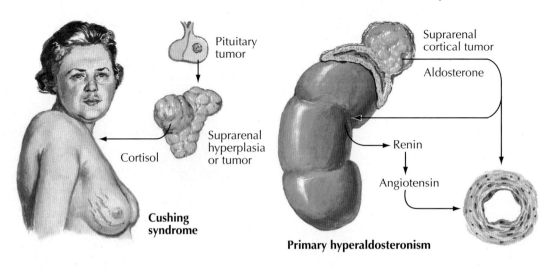

Cushing syndrome

Pituitary tumor

Cortisol

Suprarenal hyperplasia or tumor

Suprarenal cortical tumor

Aldosterone

Renin

Angiotensin

Primary hyperaldosteronism

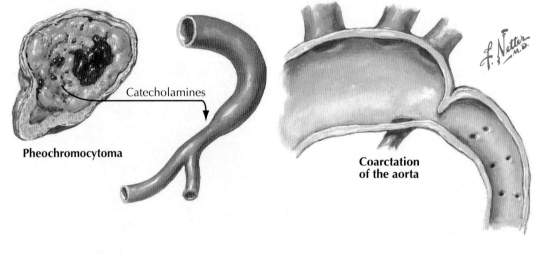

Catecholamines

Pheochromocytoma

Coarctation of the aorta

CAUSES OF SECONDARY HYPERTENSION POSSIBLY AMENABLE TO SURGERY

Hypertension secondary to obstruction to the flow of blood to the kidneys is the most common form of arterial hypertension correctable by surgery and percutaneous stenting. This form of renovascular hypertension is chiefly recognized using angiography, visualizing both large and small vessels. The most common obstruction is produced by atherosclerosis. To elicit hypertension, mean blood pressure must be substantially reduced in the renal artery. Surgical or angioplasty/stent correction of such stenosis has been notably successful and often has restored blood pressure to normal. Much less common is compression of the renal parenchyma by a connective tissue hull or by blood clots pressing on the parenchyma. Such lesions can result in malignant hypertension and are corrected by treating the condition compressing the renal parenchyma. Because of this success, even though rare, these compression conditions should not be overlooked.

Primary aldosteronism is a well-recognized cause of usually moderate arterial hypertension. The hypertension is abolished when the tumor of the adrenal cortex is surgically removed. Aldosterone secretion is determined by angiotensin from the kidneys, so increased aldosterone may be secreted in hypertension of primary renal origin. This may be one reason why low-salt diets and aldosterone antagonists are often valuable in the treatment of renovascular hypertension (Plate 6.109).

Pyelonephritis, especially in its advanced stages, is a relatively common association with arterial hypertension. Because pyelonephritis is typically bilateral, nephrectomy must not be performed in such patients unless there are indications other than treatment of the hypertension. *Polycystic kidney disease* may also be associated with hypertension, especially when the kidneys have become scarred, and pressure on the parenchyma is occurring. Draining of the cysts is rarely helpful.

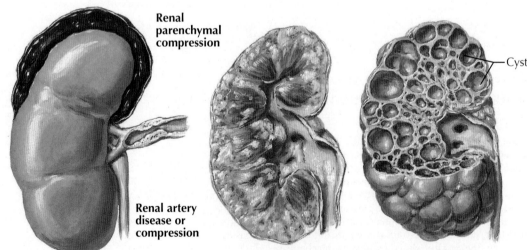

Renal parenchymal compression

Renal artery disease or compression

Cysts

Unilateral pyelonephritis or polycystic kidney

Pheochromocytoma is uncommon, but this tumor of the adrenal medulla usually produces dramatic clinical signs and symptoms; several provocative diagnostic tests are available. The tumor often occurs unilaterally, thus providing an opportunity for nephrectomy. Surgical removal of the tumor usually results in maintenance of normal blood pressure. Occasionally, the blood pressure does not return to normal because other, tiny undetected tumors are not removed, or other causes exist for the hypertension. Correction of *coarctation of the aorta* is usually followed by a decrease in blood pressure, both proximal and distal to the obstruction. This operation was one of the first to be performed in the field of cardiovascular surgery. A rare form of hypertension associated with *Cushing syndrome* is believed to be chiefly of adrenal origin, although Cushing himself thought it was primarily of pituitary origin (Plate 6.109).

Plate 6.110

Acquired Heart Disease

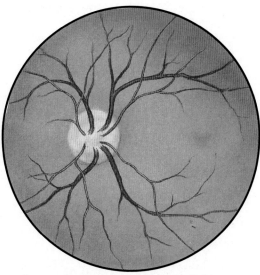

Grade I (Keith, Wagener, and Barker) mild narrowing of the retinal arteries relative to the veins

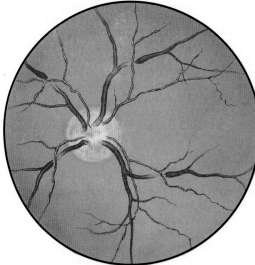

Grade II moderate sclerosis with increased light reflex and compression of veins at crossings

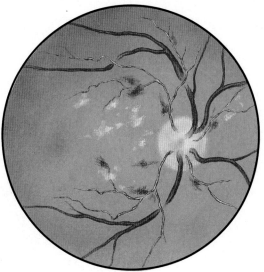

Grade III edema, exudates, and hemorrhages; sclerotic and markedly spastic ("silver-wire") arteries

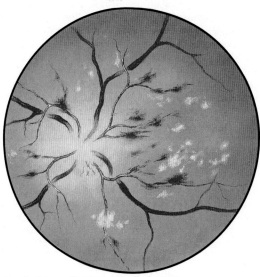

Grade IV papilledema or choked disc, extensive hemorrhages, and exudates

RETINAL CHANGES IN HYPERTENSION

Direct observation of the retina is crucial in following the course of hypertensive vascular disease. The retina is the only part of the body where *arterioles* may be seen, and the arterioles constitute the greatest locus of resistance to blood flow. Of the various grading systems for retinal changes, the earliest and most common is the classification of Keith, Wagener, and Barker, as follows:

Grade I: Retinal changes consist of mild narrowing or mild sclerosis of the arterioles that is compatible with good health for many years. The blood pressure is not excessively high and falls during rest.

Grade II: The changes in the retinal vessels are more marked than in grade I, but retinitis is not present. The disease is more progressive, and the blood pressure is higher and more sustained, but general health is good, and cardiac and renal function are satisfactory.

Grade III: Angiospastic retinitis occurs with definite sclerotic changes in the arterioles, but edema of the optic disc is not always present. The hypertension is high and sustained. Although cardiac and renal function may be adequate, alterations may occur, as indicated by dyspnea on exertion, ECG changes, and nocturia. Nervousness, headache, vertigo, and visual disturbances may occur. Proteinuria and hematuria may be present.

Grade IV: The important retinal alteration is edema of the optic discs. There is also marked spastic and organic narrowing of the arterioles with diffuse retinitis. Characteristic symptoms are nervousness, asthenia, loss of weight, headache, visual disturbances, dyspnea on exertion, and nocturia. Proteinuria, cylindruria, and red blood cells are usually present. The prognosis is poor.

The physician should become thoroughly familiar with the appearance of the retinal blood vessels during the varied stages of hypertension. For this reason, the retina should be examined repeatedly by the patient's physician rather than a consultant. The left eye often may have more extensive changes than the right eye. The normal cupping of the nerve head should be carefully noted so that, if *papilledema* occurs, it will not be overlooked. Papilledema may occur in the presence of normal or only slightly elevated cerebrospinal fluid pressure.

Under proper treatment with blood pressure control, the severe ocular and retinal changes characterizing malignant hypertension may be reversed.

Plate 6.111

Cardiovascular System: VOLUME 8

OCCLUSIVE DISEASE OF MAIN RENAL ARTERY

The recognition of a naturally occurring renovascular hypertension in humans, which parallels Goldblatt's experiments with constriction of the renal artery, has progressed rapidly during the past decade. A cause such as stenosis of a renal artery is sought because many patients with this condition can return to a normotensive state with surgery or percutaneous intervention. Howard and Poutasse did much to stimulate the search for another anatomic cause of hypertension. Development of aortography and selective renal angiography was key in diagnosing disease of the main renal artery. Constricting lesions have been demonstrated in general, and refinements have allowed recognition of exact types of renal artery disease, usually by distinguishing similar lesions that differ clinically, anatomically, and symptomatically.

ATHEROSCLEROSIS

Atherosclerosis is the most common cause of occlusive arterial disease in general and of renal artery stenosis in particular. Although this variety of renal artery disease predominates in older males, it also is found in females. Atherosclerosis usually involves the origin and first portion of the renal artery, although occasionally plaques may be found more distally in a renal artery branch. On arteriography the lesion typically appears *eccentric* as a plaque that involves only part of the renal artery's circumference. In addition to its eccentric form, the lesion also dominantly involves the intima. Thus endarterectomy can be performed because a decreased plane may be developed between the diseased part and rest of the arterial wall. (This is not true in other types of renal artery disease.) At times, the lesions may be completely *concentric,* even involving most of the media in addition to destroying the intima.

Besides hypertension and kidney damage, two other complications may be found. As in general atherosclerosis, *thrombosis* may be superimposed on the lesion. Second, the unusual morphologic problem of a *dissecting aneurysm* may occur. Blood striking an endothelial-lined channel in an abnormal manner, as must occur distal to these plaques, results in breaks in the intima, with channels of blood dissecting into the arterial wall. Frequently these channels dissect merely for short distances, forming what might be called an *intramural hematoma.* At other times, the channels dissect for appreciably greater distances along the renal artery. However, the pressure gradient distal to the plaque appears to be so much less that sufficient force is not exerted for dissection into the main aorta. As soon as blood passes beneath the occluding zone, distal pressure apparently decreases, and no more dissection occurs.

FIBROTIC LESIONS

The second general group of renal arterial lesions may be classified as fibrotic (nonatheromatous). The general term *fibromuscular hyperplasia* has been sufficient in some cases, but clinicopathologically distinct lesions also may be encountered, and because no etiologies have been found for these, a descriptive nomenclature is based primarily on the *location* of the arterial damage.

Intimal Fibroplasia

Intimal fibroplasia occurs in the main renal artery or its branches, most often in young males but also in both

VARIETIES OF RENAL ARTERY DISEASE THAT MAY INDUCE HYPERTENSION

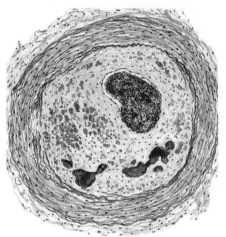

Severe concentric atherosclerosis of renal artery with lipid deposition and calcification, complicated by thrombosis (composite, ×12)

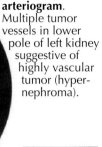

Selective left renal arteriogram. Multiple tumor vessels in lower pole of left kidney suggestive of highly vascular tumor (hypernephroma).

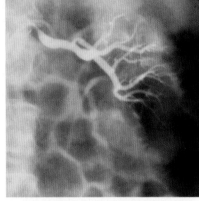

Selective arteriogram demonstrating asymmetrical narrowing of proximal left renal artery by atherosclerotic plaque

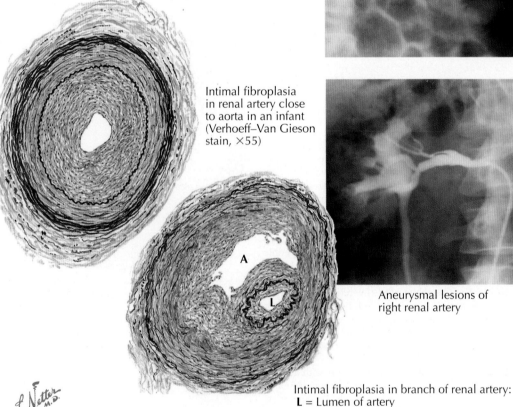

Intimal fibroplasia in renal artery close to aorta in an infant (Verhoeff–Van Gieson stain, ×55)

Aneurysmal lesions of right renal artery

Intimal fibroplasia in branch of renal artery:
L = Lumen of artery
A = Cavity of dissecting aneurysm
(Verhoeff–Van Gieson stain, ×18)

sexes at all ages. When not complicated by dissection, the lesion produces a fusiform narrowing of the renal artery. This lesion may not be limited to a renal artery and has been described in many locations; its morphology is very similar to that of *endarteritis obliterans* of the smaller arteries. Other main arteries have been involved, even in children. Microscopically, a diffuse circumferential thickening of the media most often is seen, but occasionally it seems as though a thin layer of collagen has been applied to an underlying *elastica*

interna that has been thrown into marked folds (Plates 6.111 and 6.112). In addition, the affected arteries in young patients show marked alterations of the internal elastic membrane, usually reduplication.

Medial Fibroplasia with Aneurysms

Medial fibroplasia with aneurysms was originally interpreted radiologically as fibromuscular hyperplasia. Characteristically, the angiogram resembles a string of beads, with dilated irregularities of the renal artery;

Plate 6.112

Acquired Heart Disease

OCCLUSIVE DISEASE OF MAIN RENAL ARTERY (Continued)

this beading appears larger than the diameter of the origin of the artery, which is usually spared. The disease primarily affects females and is usually bilateral. Medial fibroplasia with aneurysms does not exclusively affect the renal artery and has been reported in other locations.

The morphology is most unusual. When opened longitudinally, the affected renal artery appears similar to diverticulosis of the colon (in miniature). Small outpouchings can be seen, distorting the arterial wall (Plate 6.112). The microscopic picture reveals varying thicknesses of the arterial wall, ranging from fibrous accumulations superimposed on intact internal elastic membrane, to areas where the external elastic membrane is the only part left. The recognizable remaining media shows a marked loss of muscle and increased collagen in many areas. This increased collagen probably saves the vessel from longitudinal dissection by tethering segments of the artery to the external elastic membrane.

Subadventitial Fibroplasia

Subadventitial fibroplasia usually affects young females and may be bilateral (25% of patients in only reported series). Frequently a disease of the right renal artery, subadventitial fibroplasia usually involves variable lengths of the renal artery beyond its origin but rarely its main branches, either primarily or by extension. Microscopically, the lesion appears to be a unique involvement of the renal artery, consisting of a dense, circumferential collar of collagen external to and at times partially or completely replacing varying segments of the media (Plate 6.112). A considerable amount of the adventitial elastic tissue still remains, as well as what seems to be much of the external elastic lamellae, and thus the term *subadventitial fibroplasia*. The collagen is remarkably dense, and special stains show it to be completely mature, in contrast to some changes seen in intimal fibroplasia; this difference is best shown by techniques demonstrating acid mucopolysaccharides. In longitudinal sections the collagen appears to vary in thickness. Consequently, renal arteriograms show an irregularity in the outline of the arterial lumen. In contrast to medial fibroplasia with aneurysms, diameter of the vascular irregularity is less than that of the uninvolved proximal segment of renal artery. Here again, dissecting hematoma does not occur, and secondary thrombosis is rare.

Fibromuscular Hyperplasia

Fibromuscular hyperplasia, at least in part, is another fibrotic stenosing lesion of the main renal artery. It is the rarest of all fibrotic renal arterial problems and as such is difficult to analyze statistically. Once again, there seems to be a difference between the lesions in young children and those in adults. In young patients the lesion appears to consist predominantly of muscle, although the concentric lesion can be a uniform mixture; rarely is it bilateral. In older individuals it seems to involve primarily males and is complicated by distal dissecting hematomas. The arteriographic picture in the young group is similar to that of intimal fibroplasia, with a smooth, uniform stenosis. In older males, any narrowing is obscured by dye filling the aneurysmal dilation. In addition, children show abnormality of the aorta, which appears irregularly stenosed. This coarctation extends from above the origin of the renal arteries to, or almost to, the aortic bifurcation.

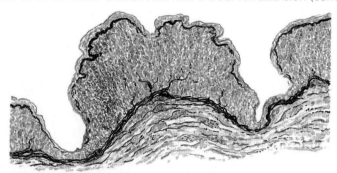

Longitudinal section of renal artery with medial fibroplasia: great variation in thickness of arterial wall, chiefly of media, with aneurysmal evagination (Verhoeff–Van Gieson stain, ×20)

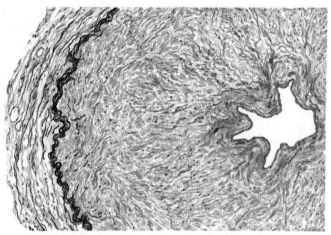

Fibromuscular hyperplasia. medial thickening consisting of fibrous and muscular tissue; internal elastic membrane not present (Verhoeff–Van Gieson stain, ×100).

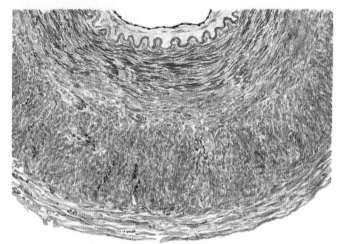

Subadventitial fibroplasia. a concentric ring of dense collagen is present between media and adventitia (Masson Trichrome stain, ×80).

Other Hypertensinogenic Changes

In addition to the rather characteristic lesions just described, other hypertensinogenic changes involve the main renal arterial vasculature. Primary dissecting aneurysms can cause partial to complete occlusion of the renal artery, as well as hypertension. Apparently, a discontinuity in the internal elastic membrane allows the intramural dissection of blood. Such lesions have been found even in children. The relationship between this lesion and the "aneurysm of the renal artery" is not clear, but the same lack of elastic-tissue continuity might be responsible for both conditions. The presence of a dissection may depend on whether the forces can pass longitudinally in the vessel or must remain contained within a pouch and form an aneurysm. *Periarterial fibroplasia* is seen as part of retroperitoneal fibrosis and can be responsible for hypertension. Large *perinephric hematomas* apparently also interfere with the main renal vasculature and possibly the small vasculature, to produce a remedial type of elevated blood pressure.

Plate 6.113

Cardiovascular System: VOLUME 8

KIDNEYS AND HYPERTENSION

Examination of a kidney problem in the patient with hypertension requires identification of specific factors. The "protected" kidney, which has been partially or completely removed from systemic circulation by alterations in renal artery flow, may show no changes but usually displays a variety of differences caused by the decreased renal blood flow. The protected kidney shows marked tubular atrophy as a result of parenchymal loss; the glomeruli appear crowded, lying much closer to each other, although their structure seems unaltered. Because this is common, even in occlusion of the main renal artery, collateral circulation from the capsular branches must be responsible for the lack of infarction.

An important variation is found in association with *atherosclerosis,* a dynamic disorder. An occlusive plaque may develop in a main renal artery after valvular change in the kidney. The vessels in this kidney can show atherosclerosis of the smaller arteries and arterioles and obliterating fibrotic and atherosclerotic changes in the medium-sized and large arteries, although these findings are not especially significant.

The changes in the kidney exposed to the full force of hypertension depend in part on the duration of disease. The first change may be a thickening of the musculature of the small arteriole. *Hyaline arteriolar sclerosis* is common in chronic hypertension, at first with only hyaline masses in arteriolar walls, but later with the arteriolosclerosis becoming thick and circumferential. The constituency of this peculiar waxy material is a conglomeration of blood constituents that have focally leaked through the vessel wall (Plate 6.113).

A more important lesion is often found in the larger arteries of the renal parenchyma and consists of marked intimal thickening (mainly collagen) in the arcuate, interlobar, and interlobular arteries. Its importance in the kidney seems related to a loss of renal parenchyma because these lesions are most likely responsible for the common granular scarring and larger wedge-shaped scars. Hypertension probably causes the intimal thickening, and hypoxia of the kidney occurs, stimulating a vasopressor mechanism to elaborate substances responsible for the maintenance of blood pressure or further increase. These fibrotic changes in the medium-sized and small arteries may be the most important alterations in renal physiology by hypertension. Although extensive in the kidney in moderate hypertension, these changes are sufficiently sparse to allow adequately functioning renal parenchyma to remain. Thus renal failure is not the usual cause of death in patients with moderate hypertension.

In contrast, the renal lesions in *malignant hypertension* are extensive, and renal failure is a common cause of death in untreated cases. The arteriole shows a wide variety of lesions. Its walls may become necrotic, with fibrin being deposited and forming minute thrombi (Plate 6.113). In addition, a peculiar *lamellar* hyperplasia that appears to be alternating collagen and elastic tissue may be seen. This is the characteristic "laminated onion" of malignant nephrosclerosis, which must not be confused with the subintimal changes in medium-sized or small arteries in hypertension. Both these

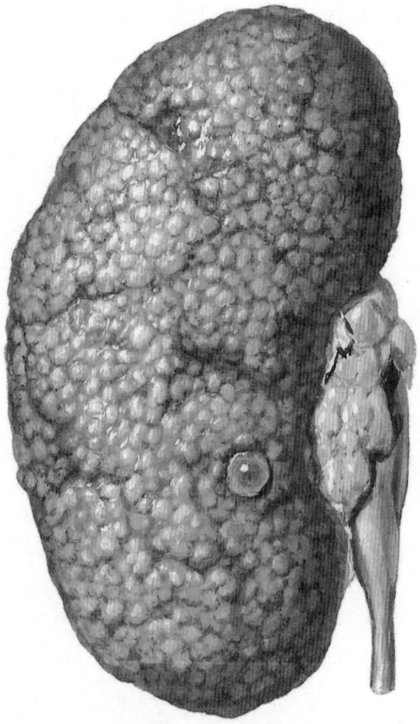

Granular arteriolosclerotic kidney. Typically found in hypertension of unknown etiology.

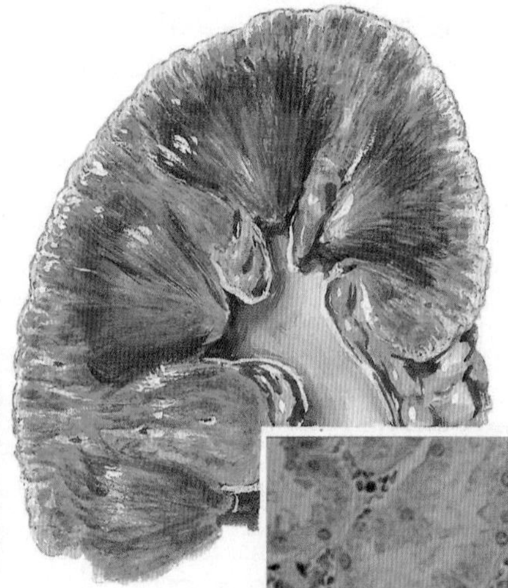

Arteriolosclerotic kidney. Cut surface

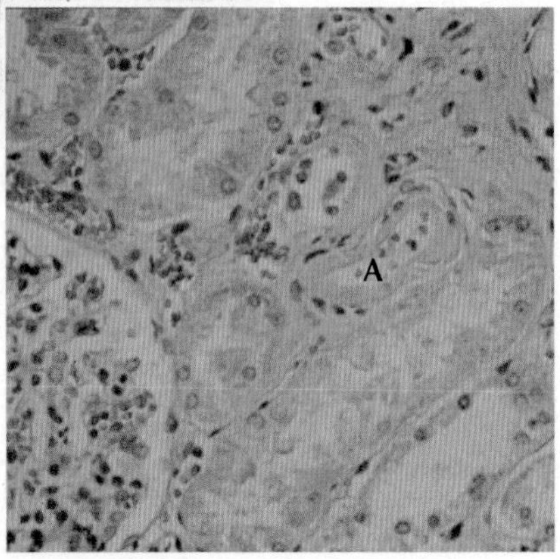

Hyalinization of an afferent arteriole (A). In arteriolosclerosis of essential hypertension.

Malignant phase of essential hypertension. Characteristic "onion skin" lamination and deterioration of a renal arteriole.

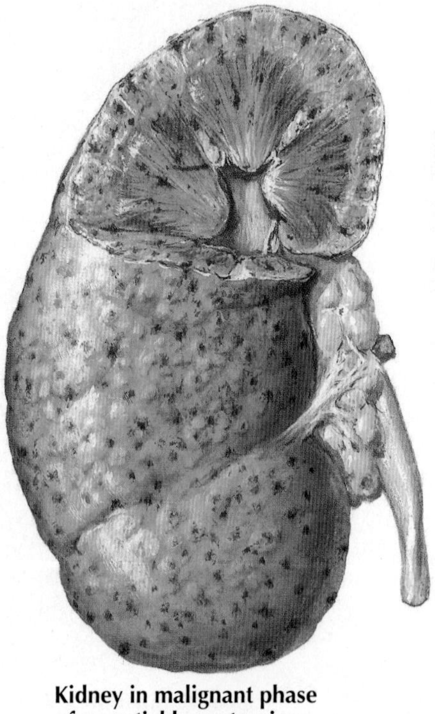

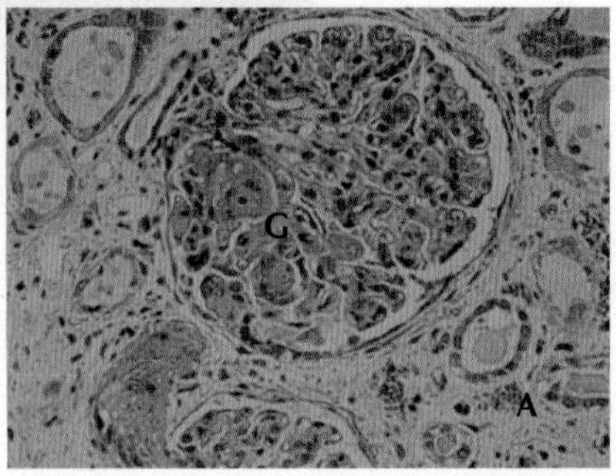

Kidney in malignant phase of essential hypertension. Numerous variegated hemorrhages

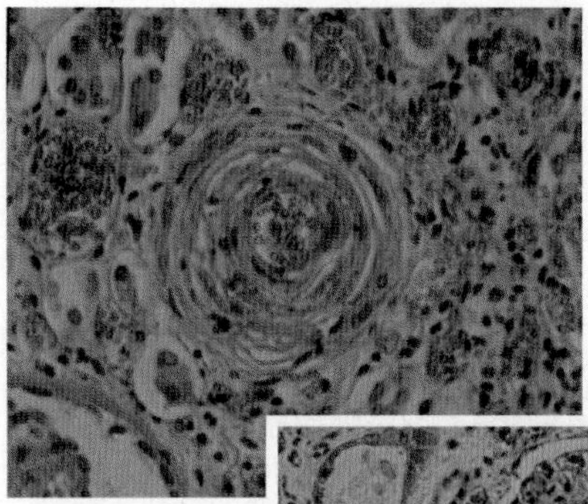

Malignant hypertension. Necrosis of a glomerulus (G) and of an afferent arteriole (A).

lesions can be responsible for changes in the glomerulus, with either partial or complete necrosis of the tuft. Whenever this extensive damage occurs, hemorrhage in the glomerulus or arteriolar wall can result.

In addition to the arteriolar changes, extensive alterations can also occur in the arteries. The extreme pressures will drive blood constituents into and beyond the arterial walls, forming large pools of fibrin and necrotic muscle. Thrombosis may be superimposed on

these lesions, and there may be small areas of infarction. Other evidence of material being driven into the arterial and arteriolar walls is the presence of *lipid* accumulations (microatheromas) within these structures. In some patients, arteries will show such major occlusive change, especially if life is prolonged by extensive antihypertensive therapy. The intimal fibroplasia in these patients has been shown to be so severe that the hypertension (and renal failure) may recur.

Plate 6.114

Acquired Heart Disease

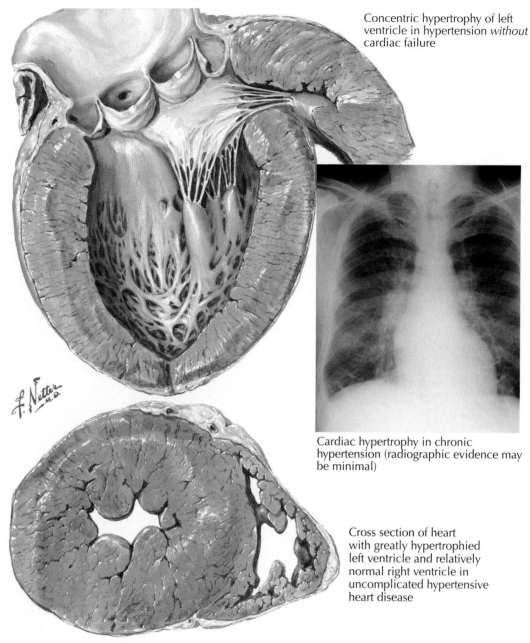

Concentric hypertrophy of left ventricle in hypertension *without* cardiac failure

Cardiac hypertrophy in chronic hypertension (radiographic evidence may be minimal)

Cross section of heart with greatly hypertrophied left ventricle and relatively normal right ventricle in uncomplicated hypertensive heart disease

HEART DISEASE IN HYPERTENSION

Although the heart often is affected adversely in patients who have various forms of elevated blood pressure, the detectable changes in the heart correlate poorly with the degree and duration of hypertension in any individual patient. Whereas 60% to 75% of patients with hypertension die with a cardiac complication, the timing, incidence, and severity of the heart disease are quite variable. The elevation of blood pressure is caused by an increased peripheral vascular resistance to blood flow in the presence of well-preserved stroke volume and cardiac output. The resulting increase in work of the heart causes *concentric hypertrophy* of the left ventricular myocardium (Plate 6.114). Thickening of the heart wall ensues over a variable period and serves as a compensatory mechanism, maintaining the normal cardiac output against the increased peripheral resistance, which in turn results from arteriolar constriction of various causes and mechanisms, depending on etiology of the hypertension.

During this phase of concentric LV hypertrophy, a high index of suspicion is necessary to make a diagnosis of *hypertensive heart disease*. The clinician may detect

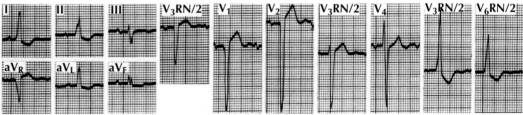

Electrocardiographic evidence of left ventricular hypertrophy may or may not be present (tall R waves in V_4, V_5, and V_6; deep S waves in V_3R, V_1, V_2, III, and aV_R; depressed ST and inverted T in V_5, V_6, I, II, aV_L, and aV_F)

increased forcefulness of the point of maximum impulse over the left precordium, with increased intensity of the S_2 aortic component (A_2), and increased palpable pulsation of the great vessels at the neck base. Chest radiograph evidence of LV enlargement and ultrasound and ECG evidence of hypertrophy may be seen. At this stage the ECG may show one of the earliest and most reliable signs of LV hypertrophy: left-axis deviation, increased amplitude of R wave in leads I, V_5, and V_6, as well as of

the S wave in leads III, V_1, V_2, and V_3; negative P wave in V_1 and depressed ST segments in leads V_5, V_6, I, II, aV_L, and aV_F; and elevated ST segments in aVR, V_1, V_2, and V_3. (The changes depicted in Plate 6.114 are indicative of more advanced LV hypertrophy.) ECG changes frequently correlate with the presence of a fourth heart sound (S_4) caused by LV stiffness. These abnormalities may disappear if effective lowering of the systemic blood pressure can be accomplished.

Plate 6.115

Cardiovascular System: VOLUME 8

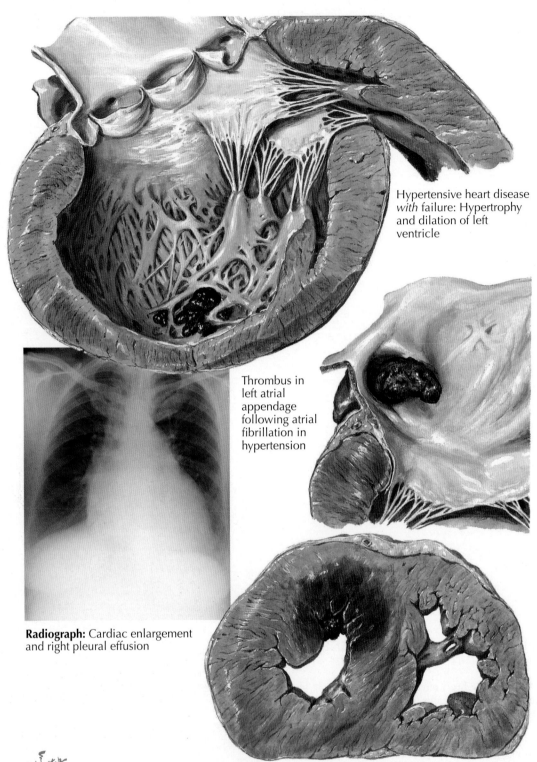

Hypertensive heart disease *with* failure: Hypertrophy and dilation of left ventricle

Thrombus in left atrial appendage following atrial fibrillation in hypertension

Radiograph: Cardiac enlargement and right pleural effusion

Hypertrophy of right as well as left ventricle in left ventricular failure due to hypertension; anteroseptal infarct

HEART DISEASE IN HYPERTENSION (Continued)

During this phase of compensated hypertensive heart disease, the patient may have no particular cardiac symptoms except fatigability and sensation of increased forcefulness of the heartbeat, particularly with excitement or exercise. Blood volume and venous pressure measurements are normal, as is cardiac output, whether measured by thermodilution or other catheterization techniques. The incidence of coronary atherosclerosis is moderately increased in patients with hypertensive heart disease, who thus develop stable angina pectoris and acute coronary syndromes (e.g., MI) more often than usual. The LV myocardium tends to outgrow its own blood supply, which is also intrinsically compromised because of the apparently traumatic effects of higher blood pressure on the coronary artery walls.

At some point in the progression of hypertensive heart disease, which cannot be accurately evaluated in an individual patient as to severity or duration of the hypertensive history; the compensatory mechanism of concentric hypertrophy is no longer sufficient. Evidence of cardiac decompensation and congestive heart failure supervenes, but this state is usually marked by coronary atherosclerosis, malignant phase of hypertension, or retention of sodium and water caused by renal function changes.

The first stage in the development of congestive heart failure is elevation of LVEDP, with the left ventricle subsequently showing dilation in addition to hypertrophy. Progressive cardiac enlargement then develops, and dilation of the mitral annulus may result in mitral regurgitation and a characteristic holosystolic murmur at the cardiac apex. A ventricular gallop sound, pulsus alternans, or increased intensity of P_2 may all be detected at the bedside. Atrial fibrillation may occur in about 25% of patients, depending on duration and degree of associated coronary atherosclerosis and age of the patient (Plate 6.115). At this stage the patient usually has definite symptoms of pulmonary congestion, with exertional dyspnea, orthopnea, and paroxysms of unprovoked nocturnal dyspnea. Frank pulmonary edema occasionally may be precipitated, requiring aggressive treatment with oxygen administration, vigorous

Plate 6.116

Acquired Heart Disease

HYPERTENSION AND CONGESTIVE HEART FAILURE

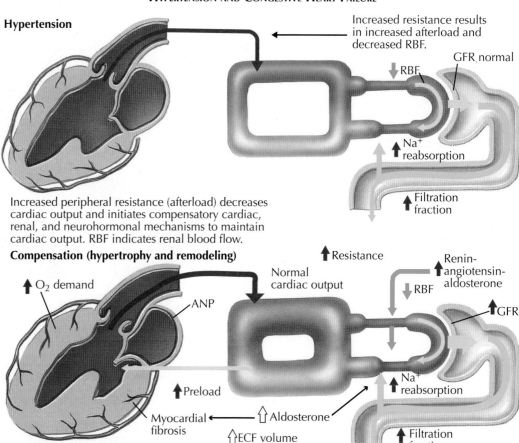

Hypertension

Increased resistance results in increased afterload and decreased RBF.

↓RBF

GFR normal

↑Na+ reabsorption

↑Filtration fraction

Increased peripheral resistance (afterload) decreases cardiac output and initiates compensatory cardiac, renal, and neurohormonal mechanisms to maintain cardiac output. RBF indicates renal blood flow.

Compensation (hypertrophy and remodeling)

↑O₂ demand

↑Resistance

Normal cardiac output

Renin-↑angiotensin-aldosterone

↓RBF

↑GFR

ANP

↑Preload

Myocardial fibrosis ← ⇧Aldosterone

⇧ECF volume

↑Na+ reabsorption

↑Filtration fraction

Concentric hypertrophy

Ventricular hypertrophy preserves cardiac output. Neurohormonal mechanisms increase vascular resistance and extracellular fluid (ECF) volume and maintain glomerular filtration rate (GFR).

Decompensation (myocardial failure–CHF)

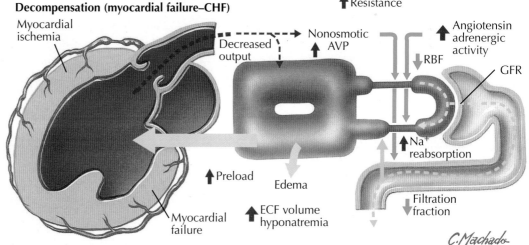

Myocardial ischemia

↑Resistance

Decreased output

↑Nonosmotic AVP

↑Angiotensin adrenergic activity

↓RBF

GFR

↑Preload

Edema

↑Na+ reabsorption

↑ECF volume hyponatremia

Myocardial failure

↓Filtration fraction

Eccentric hypertrophy

Decreased output causes increased resistance and volume. This results in marked decrease in cardiac output, renal perfusion, and GFR.

HEART DISEASE IN HYPERTENSION (Continued)

loop diuretic therapy (e.g., IV furosemide), and control of systemic hypertension with vasodilator therapy (e.g., ACE inhibitors, ARBs) or other appropriate drugs.

The subsequent course of hypertensive heart disease depends largely on the incidence and severity of the associated coronary atherosclerosis, control of blood pressure, and presence or absence of renal insufficiency. Provided the patient survives, pulmonary artery pressure rises because of vascular changes similar to those found in rheumatic mitral stenosis (i.e., secondary to elevated left atrial pressure). Hypertrophy of the right ventricle and sometimes RV failure may follow, in which dependent edema and hepatic congestion cause more symptoms (Plate 6.116).

Additional complications of hypertensive heart disease include peripheral emboli, particularly in patients with MI and in the presence of chronic atrial fibrillation. If renal failure and azotemia develop, *fibrinous pericarditis* occasionally occurs, with characteristic friction sounds heard over the precordium. If control of electrolyte imbalance becomes difficult, extra care must

be taken in the use of diuretic or hypotensive drugs as well as digitalis preparations.

The treatment of hypertensive heart disease, especially in the "decompensated stage," has improved with the more effective hypotensive agents (ACE inhibitors, ARBs, β-blockers, calcium antagonists) and more sensitive loop diuretics (e.g., metolazone). Weight reduction, control of complicating factors (e.g., diabetes mellitus), maintenance of adequate nutrition, and proper balance

of physical activity are all important features of the program for the hypertensive cardiac patient. Prognosis remains relatively satisfactory unless MI, stroke, malignant hypertension, or renal failure aggravate the overall problem.

A newer catheter-based technology is another way to manage refractory hypertension. Radiofrequency energy is used to ablate, moderate, or interrupt the efferent and afferent sympathetic nerves in the renal arteries.

Plate 6.117

Cardiovascular System: VOLUME 8

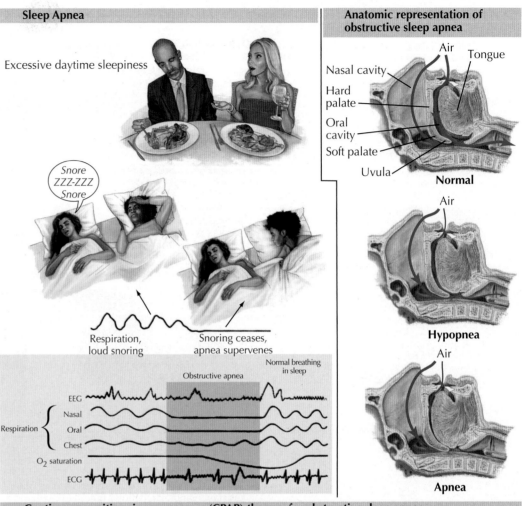

Sleep Apnea

Excessive daytime sleepiness

Snore
ZZZ-ZZZ
Snore

Respiration, loud snoring

Snoring ceases, apnea supervenes

Anatomic representation of obstructive sleep apnea

Air

Tongue

Nasal cavity

Hard palate

Oral cavity

Soft palate

Uvula

Normal

Air

Hypopnea

Air

Apnea

EEG

Respiration { Nasal, Oral, Chest }

O₂ saturation

ECG

Obstructive apnea

Normal breathing in sleep

Continuous positive airway pressure (CPAP) therapy for obstructive sleep apnea

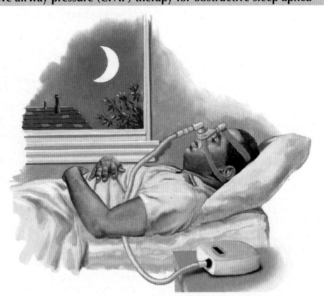

OBSTRUCTIVE SLEEP APNEA AND HYPERTENSION

The term *apnea* is used when a person has stopped breathing. The most common form of apnea is obstructive sleep apnea (OSA). OSA occurs frequently during sleep in susceptible individuals, more often in females, and incidence increases with age. Complete or partial blockage of the upper airways (nose, retroglossal or retropalatal regions, or pharynx) makes it difficult to breathe because movement of air is compromised. The apnea is temporary but can occur multiple times during the night. When patients resume normal breathing after an apneic spell, it usually occurs after some sort of gasp or body jerking or snoring loudly. A spouse or partner usually first notices the apnea because most patients with OSA snore (Plate 6.117).

Classic clinical manifestations of OSA include snoring, easy fatigability or sleepiness in midday, morning headache, and poor sleep patterns with frequent sudden awakenings. Cardiovascular manifestations include hypertension, myocardial ischemia, MI, pulmonary hypertension, heart failure, atrial fibrillation, and other arrhythmias. OSA can occur in anyone but typically occurs more often in patients with obesity. According to the US National Heart, Lung, and Blood Institute, more than 12 million Americans have sleep apnea, more than half of whom are overweight. Bariatric surgery may be necessary to achieve weight loss in a patient with morbid obesity. OSA therapy also includes use of continuous positive airway pressure (Plate 6.117).

Plate 6.118

Acquired Heart Disease

Gowers Maneuver

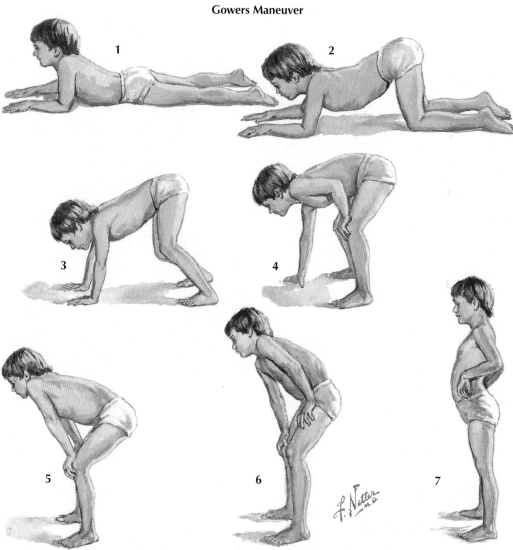

Characteristically, the child arises from prone position by pushing himself up with hands successively on floor, knees, and thighs, because of weakness in gluteal and spine muscles. He stands in lordotic posture.

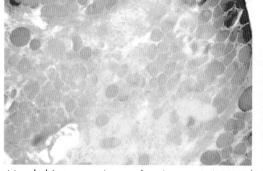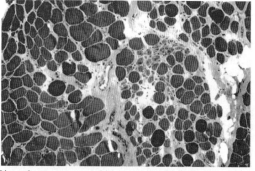

Muscle biopsy specimens showing necrotic muscle fibers being removed by groups of small, round phagocytic cells (**left**, trichrome stain) and replaced by fibrous and fatty tissue (**right**, H&E stain)

DUCHENNE MUSCULAR DYSTROPHY

Duchenne muscular dystrophy is an inherited disorder that involves muscle weakness. The genetic abnormality is sex linked, and only boys are affected. Females are carriers of the disease but have no symptoms. The incidence is 1 in 3600 male children, usually age 6 years or younger. Despite some boys with disease manifestations who have no family history of Duchenne muscular dystrophy, a family history is a risk factor for male children. Once diagnosed in children, Duchenne worsens quickly compared with other muscular dystrophies, and few patients live beyond age 25 years, usually dying of lung disorders (e.g., pneumonia). Many of these children use the Gowers maneuver to arise from the prone position, pushing the body up with the hands successively on floor, knees, and thighs because of weakness in gluteal and spinal muscles. They then stand in a lordotic posture (Plate 6.118).

Classic symptoms include easy fatigability and muscle weakness beginning in the legs and pelvis, with all of the attendant limitations. This weakness rapidly progresses and can involve other muscles (upper extremities, back of neck), and usually the patient requires a wheelchair in the teenage years. Cardiac problems generally begin in late adolescence, and physical examination reveals congestive heart failure and serious ventricular arrhythmias secondary to cardiomyopathy. Other physical abnormalities include severe scoliosis, pseudohypertrophy of muscles (muscle replaced by fat), loss of muscle mass, and pulmonary problems from aspiration of food.

Muscle biopsy reveals necrotic muscle fibers being removed by groups of small round phagocytic cells and replaced by fibrosis and fatty tissue. Muscle biopsies also reveal abnormalities of dystrophin content, which is the result of a defective gene for the protein (Plate 6.118).

There is no known cure for Duchenne muscular dystrophy. Treatment is mainly symptom control to improve quality of life. Patients are encouraged to remain active to slow disease progression. Physical therapy and speech therapy may also be useful. If cardiac or respiratory failure is prominent, assisted ventilation and standard heart failure therapies (e.g., ACE inhibitors, β-blockers, diuretics) should be used. Steroid therapy may slow the loss of muscle strength. Many other therapies have positive but unproven effects. Stem cell therapy and gene therapy are being considered. Recently, a young patient in refractory heart failure received a left ventricular assist device that seems well tolerated.

Plate 6.119

Cardiovascular System: VOLUME 8

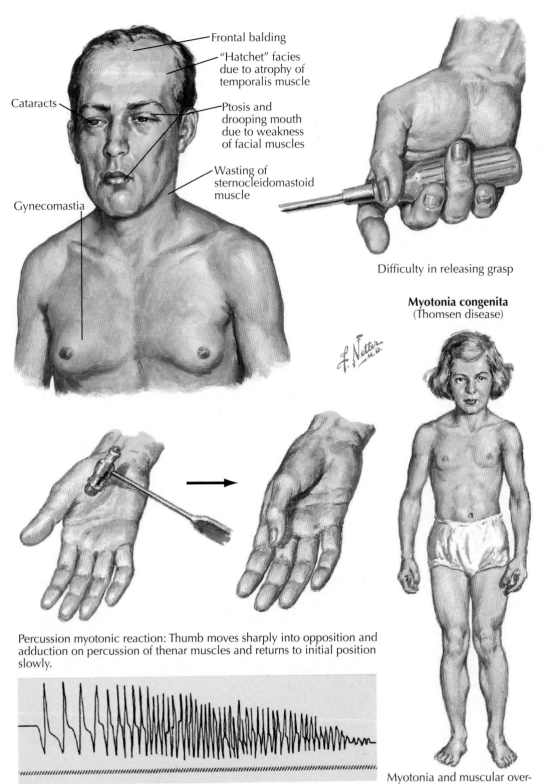

Frontal balding

"Hatchet" facies due to atrophy of temporalis muscle

Cataracts

Ptosis and drooping mouth due to weakness of facial muscles

Wasting of sternocleidomastoid muscle

Gynecomastia

Difficulty in releasing grasp

Myotonia congenita
(Thomsen disease)

Percussion myotonic reaction: Thumb moves sharply into opposition and adduction on percussion of thenar muscles and returns to initial position slowly.

Electromyogram showing spontaneous myotonic discharge evoked by needle insertion.

Myotonia and muscular over-development. Disease affects both males and females.

MYOTONIC DYSTROPHY

An autosomal dominant genetic abnormality, myotonic dystrophy occurs in about 1 in 8000 births, affects both sexes, and is the most frequently inherited neuromuscular disease of adult life. It usually occurs in young adults and progresses slowly over time. Myotonic dystrophy can also begin later in life and manifests as mild muscle weakness and myotonia, and sometimes only cataracts. This form of the dystrophy may be associated with a normal life span. Thus, although an autosomal dominant disorder, myotonic dystrophy has incomplete penetrance and variable phenotypic manifestations. This multisystem disease frequently involves the heart and may be a cause of sudden cardiac death.

Although neuromuscular alterations are usually the initial clinical manifestation of myotonic dystrophy, symptoms caused by cardiac involvement are occasionally seen. The first to appear are conduction abnormalities, ventricular and supraventricular arrhythmias, or, less often, myocardial dysfunction (e.g., cardiomyopathy). On physical examination, patients with classical myotonia have a delayed relaxation after a muscular contraction. They also have generalized muscle weakness and slowly progressive wasting of facial and axial musculature. Cataracts, frontal balding, ptosis, gynecomastia, difficulty releasing grasp, diabetes, hypogonadism, and cardiac dysfunction can accompany the muscle disorder (Plate 6.119). Myocardial biopsies and autopsy studies show various degrees of nonspecific changes, such as interstitial fibrosis, fatty infiltration, hypertrophy of cardiomyocytes, and focal myocarditis. The most common cardiac manifestation seen at autopsy is a selective and extensive impairment of the conduction system.

Respiratory failure from multiple causes (e.g., pneumonias) and cardiovascular disease caused by conduction system disease are the most prevalent causes of death, accounting for about 30% (cardiac) to 40% (respiratory) of deaths. Cardiac mortality can result from progressive LV dysfunction, ischemic heart disease (especially in older patients), pulmonary embolism, or unexpected sudden death, probably dysrhythmic in origin. Most agree that cardiac arrhythmias may represent the most prevalent cause of sudden death as a result of ventricular asystole, ventricular tachycardia, ventricular fibrillation, or atrioventricular conduction abnormalities caused by degeneration of the conduction system. An early invasive approach may be warranted in select patients with asymptomatic AV conduction delay. If electrophysiologic investigation reveals a prolonged HV (His bundle to ventricular activation) interval, prophylactic pacemaker implant should be considered, even in the absence of symptoms.

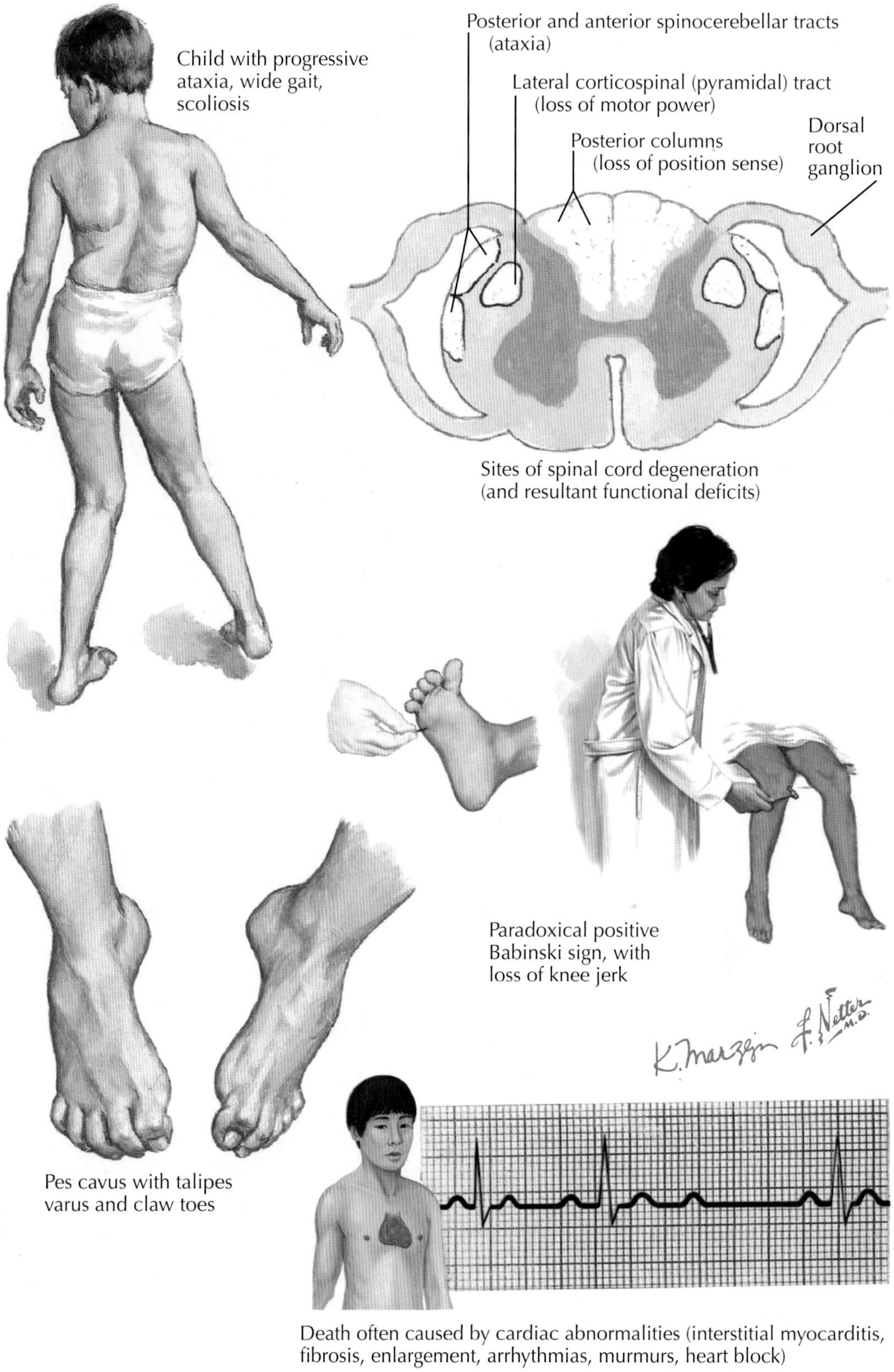

Plate 6.120

Acquired Heart Disease

Child with progressive ataxia, wide gait, scoliosis

Posterior and anterior spinocerebellar tracts (ataxia)

Lateral corticospinal (pyramidal) tract (loss of motor power)

Posterior columns (loss of position sense)

Dorsal root ganglion

Sites of spinal cord degeneration (and resultant functional deficits)

Paradoxical positive Babinski sign, with loss of knee jerk

Pes cavus with talipes varus and claw toes

Death often caused by cardiac abnormalities (interstitial myocarditis, fibrosis, enlargement, arrhythmias, murmurs, heart block)

FRIEDREICH ATAXIA

An autosomal recessive inherited disease, Friedreich ataxia has onset early in childhood, in some patients after a febrile illness in which ataxia of one lower extremity precedes that of both lower extremities. Classic Friedreich ataxia is the result of a gene mutation decreasing synthesis of frataxin protein, resulting in frataxin deficiency. *Frataxin* is essential for normal mitochondrial function, for both oxidative phosphorylation and iron homeostasis. Frataxin deficiency results in iron accumulation within mitochondria and hearts of patients with Friedreich ataxia. Increased generation of free radicals and damage to the mitochondria occur, inactivating mitochondrial enzymes essential for the production of adenosine triphosphate. Cells and tissues of the body are differentially sensitive to frataxin deficiency; cells requiring and producing more frataxin tend to be most affected by ataxia. For example, sensory neurons in the dorsal root ganglion responsible for position sense highly express the frataxin gene and are affected greatly in Friedreich ataxia.

Neuropathologically, patients with Friedreich ataxia have spinal cord degeneration at posterior and anterior spinocerebellar tracts (resulting in ataxia), lateral corticospinal (pyramidal) tracts (loss of motor power), posterior columns (loss of position sense), and dorsal root ganglia. Physical signs include severe kyphoscoliosis and progressive ataxia in children, manifested as a wide-based gait (Plate 6.120). Many have pes cavus with talipes varus and claw toes, positive Babinski sign with loss of knee jerk, and cardiac abnormalities such as interstitial myocarditis, fibrosis, cardiomegaly, hypertrophic cardiomyopathy, dilated cardiomyopathy, ventricular tachycardia, and heart block. Hypertrophic cardiomyopathy develops in more than 50% of patients. Cardiac arrhythmia and congestive heart failure contribute to a significant number of deaths in patients with Friedreich ataxia. Approximately 10% of patients develop diabetes mellitus, and a higher percentage demonstrate impaired glucose tolerance.

The risk of a child developing Friedreich ataxia is highest if parents have a blood relationship. However, most cases are sporadic and occur in nonconsanguineous families. The overall risk of a patient with Friedreich ataxia having a child with the condition is approximately 1 in 200. The risk is much higher if consanguinity is involved and much lower if not. As the disease progresses, ataxia affects the entire body, and some patients develop choreiform movements along with profound distal weakness of the legs and feet. Eventually the patient requires a wheelchair for mobility, and ultimately becoming bedbound, and may become dysarthric and dysphagic. Variability in the clinical presentation of Friedreich ataxia may be explained by the differential sensitivity of cells and tissues to frataxin deficiency and correlates with age of onset and time to end stages; myocardial muscle fibers require large amounts of frataxin and are greatly affected by ataxia.

Plate 6.121

Cardiovascular System: VOLUME 8

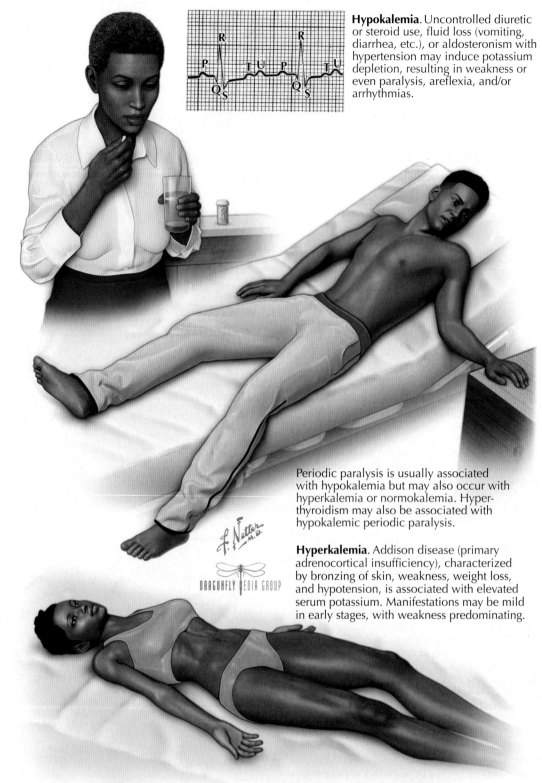

Hypokalemia. Uncontrolled diuretic or steroid use, fluid loss (vomiting, diarrhea, etc.), or aldosteronism with hypertension, may induce potassium depletion, resulting in weakness or even paralysis, areflexia, and/or arrhythmias.

Periodic paralysis is usually associated with hypokalemia but may also occur with hyperkalemia or normokalemia. Hyperthyroidism may also be associated with hypokalemic periodic paralysis.

Hyperkalemia. Addison disease (primary adrenocortical insufficiency), characterized by bronzing of skin, weakness, weight loss, and hypotension, is associated with elevated serum potassium. Manifestations may be mild in early stages, with weakness predominating.

DISORDERS OF POTASSIUM METABOLISM

Periodic paralysis is a term applied to either hyperkalemia or hypokalemia that results in temporary episodes of flaccid paralysis. This rare group of neurologic autosomal dominant disorders with variable penetrance (more common in males) results from mutations of genes responsible for regulation of sodium-potassium (Na-K) and calcium (Ca) channels in nerve cells. Onset of symptoms is usually in adolescent children. The flaccid paralysis is associated with loss of deep tendon reflexes and failure of the muscle to respond to electrical stimulation. The patient rarely becomes unconscious.

Both hypokalemia and hyperkalemia can result in periodic paralysis (Plate 6.121). Many factors induce potassium depletion (hypokalemia) that results in weakness or even paralysis, areflexia, and cardiac arrhythmias. These include uncontrolled diuretic or steroid use, fluid loss (vomiting, diarrhea), or primary aldosteronism with hypertension. Periodic paralysis was one of the first neurologic *channelopathies* characterized at a genetic and cellular level involving Na-K and Ca channel subunits. With the channel mutations, attacks often begin in adolescence, triggered by strenuous exercise, high-carbohydrate meals, and injection of insulin, glucose, or epinephrine. ECG changes in patients with very low serum potassium levels include prominent U waves, flattening of T waves, and ST depression. ECG changes during hyperkalemia include tall peaked T waves, diminished R-wave amplitude, increased QRS complex or PR intervals, and P-wave disappearance.

Periodic paralysis is usually associated with hypokalemia but may also occur with hyperkalemia and normokalemia. Hyperthyroidism may also be associated

with hypokalemic periodic paralysis. Cardiomyopathies have been reported in patients with this condition. Hyperkalemia can be caused by Addison disease (primary adrenocortical insufficiency), characterized by bronzing of the skin, weakness, weight loss, and hypotension and associated with elevated serum potassium and ventricular arrhythmias secondary to prolonged QT interval (Plate 6.121). Manifestations may be mild

in early stages, with weakness predominating. Potassium ingestion and drugs (e.g., potassium, ACE inhibitors, ARBs) must be considered in any patient with hyperkalemia.

Daily oral acetazolamide induces a mild metabolic acidosis and may prevent both hyperkalemic and hypokalemic attacks, but oral potassium may be necessary in patients with resistant hypokalemic attacks.

Plate 6.122

Acquired Heart Disease

CARDIAC TAMPONADE

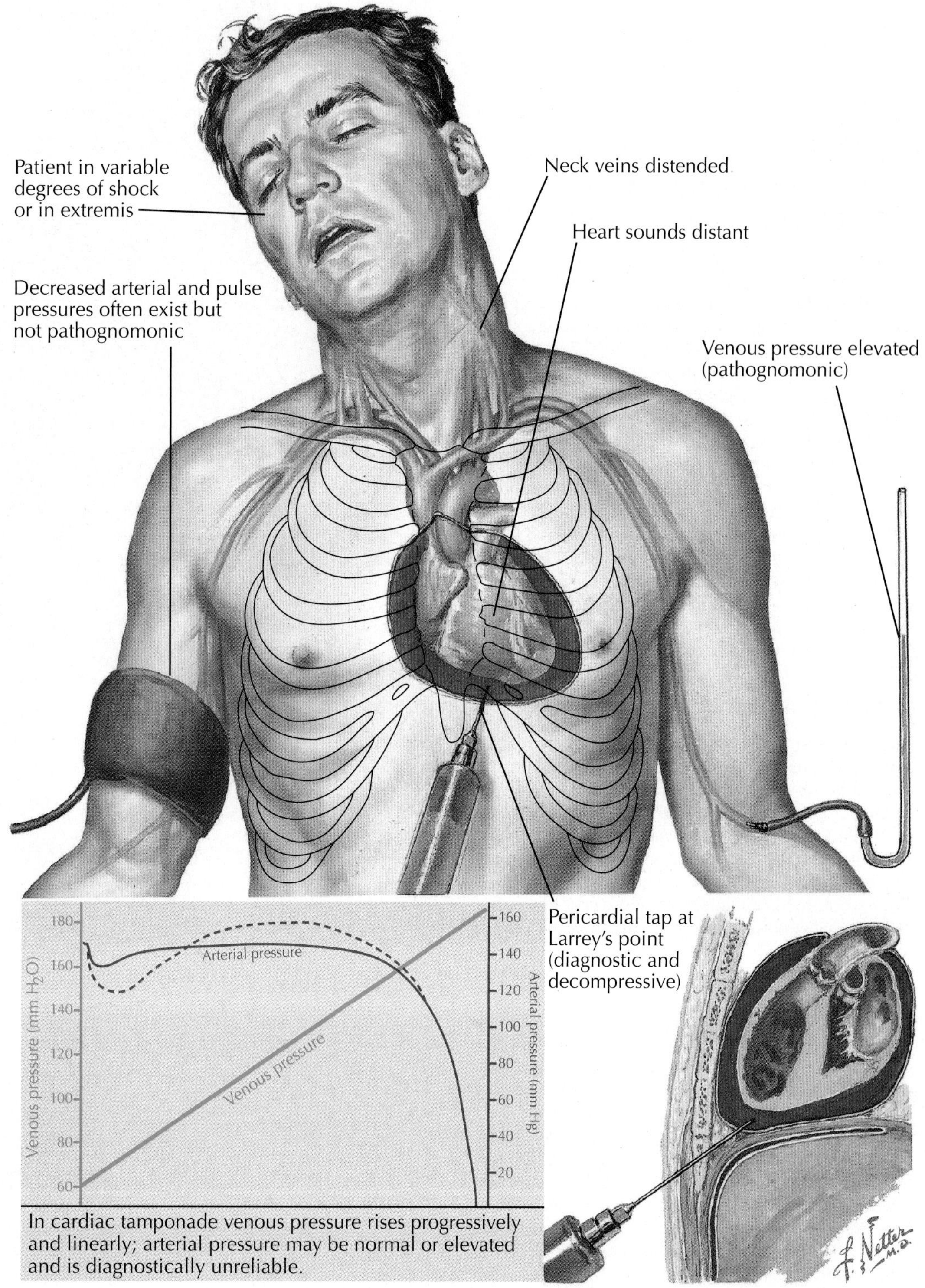

PENETRATING HEART WOUNDS

The vast majority of cardiac injuries are caused by knives, bullets, or other penetrating agents; the knife blades are about 6 inches (30 cm) long. Patients with penetrating wounds of the heart can be classified in three general groups: (1) those with extensive lacerations or large-caliber gunshot wounds, who die almost immediately as a result of rapid, voluminous blood loss; (2) those with small wounds of the heart caused by ice picks, knives, or other small objects several millimeters to 2.5 cm in length, who reach the hospital alive because *cardiac tamponade* develops; and (3) those with associated serious injuries in the chest and elsewhere that may contribute to death. The potentially lethal complication of cardiac tamponade in the second group results from a tough, fibrous, nonextensible pericardial sac encasing the heart and the roots of the great vessels. Without this sac, almost all heart wounds would present a hopeless situation because of massive blood loss, as occurs with wounds of the great vessels outside the pericardium. Cardiac tamponade, by bringing pressure to bear on the bleeding heart wall, also plays an important role in controlling the hemorrhage (Plate 6.122).

Although they may not all reach a hospital alive, patients with penetrating cardiac wounds who receive prompt definitive therapy have an 80% to 90% chance for recovery or more. The patient's condition on admission must not be used as an index of injury severity. Some moribund patients with no blood pressure and imperceptible pulse survive surgery and recover, whereas some patients with 80 mm Hg to normal systolic pressure and fair to good pulse die before surgery can be instituted. Therefore poor patient status should never suggest a "hopeless" case, and a seemingly stabilized clinical picture should never lead to a false sense of security.

The thoracic "danger area" and the approximate *relative distribution* of penetrating heart wounds are revealing (see Plate 6.123). The types of wounds vary. There may be a simple laceration (nick) in the wall of the heart, penetration into the wall without entering the cardiac chamber (intramural), penetration into the cardiac chamber (intraluminal), or actual perforation through one or more chambers. The vast majority are of the intraluminal variety. In a small percentage of patients, a solitary laceration of the pericardium exists without cardiac involvement.

The immediate cause of death is exsanguination, cardiac tamponade, or arrhythmia. The delayed causes include sepsis, massive cerebral embolism with infarction from a mural thrombus of the left ventricle, cardiac failure due to valvular or interventricular septal injury, and constrictive pericarditis. The variable course of penetrating wounds of the heart is illustrated in Plate 6.124.

CARDIAC TAMPONADE

Acute hemopericardium of sufficient size to cause cardiac tamponade constitutes the basic pathologic sequela of heart wounds, whether caused by penetrating

Patient in variable degrees of shock or in extremis

Decreased arterial and pulse pressures often exist but not pathognomonic

Neck veins distended

Heart sounds distant

Venous pressure elevated (pathognomonic)

Pericardial tap at Larrey's point (diagnostic and decompressive)

In cardiac tamponade venous pressure rises progressively and linearly; arterial pressure may be normal or elevated and is diagnostically unreliable.

or nonpenetrating trauma. Tamponade is both lethal and lifesaving; it contributes to the reduction or cessation of hemorrhage from the cardiac wound, but after a certain point produces *profound shock,* which proves fatal unless promptly relieved.

Acute cardiac tamponade results in three major physiologic alterations: (1) on the venous side the increased intrapericardial pressure restricts venous return to the right ventricle during diastole, increasing

RVEDP, which is reflected back to the right atrium as an elevated central venous pressure; (2) on the arterial side the resultant cardiac compression reduces cardiac output, decreasing blood pressure and reducing coronary filling factors that predispose to myocardial hypoxia and failure; and (3) on the systemic arterial side the reduced cardiac output leads to generalized vasoconstriction, which in turn increases peripheral vascular resistance. This third factor may be responsible for the

Plate 6.123   Cardiovascular System: VOLUME 8

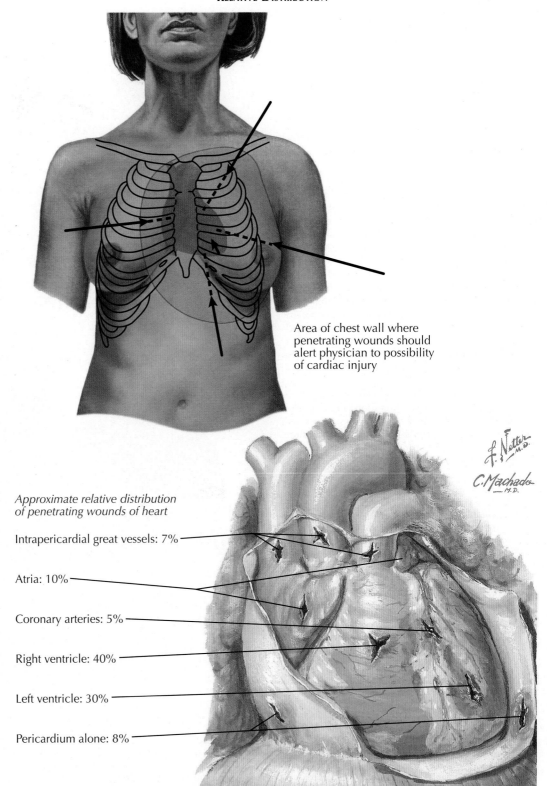

RELATIVE DISTRIBUTION

Area of chest wall where penetrating wounds should alert physician to possibility of cardiac injury

Approximate relative distribution of penetrating wounds of heart

Intrapericardial great vessels: 7%

Atria: 10%

Coronary arteries: 5%

Right ventricle: 40%

Left ventricle: 30%

Pericardium alone: 8%

PENETRATING HEART WOUNDS (Continued)

maintenance of near-normal or even higher-than-normal blood pressure during the early stage, despite a progressively falling cardiac output and a progressively rising venous pressure.

The clinical effects of small quantities of blood in the pericardial sac are negligible, but when the volume reaches 150 to 200 mL, cardiogenic shock may develop, often abruptly, because the pericardium cannot be stretched acutely. At this critical point, the addition or removal of only 10 to 20 mL of blood may improve cardiac output and mean the difference between life and death. In some patients the amount of blood in the pericardial sac is insufficient to produce detectable tamponade, and both cardiac and pericardial wounds heal spontaneously. The final outcome depends on the interplay of three important variables: cardiac wound, pericardial wound, and hemopericardium.

DIAGNOSIS OF CARDIAC INJURY

Diagnosis is generally simplified if the physician maintains a high degree of suspicion of cardiac injury in every chest wound encountered. Wounds of the upper abdomen, axillary region, posterior chest wall, and base of the neck also may be associated with heart injury. Wounds caused by ice picks or other small instruments are readily missed. Occasionally a progressive rise in blood pressure to 160 mm Hg or more over hours may occur in patients who have not only bleeding cardiac wounds but also significant hemopericardium and intrapericardial clot formation at surgery. Shock favors a diagnosis of cardiac injury when the degree of shock seems disproportionate to wound severity or blood loss. Cardiac injury may be followed by a symptom-free interval of several minutes to several hours and then deep shock, and it may be difficult to determine whether the shock is caused by tamponade or blood loss.

Tamponade can be recognized easily by history or by physical examination alone. The classic clinical features are elevated venous pressure, falling or absent arterial pressure, and muffled and distant heart tones. The circulatory collapse is out of proportion to the blood loss. When tamponade persists, the cervical veins, especially the external jugular veins, become full and tense. The aspiration of blood from the pericardial sac confirms the diagnosis of hemopericardium (see Plate 6.122). Frequently, the respiration is rapid and sighing, and the excursions usually are irregular. Dyspnea, air hunger, and extreme thirst are common. Chest radiography and venous pressure assessment may be helpful but not necessary to establish a diagnosis. Radiographs may demonstrate a widening of the cardiac silhouette. In some patients, these typical studies may be of no value, because death can occur from a hemopericardium, which is too small to cause noticeable changes in the size and contour of the cardiac

shadow. Cardiac ultrasound can be helpful in this situation. Radiography can assess the presence or absence of hemothorax and pneumothorax.

Elevated jugular venous pressure always accompanies cardiac tamponade but may be normal or even below normal when moderate to severe intrathoracic bleeding is present. Elevated venous pressure constitutes an excellent means of differentiating shock from cardiac tamponade and shock from hemorrhage.

An elevated systemic venous pressure suggests cardiac tamponade; a low systemic venous pressure in the patient with a penetrating cardiac wound may indicate significant blood loss. ECG is not particularly helpful, showing minor deviation from normal several hours after injury and thus of little value when needed most. Cardiac ultrasound is the best noninvasive way to estimate the amount of pericardial effusion and the existence of cardiac tamponade.

Plate 6.124

Acquired Heart Disease

VARIABLE COURSE OF PENETRATING WOUNDS OF HEART

PENETRATING HEART WOUNDS
(Continued)

Prompt, definitive therapy is imperative, including antishock therapy, pericardiocentesis, and thoracotomy with pericardiotomy and wound closure (Plate 6.124).

ANTISHOCK THERAPY

The patient is placed immediately in a moderate Trendelenburg position, oxygen is administered, and a rapid IV infusion of physiologic saline solution, plasma, or both is started. As soon as available, blood is substituted for these solutions. If typing and crossmatching are delayed, O-negative blood should be used. On occasion, autotransfusion is lifesaving, used only when indicated, while bank blood is being crossmatched. Narcotics, if necessary, should be used judiciously; restlessness usually reflects cerebral hypoxia, and further depression of the cardiorespiratory centers may prove fatal.

PERICARDIOCENTESIS

With tamponade, immediate aspiration is mandatory and often lifesaving. Surgical procedures should be performed if several aspirations fail to relieve tamponade, tamponade rapidly occurs after aspiration, or hemorrhage persists.

THORACOTOMY WITH PERICARDIOTOMY AND WOUND SUTURE

All surgeons agree that when the cardiac wound is complicated by persistent and profuse hemorrhage, an immediate thoracotomy is mandatory, with pericardiotomy and direct repair of the wound. Appropriate emergency care also must be provided for associated injuries to the lung and the internal mammary, intercostal, and great vessels resulting in pneumothorax, hemothorax, or hemopneumothorax, as well as life-threatening injuries of other structures. The anesthetic and technique used vary with the patient's condition. In the comatose patient, no anesthesia is required initially. In the patient with profound hypotension, regional anesthesia with oxygen therapy is preferred. In the patient with a relatively stable cardiovascular system, general anesthesia is used.

Endotracheal intubation with assisted respiration is preferred. Although this is an extremely important detail, positive airway pressure further increases intrathoracic pressure, augments the severity of tamponade of the heart and venae cavae, and converts reduced cardiac output to no output.

THORACOTOMY

Cardiac wounds, regardless of their location, are managed through a left thoracotomy to afford maximum

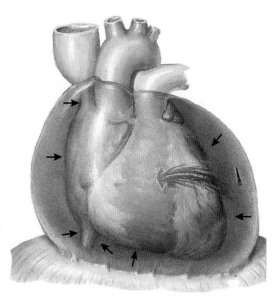

Voluminous blood loss: If wounds in myocardium and pericardium are large and both remain open, hemorrhage often leads rapidly to death; prompt cardiorrhaphy may occasionally be lifesaving.

Early tamponade: If myocardial wound remains open and pericardial wound seals off, cardiac tamponade results and may rapidly cause death unless relieved by pericardiocentesis. This may also be effective definitive therapy but cardiorrhaphy is preferred.

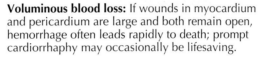

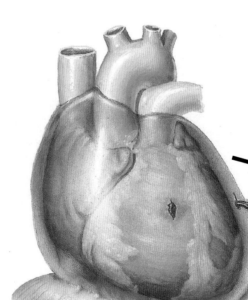

Early stabilization. If myocardial wound is sealed by clot, variable degrees of hemopericardium result, and if relieved by seepage or tap, effective heart action may continue and the patient survives.

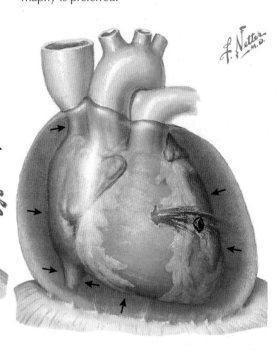

Delayed tamponade. After hours, days, or weeks, the clot may dislodge and fatal tamponade results this emphasizes desirability of prompt operative therapy.

exposure (Plate 6.125). The right-side approach may be necessary, however, when the wound of entrance indicates an injury through the right chest. Despite the urgency of exploration, a rapid, systematic routine must be followed. Unless the incisions in the skin, underlying muscles, intercostal spaces, and cartilages are separated from each other, in association with a careful chest wall closure, the complications of wound breakdown, infection, and chest wall sinus tract are

prone to occur. The most crucial moment during surgery is when cardiac compression is released. Just as the pericardial sac is opened, uncontrollable brisk bleeding and clot formation may be encountered, with blood welling up in the wound. Therefore, before the pericardium is incised, the following considerations are essential:

1. Providing adequate exposure through a *limited* thoracic incision of the structures in the pericardial

Plate 6.125

Cardiovascular System: VOLUME 8

THORACOTOMY AND CARDIORRHAPHY

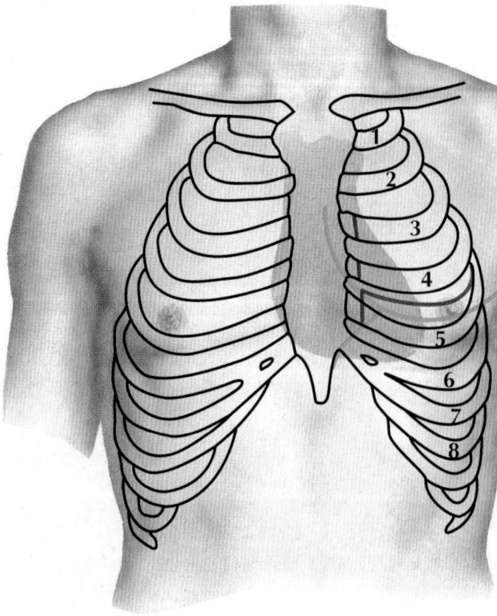

PENETRATING HEART WOUNDS (Continued)

sac is virtually impossible, and cutting ribs to improve exposure when seconds count may prove disastrous.

2. There must be a preconceived plan of action. The surgeon must pause to see that all necessary instruments (particularly rakes) are in readiness.

3. There must be sufficient amounts of blood and blood substitutes.

Attention to these three factors often makes the management of a complex and potentially lethal situation appear simple and logical.

Three crucial maneuvers spell the difference between life and death. First, soon after entry into the thoracic cavity, the first assistant elevates the *sternum* with two rakes, which places the assistant in a ready position to permit instantaneous *retraction* and fixation of the pericardium when presented to the assistant at pericardiotomy. Second, the surgeon grasps the pericardium with a Kocher clamp and opens its entire length (anterior to phrenic nerve) from its base on the diaphragm to the upper narrower part surrounding the great vessels. The edges of the pericardium are grasped with two additional Kocher clamps. As the surgeon retracts the pericardium with the Kocher clamps, to the left and then up and over the sternum, the first assistant releases the rakes from under the sternum and then reapplies them to retract the pericardium to the desired degree. This causes practically the entire heart to lie in the left hemithorax, resulting in excellent exposure. If necessary, the exposure can be enhanced further by forceful elevation of the sternum. In the third crucial maneuver, just as the pericardium is incised, the second assistant forcefully flushes out the area with copious amounts of warm saline solution. This maneuver rapidly clears the field of blood and quickly brings the bleeding point into view. With the bleeding point in view, digital compression over the wound will adequately control the hemorrhage.

The myocardial wound is closed. The heart muscle, which is soft and friable because of myocardial hypoxia, may require mattress sutures reinforced with small Teflon felt pledgets, to enhance safety in placing the sutures. A wound near a coronary vessel should be closed by passing a mattress-type suture beneath the vessel to avoid it. For an atrial wound, a noncrushing clamp is effective. Atrial wounds are closed with interrupted or continuous 4-0 or 5-0 arterial silk sutures. Lacerations of the aorta and other great vessels are clamped tangentially with a noncrushing clamp, and closure is accomplished with simple interrupted or continuous sutures of 5-0 arterial silk. The back part of the heart can be exposed by simple manual luxation, with the fingers spread apart. For torrential bleeding, some advocate temporary occlusion of the venae cavae. On the left side, the pericardial sac is left wide open to

A. Curved "Y"-shaped incision in skin and pectoralis major muscle (blue); incision of intercostal and pectoralis minor muscles and section of costal cartilages (red)

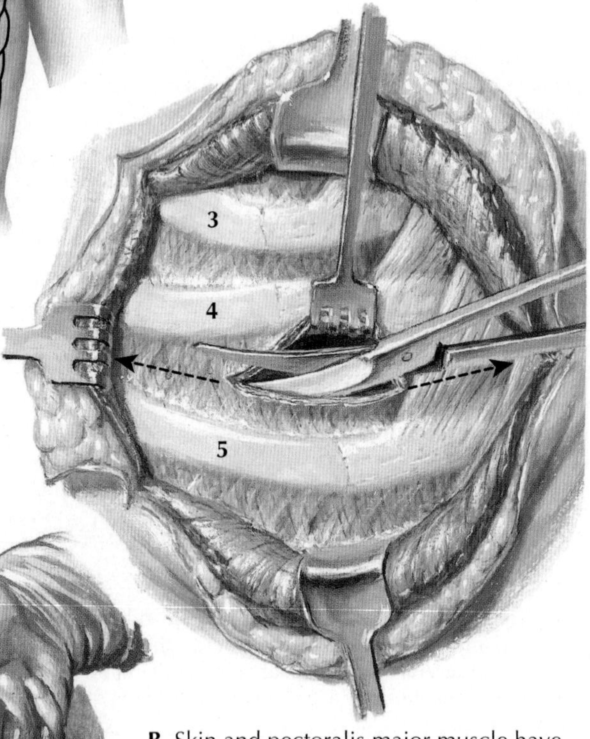

B. Skin and pectoralis major muscle have been divided and reflected; intercostal and pectoralis minor muscles are divided in 4th interspace

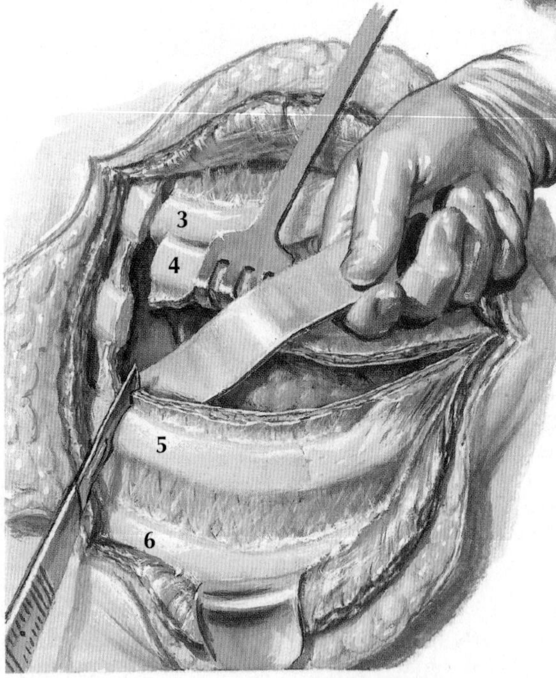

C. 3rd, 4th, and 5th costal cartilages divided over a flat ribbon retractor that protects underlying structures

allow free drainage into the pleural cavity. On the right side, the sac is closed loosely to prevent dislocation and strangulation of the heart. A catheter is placed in the pleural cavity and attached to an underwater negative-pressure drainage system.

In closure of the thoracotomy wound, the sectioned cartilages are approximated and sutured together with chromic gut (Plate 6.126). Postoperative management is similar to that of any procedure for open thoracotomy.

PERICARDIOCENTESIS VERSUS OPEN OPERATION

With pericardiocentesis as the primary method of treatment for patients with penetrating heart wounds, a large series (Beall et al.) reported that mortality in 78 patients treated was 5.5% of those requiring only aspiration. In 23 patients not responding to pericardiocentesis, mortality was only 26.7% with immediate surgery but increased to 62.5% if cardiac action was

Plate 6.126

Acquired Heart Disease

PENETRATING HEART WOUNDS (Continued)

allowed to stop before thoracotomy. For patients with more serious disease, 12 were treated primarily by surgery, with 33% mortality. These values show that a direct comparison of results would be misleading, because results after pericardiocentesis are highly selective, omitting patients with large wounds and massive hemorrhage.

A review of the literature is confusing because proponents of both pericardiocentesis and surgery report excellent results. Clearly, survival rates depend more on the nature and severity of the injury than on the form of treatment. A review of 113 patients with penetrating cardiac wounds treated surgically (June 1955–June 1963) reported a mortality of only 8.6% in 58 procedures, a considerable reduction over an earlier series (Maynard et al.). This reduction is attributable primarily to accumulated experience, improved surgical and anesthesiologic techniques, and the use of blood, plasma, and other IV fluids.

REASONS FOR FAVORING THORACOTOMY

Unquestionably, pericardial aspiration can be definitive therapy for a solitary heart wound complicated solely by hemopericardium and tamponade. Practically, however, as initial therapy for hemopericardium followed by prompt, definitive surgical intervention, pericardiocentesis is preferable to conservative management by aspiration. Pericardiocentesis used preoperatively for acute hemopericardium or tamponade helps the patient over that hazardous period of shock until surgery can be done. For excellent results, the surgical team must be skilled in thoracotomy. For the inexperienced operator confronted by a solitary heart wound complicated only by tamponade, nonoperative intervention with pericardiocentesis may be safer because some of these patients do survive with aspiration alone and sometimes even without aspiration. Nevertheless, when the problem is continuous exsanguination, thoracotomy with pericardiotomy and suture closure offers the only chance for survival. Surgery is favored over conservative aspiration as definitive therapy for the following reasons:

1. The site of injury can be determined with precision.
2. The type of injury can be adequately ascertained.
3. In about 50% of patients, large intrapericardial hemorrhagic clots are found, which prevent effective withdrawal of blood from the sac. A negative pericardiocentesis may lull the physician into a false sense of security, although cardiac ultrasound may show blood still in the pericardial space, and tamponade persists.
4. Secondary hemorrhage (delayed hemopericardium) can occur after hours, days, or even weeks in a significant number of patients.

5. The usual technique of aspiration with the patient supine is simple but risks laceration of the myocardium or left coronary artery.
6. The incomplete evacuation of hemopericardium may result in development of chronic pericardial effusions, adhesive pericarditis, or myocardial constrictive physiology.
7. A traumatic ventricular aneurysm may result near the epicardial opening, and a traumatic aneurysm of a coronary vessel may rupture.

8. The patients who do well with aspiration may survive, but the patients who do poorly or are unresponsive to aspiration either die or undergo surgery as the only recourse. Thus pericardiocentesis is fundamentally a trial; if it works, surgery may not be necessary.

Thoracotomy with pericardiotomy and direct wound repair is the most effective treatment. Pericardiocentesis should be employed as definitive therapy only in select patients and not regarded as the sole recommended procedure.

THORACOTOMY AND CARDIORRHAPHY (CONTINUED)

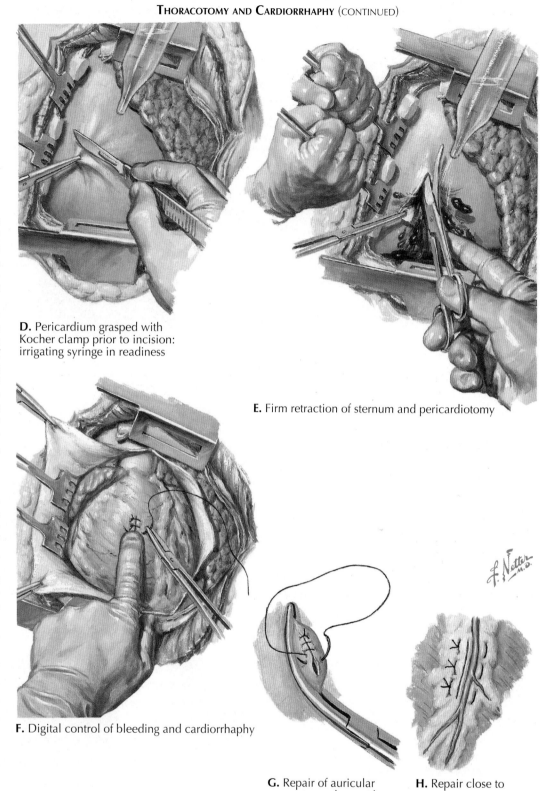

D. Pericardium grasped with Kocher clamp prior to incision: irrigating syringe in readiness

E. Firm retraction of sternum and pericardiotomy

F. Digital control of bleeding and cardiorrhaphy

G. Repair of auricular or great vessel wound

H. Repair close to coronary artery

Plate 6.127

Cardiovascular System: VOLUME 8

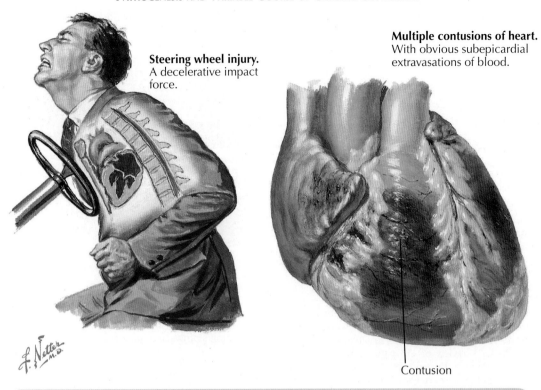

PATHOGENESIS AND VARIABLE COURSE OF CARDIAC CONTUSION

Steering wheel injury.
A decelerative impact force.

Multiple contusions of heart.
With obvious subepicardial extravasations of blood.

Contusion

NONPENETRATING HEART WOUNDS

Cardiac contusion and commotio cordis have been recorded in falls from heights or automobile steering wheel injury, or *deceleration injury*; as a result of *indirect force,* or force applied to the abdomen and extremities and transmitted to the heart through the intravascular hemodynamic route; and as incident to the passage of high-velocity bullets and missile fragments through the abdomen or chest or from blast explosions in the air or water. The latter generate pressure waves of energy damaging to the tissues. The major cause of contusion, however, is direct impact force applied violently to the precordium by a solid blunt object. Currently, the agent frequently involved is the motor vehicle crash (car accident), in which the chest wall is hurled against the *steering wheel* when the forward momentum of the vehicle is suddenly stopped. Uniquely, and more often than not, impact contusion occurs without fracture of the sternum and with an intact pericardium (Plate 6.127).

The contused heart may reveal either a discrete area or disseminated foci of hemorrhage in the heart wall. In most patients, hemorrhage apparently originates at the endocardium, ranging from subendocardial, mural, and valvular petechiae to frank hemorrhage that may remain subendocardial or may spread interstitially through and across the myocardium to the epicardium. It may be confined within the myocardium or may be complicated by lacerations of the endocardial or epicardial surfaces—lesions that are conducive to the formation of endocardial and mural thrombi and to acute hemopericardium. Contusion also includes myocardial damage, from an innocuous bruise to the disruption and separation of muscle fibers to necrosis. Vascular damage usually is restricted to the capillaries; the arterioles and coronary branches are rarely involved.

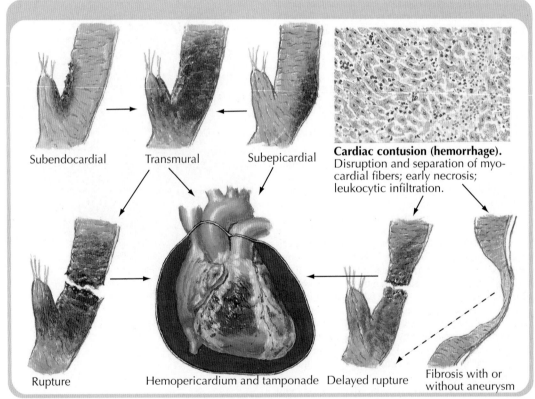

Subendocardial   Transmural   Subepicardial

Cardiac contusion (hemorrhage).
Disruption and separation of myocardial fibers; early necrosis; leukocytic infiltration.

Rupture   Hemopericardium and tamponade   Delayed rupture   Fibrosis with or without aneurysm

Although it has been suggested that contusive injury could initiate coronary thrombosis, it is generally agreed that this occurs almost exclusively to the diseased atheromatous vessel. Pericardial effusions occur, not necessarily acutely, in more than 50% of lesions uncomplicated by a pericardial tear. A fibrinous reaction at the contusion site may cause pain, a friction rub, and adhesion to the pericardium. A severe contusion projects a continuing degeneration and necrosis of damaged tissue, which may terminate in delayed rupture or a scarred (fibrotic) and weakened area that, under the intermittent intracardiac pressure, may give way to aneurysm formation.

The diagnosis of contusion has now achieved full acceptance as a clinical and legal entity, based on (1) an appropriate history, (2) clinical evidence, and (3) ECG findings and laboratory data. Pain may be immediate or may occur up to 24 hours or even days later. It is *retrosternal pain,* often simulating that of myocardial

Plate 6.128

Acquired Heart Disease

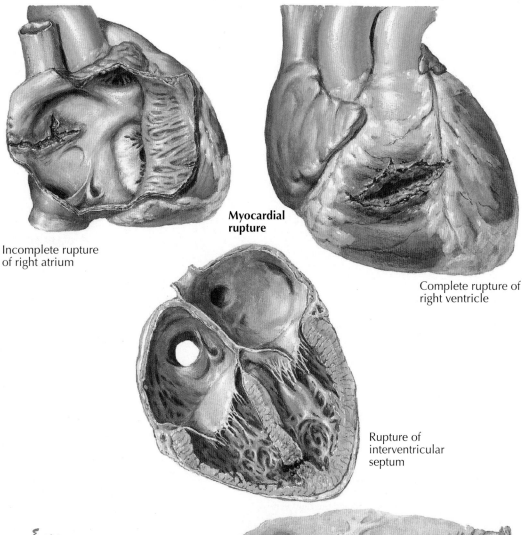

MYOCARDIAL RUPTURE AND VALVULAR INJURIES

Incomplete rupture
of right atrium

Myocardial
rupture

Complete rupture of
right ventricle

Rupture of
interventricular
septum

NONPENETRATING HEART WOUNDS (Continued)

ischemia or infarction. It may be refractory to nitroglycerin and responsive to oxygen and analgesia. Functional disturbances include tachycardia (usually paroxysmal) and rarely bradycardia. Supraventricular disturbances are evidenced by ectopic beats, atrial flutter, and atrial fibrillation. Pericardial tamponade is suspected when venous pressure increases and arterial pressure decreases.

All types of ECG alteration, including conduction disturbances, have been noted, mainly in the ventricular complex, ST segment, and T wave. The location of the lesion undoubtedly influences the type of arrhythmia and ECG alteration. Elevation of troponin T and CK enzymes suggest myocardial damage, especially if cardiac contusion is the only injury.

CARDIAC RUPTURE

With rare exceptions, cardiac or myocardial rupture involving any or all chambers causes immediate or early fatality. Interestingly, in the resilient juvenile chest, cardiac rupture has sometimes been the result of impact or compressive trauma without damage to the bony thorax and its soft tissues. In a study of 138 cases of rupture, Bright and Beck concluded that about 30 patients who lived longer than 1 hour might have been helped by surgery because their injuries were not so extensive as to preclude repair.

Interventricular Septal Rupture

An isolated interventricular septal defect is a rare lesion. When it arises from *septal rupture,* it may manifest immediately or early. It is more common, however, as a sequela to *septal myocardial contusion,* appearing late in the course after the trauma. Currently, steering wheel

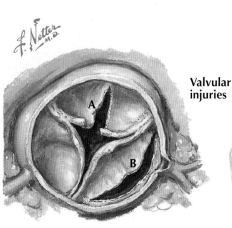

Valvular
injuries

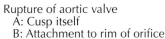

Rupture of aortic valve
A: Cusp itself
B: Attachment to rim of orifice

Rupture of chordae tendineae and/or papillary
muscle and, rarely, the valve cusps

impact is the chief etiologic agent. (Bright and Beck considered the end of diastole, with the ventricles full and the tricuspid and mitral valves closed, as the moment in the cardiac cycle most propitious for septal rupture or contusion, but this has never been proved.) Time is required for a contusion fistula to become clearly delineated, its size and anatomic pattern established, and its borders defined by scar tissue and viable myocardium. If trauma has seriously or extensively

involved the muscle surrounding the defect, progressive necrosis ultimately may produce a defect of a size incompatible with life. The defects observed at surgery have been irregular, sinuous, and even possessed of multiple orifices (Plate 6.128).

Diagnosis is made on (1) the patient history; (2) a holosystolic murmur, possibly related to tricuspid regurgitation because right ventricle is anterior and just underneath sternum, and thrill along lateral sternal border

Plate 6.129   Cardiovascular System: VOLUME 8

MECHANISM OF SUDDEN CARDIAC DEATH IN COMMOTIO CORDIS

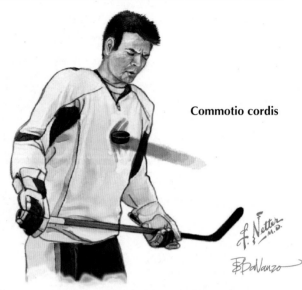

Commotio cordis

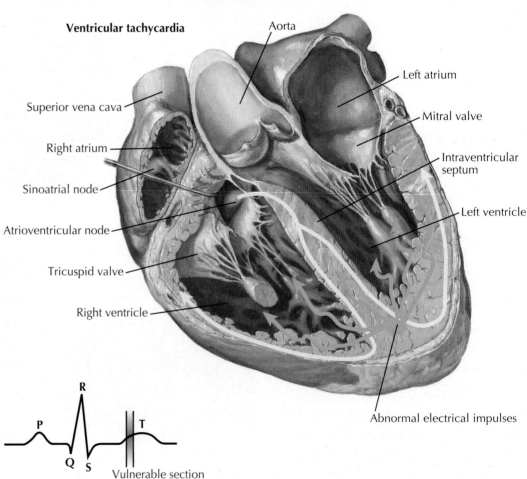

NONPENETRATING HEART WOUNDS (Continued)

at fourth or fifth interspace; and (3) a contusion defect (not always present) just above the apex. Cardiac ultrasound with Doppler imaging can evaluate the right ventricular size and function and presence or absence of tricuspid regurgitation as well as left ventricular function and presence or absence of aortic or mitral regurgitation. Doppler interrogation of the ventricular septum can detect a left-to-right shunt from a traumatic ventricular septal defect. Cardiac catheterization for the collection of hemodynamic data on pressures and oxygen saturation in the right ventricle, pulmonary artery, and superior vena cava is essential. The symptoms and course depend primarily on the volume of blood shunted into the right ventricle and the pulmonary circuit. Surgical repair is made using cardiopulmonary bypass.

Valvular Injuries

Endothelial tears, hemorrhage into the valve cusps, and most frequently rupture are the valvular injuries encountered at postmortem. Rupture results from impact force to the precordium, from indirect force, and from a specific indirect force associated with an intense or excessive physical effort mediated through the vascular route and affecting almost exclusively the aortic valve, particularly in hypertensive patients. Ruptures occur when the valves are subjected to the greatest internal pressure: at the end of systole for the aortic valves and at the beginning of ventricular systole for the mitral and tricuspid valves (see Plate 6.128).

Rupture of the aortic valve may involve the cusps themselves or the site of their attachment to the rim of the orifice. Rupture of the mitral or tricuspid valves usually implicates the chordae tendineae, papillary muscles, and rarely the cusps. The majority of ruptured valves found at autopsy have shown acute inflammation,

residual stigmata of bacterial endocarditis, valvulitis, or atherosclerotic changes. The valvular incompetence precipitated by rupture may not be sufficiently severe to induce an immediate or early fatality. With stabilization, the physical signs specific for the valvular lesion may be detected and further investigation carried out by cardiac catheterization and angiocardiography. Valve repair or replacement can then be performed as the procedure of choice.

COMMOTIO CORDIS AND SUDDEN CARDIAC DEATH

Commotio cordis is a blunt, nonpenetrating blow to the chest wall; Plate 6.129 illustrates the mechanism of sudden cardiac death (SCD) in commotio cordis. In athletes an object (e.g., puck, baseball) strikes the sternum at a time when the heart and conduction system are vulnerable to ventricular fibrillation, possibly the upward slope of the T wave.

Plate 6.130

Acquired Heart Disease

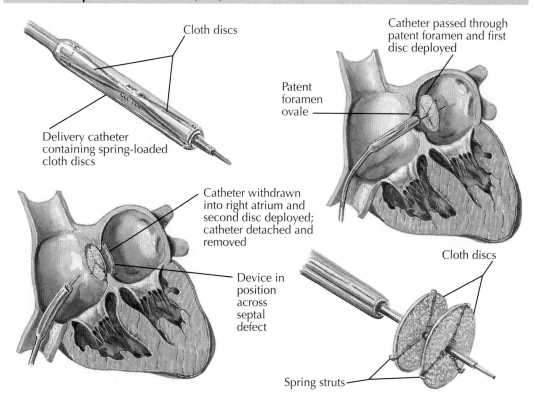

Closure of patent foramen ovale (PFO)

Cloth discs

Delivery catheter containing spring-loaded cloth discs

Catheter passed through patent foramen and first disc deployed

Patent foramen ovale

Catheter withdrawn into right atrium and second disc deployed; catheter detached and removed

Device in position across septal defect

Cloth discs

Spring struts

PERCUTANEOUS APPROACHES TO REDUCE CEREBRAL EMBOLI

LEFT ATRIAL APPENDAGE OCCLUSION

In 2013, atrial fibrillation was the most common arrhythmia responsible for hospital admission. In patients who remain in atrial fibrillation, a major concern is the risk of embolization to the central nervous system (CNS), principally from the left atrial appendage. To address this problem, anticoagulation with warfarin is the usual therapy. An international normalized ratio should be maintained between 2 and 3 to prevent cerebrovascular accident (stroke). Some patients have a contraindication to anticoagulation such as excessive bleeding, poor control of international normalized ratio, or stroke despite good control.

Recently, *percutaneous left atrial appendage transcatheter occlusion* devices have been used in these patients to prevent emboli from exiting the appendage (Plate 6.130, *bottom*). This device is delivered to the atrial appendage through a catheter passed transseptally from right atrium through patent foramen ovale or through an atrial septal puncture to left atrium and then into left atrial appendage. This is usually done under fluoroscopic and/or transesophageal guidance. All devices are variations of an expandable occlusive plug that prevents clots from embolizing from the appendage. Once released from the catheter and deployed, these devices eventually endothelialize over time, minimizing the ability of the appendage to form clots.

PATENT FORAMEN OVALE OCCLUSION

Another source of potential cerebral emboli is from the peripheral veins through a patent foramen ovale (PFO) or atrial septal defect (ASD). About 25% of healthy

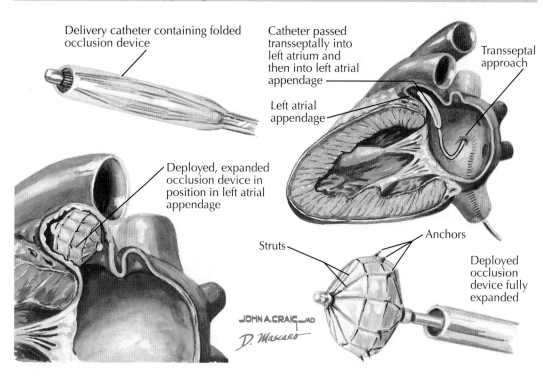

Percutaneous left atrial appendage transcatheter occlusion (PLAATO)

Delivery catheter containing folded occlusion device

Catheter passed transseptally into left atrium and then into left atrial appendage

Transseptal approach

Left atrial appendage

Deployed, expanded occlusion device in position in left atrial appendage

Struts

Anchors

Deployed occlusion device fully expanded

JOHN A. CRAIG—MD
D. Mascaro

people have PFO. Patients who present with cryptogenic stroke should have cardiac ultrasound procedures (bubble studies) to assess for atrial septal communication from right atrium to left atrium and ultrasound assessing the venous circulation of the pelvis and legs.

Percutaneous closure of the PFO or an ASD prevents clots from entering the systemic circulation and thus embolizing to the brain through a PFO. The procedure involves a delivery catheter containing spring-loaded

discs (Plate 6.130, *top*). The catheter is passed through the atrial septum and the first disc deployed. The catheter is then withdrawn into the right atrium, and the second disc is deployed and the catheter detached and removed. When the device is in position, the ASD is closed, preventing the entry of emboli from the venous circulation into the systemic circulation. Endothelialization of the device prevents clots from accumulating on the discs.

Plate 6.131

Cardiovascular System: VOLUME 8

CEREBROVASCULAR EMBOLI PROTECTION DEVICE

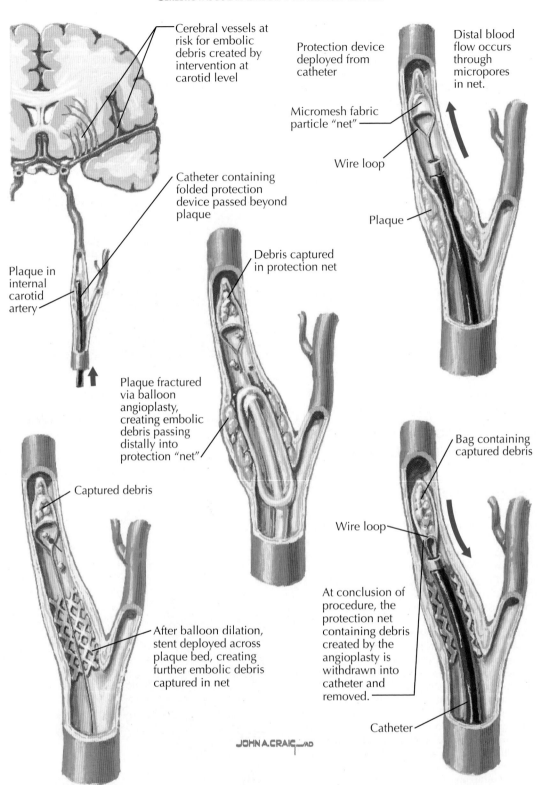

Cerebral vessels at risk for embolic debris created by intervention at carotid level

Plaque in internal carotid artery

Catheter containing folded protection device passed beyond plaque

Protection device deployed from catheter

Distal blood flow occurs through micropores in net.

Micromesh fabric particle "net"

Wire loop

Plaque

Debris captured in protection net

Plaque fractured via balloon angioplasty, creating embolic debris passing distally into protection "net"

Captured debris

After balloon dilation, stent deployed across plaque bed, creating further embolic debris captured in net

Bag containing captured debris

Wire loop

At conclusion of procedure, the protection net containing debris created by the angioplasty is withdrawn into catheter and removed.

Catheter

JOHN A. CRAIG—AD

PERIPHERAL ARTERY INTERVENTION

CAROTID STENOSES

Stroke is a dreaded event that may be the result of emboli from a carotid artery stenosis. The initial indication for using balloon dilation of a carotid stenosis was the patient at high risk for carotid endarterectomy because of comorbidities such as heart failure and severe chronic lung disease. This limited indication is now changed and includes patients at standard risk for carotid revascularization using catheter balloon dilation. In general, patients with symptomatic carotid stenoses or patients who are asymptomatic with high-grade carotid stenoses (≥80%) have indications for balloon dilation.

However, when interventional procedures are performed on a plaque in the internal carotid artery, cerebral vessels are at risk for embolic debris created by the intervention. Embolization of thromboatheromatous material to the distal circulation is always possible, and a small volume of this material can cause significant brain damage. To prevent this, catheters containing folded protection devices are passed beyond the plaque. The *protection device* is deployed from the catheter and consists of a micromesh fabric suspended by a wire loop (Plate 6.131). The device allows distal blood to

flow through the micropores in the net. The plaque is then fractured by balloon angioplasty. This creates embolic debris that flows toward the brain and is captured by the protection net. After balloon dilation of the plaque, a stent is deployed across the plaque bed, creating further embolic debris that is also captured in the net. At the conclusion of the procedure, the protection net containing debris created by the angioplasty is

withdrawn into the catheter and removed. Multiple devices are available to "catch" any debris before it embolizes to the brain.

LOWER EXTREMITY ARTERIAL DISEASE

Indications for *percutaneous transluminal angioplasty with stent* (PTAS) of lower extremity arterial disease

Plate 6.132

Acquired Heart Disease

INTERVENTIONAL APPROACHES TO PERIPHERAL ARTERIAL DISEASE

Lower extremity arterial disease (PTA or PTAS)

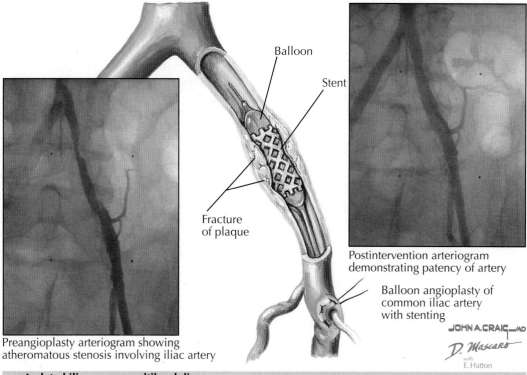

Balloon

Stent

Fracture
of plaque

Postintervention arteriogram
demonstrating patency of artery

Balloon angioplasty of
common iliac artery
with stenting

JOHN A. CRAIG—MD

D. Mascaro
with
E. Hatton

Preangioplasty arteriogram showing
atheromatous stenosis involving iliac artery

Isolated iliac versus multilevel disease

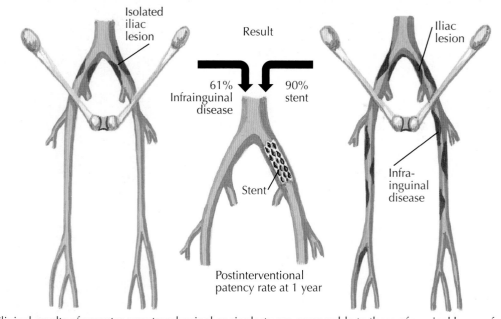

Isolated
iliac
lesion

Result

Iliac
lesion

61%
Infrainguinal
disease

90%
stent

Stent

Infra-
inguinal
disease

Postinterventional
patency rate at 1 year

PERIPHERAL ARTERY INTERVENTION (Continued)

include patients who still demonstrate progressive and limiting intermittent claudication that prevents them from doing activities even after medical therapy, including exercise programs. The decision whether to perform PTAS should be made jointly by a vascular surgeon and interventional radiologist or cardiologist. Rest pain and peripheral gangrene increase the urgency for revascularization, and these patients usually undergo surgery. Patients with localized occlusive arterial disease in the lower extremities caused primarily by atherosclerosis are candidates for PTAS. However, before performing the procedure, diagnostic studies must establish the location and extent of pathologic anatomy. Preangioplasty arteriograms can accurately illustrate atheromatous stenoses in the peripheral arterial circulation (Plate 6.132).

The procedure consists of dilating the diseased segment with a noncompliant balloon that fractures the plaque and allows deployment of a stent. Best results with PTAS are obtained when performed above the knee using iliac or femoropopliteal arteries, with iliac arteries most beneficial. The subset of patients with stenosis confined to iliac arteries benefits most from

Clinical results of percutaneous transluminal angioplasty are comparable to those of surgical bypass for above-knee (iliac or femoropopliteal) arterial disease that does not include multiple serial stenoses or long occlusions. The subset of patients with stenosis confined to iliac arteries benefits most from PTA or stenting.

PTA or stenting, with 90% patency rate at 1 year, whereas PTAS in the infrainguinal part of the femoral circulation has only 61% patency. After the procedure, angiography can demonstrate patency of the treated artery. Clinical results of PTA are comparable to surgical bypass for above-knee (iliac or femoropopliteal) arterial disease that does not include serial stenoses or long occlusions, which benefit most from surgery.

The concern for distal embolization is much less in the lower extremity than in the cerebral circulation when PTAS is performed. If a small, symptomatic embolus does occur, it probably does not require surgery. If large and causing ischemic symptoms in the leg, however, the embolus may require surgery. Other, rare complications include thrombosis at the dilation site and intimal dissection of the artery associated with occlusion.

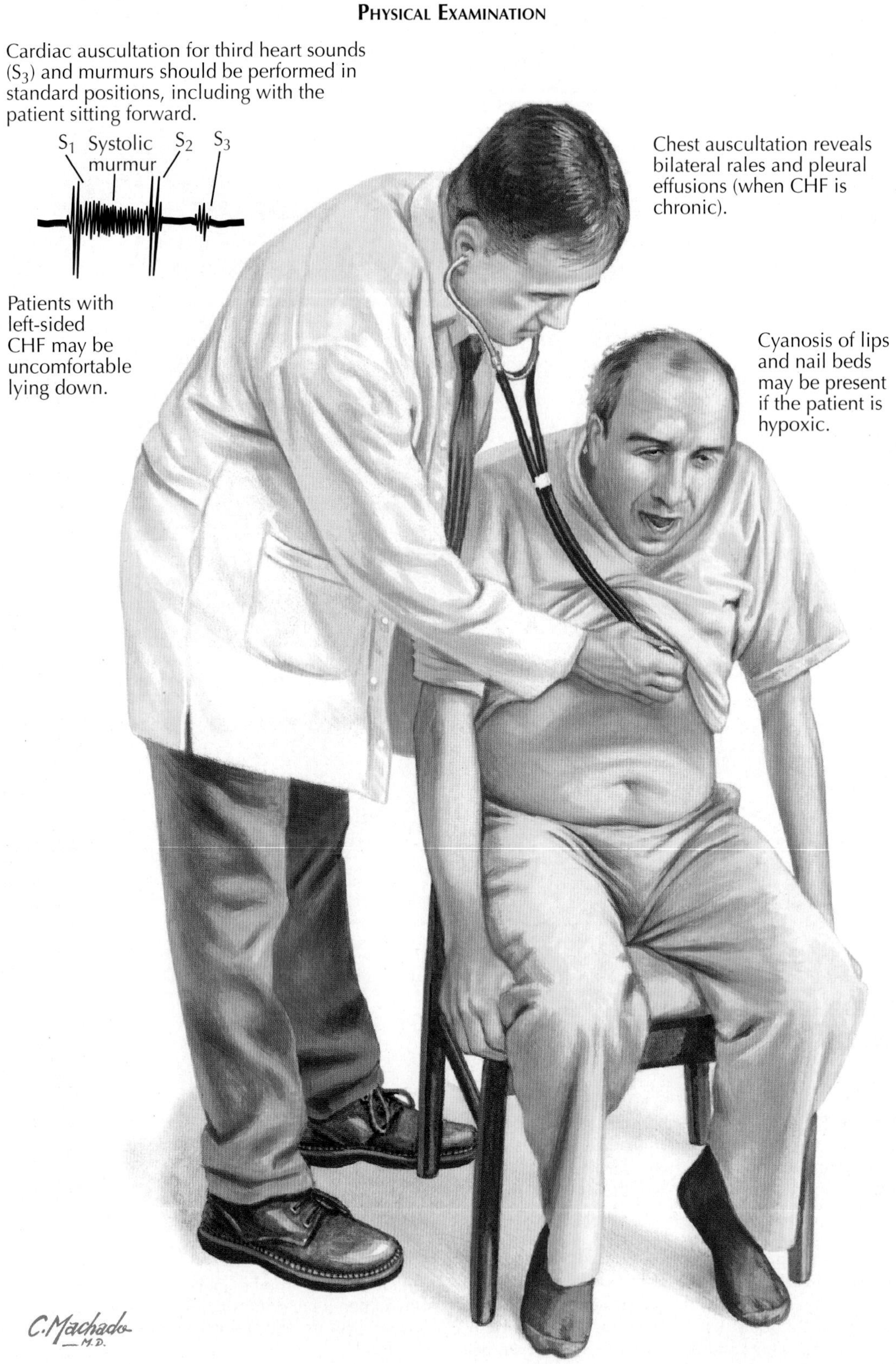

Plate 6.133

Cardiovascular System: VOLUME 8

Cardiac auscultation for third heart sounds (S₃) and murmurs should be performed in standard positions, including with the patient sitting forward.

S_1 Systolic S_2 S_3
murmur

Patients with left-sided CHF may be uncomfortable lying down.

Chest auscultation reveals bilateral rales and pleural effusions (when CHF is chronic).

Cyanosis of lips and nail beds may be present if the patient is hypoxic.

RIGHT-SIDED AND LEFT-SIDED HEART FAILURE AND SYSTEMIC CONGESTION

Physical examination of patients with left-sided congestive heart failure is performed with patient supine at a 45-degree angle and may reveal tachypnea and tachycardia with rapid and diminished peripheral pulses. Rhythm irregularity may also be present. In severe left ventricular decompensation, peripheral pulse may alternate between strong and weak beats at regular intervals (pulsus alternans). On precordial palpation, the apical impulse may be prominent and inferolaterally displaced. Auscultation of the heart, with clothes removed, may reveal systolic murmurs of mitral or tricuspid valve regurgitation or aortic stenosis, as well as an S_3 or S_4 gallop. Auscultation of the lungs may reveal crackles or decreased breath sounds at the bases, suggesting pleural effusions. Peripheral edema may be present but not necessarily in patients with heart failure (Plate 6.133).

RIGHT-SIDED HEART FAILURE AND CARDIOMYOPATHY

Systemic congestion is often caused by RV failure, which leads to an increase in diastolic pressure (RVEDP) and increased right atrial and systemic venous pressures. As a result, the visible veins, especially the jugular veins, become engorged and actively pulsate. The liver becomes enlarged and tender and, if significant tricuspid regurgitation is present, may be pulsatile to palpation. In severe or prolonged failure, ascites will develop (see Plate 6.134). Cyanosis and dependent edema can be severe. Inspection and palpation reveal these features, documented by chest radiograph (right-sided dilation), measurement of venous pressure (increased), cardiac ultrasound (large right atrium/ventricle, dilated IVC), and right-sided heart catheterization (increased RVEDP).

In the common patient presentation in which right-sided heart failure follows left-sided failure, the lungs will become less congested, dyspnea and orthopnea will decrease, the liver will become severely engorged, the systemic veins will be turgid, and peripheral (dependent) edema will appear.

A common result of right-sided heart failure is relative *tricuspid insufficiency*, caused by dilation of the tricuspid ring and stretching of the RV papillary muscles. This is revealed by large systolic pulsations of the jugular veins and the liver and by a right-sided pansystolic murmur. Right atrial distention may be followed by atrial fibrillation. as manifested by an irregular

rhythm detected by examining the peripheral pulse. Similar manifestations may be related to chronic obstruction of the jugular veins or tricuspid valve or to impaired RV filling, as with constrictive pericarditis and infiltrative cardiomyopathies (e.g., amyloid). Cardiac catheterization may show a restrictive right-sided filling pattern, with prominent x and y descents and absent respiratory variation of the right atrial waveform, as a sharp early filling wave of the right ventricle

followed by a plateau, due to severely impaired late mid and late diastolic filling. If the tricuspid valve is narrowed, a diastolic pressure gradient is observed between right atrium and right ventricle.

Dependent edema is a common result of right-sided heart failure. This is particularly obvious in the lower extremities and the sacrum. In an advanced stage the edema is massive and diffuse and associated with effusion of various sites, particularly in the right pleural

C. Machado
— M.D.

Plate 6.134

Acquired Heart Disease

RIGHT-SIDED AND LEFT-SIDED HEART FAILURE IN PATIENT WITH DILATED CARDIOMYOPATHY

Right-sided heart failure

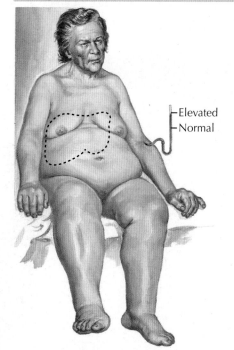

—Elevated
—Normal

Right-sided heart failure. Cyanosis, engorgement of jugular veins, enlargement of liver, ascites, dependent edema, elevated venous pressure.

RIGHT-SIDED AND LEFT-SIDED HEART FAILURE AND SYSTEMIC CONGESTION (Continued)

cavity and peritoneal cavity (ascites). Another frequent result is oliguria, probably related to high renal venous pressure with frequent episodes of nocturia.

Right ventricular failure manifests as a rise in RVEDP (normal increase, 0–5 mm Hg; abnormal, 8–20 mm Hg). RV failure frequently causes a relative tricuspid insufficiency, which can be recognized by systolic pulsations in the jugular veins and reflux of blood from the right ventricle to the right atrium, using cardiac ultrasound (Doppler) and other imaging (angiography, MRI).

LEFT-SIDED HEART FAILURE AND PULMONARY CONGESTION

Pulmonary congestion often is caused by left-sided heart failure, which leads to an increase in diastolic pressure (LVEDP) and increased left atrial and pulmonary venous pressures. As a result, the pulmonary veins and capillaries become engorged. Exertional and positional orthopnea and finally continuous dyspnea occur, and there may be paroxysmal nocturnal dyspnea (see Plate 6.134). These acute, occasional, or continuous disturbances can be readily ascertained by observing the patient in various positions (sitting vs lying supine).

The chest radiograph reveals a dilation of the left-sided heart chambers and an increased opacity of the pulmonary vasculature. Left-sided and right-sided heart catheterization shows an increase in LVEDP as well as increased left atrial, pulmonary wedge, and pulmonary arterial pressures. The RV pressure is elevated in systole because of increased pulmonary artery pressure but may remain normal in diastole. Importantly, all these manifestations of pulmonary venous congestion are paralleled by the less obvious decrease in cardiac output. The LV output decreases, also decreasing RV output. Although this decrease is partly compensated by peripheral vasoconstriction, so that no marked changes of blood pressure occur, the systemic circulation to organs tends to decrease, resulting in ischemic organs. The most common results are weakness and oliguria. If some peripheral arteries are narrowed because of segmental lesions, ischemia becomes particularly obvious in these areas (e.g., bowel, brain, kidney, heart, legs).

A common result of LV failure is mitral insufficiency, caused by dilation of the mitral ring and splaying of the LV papillary muscles. This is associated with a holosystolic murmur and with systolic expansion of the left

Left-sided heart failure and pulmonary congestion

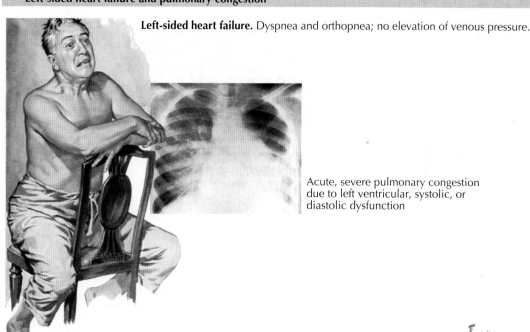

Left-sided heart failure. Dyspnea and orthopnea; no elevation of venous pressure.

Acute, severe pulmonary congestion due to left ventricular, systolic, or diastolic dysfunction

atrium on cardiac ultrasound, angiography, or MRI. Atrial fibrillation often occurs, exacerbating pulmonary congestion. Similar manifestations may occur in patients with chronic obstruction at the level of the pulmonary veins (e.g., mediastinal collagenosis, left atrial myxoma, cor triatriatum) and mitral valve (mitral stenosis) or in patients with pericardial or myocardial diseases that decrease or impair LV filling (e.g., constrictive pericarditis, infiltrative myocardial disease).

Cardiac ultrasound or left-sided and right-sided heart catheterization reveals the existence of a diastolic pressure gradient between left atrium and left ventricle and may also reveal atrial lesions obstructing flow across the mitral valve.

Left ventricular failure manifests as a rise in LVEDP (normal increase, 3–9 mm Hg; abnormal, 10–25 mm Hg) and a decrease in ejection fraction, as seen on cardiac ultrasound or left ventriculography.

Plate 6.135

Cardiovascular System: VOLUME 8

PULMONARY CONGESTION OR EDEMA OF CARDIAC ORIGIN

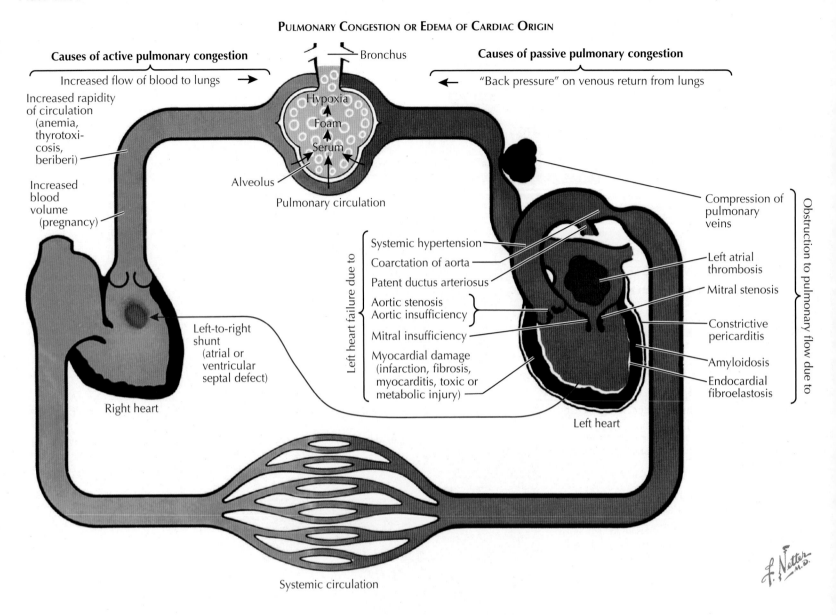

Causes of active pulmonary congestion

Increased flow of blood to lungs →

Increased rapidity of circulation (anemia, thyrotoxicosis, beriberi)

Increased blood volume (pregnancy)

Bronchus

Hypoxia

Foam

Serum

Alveolus

Pulmonary circulation

Causes of passive pulmonary congestion

← "Back pressure" on venous return from lungs

Compression of pulmonary veins

Left atrial thrombosis

Mitral stenosis

Constrictive pericarditis

Amyloidosis

Endocardial fibroelastosis

Obstruction to pulmonary flow due to

Left heart failure due to:
- Systemic hypertension
- Coarctation of aorta
- Patent ductus arteriosus
- Aortic stenosis / Aortic insufficiency
- Mitral insufficiency
- Myocardial damage (infarction, fibrosis, myocarditis, toxic or metabolic injury)

Left-to-right shunt (atrial or ventricular septal defect)

Right heart

Left heart

Systemic circulation

PULMONARY CONGESTION OR EDEMA OF CARDIAC AND OTHER ORIGINS

PULMONARY CONGESTION

Pulmonary congestion can be defined as an increase in the blood present in the vessels of the lungs. This can result from increased pulmonary flow (e.g., ASD), anemia, thyrotoxicosis, beriberi, heart disease, or any condition associated with increased rapidity of the circulation or with increased blood volume (e.g., pregnancy), with or without an arteriocapillary increase of pressure. Congestion also results from increased pulmonary venous capillary pressure caused by left-sided conditions, including heart failure (passive congestion).

Passive pulmonary congestion is found in any condition in which there is obstruction to flow at any point from the capillary bed of the lungs to the aortic valve and beyond. Elevation of the LV diastolic pressure caused by LV hypertrophy, ischemia, or hypertrophic cardiomyopathy will result in increased left atrial pressure and pulmonary capillary wedge pressure. One typical cause of passive congestion is chronic LV failure caused by extremely severe LV systolic overload (systemic hypertension, coarctation of aorta, aortic stenosis), extremely severe LV volume overload (mitral insufficiency, patent ductus arteriosus, aortic insufficiency), myocardial damage (myocarditis, fibrosis, infarction, toxic effects on myocardium, metabolic alterations), and formation of an LV aneurysm, usually secondary to MI because this lesion interferes with normal LV contraction (Plate 6.135).

Another typical cause of passive congestion is impaired ventricular diastolic filling by constrictive pericarditis or infiltrative myocardial disease (e.g., amyloidosis); mitral stenosis, left atrial thrombosis, left atrial myxoma, or endocardial fibroelastosis; compression of pulmonary veins by tumor or mediastinal collagenosis; or impaired flow caused by pulmonary vein stenosis. Pulmonary vein radiofrequency ablation for atrial fibrillation has resulted in pulmonary venous stenosis.

PULMONARY EDEMA

Pulmonary edema is the infiltration of serum in the thin, interalveolar septa, with immediate transudation into the alveoli. This is followed by churning of the fluid with air and formation of bubbling foam, which may be eliminated through the air passages but also impairs respiration, resulting in hypoxia (see Plate 6.136). Pulmonary edema is found in association with many disease states, as follows:

- Of cardiovascular diseases, including all possible causes of active and passive pulmonary congestion as well as shock, the most common are mitral valve disease, aortic stenosis or insufficiency, coarctation of aorta, systemic hypertension, acute myocarditis, thyrotoxic heart disease, and MI.
- Among diseases of the CNS, the most common causes are stroke, including cerebral hemorrhage,

Plate 6.136

Acquired Heart Disease

CAUSES AND PATHOGENESIS OF PULMONARY EDEMA

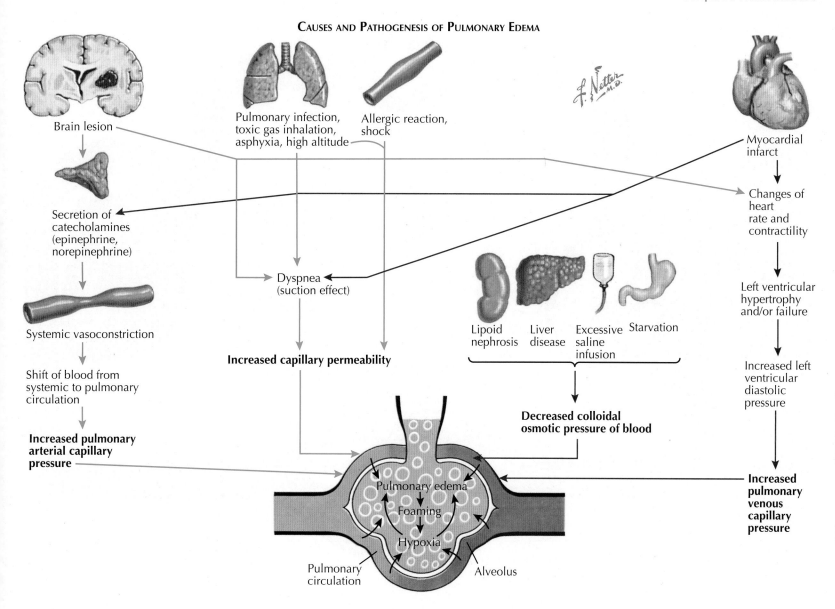

Brain lesion

Pulmonary infection, toxic gas inhalation, asphyxia, high altitude

Allergic reaction, shock

Myocardial infarct

Secretion of catecholamines (epinephrine, norepinephrine)

Changes of heart rate and contractility

Dyspnea (suction effect)

Systemic vasoconstriction

Lipoid nephrosis

Liver disease

Excessive saline infusion

Starvation

Left ventricular hypertrophy and/or failure

Shift of blood from systemic to pulmonary circulation

Increased capillary permeability

Increased left ventricular diastolic pressure

Increased pulmonary arterial capillary pressure

Decreased colloidal osmotic pressure of blood

Pulmonary edema

Foaming

Hypoxia

Pulmonary circulation

Alveolus

Increased pulmonary venous capillary pressure

PULMONARY CONGESTION OR EDEMA OF CARDIAC AND OTHER ORIGINS (Continued)

cerebral thrombosis, subarachnoid hemorrhage, and trauma to the skull. Poliomyelitis and tetanus may also lead to pulmonary edema but now are rare causes.

- Diseases of the lungs, including pulmonary infections, pulmonary embolism, toxic gas inhalation, and asphyxia, may cause pulmonary edema. Drowning, in fresh or salt water, is also associated with pulmonary edema. A special condition is high-altitude pulmonary edema.
- Several toxic or allergic states may be factors, especially associated with laryngeal edema.
- Pulmonary edema may follow excessive infusions, particularly in surgical or obstetric patients and those with structural heart disease.

The following three elements are especially important in the pathogenesis of pulmonary edema:

1. High pressure in the pulmonary capillaries occurs mostly by passive congestion. Whatever the etiology, the rapid shift of a large volume of blood from the periphery to the lungs may be the result of systemic vasoconstriction, spontaneous or drug induced, or may be caused by sympathetic stimuli usually increased by sympathomimetic amines (epinephrine, norepinephrine). Typical examples are found in sudden LV overload (paroxysmal hypertension) and when a sudden increase of venous return aggravates the effect of mitral valve obstruction or chronic LV failure. Sympathetic stimuli cause LV stiffness and elevate LV diastolic pressure.

2. In addition to the increase related to capillary dilation, conditions such as shock, allergic reaction, inhalation of toxic gases, respiratory burns, asphyxia, and hypoxia are possible causes of increased capillary *permeability*. Certain substances

(still unidentified) may contribute to the more common types of edema by increasing permeability, most likely histamine.

3. A decreased osmotic pressure of the blood occurs after excessive fluid infusions and in nephrotic syndrome, starvation, or liver diseases. Pulmonary edema caused by decreased osmotic pressure is either part of diffuse anasarca or related to mechanical factors acting on the lungs.

Most elements of pulmonary edema are interrelated: Chemical and endocrine products may cause systemic arterial or pulmonary venous constriction and also may induce changes in lung permeability. Blood pressure changes may cause a reflex release of hormones or chemicals. Neurogenic stimuli modify the caliber of the systemic vessels, cause the release of catecholamines, and influence heart contractility.

Even though pulmonary congestion may be followed by acute pulmonary edema, the two conditions, although related, should not be confused.

Plate 6.137

Cardiovascular System: VOLUME 8

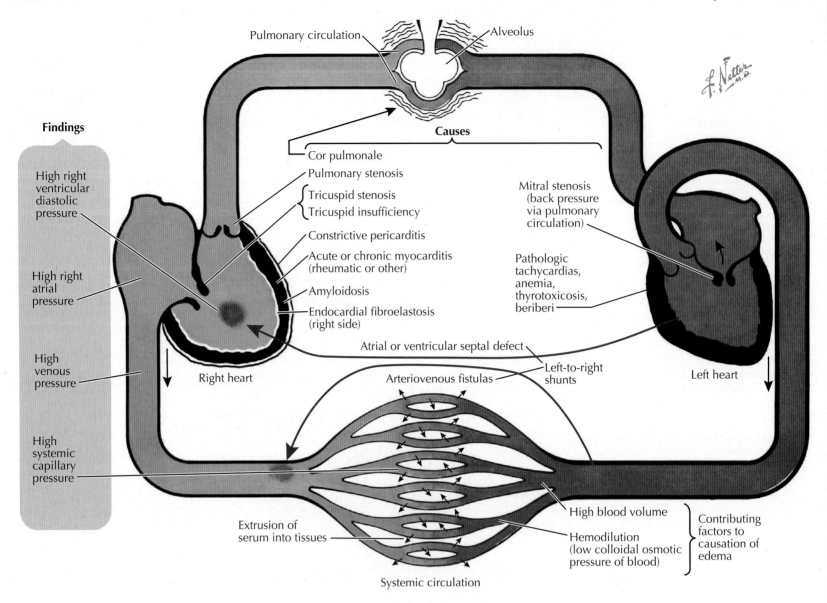

Pulmonary circulation — Alveolus

Findings

High right ventricular diastolic pressure

High right atrial pressure

High venous pressure

High systemic capillary pressure

Causes

Cor pulmonale

Pulmonary stenosis

Tricuspid stenosis

Tricuspid insufficiency

Constrictive pericarditis

Acute or chronic myocarditis (rheumatic or other)

Amyloidosis

Endocardial fibroelastosis (right side)

Mitral stenosis (back pressure via pulmonary circulation)

Pathologic tachycardias, anemia, thyrotoxicosis, beriberi

Atrial or ventricular septal defect

Left-to-right shunts

Arteriovenous fistulas

Right heart

Left heart

Extrusion of serum into tissues

High blood volume

Hemodilution (low colloidal osmotic pressure of blood)

Contributing factors to causation of edema

Systemic circulation

Cardiac Origins of Peripheral or Systemic Congestion or Edema

Peripheral congestion or edema is caused by an increase of systemic venous and capillary pressures. In addition to a local increase (thrombophlebitis, varicose veins, or compression of the IVC by a pregnant uterus or an abdominal mass), the most common cause of symmetric diffuse edema is found in the mediastinal organs, primarily the heart (Plate 6.137).

RIGHT VENTRICULAR FAILURE

Absolute right ventricular failure is found in acute or chronic myocarditis (e.g., acute rheumatic fever), which causes inflammation of the RV muscle, altering contractility. *Relative* RV failure occurs in patients with cardiac issues having severe RV overloading caused by pulmonary or left-sided valve lesions, left-to-right shunts, or RV outflow obstruction. *Overloading* caused by increased cardiac dynamics occurs in pathologic

tachycardias, anemia, thyrotoxicosis, and beriberi heart. The heart beats faster, and cardiac output increases. Relative failure may follow. Over time, patients with persistent tachycardia of any etiology can develop a *tachycardia-induced cardiomyopathy*. Diastolic or volume overloading occurs in congenital or acquired shunts such as atrial or ventricular septal defects and arteriovenous fistula. The volume overload of the right side of the heart may be followed by right-sided failure and systemic congestion. Systolic or pressure overloading occurs in patients with large pulmonary embolism (which results in acute cor pulmonale), chronic cor pulmonale, mitral stenosis, and pulmonary stenosis. The increase in work of the right ventricle may result in RV failure.

Mechanical impairment of RV diastole is seen in constrictive pericarditis and infiltrative myocardial disease such as amyloid heart disease or endocardial fibroelastosis of the right side of the heart. Mechanical obstruction occurs in tricuspid stenosis of any etiology, including congenital tricuspid atresia. When tricuspid insufficiency occurs, especially in patients with pulmonary hypertension, the right ventricle and right atrium distend because of volume overloading.

Right-sided heart failure is further complicated by an increase in blood volume through a pituitary–corticoadrenal–renal mechanism and hemodilution caused by water retention or a hepatic disturbance. The chronically congested liver and kidney frequently contribute hypoproteinemia to the picture of failure, and nephrotic syndrome or cirrhosis may decrease colloidal osmotic pressure to such a degree that diffuse edema occurs, related to these effects of right-sided heart failure. Peripheral edema from cardiac causes is associated with elevated venous pressure; other causes may not be associated with elevated venous pressure.

The usual RV failure can be corrected by stimulating the myocardium or removing the cause. A decrease in the volume overload may help temporarily. Relative RV failure is best corrected by removing the cause; cardiac stimulants have only secondary or collateral importance. Any obstruction to flow causing congestion does not usually respond to drug therapy, although drugs that decrease blood volume—loop diuretics combined with metolazone, a potent hydrochlorothiazide-like diuretic—may greatly reduce peripheral edema. In some patients, ultrafiltration may be required. For any obstruction to flow, however, corrective surgery is the treatment of choice.

Plate 6.138

Acquired Heart Disease

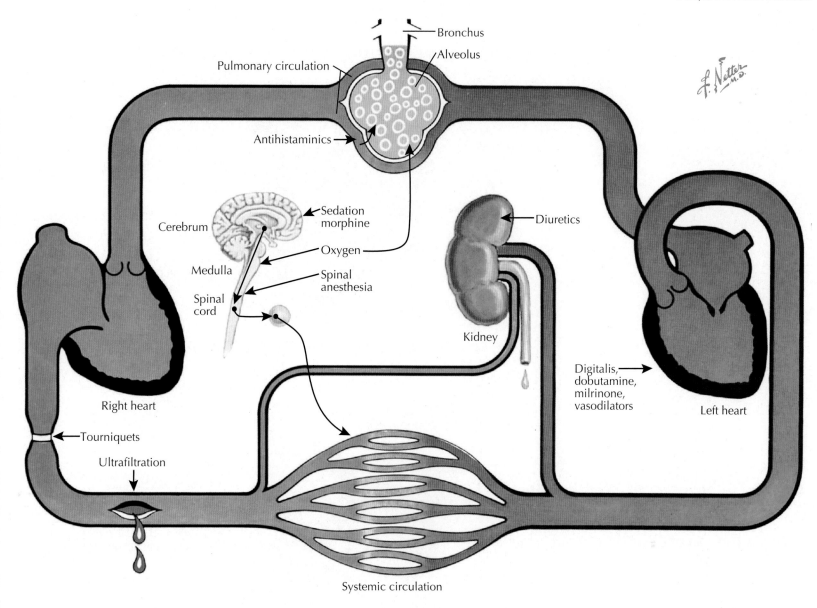

Bronchus
Alveolus
Pulmonary circulation
Antihistaminics
Cerebrum
Sedation morphine
Oxygen
Medulla
Spinal anesthesia
Spinal cord
Kidney
Diuretics
Right heart
Digitalis, dobutamine, milrinone, vasodilators
Left heart
Tourniquets
Ultrafiltration
Systemic circulation

THERAPY FOR PULMONARY EDEMA AND PAROXYSMAL DYSPNEA

REDUCTION OF ACUTE PULMONARY CONGESTION

Pulmonary congestion can be reduced in various ways. The IV infusion of rapid-acting loop diuretics (e.g., furosemide) reduces the blood volume. IV infusion of dobutamine or milrinone may decrease the level of LV diastolic pressure as a result of the stimulation of LV contraction and vasodilation of the systemic arterial system. Patients with mitral stenosis have moderate improvement with drugs to slow the heart (e.g., digitalis) and prolong diastole, particularly patients in atrial fibrillation, although correction of the mechanical defect is the treatment of choice (Plate 6.138).

The application of tourniquets will decrease venous return. Before IV diuretics and other vasodilators were available, this was a treatment of choice, but the tourniquet technique is no longer used. The positive effect of endotracheal intubation and positive-pressure ventilation is partly related to a similar mechanism; the IV injection of diuretics obtains the same result by decreasing venous return to the lungs and heart and decreasing central blood volume. Nitroprusside, nitrates, ACE inhibitors, and ARBs are also used to decrease venous return. By causing peripheral vasodilation, blood can be shifted from the lungs to the periphery using vasodilator therapy. *Hypoxia*, an important element in pulmonary edema, can be treated with oxygen administration and, in certain cases, intermittent positive-pressure respiration (or breathing). Reduction of venous return or systemic vasodilation may be dangerous in patients with mitral stenosis and shock; even though the pulmonary edema decreases, these patients may develop significant hypotension. Therefore the methods previously cited should be used with an understanding that treatment may have detrimental effects in some patients.

Mechanical obstruction to blood flow across a cardiac valve is a common cause of pulmonary edema. Definitive therapy can be obtained only by correction of the mechanical defect.

Plate 6.139

Cardiovascular System: VOLUME 8

BENEFIT OF BIVENTRICULAR PACING

Delayed ventricular activation

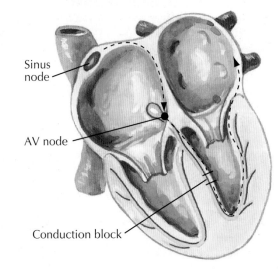

Sinus node

AV node

Conduction block

- Delayed lateral wall contraction

- Disorganized ventricular contraction

- Decreased pumping efficiency

- Increased mitral regurgitation

JOHN A. CRAIG—MD
D. Mascaro

Ventricular resynchronization

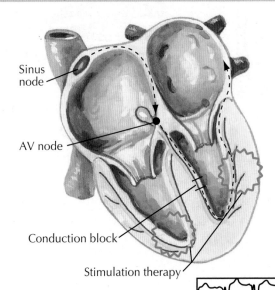

Sinus node

AV node

Conduction block

Stimulation therapy

- Organized ventricular activation sequence

- Coordinated septal and free-wall contraction

- Improved pumping efficiency

- Less mitral regurgitation

BIVENTRICULAR PACING AND INTRACARDIAC DEFIBRILLATOR

BIVENTRICULAR PACING FOR HEART FAILURE

Patients with left ventricular failure often have asynchrony of the left ventricle that results in delayed lateral-wall electrical activation and mechanical contraction of the lateral LV wall, disorganized LV contraction, decreased efficiency of the LV pumping chamber, and often mitral regurgitation. ECG reveals a conduction block manifested as left bundle branch block. When this asynchrony is related to impaired conduction, the septum may contract normally but the LV free wall may not. In general, the wider the QRS complex in left bundle branch block, the better the results of biventricular (BiV) pacing. The purpose of BiV pacing is to synchronize contraction of the septum and the LV free wall (Plate 6.139).

Thus the BiV pacing device, when working properly, is responsible for *cardiac resynchronization therapy*. Cardiac resynchronization therapy organizes the ventricular activation sequence by coordinating septal free wall contraction, which improves pumping efficiency of the left ventricle, diminishes mitral regurgitation and increases cardiac output, and facilitates management of patients in severe cardiac failure. For this device to work properly, the septum and the lateral LV

In patients with conduction block (e.g., left bundle branch block), there is delayed lateral wall electrical activation and mechanical contraction leading to decreased pumping efficiency. By simultaneously pacing the septal and lateral walls of the left ventricle with right ventricular and left ventricular leads (via the coronary sinus), the ventricular walls are "resynchronized," thereby improving pumping efficiency.

wall must be viable. Thus failure to improve ventricular function can occur in patients with lateral wall or septal MIs.

The generator for endocardial pacing systems is inserted into a pocket commonly made below the midclavicle. The endocardial lead system of an AV dual-chamber pacemaker is usually introduced through the subclavian vein, which becomes the basic pacing unit. An additional lead system is added to pace the LV free wall. The new catheter lead is introduced into the coronary sinus and

then advanced to a marginal vein so that it paces the epicardial surface of the LV free wall. Thus the septum is paced by the intraventricular route from the right ventricle, and the LV lateral wall is paced epicardially.

INTRACARDIAC DEFIBRILLATOR IN PATIENTS WITH HEART FAILURE

Patients in heart failure who are to receive a biventricular pacing device also often receive a BiV intracardiac

Plate 6.140

Acquired Heart Disease

BIVENTRICULAR PACING AND IMPLANTABLE CARDIAC DEFIBRILLATOR

Cardiac resynchronization (biventricular) pacing

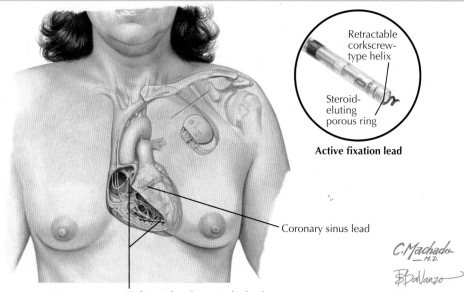

Retractable corkscrew-type helix

Steroid-eluting porous ring

Active fixation lead

Coronary sinus lead

Right atrial and ventricular leads

The leads connecting the pulse generator to the endocardium can be different types: unipolar or bipolar and of active fixation or passive fixation. The unipolar system has a single electrode (cathode, negative pole) in contact with the endocardium, and the anode is the pulse generator itself. The bipolar system lead has both a cathode and an anode at the tip of the same lead. Passive fixation leads have tines, barbs that anchor the lead to the endocardial trabecular muscle of the chamber in which it is implanted. Active fixation leads have a corkscrew-type device or helix that is placed into the myocardium. Both types irritate the myocardium, causing inflammatory reaction and cellular growth around the lead. To minimize the inflammatory reaction, most leads have steroid-eluting tips. The coronary sinus lead allows for "resynchronization" of disorganized ventricular contraction in selected patients with impaired cardiac function and conduction block.

Implantable Cardiac Defibrillator (Dual-Chamber Leads)

In all aspects, the surgical procedure for ICD implantation is very similar to that of cardiac pacemaker implantation. The venous access and the "pocket" for the pulse generator in the subcutaneous region above the prepectoralis fascia or in the submuscular region below the midclavicle are the same as those used for pacemaker implants.

Due to the number of functions the ICD can perform (cardioverter, defibrillator, and pacemaker), the ICD is usually slightly larger than a pacemaker. The surface of the ICD functions as one of the electrodes of the defibrillation system.

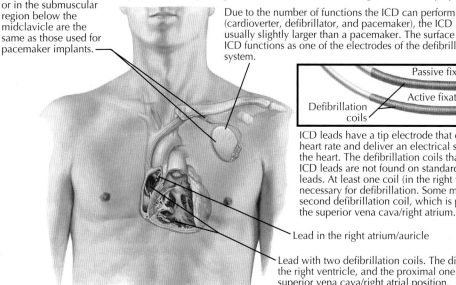

Passive fixation lead

Active fixation lead

Defibrillation coils

ICD leads have a tip electrode that can sense the heart rate and deliver an electrical stimulus to pace the heart. The defibrillation coils that are part of ICD leads are not found on standard pacemaker leads. At least one coil (in the right ventricle) is necessary for defibrillation. Some models have a second defibrillation coil, which is positioned in the superior vena cava/right atrium.

Lead in the right atrium/auricle

Lead with two defibrillation coils. The distal coil is in the right ventricle, and the proximal one is in the superior vena cava/right atrial position.

BIVENTRICULAR PACING AND INTRACARDIAC DEFIBRILLATOR (Continued)

defibrillator, or implantable cardioverter-defibrillator (ICD), because most have poor LV function (EF <35%) and are at high risk for sudden cardiac death. The ICD has become the dominant therapy for the treatment of these patients. Randomized trials have shown that ICDs reduce mortality from sudden cardiac death in those patients resuscitated from a cardiac arrest caused by ventricular tachycardia (VT). Antiarrhythmic drugs (e.g., amiodarone, sotalol) are used as adjunctive therapy to reduce frequent ICD shocks in these patients.

The ICD is similar to a typical pacemaker, but the generator is slightly larger than the usual pacemaker generator. In all aspects, the implantation procedure is similar to that of standard pacemaker implantation. The venous access and pocket for the device are the same as for a dual-chamber pacemaker: the subcutaneous region below the midclavicle. Because of the numerous functions of an implantable cardiac defibrillator (e.g., cardioverter, defibrillator, and pacemaker), the device is slightly larger than a standard pacemaker. All ICD leads have tip electrodes than can sense the heart rate and deliver an electrical stimulus to pace the heart (Plate 6.140).

Various models of defibrillators are available. In general, when a serious arrhythmia (e.g., VT) is detected, the ICD can be programmed to "burst pace" at a rate higher than the VT. The burst pacing is then abruptly terminated, and often the VT is converted to sinus rhythm. If the device fails to convert the arrhythmia, the energy required for defibrillation will ramp up, and the patient will be shocked. All ICDs have the built-in ability to interpret the device for rhythm disturbances, to determine which arrhythmia was cardioverted or shocked. Most often the device is programmed to detect a heart rate, above which the device will activate with burst pacing or shocks. Until recently, pacemakers and ICDs were not magnetic resonance compatible, but most manufacturers now have MR-compatible ICDs.

Plate 6.141

Cardiovascular System: VOLUME 8

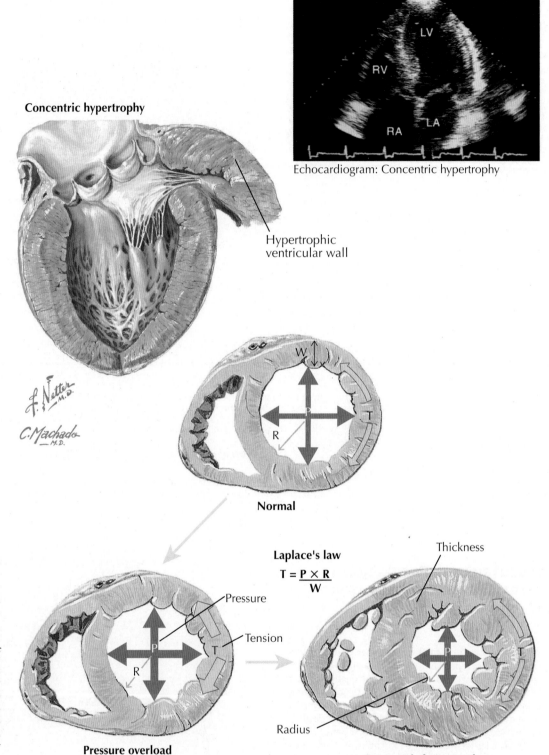

Concentric hypertrophy

Echocardiogram: Concentric hypertrophy

Hypertrophic
ventricular wall

Normal

Laplace's law

$$T = \frac{P \times R}{W}$$

Thickness

Pressure

Tension

Radius

Pressure overload

Concentric hypertrophy

Elevated pressure (P) increases wall thickness (W) relative to radius (R); wall tension (T) remains normal.

DIASTOLIC HEART FAILURE

Diastolic heart failure (heart failure symptoms with "preserved ventricular function") has become a common problem, especially in elderly females with hypertension. Patients usually have normal LV volume and normal or near-normal systolic function. Often the patient exhibits LV hypertrophy on ECG and ultrasound. Ischemic heart disease can also result in diastolic dysfunction because of the decreased relaxation of the stiff left ventricle due to myocardial ischemia. Patients with hypertrophic and restrictive cardiomyopathies as well as patients with constrictive pericarditis have impaired ventricular relaxation, high LVEDP, and high left atrial pressure, which may result in pulmonary congestion despite a normal, hypernormal, or near-normal ejection fraction. The impediment to diastolic filling probably results from fibrosis, scarring, or infiltration of the ventricle. At autopsy, typical findings include hypertrophy of LV wall that is disproportionate to the LV cavity. During life, cardiac ultrasound reveals signs of concentric LV hypertrophy (Plate 6.141).

Approximately 50% of patients with clinical heart failure (HF) have a preserved LV ejection fraction (PEF), and thus HF-PEF ("hefpef") is now used instead of "diastolic dysfunction." This condition is not benign. Patients with repeated admissions for HF, regardless of their EF, are a high-risk group for readmission and should be a population targeted in designing future trials of HF-PEF. The relationship of heart rate to morbidity and mortality is well known in coronary artery disease and in HF with low EF. The relationship

between heart rate and poor outcome is also present in patients with HF-PEF.

Current management strategies for patients with pulmonary congestion related to hypertension and HF-PEF should consist of diligent observation of the patients by frequent office visits, home health professional visits, or telemedicine protocols in which patients weigh themselves daily and control hypertension, diabetes, salt intake, heart rate, and state of hydration. It is important to treat comorbid conditions.

Current guidelines suggest using diuretics for symptom relief from congestion. Sodium glucose cotransporter 2 (SGLT2) inhibitors may help diuresis and provide benefits in energy, metabolism, vascular function, and blood pressure that lead to a mortality benefit in HF-PEF. The use of angiotensin receptors, neprilysin inhibition, or angiotensin 2 receptor blockers and mineralocorticoid receptor antagonists can be used to provide symptomatic relief and reduce heart failure hospitalizations.

Plate 6.142

Acquired Heart Disease

TECHNIQUE OF ORTHOTOPIC BIATRIAL CARDIAC TRANSPLANTATION

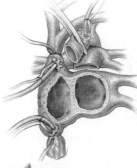

1. The recipient is placed on cardiopulmonary bypass support with venous drainage cannulas placed into the superior and inferior venae cavae. The cardiopulmonary bypass circuit returns oxygenated blood with controlled perfusion into the ascending aorta through a cannula placed distal to the aortic cross-clamp. Cardiopulmonary bypass provides systemic perfusion allowing excision of the recipient heart, retaining the posterior cuff of the right and left atria as well as the ascending aorta and main pulmonary artery.

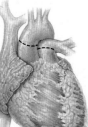

2. Dashed markings represent excision lines for removal of the donor heart.

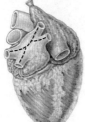

3. The donor heart is excised across the pulmonary veins, followed by preparation for transplantation by opening the posterior wall of the left atrium.

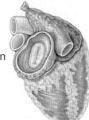

4. View of the donor mitral valve through the surgically opened left atrial posterior wall.

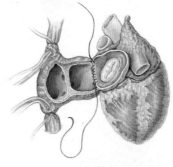

5. Initiation of cardiac implantation with anastomosis of left atrium of recipient to donor using a continuous mono-filament suture line.

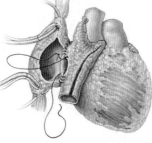

6. The left atrial anastomosis is completed, and the donor right atrium is opened from the inferior vena cava extending to the right atrial appendage.

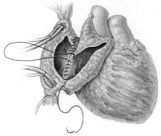

7. The right atrial cuff of the donor is anastomosed to the recipient right atrial cuff directly over the left atrial suture line reinforcing the edge of the interatrial septum.

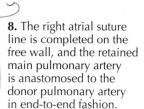

8. The right atrial suture line is completed on the free wall, and the retained main pulmonary artery is anastomosed to the donor pulmonary artery in end-to-end fashion.

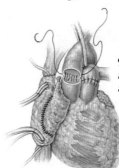

9. The fourth and final anastomosis aligns the ascending aorta of donor and recipient in end-to-end fashion.

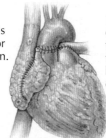

10. Completed biatrial orthotopic cardiac transplant with separation from cardiopulmonary bypass and removal of cannulas.

S. Moon, M.S.

HEART TRANSPLANTATION

Transplantation of the heart has been surgically feasible since 1960, when the essence of the surgical method was propounded. The important restrictions of the immune reaction and recipient selection remain, even though clinical experience was begun with the work of Barnard in South Africa and Kantrowitz in New York. Several early problems (e.g., surgical method) required solution before any animal could survive orthotopic homotransplantation of the heart. Another problem was protection of the donor heart against irreversible damage from its removal to reestablishment of coronary circulation. Also, the heart transplantation physiologic process involved assessment of the effect of total cardiac denervation. Drugs such as digoxin had no effect on the AV node, atropine had no chronotropic effect, nifedipine had no reflex tachycardia, and verapamil and β-blockers were still useful to treat supraventricular tachycardia.

The midline sternotomy provides optimal exposure. Protection of the heart transplant is achieved by cooling with physiologic saline solution at 2°C to 4°C.

Plate 6.142 illustrates the surgical method of biatrial transplantation, which depends on retention in the host of parts of both atria and the interatrial septum to which the transplant is sutured. Accordingly, after division of the aorta and pulmonary trunk immediately above their respective semilunar valves, the atria are incised to leave intact parts of the right and left atrial walls and the atrial septum of the recipient. Because of the disproportion between the normal donor heart and the larger recipient organ, the donor heart is removed by individual division of each of the six inflow veins. Conceivably, in infants and children, the donor heart may be of the same size as that of the recipient; if so, individual sectioning of donor inflow vessels would not be necessary. Plate 6.143 illustrates the technique of bicaval transplantation.

Resuscitation of the donor heart is mandatory before proceeding with thoracotomy in the recipient. The explanted donor heart is infused with cardioplegia and cooled. Ventricular fibrillation of the donor heart routinely develops, and no attempt is made to convert this arrhythmia to an effective contraction.

Plate 6.143

Cardiovascular System: VOLUME 8

TECHNIQUE OF BICAVAL CARDIAC TRANSPLANTATION

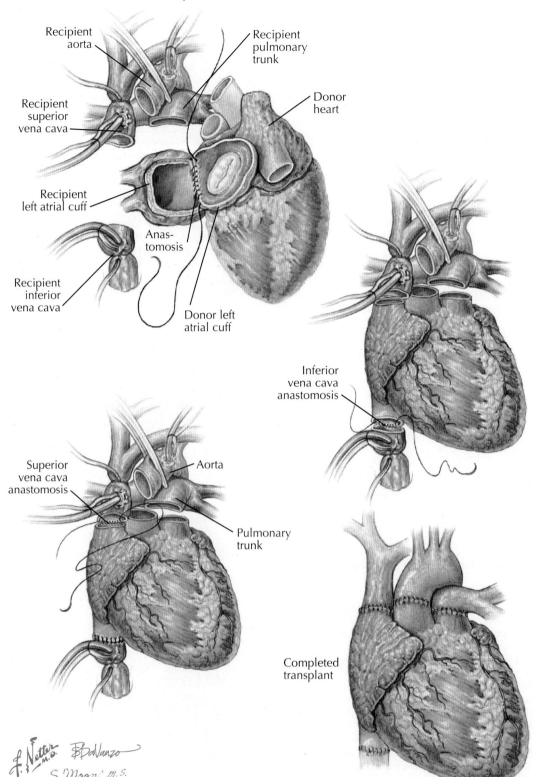

Recipient aorta

Recipient pulmonary trunk

Recipient superior vena cava

Donor heart

Recipient left atrial cuff

Anastomosis

Recipient inferior vena cava

Donor left atrial cuff

Inferior vena cava anastomosis

Superior vena cava anastomosis

Aorta

Pulmonary trunk

Completed transplant

HEART TRANSPLANTATION (Continued)

FOLLOW-UP OF TRANSPLANT PATIENT

After cardiac transplantation, the patient requires follow-up by physicians expert in heart failure and knowledgeable in immunology and infectious disease, with a focus on cardiac function, cardiac rejection, anticipation of possible rejection, and treatment of rejection and other aspects of immunosuppression, such as drug interaction. In addition, recipients must recognize their responsibility to take care of the transplanted heart. When all this is accomplished, the average survival of a transplant recipient is 10 years. Late deaths are usually from transplant coronary artery vasculopathy or malignancy. A few patients live 20 years or more, possibly related to their course, which had few episodes of rejection, infection, or malignancy.

MORAL, ETHICAL, AND SOCIAL IMPLICATIONS

The several years' delay for the successful application of orthotopic homotransplantation of the heart in humans was the result of the necessary experience with immune suppression in the initiation of heart transplants as well as the long-term laboratory observations determining whether absent CNS reflexes had prohibitively deleterious effects on cardiac performance. Also experimentally, a demand form of immunosuppression was formulated to cope specifically with heart transplants. Merely transposing accepted immune chemotherapy from kidney transplants to heart transplants tended to oversimplify the problem.

One of the most challenging and difficult aspects of human heart homotransplantation is selection of the recipient. Any patient whose heart has failed to the point where replacement is indicated may have irreversible damage of other organ systems. Cardiac transplantation has little to offer the patient at risk for sudden cardiac death from any cause. Acute cardiac care units have greatly reduced early mortality from ventricular fibrillation and other arrhythmias secondary to acute myocardial infarction. Modern therapy of heart failure and acute MI may have reduced the need for heart transplant, even though severe heart failure from MI is still a prominent indication for transplant.

Plate 6.144

Acquired Heart Disease

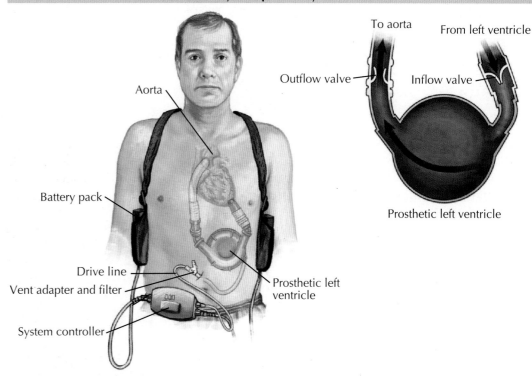

HeartMate XVE and II Left Ventricular Assist Systems

HeartMate XVE left ventricular assist system: pulsatile system

Aorta

Battery pack

Drive line

Vent adapter and filter

System controller

Prosthetic left ventricle

To aorta

From left ventricle

Outflow valve

Inflow valve

Prosthetic left ventricle

HeartMate II left ventricular assist system: continuous-flow (axial) system

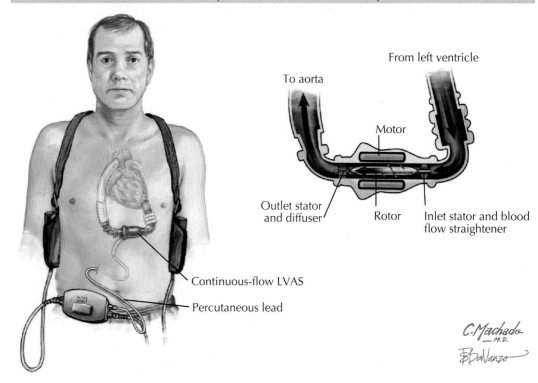

Continuous-flow LVAS

Percutaneous lead

From left ventricle

To aorta

Motor

Outlet stator and diffuser

Rotor

Inlet stator and blood flow straightener

Heart Transplantation
(Continued)

Probably the most appropriate adult candidate for heart transplantation is the patient with severe nonischemic cardiomyopathy. These patients often present a relatively long history of marginal compensation, but with increasingly frequent episodes of decompensation. The patient does not rally, unlike the typical patient with coronary artery disease. In the last stages of nonischemic cardiomyopathy, heart transplantation may be the only therapeutic application of choice. The secondary effects of CAD, such as ventricular aneurysm, mitral valve insufficiency, or ventricular septal defect, frequently are well treated by conventional open heart surgery, but no such program is available for the patient in the terminal phases of nonischemic cardiomyopathy. The etiologic factors in unrelenting heart failure are not well understood, but viral infections may play a role.

Another important application of heart transplantation is in the infant with a congenital cardiac anomaly for whom there is no corrective operation or palliative procedure. Great difficulty is encountered in this group of patients because of a paucity of donors and technical surgical problems.

The successful transplantation of the liver by Starzl and associates established the transplantation of unpaired organs. The general public appeared ready for the concept

that death of the individual occurs stepwise, with the brain dying first and then the heart, liver, and kidneys undergoing irreversible damage. These organs clearly cannot be transplanted, and various methods are necessary to resuscitate the heart in a prospective donor who had brain death. Recipient selection may be more controversial than donor selection. Time and practice have permitted the evolution of satisfactory criteria for transplant recipients.

The advent of clinical heart transplantation does not relegate the development of ventricular assist devices to total obscurity. At this time, ventricular assist devices are used as a bridge to transplant and in some patients as "destination therapy" (Plate 6.144). The future of heart replacement has by no means been settled with the initial application of homotransplantation. Future strides will consist of important research in the area of rejection, including better monitoring, better immunosuppression, and better organ preservation. If the issue of immune tolerance can be overcome, cardiac transplant patients may live normal life spans.

Plate 6.145

Cardiovascular System: VOLUME 8

SUDDEN DEATH IN HYPERTROPHIC CARDIOMYOPATHY

Although not always the case, massive hypertrophy of the intraventricular septum is common in hypertrophic cardiomyopathy.

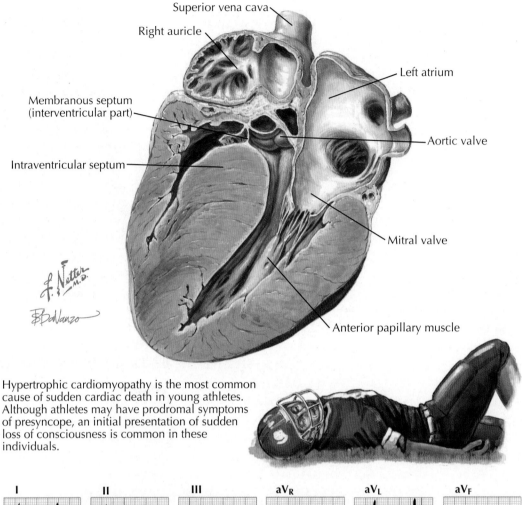

Hypertrophic cardiomyopathy is the most common cause of sudden cardiac death in young athletes. Although athletes may have prodromal symptoms of presyncope, an initial presentation of sudden loss of consciousness is common in these individuals.

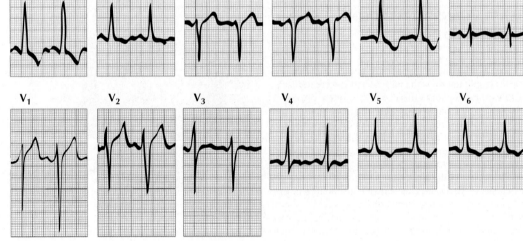

SUDDEN DEATH IN YOUNG ATHLETES

The most common cause of SCD in young athletes in the United States is hypertrophic cardiomyopathy (HCM). Many athletes may have prodromal symptoms (e.g., near-syncope), but often the initial presentation is SCD. Massive hypertrophy of the ventricular septum (asymmetric septal hypertrophy) of 30 mm or more is a common feature of SCD. HCM is autosomal dominant and occurs in 1 of 500 persons. The genotype is present from birth, but the phenotype may not be apparent until adolescence.

Other potential causes of SCD in young persons include congenital coronary anomalies, commotio cordis, Marfan syndrome, and long QT syndrome. Genetic and environmental factors such as smoking, medications, diet, lifestyle, electrolyte abnormalities, and myocardial infarction are associated with both HCM and long QT syndrome. The phenotype for long QT syndrome is prolongation of the QT interval.

Medical management of Marfan aortic disease consists of β-blockade to decrease the force and velocity of left ventricular contraction on the proximal aorta in Marfan syndrome. The rationale is that β-blocker therapy reduces the stress on the weakened tissue of the aorta and thus slows the progression of aortic dilation. Nondihydropyridine calcium channel antagonists may provide similar results.

Surgical therapy of Marfan syndrome is considered when the risk of aortic dissection is apparent, with progressive enlargement of the aortic root. Two methods are used. With the traditional method, the surgeon replaces the aorta with a graft and the aortic valve with a mechanical valve. With the valve-sparing method, the ascending aorta is replaced with a graft and the valve reimplanted.

Plate 6.146

Acquired Heart Disease

SYNCOPE: FOUR-STEP MANAGEMENT APPROACH

Step 1: Electrocardiogram

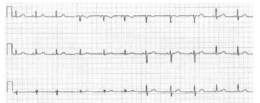

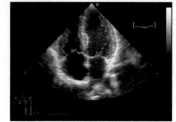

JOHN A. CRAIG—AD
D. Mascaro

All patients with syncope should undergo electrocardiography. If ECG is abnormal, confirmatory testing and appropriate therapy should be instituted.

Step 2: Echocardiography

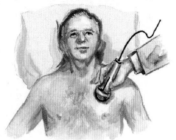

In most patients without a diagnosis, a structural evaluation with echocardiogram is required.

Step 3: Head-up tilt-table test

Should be considered if steps 1 and 2 are negative

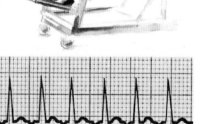

Step 4: Monitoring for symptom–rhythm correlation

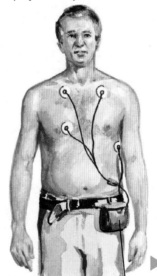

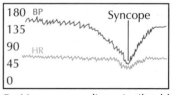

Positive neurocardiogenic tilt-table test shows drop in BP and heart rate.

Normal tilt-table test shows maintenance of normal BP and heart rate.

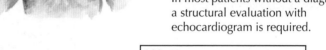

Holter monitor

Ambulatory monitoring recommended for patients with negative evaluation; duration of monitoring dependent on frequency of episodes; for daily symptoms, 48-hour monitor is adequate.

MANAGEMENT OF SYNCOPE

Syncope is defined as temporary loss of consciousness caused by decreased cerebral perfusion. The etiology of syncope may be difficult to discern and is best identified by taking a detailed history of the event. All patients with syncope should undergo electrocardiography and, if abnormal, appropriate therapy should be instituted. All patients should undergo cardiac ultrasound to assess the presence or absence of structural heart disease. If nothing is found, tilt-table testing should be performed. If still negative, ambulatory ECG should be performed. Duration of monitoring depends on how often the patient has symptoms.

In general, several categories of syncope are found. Neurally mediated syncope is common and takes the form of *reflex syncope, neurocardiogenic syncope,* or *vasovagal syncope.* Neurocardiogenic syncope or vasovagal syncope can occur in persons standing for long periods (e.g., military personnel) or in some persons at the sight of blood. Normally, if blood pressure falls, heart rate increases to maintain cardiac output. With neurocardiogenic syncope, blood pressure falls as well as heart rate, resulting in decreased cerebral perfusion and fainting. A tilt-table test is often used to confirm this form of syncope. If the etiology of syncope is not determined initially, long-term ECG or event monitoring may reveal the cause.

Carotid sinus sensitivity is similar to neurocardiogenic syncope and associated with exquisite sensitivity of the carotid sinus to manipulation; a tight shirt at the neck can precipitate syncope. Avoidance of these situations can generally prevent the syncope. Permanent pacemakers are also successful in preventing an attack.

Orthostatic hypotension and bradycardia result in a fainting spell when the patient rapidly stands up (also called *postural hypotension*), resulting in dizziness, lightheadedness, and fainting (syncope). Rare autonomic nervous system disease can result in orthostatic hypotension and may also be drug related (e.g., antihypertensives) or related to dehydration from any cause. Cardiovascular disease may also be associated with syncope, including conduction system disease resulting in arrhythmia (bradycardia, tachycardia); drug-related effects (bradycardia caused by β-blockers, tachycardias from arrhythmogenic effects of antiarrhythmics), and cardiac disease (e.g., during exercise in patients with aortic stenosis).

Plate 6.147

Cardiovascular System: VOLUME 8

TRICHINOSIS (PARASITIC HEART DISEASE)

Trichinosis is caused by the roundworm *Trichinella spiralis*. When raw or incompletely cooked pork or a pork product containing living trichina larvae is eaten, the walls of the cysts are digested, liberating the microscopic larvae. Within the small intestine of the host, the freed larvae maturate during the next 2 days to adult male or female worms and copulate. Beginning 5 days after ingestion of the infected meat and, in humans, continuing for as long as 12 weeks, the gravid adult female worms, which are partially embedded in the mucosal wall of the small bowel, give birth to larvae. The latter successively enter the lacteals of the intestinal villi, right ventricular cavity, pulmonary capillaries, and systemic circulation. By predilection, the larvae penetrate skeletal muscle fibers, where they enlarge progressively, simultaneously causing degeneration of the fibers and provoking a local reaction characterized by edema, hyperemia, and granulomatous and eosinophilic inflammation. Approximately 30 days after invasion of the muscle fibers, the larvae, which now have assumed a characteristic coiled appearance, attain their maximal size and become encapsulated. In nature, the life cycle of the parasite is completed when a carnivorous mammal becomes infected with the parasite as the result of ingesting the flesh of another animal containing living larvae (Plate 6.147).

The incubation period usually ranges between 7 and 10 days but may be as short as 1 day or as long as 28 days. As a rule, the first symptoms are intestinal; the small bowel mucosa is irritated by partial penetration of the larvae and then excysted from the digested infected meat, and the adult worms develop. Symptoms include nausea, vomiting, abdominal cramps, and diarrhea or constipation and usually last about 1 week. Symptoms of the muscular phase generally begin about 1 week after infection. As a rule, the first symptom noted by the patient is edema of the eyelids, followed by pain, tenderness, and swelling of the face and then pain on movement of any voluntary muscle. The severity of this phase depends on the number of second-generation larvae invading the tissues of the host. In a severe or moderately severe infection, this phase lasts from 4 to 8 weeks and is accompanied by fever up to 104°F (40°C) and weakness. Incidental involvement of other organs may cause bronchitis or bronchopneumonia, encephalitis or meningismus, a cutaneous rash, the sensation of insects or worms crawling beneath the skin, myocarditis, or arterial thrombosis. Mortality in patients hospitalized because of trichinosis is approximately 5%. The stage of convalescence usually is rapid.

The most frequent serious complication of trichinosis is *granulomatous myocarditis*, attended by congestive heart failure or terminated by sudden unexpected death during the sixth to eighth week of the infection. The heart is regularly involved, with young larvae invading the myocardium, although they never encyst there. As a rule, ECG changes appear during the second month of the infection. Occasionally, large arteries of the brain or an extremity become thrombosed, apparently from hypercoagulability of the blood. Recovery from myocarditis is usually complete.

Eosinophilia begins about 10 days after trichina infection, reaches its peak during the third week, and usually disappears after 6 months. Although moderately severe

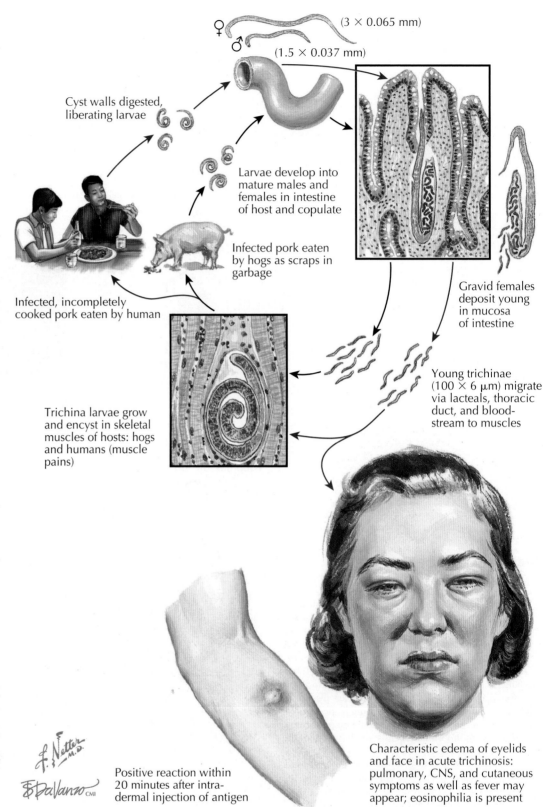

Cyst walls digested, liberating larvae

Larvae develop into mature males and females in intestine of host and copulate

Infected pork eaten by hogs as scraps in garbage

Infected, incompletely cooked pork eaten by human

Gravid females deposit young in mucosa of intestine

Young trichinae (100 × 6 μm) migrate via lacteals, thoracic duct, and bloodstream to muscles

Trichina larvae grow and encyst in skeletal muscles of hosts: hogs and humans (muscle pains)

Positive reaction within 20 minutes after intradermal injection of antigen

Characteristic edema of eyelids and face in acute trichinosis: pulmonary, CNS, and cutaneous symptoms as well as fever may appear; eosinophilia is present

infections are often attended by eosinophilia of 35% or as much as 70% or more, the degree of eosinophilia does not parallel the severity of infection. An abrupt fall from a high level to 1% or zero is ominous. In the diagnosis, a skin test is performed by intradermal injection of an antigen prepared from an extract of powdered larvae. A positive immediate reaction (evoked beginning 17 days after infection) consists of a soft wheal, 7 to 10 mm in diameter, appearing within 15 to 20 minutes;

it is surrounded by an area of bright erythema and disappears within 1 hour. Other diagnostic techniques include precipitin, flocculation, hemagglutination, complement fixation, and fluorescent antibody tests, most of which yield positive reactions beginning 17 to 30 days after infection. Biopsy is diagnostic if encysting larvae accompanied by a characteristic myositis are found.

Management of the patient with trichinosis includes bed rest, symptomatic treatment, and steroid therapy.

Plate 6.148

Acquired Heart Disease

CHAGAS DISEASE (TRYPANOSOMIASIS)

Chagas disease, also called South American (or American) *trypanosomiasis,* is a menace to millions of people in South-Central America. The parasite *Trypanosoma cruzi* enters the body, usually through the bite of a reduviid (assassin or kissing bug), or by the transfusion or inoculation of contaminated blood. The parasite circulates only in its trypanosomal form. It enters a body cell, transforms to a leishmania, and multiplies to form a leishmanial cyst, which ruptures the invaded cell. In this stage the parasites are released and transformed into *trypanosomes,* which circulate in the blood and invade other cells, thus continuing the cycle. The cardiac muscle cells are targeted in most cases, but with some strains in particular areas, there is equal or greater proclivity for the peripheral ganglion cells to be invaded or destroyed. In the rarer acute cases, all cells and tissues may be invaded, but in chronic cases, major damage is to the cardiac muscle cells and peripheral ganglion cells (Plate 6.148).

In the myocardium there is a parasitic myocarditis, although demonstrating the actual parasite may require a prolonged search. Foci of cell necrosis with an inflammatory cell infiltrate are found, including many eosinophils in the early cases. Some ruptured fibers probably recover, but others die and are replaced by fibrous tissue. The invasion is likely reduced as immunity develops, as manifested by the complement fixation reaction so important in diagnosis. A positive reaction generally indicates the presence in the body of living parasites, and with lifelong serum positivity typical, persisting damage is likely being done to the body cells. The heart becomes grossly enlarged and heavy but rather feeble in action. In patients who develop congestive failure, death may result at any time. Chagas disease is much dreaded because sudden death can occur in affected individuals who are in apparent good health but unaware of their infection. This is particularly common in young adult males and is often but not necessarily brought on by exertion. The precise cause is obscure.

Chagas disease in some geographic areas seems mainly a parasitic myocarditis with variable progression, whereas in other areas it is accompanied by a variety of lesions in other organs, apparently resulting from destruction of peripheral ganglion cells. In hollow organs the lesions manifest as tubular dilations; thus megaesophagus, megacolon, or a comparable lesion of any part of the gastrointestinal tract, including the gallbladder or bile duct, may be found. There also may be comparable dilations of the urinary bladder and ureters. Much of the ganglion cell destruction takes place in the early stages of infestation, with the dilations occurring at variable intervals thereafter.

Studies show that the cardiac ganglion cells may also be destroyed. As in other organs, this cell loss results in parasympathetic deprivation, the effects of which have not been fully explored. One cardiac lesion that develops is a loosening and slackening of the myocardial muscle bundles, producing dilation of the pulmonary conus and thinning of the ventricular vessels at the apex, so that the endocardium herniates and becomes

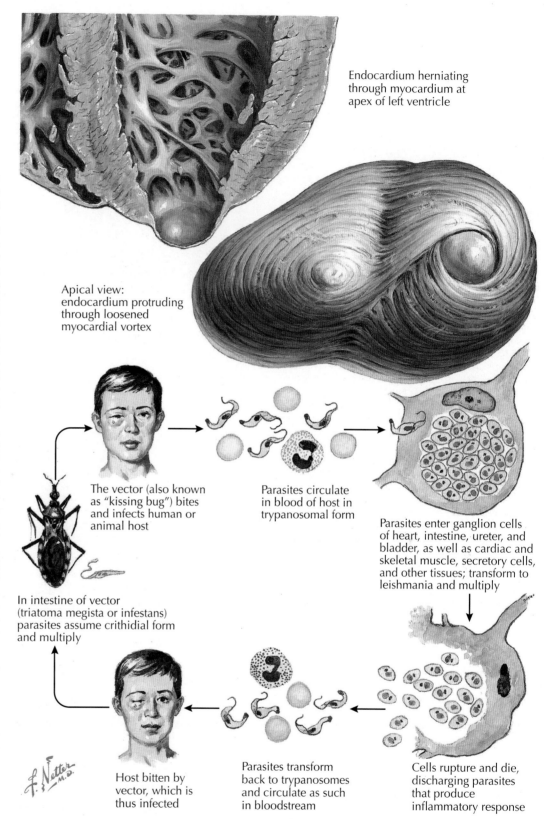

Endocardium herniating through myocardium at apex of left ventricle

Apical view: endocardium protruding through loosened myocardial vortex

The vector (also known as "kissing bug") bites and infects human or animal host

Parasites circulate in blood of host in trypanosomal form

Parasites enter ganglion cells of heart, intestine, ureter, and bladder, as well as cardiac and skeletal muscle, secretory cells, and other tissues; transform to leishmania and multiply

In intestine of vector (triatoma megista or infestans) parasites assume crithidial form and multiply

Host bitten by vector, which is thus infected

Parasites transform back to trypanosomes and circulate as such in bloodstream

Cells rupture and die, discharging parasites that produce inflammatory response

attached to the epicardium. The apical lesions in either or both ventricles may range from a deep, narrow cleft to a smooth-domed protrusion 2 to 3 cm in diameter and often filled with a thrombus. Curiously, these aneurysms rarely rupture, perhaps because the muscle tautens during systole, protecting them from the force, feeble though it may be, of ventricular ejection.

Chagas disease is controversial in many areas, and much remains to be discovered despite it being the most common parasitic myocarditis recognized in the world. A history of exposure to infection, residence in an affected area, cardiomegaly, and presence of a positive complement fixation reaction are important points in the clinical diagnosis. The presence of a myocarditis, chronic in type with variable degrees of fibrosis in a large heavy heart, should lead to a search for the parasite. Apical aneurysms appear unique to this disease. The existence of a megasyndrome in a patient with possible exposure to infection should alert the clinician to the possibility of coexistent cardiac damage.

Plate 6.149

Cardiovascular System: VOLUME 8

AMEBIC PERICARDITIS

AMEBIASIS

Amebiasis, transmitted by the protozoan *Entamoeba histolytica,* is considered initially and predominantly an intestinal disease, but it involves the liver in a substantial proportion of patients. The infective encysted form of the parasite, communicated person to person without an intermediate host and usually by water or food contaminated by human fecal material, enters the intestinal tract by the mouth, passes through the stomach, and loses its cystic wall in the small intestine. There the *cyst,* 5 to 20 μm in diameter, having matured during its passage, releases from one to four *trophozoites* (vegetative form), which, in contrast to the cyst, are mobile but do not survive outside the host's body. The *amoebas,* which have attached themselves to the colonic wall, migrate into the crypts and penetrate the epithelium and muscularis. From the submucosa, the amoebas move along to other organs, particularly the liver, creating there the *chronic nonsuppurative* form of amebic hepatitis or producing *abscesses.* Other trophozoites are excreted in the encysted form, thus maintaining the life cycle.

These events may proceed with only mild symptoms (not necessarily associated with the bowels) and thus may account for the *carrier stage.* On careful examination of the feces, however, this stage may be detected in up to 10% of the population in endemic US areas. Some disturbances of the host-parasite relationship result in the activation of the dormant form of the amoeba, causing the clinical picture of colitis, dysentery, or liver abscess.

AMEBIC PERICARDITIS

Another manifestation of amebiasis is amebic pericarditis. Until 1964, only 65 cases of this rare condition had been recorded in the world's medical literature. More recently, another 25 cases have been reported in South Africa. Pericardial involvement in amebiasis occurs by direct extension from an amebic abscess of the *left lobe* of the liver, only occasionally resulting from a lung abscess or an abscess in the right lobe of the liver (Plate 6.149). The salient features of amebic pericarditis are epigastric pain, a palpable mass in the epigastrium or left hypochondrium, tenderness over the liver area, dyspnea, pericardial friction rub, and high temperature. Radiography usually shows an elevated left diaphragm and enlargement of the heart shadow. Mild anemia and polymorphonuclear leukocytosis are usually present. The ECG shows the usual signs of pericarditis (e.g., generalized ST-segment elevation, inverted T waves, low voltage). Emetine and chloroquine administration is the treatment of choice; however, pericardial aspiration, often repeated, is usually necessary.

Amebic pericarditis is a fatal disease in more than 50% of patients. Even the patient who survives has a

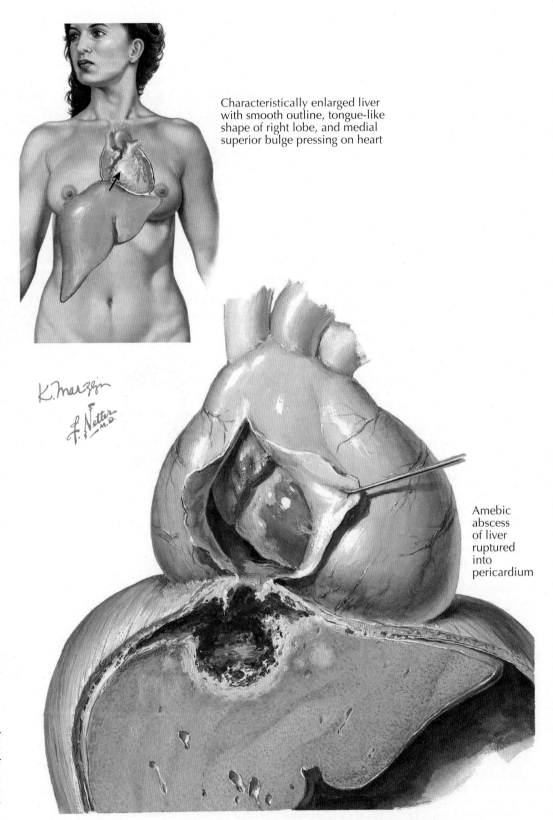

Characteristically enlarged liver with smooth outline, tongue-like shape of right lobe, and medial superior bulge pressing on heart

Amebic abscess of liver ruptured into pericardium

high risk of developing constrictive pericarditis, necessitating pericardiectomy. Another diagnostic link between amebiasis and the heart is penetrating precordial pain or discomfort often seen in chronic amebiasis and likely caused by heart disease. Radiographs show a characteristic configuration of the liver consisting of a tongue-like descending enlargement of the right lobe, with or without elevation of the right dome or bulging near the cardiac shadow. This bulging is probably responsible for the complaints related to the heart. In fact, these symptoms are caused by the elevation of the diaphragm resulting from hepatomegaly, which is extremely common in amebiasis. Another association between the heart and amebic infection is from the toxic effect of emetine on the heart. Treatment with emetine often causes ECG abnormalities, mainly flattening and inversion of the P and T waves, which are reversible and should cause no concern. Emetine is contraindicated only in the presence of serious cardiac disease.

Plate 6.150

Acquired Heart Disease

ECHINOCOCCUS INFECTION AND HYDATID PERICARDITIS

CARDIAC ECHINOCOCCUS INFECTION

Even in endemic regions, the heart is rarely affected by *Echinococcus* disease; the incidence of primary myocardial involvement is less than 2% in human echinococciasis (echinococcosis). The parasitic six-hooked embryo reaches the myocardium through the coronary circulation, having passed through the gastric or intestinal mucosa into the portal circulation, and through both the hepatic and the pulmonary capillary bed. It can establish itself and develop into an echinococcus *cyst* in almost any part of the myocardium, but cysts are mostly located in the walls of the ventricles (Plate 6.150). There is a higher incidence of cysts in the myocardium of the left ventricle because its vascular bed is more abundant. The developing parasitic membranous cyst is surrounded by a fibrous *sac* or capsule, the adventitia. When it grows larger, the cyst may protrude into a cardiac cavity, the pericardial sac, or both, its greater and more prominent part usually projecting toward the pericardium.

Primary echinococcus cyst of the heart is mostly single and slow growing. Less often, more than one cyst and rarely multiple cysts may develop. A single cyst infrequently remains univesicular and intact. In addition to free hydatid fluid, the adventitial capsule usually contains degenerated fragments of the ruptured original membranous cyst—the *mother* cyst—and multiple, even hundreds of, *daughter* cysts, both unruptured and ruptured and varying in size. Rupture of the membranous cyst is likely because of the repeated trauma of continuous heart movement. On rupture, the membranous cysts may die, the content of the adventitia becomes caseous and inspissated, and the adventitial capsule may calcify.

HYDATID PERICARDITIS

During the progressive enlargement of the echinococcus cyst, disastrous complications can occur. The cyst may rupture into a cardiac cavity or into the pericardial sac. Such ruptures may cause sudden death from anaphylactic shock and hydatid embolism, which is usually cerebral (less often, pulmonary). If the person survives, hematogenous dissemination occurs (more often in the CNS), with the eventual development of multiple metastatic or secondary cysts in the brain, usually with a fatal outcome. Rupture into the pericardial sac produces acute hydatid pericarditis (hydatid disease). Implantation of brood capsules and scolices in the pericardium leads to chronic hydatid pericarditis (hydatidopericardium) with fibrous tissue reaction and secondary cyst formation.

Clinically, the uncomplicated single cyst, when small and particularly if dead, may be asymptomatic. As it grows larger, atypical or even undetermined symptoms may appear, although these do not lead to the diagnosis. Radiographs show an eccentric deformity protruding from the contour of the cardiac shadow, generally as a circular or ovoid, homogeneous, well-defined opacity continuous with the outline of the heart silhouette. Calcification may also appear and is

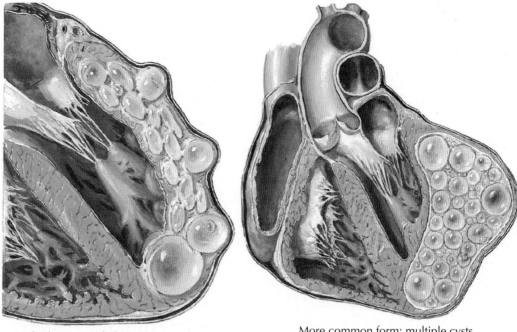

Multiple myocardial cysts intramurally located

More common form: multiple cysts within unilocular sac in heart wall

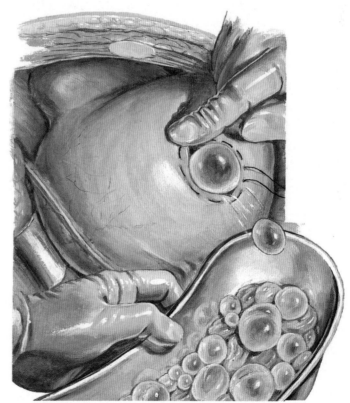

Expulsion of cysts via carefully guarded small opening prior to removal of entire external wall of common sac

more distinct on CT. Transmitted cardiac pulsation in the opacity is demonstrated on fluoroscopy. The ECG may be useful in diagnosis and more accurate localization of the cyst, showing myocardial ischemia and conduction changes more often than with other imaging. Angiocardiography is a valuable adjunct to the radiologic investigation, whereas heart catheterization is of no diagnostic value. Casoni intradermal and Weinberg tests add greatly to the establishment of the diagnosis. The correlation of radiographic and angiocardiographic findings with ECG changes, supplemented by positive biologic tests and eosinophilia, in a person living in an endemic region should lead to the diagnosis of cardiac echinococcus disease.

Treatment of cardiac *Echinococcus* infection (echinococciasis, echinococcosis, hydatid disease, hydatid pericarditis) should remove the cyst. In select patients, surgery should be performed under extracorporeal circulation. If the cyst has not ruptured into a heart chamber, surgery probably will result in cure.

Section 1: Anatomy

Anderson RH, Razavi R, Taylor AM. Cardiac anatomy revisited. *J Anat.* 2004;205:159–77.

Anderson RH, Yanni J, Boyett MR, et al. The anatomy of the cardiac conduction system. *Clin Anat.* 2009;22:99–113.

Fiss D. Normal coronary anatomy and anatomical variations. *Appl Radiol.* 2007;36:14–26.

James TJ. Anatomy of the sinus node of the dog. *Anat Rec.* 1962;143:251.

Section 2: Physiology

Bayes de Luna A. *Clinical Electrocardiography: A Textbook.* 4th ed. New York: Wiley-Blackwell; 2012.

Kameswari M, Rigolin VH, Sarano ME, Bonow RO. Valvular heart disease: diagnosis and management. *Mayo Clin Proc.* 2010;85: 483–500.

Pepine C, Hill J, Lambert C, editors. *Diagnostic and Therapeutic Cardiac Catheterization.* 3rd ed. Lippincott Williams & Wilkins; 1997.

Stub D, Bernard S, Duffy S, Kaye D. Contemporary reviews in cardiovascular medicine. Post cardiac arrest syndrome: a review of therapeutic strategies. *Circulation.* 2011;123:1428–35.

Section 3: Imaging

Choi EK, Choi SI, Rivera JJ, et al. Coronary computed tomography angiography as a screening tool for the detection of occult coronary artery disease in asymptomatic individuals. *J Am Coll Cardiol.* 2008;52:357–65.

Conti CR. Hemodynamics, coronary angiography, and ventriculography can obviate the need for noninvasive studies in many patients with ischemic heart disease. *Clin Cardiol.* 1997;20:827–8.

Jones DA, Rathod KS, Koganti S, et al. Angiography alone versus angiography plus optical coherence tomography to guide percutaneous coronary intervention: outcomes from the Pan-London PCI Cohort. *JACC Cardiovasc Interv.* 2018;11:1313–21.

Mieres JH, Makaryus AN, Redberg RF, Shaw LJ. Noninvasive cardiac imaging. *Am Fam Physician.* 2007;75:1219–28.

Pennel DJ. Contemporary reviews in cardiovascular medicine. Cardiovascular magnetic resonance. *Circulation.* 2010;121: 692–705.

Prati F, Di Vito L, Biondi-Zoccai G, et al. Angiography alone versus angiography plus optical coherence tomography to guide decision-making during percutaneous coronary intervention: the Centro per la Lotta contro l'Infarto-Optimisation of Percutaneous Coronary Intervention (CLI-OPCI) study. *EuroIntervention.* 2012;8:823–9.

Serruys PW, Hara H, Garg S, et al. Coronary computed tomographic angiography for complete assessment of coronary artery disease: JACC state-of-the-art review. *J Am Coll Cardiol.* 2021;78:713–36.

Section 4: Embryology

Abdulla R, Blew GA, Holterman MJ. Cardiovascular embryology. *Pediatr Cardiol.* 2004;25:191–200.

Angelini P. Embryology and congenital heart disease. *Tex Heart Inst J.* 1995;22:1–12.

Cochard LR. *Netter's Atlas of Human Embryology.* Elsevier; 2012.

Section 5: Congenital Heart Disease

Dybro AM, Rasmussen TB, Nielsen RR, et al. Randomized trial of metoprolol in patients with obstructive hypertrophic cardiomyopathy. *J Am Coll Cardiol.* 2021;78:2505–17.

Gersony WM, Rosenbaum MS. *Congenital Heart Disease in the Adult.* McGraw-Hill; 2002.

Lewin MB, Stout K. *Echocardiography in Congenital Heart Disease.* Elsevier; 2013.

Ommen SR, Shah PM, Tajik AJ. Left ventricular outflow tract obstruction in hypertrophic cardiomyopathy: past, present and future. *Heart.* 2008;94:1276–81.

Rudolph A. *Congenital Diseases of the Heart: Clinical–Physiological Considerations.* Wiley-Blackwell; 2009.

Section 6: Acquired Heart Disease

Conti CR, editor. *Coronary Artery Spasm.* Marcel Dekker; 1986.

Khandaker MH, Espinosa RE, Nishimura RA, et al. Pericardial disease: diagnosis and management. *Mayo Clin Proc.* 2010;85: 572–93.

Kirchhoff LV, Weiss LM, Wittner M, Tanowitz HB. Parasitic diseases of the heart. *Front Biosci.* 2004;9:706–23.

Maron BJ, Towbin JA, Thiene G, et al. Contemporary definitions and classification of the cardiomyopathies: AHA scientific statement. *Circulation.* 2006;113:1807–16.

Maseri A. *Ischemic Heart Disease: A Rational Basis for Clinical Practise and Clinical Research.* Churchill Livingstone; 1995.

Remetz MS, Matthay RA. Cardiovascular manifestations of connective tissue disorders. *J Thorac Imaging.* 1992;7:49–63.

Roberts K, Colquhoun S, Steer A, et al. Screening for rheumatic heart disease: current approaches and controversies. *Nat Rev Cardiol.* 2013;10:49–58.

Yeh ET, Bickford CL. Cardiovascular complications of cancer therapy: incidence, pathogenesis, diagnosis, and management. *J Am Coll Cardiol.* 2009;53:2231–47.

Tricuspid valve *(Continued)*
posterior cusp of, 12
regurgitation, 21f, 200
retracted, 120f
septal cusp of, 8f
stenosis, 110, 200, 200f, 201f
in tetralogy of Fallot, 117f
Tricuspid valve ring
frontal projection, 54f
LAO projection, 56f
lateral projection, 57f
RAO projection, 55f
Trileaflet aortic valve, 198, 198f
Trophoblast, 80
Troponin T, 164
Trousseau sign, 102
Truncus arteriosus, 84, 84f, 87f
at 20-somite stage, 85f
formation of, 89–90, 90f
repair, 130, 130f
Truncus septum anomalies, 130, 130f
aorticopulmonary septal defect, 130
truncus arteriosus repair, 130, 130f
Truncus swelling, 87f, 88f, 92f
Trypanosoma cruzi, 289
Trypanosomiasis, 289, 289f
Tuberculous pericarditis, 214, 215f, 216
Tunica media, 142
20-Somite stage, 85, 85f
Two-dimensional echocardiogram, 65
Two-somite stage, 82–83, 82f

U
Ultrasound
cardiac, 264
intravascular, 64, 64f
transthoracic cardiac, 65
Umbilical arteries, 85f, 95f, 96f, 97f, 98f
Umbilical cord, 98f
Umbilical vein, 83f, 84f, 85f, 95, 95f, 97f, 98f
Umbilical vesicle, primitive, 80
Unilateral pyelonephritis, hypertension and, 250, 250f
Unstable plaque formation, 147
Upper esophageal position of transducer, 67f
Uremia, 146f
Uterine arcuate arteries, 97f
Uterine arteries, 97f
Uterine epithelium, 80f
Uterine radial arteries, 97f

V
Vagal (parasympathetic) cardiac branches, 16
Vagus nerve, 3f, 17
Valve of foramen ovale, 108f
Valve replacement
aortic, 195–197, 195f
transcutaneous, 188, 188f

Valve replacement *(Continued)*
mitral, 194–195, 194f
multiple, 197, 197f
Valve swelling, 88f, 92f
Valves, 11–12
biologic, 193, 193f
prosthetic
first-generation valves, 192–193, 192f
second-generation valves, 193
Valvular apparatus, 182f
Valvular injuries, 269f, 270
Valvular insufficiency, dilation of aortic ring with, 234f
Valvular involvement, acute, in rheumatic heart disease, 170
Valvuloplasty, balloon
catheter-based, 122
mitral, 178, 178f
Vasa vasorum, 142f, 143f
Vascular access, right-sided heart catheterization and, 27
Vascular disease, end-organ damage by, 146
Vascular sling, 137, 137f
Vascular zone, 142f
Vasculitis, aortic, 191
Vasculogenesis, early intraembryonic, 81
Vasoconstriction, hypertension and, 249
Vasospasm, pulmonary arteriolar, 175
Vasovagal syncope, 287
Vegetations
of bacterial arteritis, 225f
early, of bacterial endocarditis, 223f
marantic, 229
rheumatic, on mitral valve, 170f
Venae cavae, cannulated, 195f
Venous pressure, elevated, 173f, 264
Venous pulses, 21f
Venous trunk anomalies, 101
Ventricles, 8–10, 10f, 83f, 84f, 160f
common, 115f, 116
development of, 86f, 88–89
left. *See* Left ventricle
in mitral valve replacement, 194f
primitive, 85f, 87f
primordial, 84
right. *See* Right ventricle
trabecular walls of, 90f
Ventricular aneurysmectomy, 157
Ventricular depolarization, 40f
Ventricular fibrillation, 47f, 48
in cardiopulmonary arrest, 230
Ventricular hypertrophy, 40
Ventricular pressures, normal, 29–30
Ventricular repolarization, 37
Ventricular resynchronization, 280f
Ventricular septal defects (VSDs), 23f, 30, 110f, 114–115
abnormal findings in, 30
aneurysm of membranous septum, 114f, 116
common ventricle, 115f, 116
large defects, 114–115

Ventricular septal defects *(Continued)*
moderate-sized defects, 115
murmur caused by, 24
muscular interventricular septal defect, 115f, 116
pulmonary hypertension, 115
small defects and shunts, 114
subpulmonic defect, 115f
in tetralogy of Fallot, 117f
transatrial repair of, 116f
Ventricular septum, 10, 160f
anomalies of, 114–116
regurgitant lesion on, 191f
Ventricular tachycardia, 47, 47f, 270f
Ventriculography, 72, 72f, 154
Verrucous angiitis, 209
Verrucous lesions, 209f
Vertebra, thoracic, in acromegaly, 238f
Vertebral artery, 16f, 17f, 137f, 146f
development of, 94f
Vertebral ganglion, 16f, 17, 17f
Viral myocarditis, 204, 204f
Vitelline artery, 98f
Vitelline vascular system, 98f
Vitelline veins, 83f, 84f, 85f, 94, 95f
Vitelloumbilical veins, 82f
Voluminous blood loss, in penetrating heart wounds, 265f
VSDs. *See* Ventricular septal defects

W
Walker-Murdoch wrist sign, 100f
Wandering pacemaker, 44
Waterston operation, for tetralogy of Fallot, 119
Wave reflection, hypertension and, 249f
Weakness, in pheochromocytoma, 243f
Wedge pressure
elevated
in mitral regurgitation, 180f
in mitral stenosis, 173f
normal, 29
"White coat hypertension," 249
White rami communicantes, 17
Wolff-Parkinson-White syndrome, 42

X
Xenografts, 193
Xiphoid cartilage, 2
Xiphoid process, 2, 2f

Y
Yolk sac, 80, 80f, 81f, 82f, 84f, 85f, 98f

Z
Zone of infarction, 164f
Zone of injury, 164f
Zone of ischemia, 164f
Zygote, 80